Artificial Intelligence in Gastrointestinal Disease: Diagnosis and Management

Artificial Intelligence in Gastrointestinal Disease: Diagnosis and Management

Editors

Eun-Sun Kim
Kwang-Sig Lee

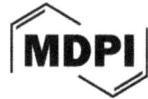

Basel • Beijing • Wuhan • Barcelona • Belgrade • Novi Sad • Cluj • Manchester

Editors
Eun-Sun Kim
Department of Internal
Medicine, Korea University
College of Medicine, Anam
Hospital
Seoul
Republic of Korea

Kwang-Sig Lee
AI Center, Korea University
College of Medicine, Anam
Hospital
Seoul
Republic of Korea

Editorial Office
MDPI
St. Alban-Anlage 66
4052 Basel, Switzerland

This is a reprint of articles from the Special Issue published online in the open access journal *Diagnostics* (ISSN 2075-4418) (available at: https://www.mdpi.com/journal/diagnostics/special_issues/gastrointest_dis).

For citation purposes, cite each article independently as indicated on the article page online and as indicated below:

Lastname, A.A.; Lastname, B.B. Article Title. *Journal Name* **Year**, *Volume Number*, Page Range.

ISBN 978-3-7258-0653-9 (Hbk)
ISBN 978-3-7258-0654-6 (PDF)
doi.org/10.3390/books978-3-7258-0654-6

© 2024 by the authors. Articles in this book are Open Access and distributed under the Creative Commons Attribution (CC BY) license. The book as a whole is distributed by MDPI under the terms and conditions of the Creative Commons Attribution-NonCommercial-NoDerivs (CC BY-NC-ND) license.

Contents

Masayuki Tsuneki and Fahdi Kanavati
Deep Learning Models for Poorly Differentiated Colorectal Adenocarcinoma Classification in Whole Slide Images Using Transfer Learning
Reprinted from: *Diagnostics* **2021**, *11*, 2074, doi:10.3390/diagnostics11112074 1

Eyal Klang, Robert Freeman, Matthew A. Levin, Shelly Soffer, Yiftach Barash and Adi Lahat
Machine Learning Model for Outcome Prediction of Patients Suffering from Acute Diverticulitis Arriving at the Emergency Department—A Proof of Concept Study
Reprinted from: *Diagnostics* **2021**, *11*, 2102, doi:10.3390/diagnostics11112102 12

Rohee Park, Seungsoo Lee, Yusub Sung, Jeeseok Yoon, Heung-Il Suk, Hyoungjung Kim, et al.
Accuracy and Efficiency of Right-Lobe Graft Weight Estimation Using Deep-Learning-Assisted CT Volumetry for Living-Donor Liver Transplantation
Reprinted from: *Diagnostics* **2022**, *12*, 590, doi:10.3390/diagnostics12030590 22

Yen-Po Wang, Ying-Chun Jheng, Kuang-Yi Sung, Hung-En Lin, I-Fang Hsin, Ping-Hsien Chen, et al.
Use of U-Net Convolutional Neural Networks for Automated Segmentation of Fecal Material for Objective Evaluation of Bowel Preparation Quality in Colonoscopy
Reprinted from: *Diagnostics* **2022**, *12*, 613, doi:10.3390/diagnostics12030613 33

Athanasios G. Pantelis, Panagiota A. Panagopoulou and Dimitris P. Lapatsanis
Artificial Intelligence and Machine Learning in the Diagnosis and Management of Gastroenteropancreatic Neuroendocrine Neoplasms—A Scoping Review
Reprinted from: *Diagnostics* **2022**, *12*, 874, doi:10.3390/diagnostics12040874 47

Alba Nogueira-Rodríguez, Miguel Reboiro-Jato, Daniel Glez-Peña and Hugo López-Fernández
Performance of Convolutional Neural Networks for Polyp Localization on Public Colonoscopy Image Datasets
Reprinted from: *Diagnostics* **2022**, *12*, 898, doi:10.3390/diagnostics12040898 61

Chia-Pei Tang, Chen-Hung Hsieh and Tu-Liang Lin
Computer-Aided Image Enhanced Endoscopy Automated System to Boost Polyp and Adenoma Detection Accuracy
Reprinted from: *Diagnostics* **2022**, *12*, 968, doi:10.3390/diagnostics12040968 78

Miguel Mascarenhas, João Afonso, Tiago Ribeiro, Hélder Cardoso, Patrícia Andrade, João P. S. Ferreira, et al.
Performance of a Deep Learning System for Automatic Diagnosis of Protruding Lesions in Colon Capsule Endoscopy
Reprinted from: *Diagnostics* **2022**, *12*, 1445, doi:10.3390/diagnostics12061445 95

Sarah Moen, Fanny E. R. Vuik, Ernst J. Kuipers and Manon C. W. Spaander
Artificial Intelligence in Colon Capsule Endoscopy—A Systematic Review
Reprinted from: *Diagnostics* **2022**, *12*, 1994, doi:10.3390/diagnostics12081994 106

Meryem Souaidi and Mohamed El Ansari
Multi-Scale Hybrid Network for Polyp Detection in Wireless Capsule Endoscopy and Colonoscopy Images
Reprinted from: *Diagnostics* **2022**, *12*, 2030, doi:10.3390/diagnostics12082030 120

Filipe Vilas-Boas, Tiago Ribeiro, João Afonso, Hélder Cardoso, Susana Lopes, Pedro Moutinho-Ribeiro, et al.
Deep Learning for Automatic Differentiation of Mucinous versus Non-Mucinous Pancreatic Cystic Lesions: A Pilot Study
Reprinted from: *Diagnostics* 2022, 12, 2041, doi:10.3390/diagnostics12092041 143

Sultan Imangaliyev, Jörg Schlötterer, Folker Meyer and Christin Seifert
Diagnosis of Inflammatory Bowel Disease and Colorectal Cancer through Multi-View Stacked Generalization Applied on Gut Microbiome Data
Reprinted from: *Diagnostics* 2022, 12, 2514, doi:10.3390/diagnostics12102514 153

Kwang-Sig Lee and Eun Sun Kim
Explainable Artificial Intelligence in the Early Diagnosis of Gastrointestinal Disease
Reprinted from: *Diagnostics* 2022, 12, 2740, doi:10.3390/diagnostics12112740 174

Joel Raymann and Ratnavel Rajalakshmi
GAR-Net: Guided Attention Residual Network for Polyp Segmentation from Colonoscopy Video Frames
Reprinted from: *Diagnostics* 2023, 13, 123, doi:10.3390/diagnostics13010123 185

Meryem Souaidi, Samira Lafraxo, Zakaria Kerkaou, Mohamed El Ansari and Lahcen Koutti
A Multiscale Polyp Detection Approach for GI Tract Images Based on Improved DenseNet and Single-Shot Multibox Detector
Reprinted from: *Diagnostics* 2023, 13, 733, doi:10.3390/diagnostics13040733 203

Alba Nogueira-Rodríguez, Daniel Glez-Peña, Miguel Reboiro-Jato and Hugo López-Fernández
Negative Samples for Improving Object Detection—A Case Study in AI-Assisted Colonoscopy for Polyp Detection
Reprinted from: *Diagnostics* 2023, 13, 966, doi:10.3390/diagnostics13050966 224

Pei-Yuan Su, Yang-Yuan Chen, Chun-Yu Lin, Wei-Wen Su, Siou-Ping Huang and Hsu-Heng Yen
Comparison of Machine Learning Models and the Fatty Liver Index in Predicting Lean Fatty Liver
Reprinted from: *Diagnostics* 2023, 13, 1407, doi:10.3390/diagnostics13081407 239

Adi Lahat, Eyal Shachar, Benjamin Avidan, Benjamin Glicksberg and Eyal Klang
Evaluating the Utility of a Large Language Model in Answering Common Patients' Gastrointestinal Health-Related Questions: Are We There Yet?
Reprinted from: *Diagnostics* 2023, 13, 1950, doi:10.3390/diagnostics13111950 250

Ioannis K. Gallos, Dimitrios Tryfonopoulos, Gidi Shani, Angelos Amditis, Hossam Haick and Dimitra D. Dionysiou
Advancing Colorectal Cancer Diagnosis with AI-Powered Breathomics: Navigating Challenges and Future Directions
Reprinted from: *Diagnostics* 2023, 13, 3673, doi:10.3390/diagnostics13243673 260

Gi Pyo Lee, Young Jae Kim, Dong Kyun Park, Yoon Jae Kim, Su Kyeong Han and Kwang Gi Kim
Gastro-BaseNet: A Specialized Pre-Trained Model for Enhanced Gastroscopic Data Classification and Diagnosis of Gastric Cancer and Ulcer
Reprinted from: *Diagnostics* 2024, 14, 75, doi:10.3390/diagnostics14010075 281

Ali Sahafi, Anastasios Koulaouzidis and Mehrshad Lalinia
Polypoid Lesion Segmentation Using YOLO-V8 Network in Wireless Video Capsule Endoscopy Images
Reprinted from: *Diagnostics* **2024**, *14*, 474, doi:10.3390/diagnostics14050474 . . . . **297**

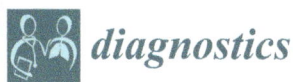

Article

Deep Learning Models for Poorly Differentiated Colorectal Adenocarcinoma Classification in Whole Slide Images Using Transfer Learning

Masayuki Tsuneki *,† and Fahdi Kanavati †

Medmain Research, Medmain Inc., Fukuoka 810-0042, Japan; fkanavati@medmain.com
* Correspondence: tsuneki@medmain.com; Tel.: +81-92-707-1977
† These authors contributed equally to this work.

Abstract: Colorectal poorly differentiated adenocarcinoma (ADC) is known to have a poor prognosis as compared with well to moderately differentiated ADC. The frequency of poorly differentiated ADC is relatively low (usually less than 5% among colorectal carcinomas). Histopathological diagnosis based on endoscopic biopsy specimens is currently the most cost effective method to perform as part of colonoscopic screening in average risk patients, and it is an area that could benefit from AI-based tools to aid pathologists in their clinical workflows. In this study, we trained deep learning models to classify poorly differentiated colorectal ADC from Whole Slide Images (WSIs) using a simple transfer learning method. We evaluated the models on a combination of test sets obtained from five distinct sources, achieving receiver operating characteristic curve (ROC) area under the curves (AUCs) up to 0.95 on 1799 test cases.

Keywords: deep learning; transfer learning; poorly differentiated adenocarcinoma; colon

1. Introduction

According to global cancer statistics in 2020 [1,2], colorectal cancer (CRC) is amongst the most common leading causes of cancer deaths in the world and the second most common in the United States [1]. In 2020, approximately 147,950 individuals were diagnosed with CRC, and 53,200 died from the disease. Screening and high-quality treatment can help in improving survival prospects. This is evidenced by the decrease in CRC death rates from 2008 to 2017 by 3% annually in individuals aged 65 years and older and by 0.6% annually in individuals aged 50 to 64 years. However, as the incidence of CRC in young and middle-aged adults (younger than 50 years) has been increasing (by 1.3% annually [1]), the American Cancer Society lowered the recommended age for screening initiation for individuals at average risk from 50 to 45 years in 2018 [2,3]. The development of endoscopy provided a major impact on the diagnosis and treatment of CRC, especially colonoscopy which allows observation of the colonic mucosal surface with biopsies of identified and/or suspicious lesions [4].

Deep learning has been successfully applied in computational pathology in the past few years for tasks such cancer classification, cell segmentation, and outcome prediction for a variety of organs and diseases [5–18]. For the classification of tumour in colorectal WSI, Iizuka et al. [18] trained a model on a large dataset of colorectal WSIs for the classification of well differentiated ADC; however, it did not include poorly differentiated ADC.

Histopathologically, adenocarcinoma (ADC) account for more than 90% of CRCs. Most colorectal ADCs are well to moderately differentiated types with gland-forming and configuration of the glandular structures. If more than 50% of the tumor is formed by non-gland forming carcinoma cells, the tumor is classified as poorly differentiated (or high grade) ADC [19–21]. The frequency of poorly differentiated ADC is relatively low (3.3% to 18% of all CRCs) [22–26]. The 5-year survival rate for patients with colorectal

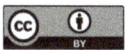

poorly differentiated ADC is 20% to 45.5%, which indicates that poorly differentiated ADC has a less favorable prognosis compared with that of well or moderately differentiated ADC [23,26–28].

In this paper, we trained deep learning models for the classification of diffuse-type ADC in endoscopic biopsy specimen whole slide images (WSIs). We have used the partial transfer learning method [29] to fine-tune the models. We obtained models with ROC AUCs up to 0.95 for on the combined test set with a total of 1799 WSIs, demonstrating the potential of such methods for aiding pathologists in their workflows.

2. Methods

2.1. Clinical Cases and Pathological Records

For the present retrospective study, a total of 2547 endoscopic biopsy cases of human colorectal epithelial lesions HE (hematoxylin & eosin) stained histopathological specimens were collected from the surgical pathology files of five hospitals: International University of Health and Welfare, Mita Hospital (Tokyo) and Kamachi Group Hospitals (consisting of Wajiro, Shinmizumaki, Shinkomonji, and Shinyukuhashi hospitals) (Fukuoka) after histopathological review of those specimens by surgical pathologists. The experimental protocol was approved by the ethical board of the International University of Health and Welfare (No. 19-Im-007) and Kamachi Group Hospitals. All research activities complied with all relevant ethical regulations and were performed in accordance with relevant guidelines and regulations in the all hospitals mentioned above. Informed consent to use histopathological samples and pathological diagnostic reports for research purposes had previously been obtained from all patients prior to the surgical procedures at all hospitals, and the opportunity for refusal to participate in research had been guaranteed by an opt-out manner. The test cases were selected randomly, so the obtained ratios reflected a real clinical scenario as much as possible. All WSIs were scanned at a magnification of $\times 20$, and the average dimension was 30 K $\times$ 15 K pixels. This protocol is similar to [18,30–32].

2.2. Dataset and Annotations

Prior to this study, the diagnosis of each WSI was verified by at least two pathologists, and they excluded cases that were inappropriate or of poor scanned quality. In particular, about 20% of poorly differentiated ADC cases were excluded due to disagreement between pathologists. Table 1 breaks down the distribution of the dataset into training, validation, and test sets. Hospitals which provided histopathological cases were anonymised (e.g., Hospital 1–5). The training and test sets were solely composed of WSIs of endoscopic biopsy specimens. The patients' pathological records were used to extract the WSIs' pathological diagnoses. In total, 36 WSIs from the training and validation sets had a poorly differentiated ADC diagnosis. They were manually annotated by a group of two surgical pathologists who perform routine histopathological diagnoses. The pathologists carried out detailed cellular-level annotations by free-hand drawing around poorly differentiated ADC cells. The well to moderately differentiated ADC ($n = 71$), adenoma ($n = 110$) and non-neoplastic subsets ($n = 531$) of the training and validation sets were not annotated and the entire tissue areas within the WSIs were used. Each annotated WSI was observed by at least two pathologists, with the final checking and verification performed by a senior pathologist. This dataset preparation is similar to [18,30–32].

2.3. Deep Learning Models

We trained all the models using the partial fine-tuning approach [29]. This method simply consists of using the weights of an existing pre-trained model and only fine-tuning the affine parameters of the batch normalisation layers and the final classification layer. We used the EfficientNetB1 [33] model starting with pre-trained weights on ImageNet. The total number of trainable parameters was only 63,329.

The training method that we have used in this study is exactly the same as reported in a previous study [30]. For completeness, we repeat the method here. To apply the CNN on the WSIs, we performed slide tiling by extracting square tiles from tissue regions. On a given WSI, we detected the tissue regions and eliminated most of the white background by performing a thresholding on a grayscale version of the WSI using Otsu's method [34]. During prediction, we performed the tiling in a sliding window fashion, using a fixed-size stride, to obtain predictions for all the tissue regions. During training, we initially performed random balanced sampling of tiles from the tissue regions, where we tried to maintain an equal balance of each label in the training batch. To do so, we placed the WSIs in a shuffled queue such that we looped over the labels in succession (i.e., we alternated between picking a WSI with a positive label and a negative label). Once a WSI was selected, we randomly sampled $\frac{\text{batch size}}{\text{num labels}}$ tiles from each WSI to form a balanced batch. To maintain the balance on the WSI, we oversampled from the WSIs to ensure the model trained on tiles from all of the WSIs in each epoch. We then switched into hard mining of tiles once there was no longer any improvement on the validation set after two epochs. To perform the hard mining, we alternated between training and inference. During inference, the CNN was applied in a sliding window fashion on all of the tissue regions in the WSI, and we then selected the k tiles with the highest probability for being positive if the WSI was negative and the k tiles with the lowest probability for being positive if the WSI was positive. This step effectively selected the hard examples with which the model was struggling. The selected tiles were placed in a training subset, and once that subset contained N tiles, the training was run. We used $k = 16$, $N = 256$, and a batch size of 32.

From the WSIs with poorly-differentiated ADC, we sampled tiles based on the free-hand annotations. If the WSI contained annotations for cancer cells, then we only sampled tiles from the annotated regions as follows: if the annotation was smaller than the tile size, then we sampled the tile at the centre of the annotation regions; otherwise, if the annotation was larger than the tile size, then we subdivided the annotated regions into overlapping grids and sampled tiles. Most of the annotations were smaller than the tile size. On the other hand, if the WSI did not contain diffuse-type ADC, then we freely sampled from the entire tissue regions.

The models were trained on WSIs at ×20 magnification. To obtain a prediction on a WSI, the model was applied in a sliding window fashion using a tile size of 512 × 512 px and a stride of 256 × 256 px, generating a prediction per tile. The WSI prediction was then obtained by taking the maximum from all of the tiles. The prediction output for the ensemble model was obtained as simply the average output of the three models used.

We trained the models with the Adam optimisation algorithm [35] with the following parameters: $beta_1 = 0.9$, $beta_2 = 0.999$, and a batch size of 32. We used a learning rate of 0.001 when fine-tuning. We applied a learning rate decay of 0.95 every 2 epochs. We used the binary cross entropy loss function. We used early stopping by tracking the performance of the model on a validation set, and training was stopped automatically when there was no further improvement on the validation loss for 10 epochs. The model with the lowest validation loss was chosen as the final model.

2.4. Software and Statistical Analysis

We implemented the models using TensorFlow [36]. We calculated the AUCs in python using the scikit-learn package[37] and performed the plotting using matplotlib [38]. We performed image processing, such as the thresholding with scikit-image [39]. We computed the 95% CIs estimates using the bootstrap method [40] with 1000 iterations. We used openslide [41] to perform realtime slide tiling.

3. Results

The aim of this study was to train a deep learning model based on convolutional neural networks (CNNs) to classify poorly differentiated ADC in WSIs of colorectal biopsy specimens. We had a total of 748 WSIs which were available for training of which only 36 WSIs had poorly differentiated ADC. Given the small number of WSIs, we opted for using a transfer learning method which was suitable for such a task. Transfer learning consists of fine-tuning the weights of a model that was pre-trained on another dataset for which a larger number of images were available for training. To this end, we evaluated four models: (1) a model that was fine-tuned starting with pre-trained weights on ImageNet [42], (2) a model that was fine-tuned starting with pre-trained weights on a stomach WSIs dataset [30], (3) a model that was pre-trained for the classification of gastric poorly differentiated ADC which we did not fine-tune [30], and (4) a model which consisted of an ensemble [43] of the previous three models. Figure 1 shows an overview of our training method.

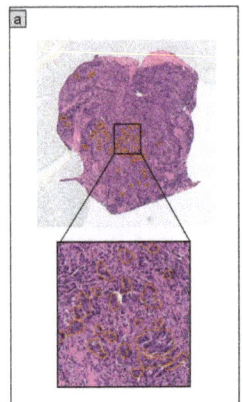
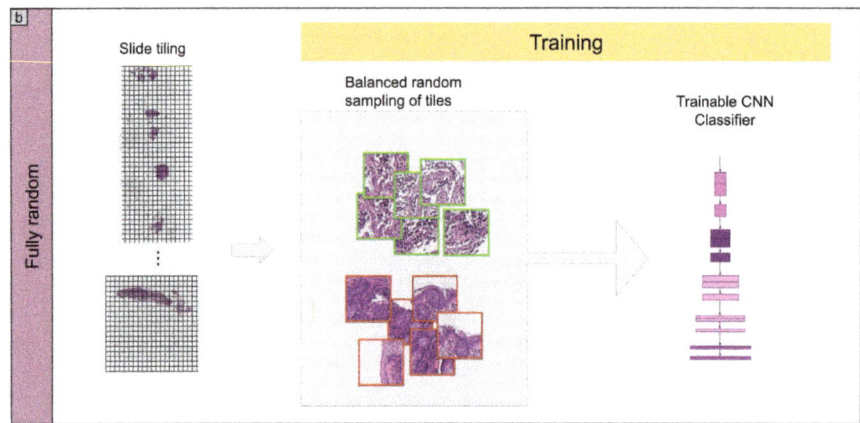
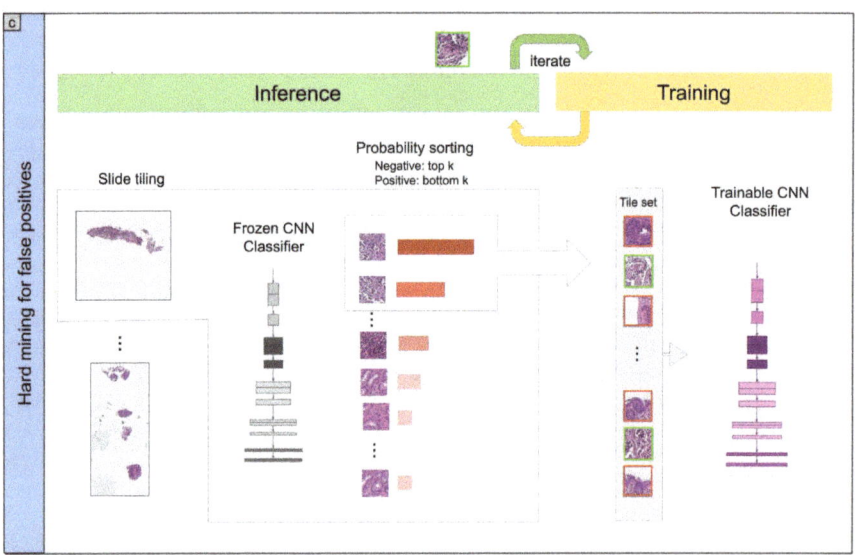

Figure 1. Method overview. (**a**) An example of poorly differentiated ADC annotation that was carried out on the WSIs by pathologists using in an in-house web-based application. (**b**) The initial training consisted in fully-random balanced sampling of positive (poorly differentiated ADC) and negative tiles to fine-tune the models. (**c**) After a few epochs of random sampling, the training switched into iterative hard mining of tiles that alternates between training and inference. During the inference step, we applied the model in a sliding window fashion on all of the WSI and selected the k tiles with the highest probabilities if the WSI was negative, and k tiles with the lowest probabilities if the WSI was positive. The tiles were collected in a subset that was batched and used for training. This process allows training to reduce false positives.

Evaluation on Five Independent Test Sets from Different Sources

We evaluated our models on five distinct test sets consisting of biopsy specimens, three of which were from hospitals not in the training set. Table 1 breaks down the distribution of the WSIs in each test set. For each test set for for their combination, we computed the ROC AUC and log loss for the WSI classification of poorly differentiated ADC as well as the log loss, and we have summarised the results in Table 2 and Figure 2. Figures 3 and 4 show true positive and false positive example heatmap outputs, respectively. Table 3 shows a confusion matrix for the combined test set using the ensemble model and a probability threshold of 0.5. When operating with a high sensitivity threshold (sensitivity 100%), the specificity for the best model on the combined test set was 75%.

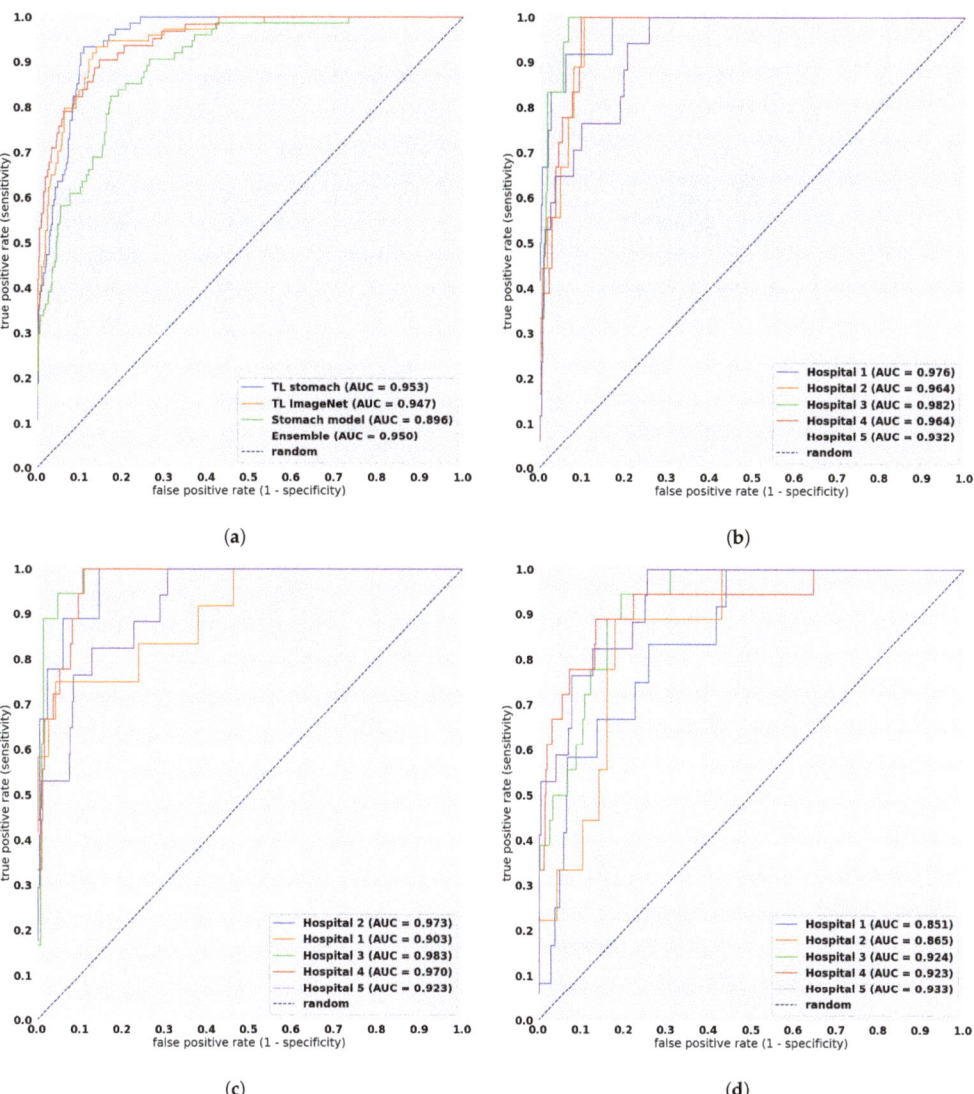

Figure 2. ROC curves for the four models as evaluated on the combined test sets and each test set separately. (**a**) Evaluation of the four models on the combined test set ($n = 1741$), (**b**) TL stomach model on the test sets that had poorly differentiated ADC, (**c**) TL ImageNet model on the test sets that had poorly ADC, (**d**) Stomach model on the test sets that had poorly differentiated ADC.

Table 1. Distribution of WSIs in the training, validation, and test sets.

		Poorly Diff. ADC	Well-to-Moderately-Diff. ADC	Adenoma	Non-Neoplastic	Total
Test	Hospital 1	12	125	61	251	449
	Hospital 2	9	41	78	44	172
	Hospital 3	18	20	210	39	287
	Hospital 4	18	74	239	158	489
	Hospital 5	17	144	55	186	402
Training	Hospital 1 & 5	30	60	90	500	680
Validation	Hospital 1 & 5	6	11	20	31	68

Table 2. ROC and log loss results on the different test sets using the different transfer learning methods.

Method	Source	ROC AUC	Log Loss
Ensemble	combined	0.950 [0.925, 0.971]	0.135 [0.122, 0.148]
TL stomach	combined	0.953 [0.937, 0.966]	0.466 [0.426, 0.506]
TL ImageNet	combined	0.947 [0.923, 0.968]	0.555 [0.511, 0.594]
Stomach model	combined	0.896 [0.862, 0.923]	0.863 [0.814, 0.911]
TL stomach	Hospital 1	0.976 [0.936, 0.997]	0.236 [0.196, 0.271]
TL stomach	Hospital 2	0.964 [0.927, 0.991]	0.459 [0.347, 0.576]
TL stomach	Hospital 3	0.982 [0.966, 0.995]	0.195 [0.143, 0.244]
TL stomach	Hospital 4	0.964 [0.94, 0.983]	0.44 [0.36, 0.515]
TL stomach	Hospital 5	0.932 [0.886, 0.97]	0.949 [0.855, 1.081]
TL ImageNet	Hospital 1	0.903 [0.774, 0.993]	0.325 [0.284, 0.367]
TL ImageNet	Hospital 2	0.973 [0.939, 0.999]	0.613 [0.468, 0.72]
TL ImageNet	Hospital 3	0.983 [0.965, 0.997]	0.268 [0.209, 0.326]
TL ImageNet	Hospital 4	0.97 [0.948, 0.987]	0.48 [0.398, 0.549]
TL ImageNet	Hospital 5	0.923 [0.868, 0.969]	1.085 [0.972, 1.219]
Stomach model	Hospital 1	0.851 [0.739, 0.928]	1.055 [0.953, 1.167]
Stomach model	Hospital 2	0.865 [0.768, 0.951]	0.882 [0.722, 1.032]
Stomach model	Hospital 3	0.924 [0.864, 0.96]	0.607 [0.506, 0.716]
Stomach model	Hospital 4	0.923 [0.843, 0.981]	0.554 [0.475, 0.62]
Stomach model	Hospital 5	0.933 [0.881, 0.972]	1.2 [1.102, 1.326]

Table 3. Confusion matrix for the ensemble model with a threshold of 0.5.

		Predicted Label	
		Other	Poorly ADC
True label	Other	1572	153
	Poorly ADC	11	63

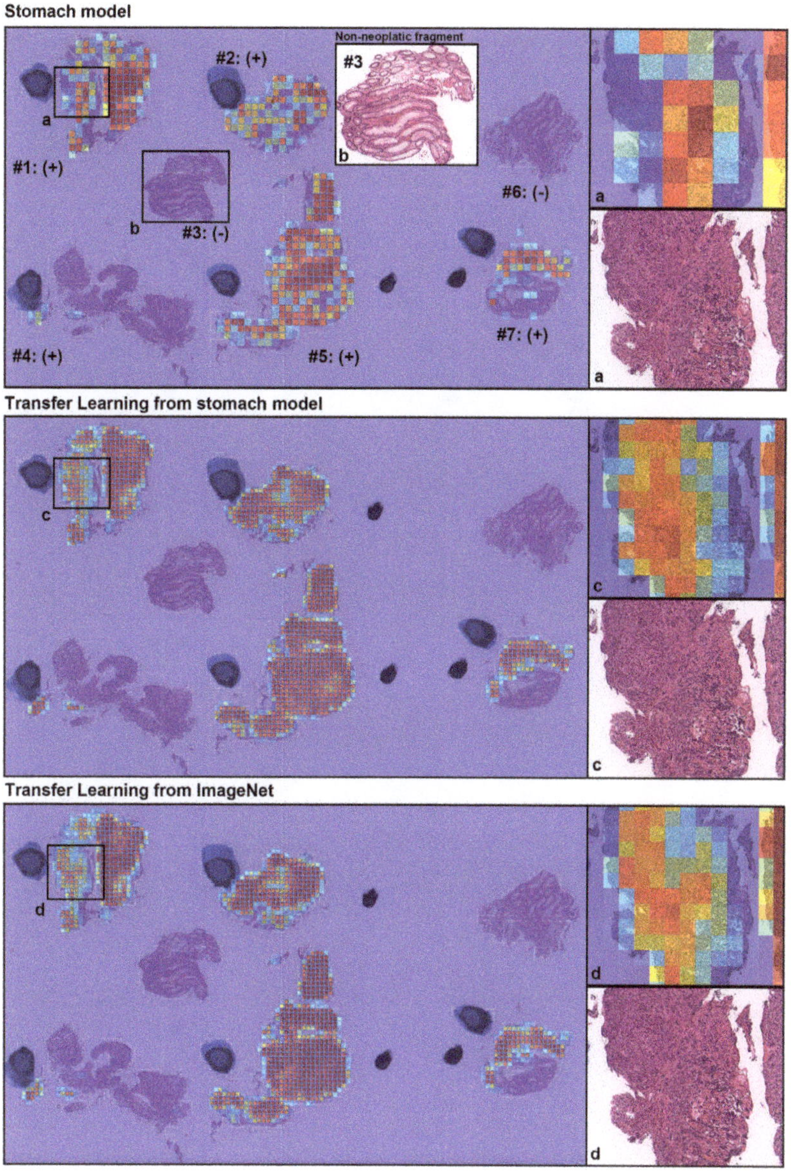

Figure 3. A representative true positive poorly differentiated colorectal ADC case from the endoscopic biopsy test set. Heatmap images show true positive predictions of poorly differentiated ADC cells and they correspond, respectively, to H&E histopathology (a, c, d) using stomach model (**upper panel**), transfer learning from stomach model (**middle panel**), and transfer learning from ImageNet model (**lower panel**). According to the pathological diagnosis provided by surgical pathologists, histopathological evaluation for each tissue fragment is as follows: #1, #2, #4, #5, and #7 were positive for poorly differentiated ADC; #3 and #6 were negative for poorly differentiated ADC. The high magnification image (b) shows representative H&E histology (#3 fragment), which is negative for poorly differentiated ADC.

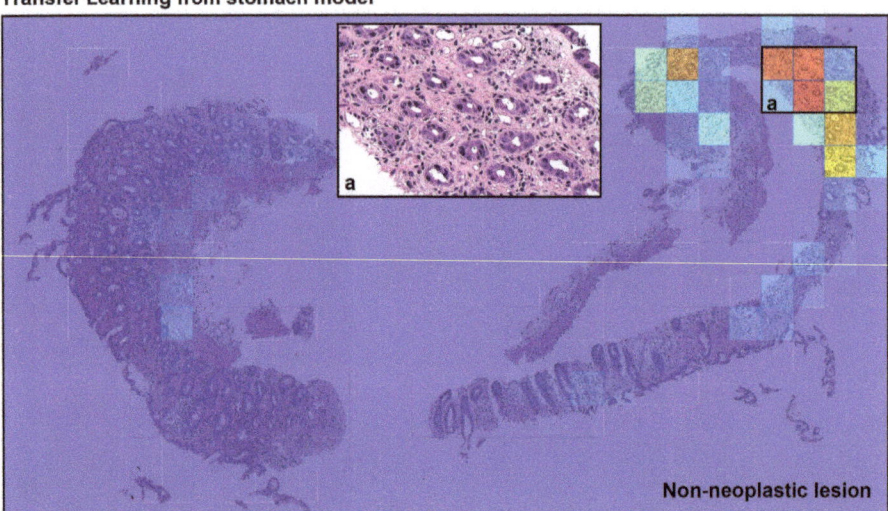
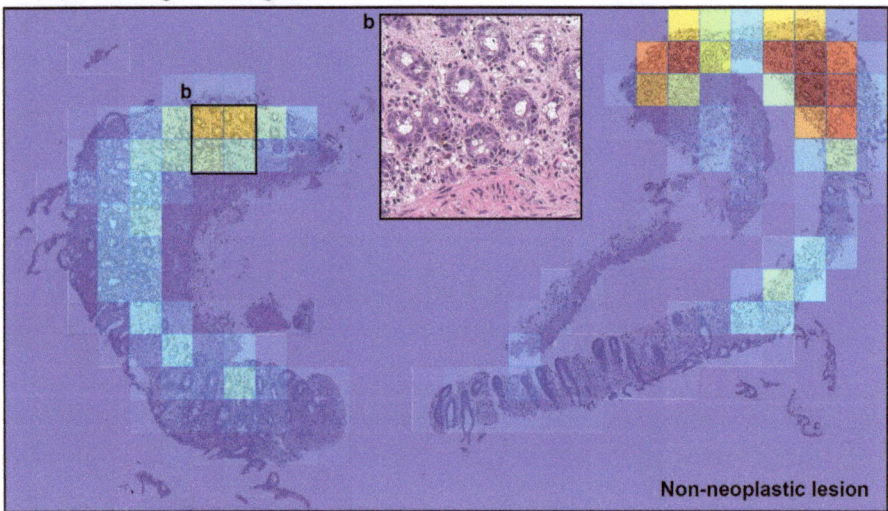

Figure 4. A representative example of poorly differentiated colorectal adenocarcinoma (ADC) false positive prediction output on a case the from endoscopic biopsy test set. Histopathologically, this case is a non-neoplastic lesion (colitis). Heatmap images exhibited false positive prediction of poorly differentiated ADC using transfer learning from stomach model (**upper panel**) and transfer learning from ImageNet model (**lower panel**). The inflammatory tissue with plasma cell infiltration (a and b) is the primary cause of false positive due to its analogous nuclear and cellular morphology to poorly differentiated ADC cells.

4. Discussion

In this study, we trained deep learning models for the classification of poorly differentiated ADC from colorectal biopsy WSIs. We used transfer learning with a hard mining of false positives to train the models on a training set obtained from two hospitals. We evaluated four models—one of which was an ensemble of the other three—on five different test sets originating from different hospitals, and on the combination of all five, given the small number of cases with poorly differentiated ADC. Overall, we obtained high ROC AUC of about 0.95.

Given the histopathological similarity between gastric and colonic ADC, the stomach model—which was previously trained on poorly differentiated cases of gastric ADC—was still able to perform well on the colonic cases. There was improvement in further fine-tuning the model, where the ROC AUC increased from 0.89 to 0.95. However, the result is similar to having fine-tuned a model that was previously only trained on ImageNet. The ensemble model had similar AUC, albeit with the lowest log loss of all the models.

The primary limitation of this study was the small number of poorly differentiated ADC cases; overall, there were only 36 in the training set and 74 in the test set. The small number of poorly differentiated ADC is to be expected given that well to moderately differentiated ADC is typically more common. The combined test set contained a large number of well to moderately differentiated ADC and non-neoplastic, which increases the chances of false positives. Nonetheless, the models performed well and did not have a high false positive rate across a wide range of thresholds, based on the ROC curves in Figure 2.

Most ADCs in colon are moderately to well differentiated types. On the other hand, because poorly differentiated ADC exhibits the worst prognoses among the various types of colorectal cancer, it is important to classify on endoscopic biopsy specimens [26]. In this study, we have shown that deep learning models could potentially be used for the classification of poorly differentiated ADC. Using a simple transfer learning method, it was possible to train a high performing model relatively quickly compared to having to train a model from scratch. Deep learning models show high potential for aiding pathologists and improving the efficiency of their workflow systems.

Poorly differentiated ADC tends to grow and spread more quickly than well and moderately differentiated ADC, and this makes early screening critical for improving patient prognosis. The promising results of this study add to the growing evidence that deep learning models could be used as a tool to aid pathologists in their routine diagnostic workflows, potentially acting as a second screener. One advantage of using an automated tool is that it can systematically handle large amounts of WSIs without potential bias due to fatigue commonly experienced by surgical pathologists. It could also drastically alleviate the heavy clinical burden of daily pathology diagnosis. AI is considered a valuable tool that could transform the future of healthcare and precision oncology.

Author Contributions: M.T. and F.K. contributed equally to this work; M.T. and F.K. designed the studies, performed experiments, analysed the data, and wrote the manuscript; M.T. supervised the project. All authors reviewed the manuscript. All authors have read and agreed to the published version of the manuscript.

Funding: This research received no external funding.

Institutional Review Board Statement: The experimental protocol was approved by the ethical board of the International University of Health and Welfare (No. 19-Im-007) and Kamachi Group Hospitals. All research activities complied with all relevant ethical regulations and were performed in accordance with relevant guidelines and regulations in the all hospitals mentioned above.

Informed Consent Statement: Informed consent to use histopathological samples and pathological diagnostic reports for research purposes had previously been obtained from all patients prior to the surgical procedures at all hospitals, and the opportunity for refusal to participate in research had been guaranteed by an opt-out manner.

Data Availability Statement: Due to specific institutional requirements governing privacy protection, datasets used in this study are not publicly available.

Acknowledgments: We are grateful for the support provided by Takayuki Shiomi and Ichiro Mori at the Department of Pathology, Faculty of Medicine, International University of Health and Welfare; Ryosuke Matsuoka at the Diagnostic Pathology Center, International University of Health and Welfare, Mita Hospital; pathologists at Kamachi Group Hospitals (Fukuoka). We thank the pathologists who have been engaged in the annotation, reviewing cases, and pathological discussion for this study.

Conflicts of Interest: M.T. and F.K. are employees of Medmain Inc.

References

1. Siegel, R.L.; Miller, K.D.; Goding Sauer, A.; Fedewa, S.A.; Butterly, L.F.; Anderson, J.C.; Cercek, A.; Smith, R.A.; Jemal, A. Colorectal cancer statistics, 2020. *CA Cancer J. Clin.* **2020**, *70*, 145–164. [CrossRef]
2. Sung, H.; Ferlay, J.; Siegel, R.L.; Laversanne, M.; Soerjomataram, I.; Jemal, A.; Bray, F. Global cancer statistics 2020: GLOBOCAN estimates of incidence and mortality worldwide for 36 cancers in 185 countries. *CA Cancer J. Clin.* **2021**, *71*, 209–249. [CrossRef]
3. Wolf, A.M.; Fontham, E.T.; Church, T.R.; Flowers, C.R.; Guerra, C.E.; LaMonte, S.J.; Etzioni, R.; McKenna, M.T.; Oeffinger, K.C.; Shih, Y.C.T.; et al. Colorectal cancer screening for average-risk adults: 2018 guideline update from the American Cancer Society. *CA Cancer J. Clin.* **2018**, *68*, 250–281. [CrossRef]
4. Winawer, S.J.; Zauber, A.G. The advanced adenoma as the primary target of screening. *Gastrointest. Endosc. Clin. N. Am.* **2002**, *12*, 1–9. [CrossRef]
5. Yu, K.H.; Zhang, C.; Berry, G.J.; Altman, R.B.; Ré, C.; Rubin, D.L.; Snyder, M. Predicting non-small cell lung cancer prognosis by fully automated microscopic pathology image features. *Nat. Commun.* **2016**, *7*, 12474. [CrossRef]
6. Hou, L.; Samaras, D.; Kurc, T.M.; Gao, Y.; Davis, J.E.; Saltz, J.H. Patch-based convolutional neural network for whole slide tissue image classification. In Proceedings of the IEEE Conference on Computer Vision and Pattern Recognition, Las Vegas, NV, USA, 27–30 June 2016; pp. 2424–2433.
7. Madabhushi, A.; Lee, G. Image analysis and machine learning in digital pathology: Challenges and opportunities. *Med. Image Anal.* **2016**, *33*, 170–175. [CrossRef]
8. Litjens, G.; Sánchez, C.I.; Timofeeva, N.; Hermsen, M.; Nagtegaal, I.; Kovacs, I.; Hulsbergen-Van De Kaa, C.; Bult, P.; Van Ginneken, B.; Van Der Laak, J. Deep learning as a tool for increased accuracy and efficiency of histopathological diagnosis. *Sci. Rep.* **2016**, *6*, 26286. [CrossRef] [PubMed]
9. Kraus, O.Z.; Ba, J.L.; Frey, B.J. Classifying and segmenting microscopy images with deep multiple instance learning. *Bioinformatics* **2016**, *32*, i52–i59. [CrossRef] [PubMed]
10. Korbar, B.; Olofson, A.M.; Miraflor, A.P.; Nicka, C.M.; Suriawinata, M.A.; Torresani, L.; Suriawinata, A.A.; Hassanpour, S. Deep learning for classification of colorectal polyps on whole-slide images. *J. Pathol. Inform.* **2017**, *8*, 30. [PubMed]
11. Luo, X.; Zang, X.; Yang, L.; Huang, J.; Liang, F.; Rodriguez-Canales, J.; Wistuba, I.I.; Gazdar, A.; Xie, Y.; Xiao, G. Comprehensive computational pathological image analysis predicts lung cancer prognosis. *J. Thorac. Oncol.* **2017**, *12*, 501–509. [CrossRef] [PubMed]
12. Coudray, N.; Ocampo, P.S.; Sakellaropoulos, T.; Narula, N.; Snuderl, M.; Fenyö, D.; Moreira, A.L.; Razavian, N.; Tsirigos, A. Classification and mutation prediction from non–small cell lung cancer histopathology images using deep learning. *Nat. Med.* **2018**, *24*, 1559–1567. [CrossRef] [PubMed]
13. Wei, J.W.; Tafe, L.J.; Linnik, Y.A.; Vaickus, L.J.; Tomita, N.; Hassanpour, S. Pathologist-level classification of histologic patterns on resected lung adenocarcinoma slides with deep neural networks. *Sci. Rep.* **2019**, *9*, 3358. [CrossRef] [PubMed]
14. Gertych, A.; Swiderska-Chadaj, Z.; Ma, Z.; Ing, N.; Markiewicz, T.; Cierniak, S.; Salemi, H.; Guzman, S.; Walts, A.E.; Knudsen, B.S. Convolutional neural networks can accurately distinguish four histologic growth patterns of lung adenocarcinoma in digital slides. *Sci. Rep.* **2019**, *9*, 1483. [CrossRef]
15. Bejnordi, B.E.; Veta, M.; Van Diest, P.J.; Van Ginneken, B.; Karssemeijer, N.; Litjens, G.; Van Der Laak, J.A.; Hermsen, M.; Manson, Q.F.; Balkenhol, M.; et al. Diagnostic assessment of deep learning algorithms for detection of lymph node metastases in women with breast cancer. *JAMA* **2017**, *318*, 2199–2210. [CrossRef] [PubMed]
16. Saltz, J.; Gupta, R.; Hou, L.; Kurc, T.; Singh, P.; Nguyen, V.; Samaras, D.; Shroyer, K.R.; Zhao, T.; Batiste, R.; et al. Spatial organization and molecular correlation of tumor-infiltrating lymphocytes using deep learning on pathology images. *Cell Rep.* **2018**, *23*, 181–193. [CrossRef]
17. Campanella, G.; Hanna, M.G.; Geneslaw, L.; Miraflor, A.; Silva, V.W.K.; Busam, K.J.; Brogi, E.; Reuter, V.E.; Klimstra, D.S.; Fuchs, T.J. Clinical-grade computational pathology using weakly supervised deep learning on whole slide images. *Nat. Med.* **2019**, *25*, 1301–1309. [CrossRef]
18. Iizuka, O.; Kanavati, F.; Kato, K.; Rambeau, M.; Arihiro, K.; Tsuneki, M. Deep learning models for histopathological classification of gastric and colonic epithelial tumours. *Sci. Rep.* **2020**, *10*, 1504. [CrossRef]
19. Hamilton, S.; Vogelstein, B.; Kudo, S.; Riboli, E.; Nakamura, S.; Hainaut, P. Carcinoma of the colon and rectum. Pathology and genetics of tumours of the digestive system. In *World Health Organization Classification of Tumours*; IARC Press: Lyon, France, 2000; pp. 103–119.
20. Ogawa, M.; Watanabe, M.; Eto, K.; Kosuge, M.; Yamagata, T.; Kobayashi, T.; Yamazaki, K.; Anazawa, S.; Yanaga, K. Poorly differentiated adenocarcinoma of the colon and rectum: Clinical characteristics. *Hepato-gastroenterology* **2008**, *55*, 907–911.
21. Winn, B.; Tavares, R.; Matoso, A.; Noble, L.; Fanion, J.; Waldman, S.A.; Resnick, M.B. Expression of the intestinal biomarkers Guanylyl cyclase C and CDX2 in poorly differentiated colorectal carcinomas. *Hum. Pathol.* **2010**, *41*, 123–128. [CrossRef]
22. Kazama, Y.; Watanabe, T.; Kanazawa, T.; Tanaka, J.; Tanaka, T.; Nagawa, H. Poorly differentiated colorectal adenocarcinomas show higher rates of microsatellite instability and promoter methylation of p16 and hMLH1: A study matched for T classification and tumor location. *J. Surg. Oncol.* **2008**, *97*, 278–283. [CrossRef]
23. Takeuchi, K.; Kuwano, H.; Tsuzuki, Y.; Ando, T.; Sekihara, M.; Hara, T.; Asao, T. Clinicopathological characteristics of poorly differentiated adenocarcinoma of the colon and rectum. *Hepato-gastroenterology* **2004**, *51*, 1698–1702. [PubMed]

24. Secco, G.; Fardelli, R.; Campora, E.; Lapertosa, G.; Gentile, R.; Zoli, S.; Prior, C. Primary mucinous adenocarcinomas and signet-ring cell carcinomas of colon and rectum. *Oncology* **1994**, *51*, 30–34. [CrossRef] [PubMed]
25. Taniyama, K.; Suzuki, H.; Matsumoto, M.; Hakamada, K.; Toyam, K.; Tahara, E. Flow Cytometric DNA Analysis of Poorly Differentialted Adenocarcinoma of the Colorectum. *Jpn. J. Clin. Oncol.* **1991**, *21*, 406–411. [PubMed]
26. Kawabata, Y.; Tomita, N.; Monden, T.; Ohue, M.; Ohnishi, T.; Sasaki, M.; Sekimoto, M.; Sakita, I.; Tamaki, Y.; Takahashi, J.; et al. Molecular characteristics of poorly differentiated adenocarcinoma and signet-ring-cell carcinoma of colorectum. *Int. J. Cancer* **1999**, *84*, 33–38. [CrossRef]
27. Sugao, Y.; Yao, T.; Kubo, C.; Tsuneyoshi, M. Improved prognosis of solid-type poorly differentiated colorectal adenocarcinoma: A clinicopathological and immunohistochemical study. *Histopathology* **1997**, *31*, 123–133. [CrossRef] [PubMed]
28. Komori, K.; Kanemitsu, Y.; Ishiguro, S.; Shimizu, Y.; Sano, T.; Ito, S.; Abe, T.; Senda, Y.; Misawa, K.; Ito, Y.; et al. Clinicopathological study of poorly differentiated colorectal adenocarcinomas: Comparison between solid-type and non-solid-type adenocarcinomas. *Anticancer Res.* **2011**, *31*, 3463–3467. [PubMed]
29. Kanavati, F.; Tsuneki, M. Partial transfusion: On the expressive influence of trainable batch norm parameters for transfer learning. *arXiv* **2021**, arXiv:2102.05543.
30. Kanavati, F.; Tsuneki, M. A deep learning model for gastric diffuse-type adenocarcinoma classification in whole slide images. *arXiv* **2021**, arXiv:2104.12478.
31. Kanavati, F.; Toyokawa, G.; Momosaki, S.; Rambeau, M.; Kozuma, Y.; Shoji, F.; Yamazaki, K.; Takeo, S.; Iizuka, O.; Tsuneki, M. Weakly-supervised learning for lung carcinoma classification using deep learning. *Sci. Rep.* **2020**, *10*, 9297. [CrossRef]
32. Kanavati, F.; Toyokawa, G.; Momosaki, S.; Takeoka, H.; Okamoto, M.; Yamazaki, K.; Takeo, S.; Iizuka, O.; Tsuneki, M. A deep learning model for the classification of indeterminate lung carcinoma in biopsy whole slide images. *Sci. Rep.* **2021**, *11*, 8110. [CrossRef]
33. Tan, M.; Le, Q. Efficientnet: Rethinking model scaling for convolutional neural networks. In Proceedings of the International Conference on Machine Learning, Long Beach, CA, USA, 9–15 June 2019; pp. 6105–6114.
34. Otsu, N. A threshold selection method from gray-level histograms. *IEEE Trans. Syst. Man Cybern.* **1979**, *9*, 62–66. [CrossRef]
35. Kingma, D.P.; Ba, J. Adam: A method for stochastic optimization. *arXiv* **2014**, arXiv:1412.6980.
36. Abadi, M.; Agarwal, A.; Barham, P.; Brevdo, E.; Chen, Z.; Citro, C.; Corrado, G.S.; Davis, A.; Dean, J.; Devin, M.; et al. TensorFlow: Large-Scale Machine Learning on Heterogeneous Systems. 2015. Available online: tensorflow.org (accessed on 24 January 2020).
37. Pedregosa, F.; Varoquaux, G.; Gramfort, A.; Michel, V.; Thirion, B.; Grisel, O.; Blondel, M.; Prettenhofer, P.; Weiss, R.; Dubourg, V.; et al. Scikit-learn: Machine Learning in Python. *J. Mach. Learn. Res.* **2011**, *12*, 2825–2830.
38. Hunter, J.D. Matplotlib: A 2D graphics environment. *Comput. Sci. Eng.* **2007**, *9*, 90–95. [CrossRef]
39. van der Walt, S.; Schönberger, J.L.; Nunez-Iglesias, J.; Boulogne, F.; Warner, J.D.; Yager, N.; Gouillart, E.; Yu, T.; the scikit-image contributors. scikit-image: Image processing in Python. *PeerJ* **2014**, *2*, e453. [CrossRef]
40. Efron, B.; Tibshirani, R.J. *An Introduction to the Bootstrap*; CRC Press: Boca Raton, FL, USA, 1994.
41. Goode, A.; Gilbert, B.; Harkes, J.; Jukic, D.; Satyanarayanan, M. OpenSlide: A vendor-neutral software foundation for digital pathology. *J. Pathol. Inform.* **2013**, *4*, 27.
42. Deng, J.; Dong, W.; Socher, R.; Li, L.J.; Li, K.; Fei-Fei, L. Imagenet: A large-scale hierarchical image database. In Proceedings of the 2009 IEEE Conference on Computer Vision and Pattern Recognition, Miami, FL, USA, 20–25 June 2009; pp. 248–255.
43. Zhang, C.; Ma, Y. *Ensemble Machine Learning: Methods and Applications*; Springer: Berlin/Heidelberg, Germany, 2012.

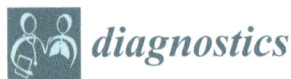

Article

Machine Learning Model for Outcome Prediction of Patients Suffering from Acute Diverticulitis Arriving at the Emergency Department—A Proof of Concept Study

Eyal Klang [1,2], Robert Freeman [3], Matthew A. Levin [3,4], Shelly Soffer [5,6], Yiftach Barash [1] and Adi Lahat [7,8,*]

1. Sheba Medical Center, Department of Diagnostic Imaging, Tel Hashomer, Israel, and Sackler Medical School, Tel Aviv University, Tel Aviv 52621, Israel; eyalkla@hotmail.com (E.K.); yibarash@gmail.com (Y.B.)
2. Sheba Talpiot Medical Leadership Program, Tel Hashomer, Israel, and Sackler Medical School, Tel Aviv University, Tel Aviv 52621, Israel
3. Department of Population Health Science and Policy, Institute for Healthcare Delivery Science, Icahn School of Medicine at Mount Sinai, New York, NY 10029, USA; Robert.Freeman@mountsinai.org (R.F.); Matthew.Levin@mssm.edu (M.A.L.)
4. Department of Anesthesiology, Perioperative and Pain Medicine, Icahn School of Medicine at Mount Sinai, New York, NY 10029, USA
5. Assuta Medical Center, Ashdod 7747629, Israel; soffer.shelly@gmail.com
6. Ben-Gurion University of the Negev, Be'er Sheba 69710, Israel
7. Chaim Sheba Medical Center, Department of Gastroenterology, Sackler Medical School, Tel Aviv University, Tel Hashomer 52620, Israel
8. Sackler Medical School, Tel Aviv University, Tel Aviv 67011, Israel
* Correspondence: zokadi@gmail.com

Citation: Klang, E.; Freeman, R.; Levin, M.A.; Soffer, S.; Barash, Y.; Lahat, A. Machine Learning Model for Outcome Prediction of Patients Suffering from Acute Diverticulitis Arriving at the Emergency Department—A Proof of Concept Study. *Diagnostics* **2021**, *11*, 2102. https://doi.org/10.3390/diagnostics11112102

Academic Editors: Eun-Sun Kim and Kwang-Sig Lee

Received: 13 October 2021
Accepted: 11 November 2021
Published: 13 November 2021

Publisher's Note: MDPI stays neutral with regard to jurisdictional claims in published maps and institutional affiliations.

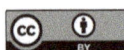

Copyright: © 2021 by the authors. Licensee MDPI, Basel, Switzerland. This article is an open access article distributed under the terms and conditions of the Creative Commons Attribution (CC BY) license (https://creativecommons.org/licenses/by/4.0/).

Abstract: Background & Aims: We aimed at identifying specific emergency department (ED) risk factors for developing complicated acute diverticulitis (AD) and evaluate a machine learning model (ML) for predicting complicated AD. Methods: We analyzed data retrieved from unselected consecutive large bowel AD patients from five hospitals from the Mount Sinai health system, NY. The study time frame was from January 2011 through March 2021. Data were used to train and evaluate a gradient-boosting machine learning model to identify patients with complicated diverticulitis, defined as a need for invasive intervention or in-hospital mortality. The model was trained and evaluated on data from four hospitals and externally validated on held-out data from the fifth hospital. Results: The final cohort included 4997 AD visits. Of them, 129 (2.9%) visits had complicated diverticulitis. Patients with complicated diverticulitis were more likely to be men, black, and arrive by ambulance. Regarding laboratory values, patients with complicated diverticulitis had higher levels of absolute neutrophils (AUC 0.73), higher white blood cells (AUC 0.70), platelet count (AUC 0.68) and lactate (AUC 0.61), and lower levels of albumin (AUC 0.69), chloride (AUC 0.64), and sodium (AUC 0.61). In the external validation cohort, the ML model showed AUC 0.85 (95% CI 0.78–0.91) for predicting complicated diverticulitis. For Youden's index, the model showed a sensitivity of 88% with a false positive rate of 1:3.6. Conclusions: A ML model trained on clinical measures provides a proof of concept performance in predicting complications in patients presenting to the ED with AD. Clinically, it implies that a ML model may classify low-risk patients to be discharged from the ED for further treatment under an ambulatory setting.

Keywords: machine learning; artificial intelligence; acute diverticulitis; outcome prediction; emergency; complications

1. Introduction

Diverticulosis of the colon is a common condition in Western societies; by the age of 85, two-thirds of Western countries' populations will have developed colonic diverticula [1,2].

While most patients remain asymptomatic, a minor portion will suffer from diverticular disease, most commonly acute diverticulitis (AD) occurring in 10–25% of patients [2–6] or even less—up to 4% according to recent literature [7].

Data from recent years show an increase in hospitalization rates for AD in most countries. In the US, more than 216,000 hospital admissions due to AD were reported in 2012, an increase of 21% from 2003 [8]. In Europe, a yearly increase in the admission rate of approximately 2% was shown in Italy between 2008–2015 [9], with a similar increase in the admission rate in the UK between 1996 to 2006 from 0.56 per 1000 person-years to 1.2 per 100 person-years [10].

Complications of AD affect 10–12% of patients [11]. The most common complication affecting 70% of patients is abscess formation, followed by peritonitis, obstruction, and fistula.

Patients suffering from complicated AD are at an increased risk of mortality compared to patients with an uncomplicated disease [11,12]. A population-based study from the UK found a 20% one-year mortality for patients suffering from complicated diverticulitis, compared to 4% in age- and sex-matched controls [12].

On the other hand, patients with an uncomplicated disease can safely be managed in an ambulatory setting [13–15].

Therefore, it is clear that assessing patients' risk factors for developing a complicated disease is highly important during the clinical decision-making process.

Few recent studies found a correlation between either CRP levels and the white blood cell count (WBC) and severe disease [14,16–21]. Other reporter risk factors were the comorbidity index (ASA) [20], body mass index [22], and diabetes mellitus [23]. Most of the studies were relatively small, and a recent literature review concluded that evidence in the current literature of risk factors for complicated AD is not strong [13].

In the last decade, there has been much progress in the field of machine learning. Various machine learning applications are being investigated for optimizing healthcare. Emphasis is placed on the use of algorithms for predicting the clinical course [24,25]. Such decision support tools can affect the diagnostic workup and treatment plan.

Therefore, in our current multi-site study assessing 4997 emergency department (ED) visits during the years 2011–2021, we aimed at identifying specific risk factors for developing complicated AD and evaluating different machine learning models for predicting complicated AD.

2. Materials and Methods

2.1. Study Design

We retrieved data for consecutive patients with acute diverticulitis, as defined by a computerized data system using the ICD-10 diagnosis code. Data came from 5 hospital campuses serving different geographic populations: Mount Sinai Hospital (MSH), Mount Sinai Brooklyn (MSB), Mount Sinai Queens (MSQ), Mount Sinai Morningside (MSM), and Mount Sinai West (MSW). The Mount Sinai Institutional Review Board (IRB) approved this study. The IRB committee waived informed consent. The time frame of the study was between 1 January 2011 and 29 March 2021.

Data were retrieved from the Epic electronic medical records (EMR) system, which is unified for the five included hospitals (Epic Systems Corporation, Verona, WI, USA).

Variables included demographics; comorbidities; arrival mode (walk-in, by ambulance, or by intensive care ambulance); chief complaints; vital signs measurements at admission; acuity level, also called emergency severity index (ESI), which is a five-level acuity score assigned by the triage nurse and which provides a clinically relevant stratification of patients into five groups from 1 (most urgent) to 5 (least urgent) on the basis of acuity and resource needs; and laboratory results obtained at admission.

All patients included transit through the ER, and the lab results were collected in the ER. Thus, patients' evaluation was performed in the ER setting.

Complicated diverticulitis was defined as a need for intervention (surgical or drainage) or in-hospital mortality. All complications necessitating intervention were CT-proven and showed an overt abscess and/or free perforation. All patients were followed for recurrent ER visits. A recurrent visit within 7 days from discharge was regarded as a same visit. Data were split into training, internal validation (MSH, MSB, MSM, MSW), and external testing (MSQ) sets. Machine learning models were trained on the data to predict a complicated diverticulitis.

2.2. Inclusion and Exclusion Criteria

We included adult patients ($\geq$18) diagnosed with acute large bowel diverticulitis in the emergency department (ED) or hospital wards. We excluded patients younger than 18 and patients with small bowel diverticulitis.

2.3. Machine Learning Models

Comorbidities were coded as International Classification of Diseases (ICD-10) records and grouped using the diagnostic clinical classification software (CCS). Categorical factors were one-hot-encoded. Missing values were imputed using the training cohort median.

We have compared two machine learning model: gradient boosting (GB) and random forest (RF). The GB model was implemented using the XGBoost library. The RF algorithm was implemented using the scikit-learn library. Recursive feature selection was used to find an estimate of the number of features in the models. The recursive feature selection experiments were conducted in the training/internal validation cohort (MSH, MSB, MSM, MSW), using the bootstrapping of 100 random 90/10 split. Model hyper-parameters were also tuned in the training/internal validation cohort, using the same split method. (GB—number of estimators: 25, eta: 0.3, max depth: 3, RF: number of estimators: 200, criterion: "gini", max depth: "None"). Data balancing techniques using scale weighting did not improve the models' accuracies and thus were not employed. The final GB and RF models were trained on the entire internal validation cohort and tested on the external validation cohort. SHAP summary explainability plots were constructed to assess the final GB and RF models' feature importance.

Programming was done with Python (Version 3.6.5 64 bits).

2.4. Statistical Analysis

Categorical variables were compared using the χ^2 test. Continuous variables were compared using Student's *t*-test.

The area under the receiver curve (AUC) metric assesses the models' performance on the external validation cohort. Further metrics were evaluated for the GB final model. Youden's index was used to find an optimal sensitivity-specificity cutoff point on the receiver operating characteristic (ROC) curve. Different metrics were also evaluated for fixed specificities of 90%, 95%, and 99%. Metrics included sensitivity, specificity, false-positive rate (FPR), negative predictive value (NPV), positive predictive value (PPV), and F1 score. Bootstrapping validations (1000 bootstrap resamples) were used to calculate 95% confidence intervals (CI) for the different metrics.

3. Results

The study's inclusion flow diagram is presented in Figure 1. The final cohort included 4997 visits with large bowel diverticulitis. These corresponded to 3600 unique patients. Of the 4997 visits, 1821 (40.5%) were admitted to the hospital from the ED. Five (0.1%) patients returned to the hospital with complicated AD within a week from discharge from a noncomplicated AD visit.

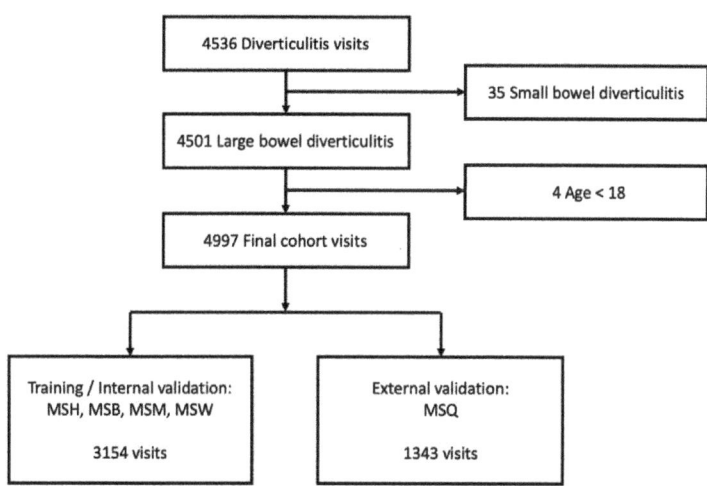

Figure 1. Study flow chart. Abbreviations: Mount Sinai Hospital MSH; Mount Sinai Brooklyn MSB; Mount Sinai Morningside MSM; Mount Sinai West MSW; Mount Sinai Queens MSQ.

Overall, 129 (2.9%) visits had complicated diverticulitis (59 surgical intervention, 71 drainage intervention, seven mortality cases; with overlap). Table 1 presents the characteristics of the entire cohort, stratified by complicated diverticulitis status.

Table 1. Baseline characteristics of the study cohort comparing the complicated AD group to the uncomplicated AD group.

	Uncomplicated AD (n = 4368, 97.1%)	Complicated AD (n = 129, 2.9%)	p Value
	Demographics		
Age, median (IQR), y	58.0 (48.0–69.0)	56.0 (48.0–67.0)	0.348
Female, N. (%)	2561 (58.6)	57 (44.2)	0.001
Black, N. (%)	750 (17.2)	34 (26.4)	0.010
White, N. (%)	1390 (31.8)	45 (34.9)	0.523
	ED Triage		
Arrival Mode: EMS, N. (%)	466 (10.7)	25 (19.4)	0.003
Arrival Mode: BLS, N. (%)	254 (5.8)	19 (14.7)	<0.001
ESI, median (IQR), Acuity level (1–5)	3.0 (3.0–3.0)	3.0 (3.0–3.0)	<0.001
	Vital Signs		
SBP, median (IQR), mmHg	135.0 (122.0–150.0)	132.0 (117.0–148.0)	0.171
DBP, median (IQR), mmHg	78.0 (70.0–86.0)	77.0 (66.0–88.0)	0.511
Heart rate, median (IQR), b/min	87.0 (76.0–98.0)	98.0 (86.0–110.0)	<0.001
Temperature, median (IQR), Celsius	36.7 (36.4–37.1)	36.8 (36.5–37.2)	0.026
Respirations, median (IQR), num/min	18.0 (18.0–19.0)	18.0 (18.0–19.0)	0.295
O2 saturation, median (IQR)%	98.0 (97.0–99.0)	98.0 (97.0–99.0)	0.042
Pain scale, median (IQR), (0–10)	7.0 (5.0–9.0)	7.0 (5.0–10.0)	0.652
	Comorbidities		
CAD, N. (%)	452 (10.3)	11 (8.5)	0.600
CHF, N. (%)	262 (6.0)	13 (10.1)	0.086
DM, N. (%)	933 (21.4)	27 (20.9)	0.993
HTN, N. (%)	1443 (33.0)	46 (35.7)	0.597
CKD, N. (%)	270 (6.2)	6 (4.7)	0.598
COPD, N. (%)	305 (7.0)	10 (7.8)	0.871
NEOPLASTIC, N. (%)	873 (20.0)	21 (16.3)	0.353
Past or present smoking, N. (%)	1455 (33.3)	47 (36.4)	0.518
BMI, median (IQR), kg/m^2	28.3 (24.9–32.7)	28.7 (25.1–34.0)	0.455

Table 1. Cont.

	Uncomplicated AD (n = 4368, 97.1%)	Complicated AD (n = 129, 2.9%)	p Value
	Laboratory values		
WBC, median (IQR), x10^3/uL	10.5 (8.1–13.2)	13.9 (11.1–17.7)	<0.001
NEUT, median (IQR), ×10^3/uL	7.6 (5.4–10.1)	11.6 (8.5–15.1)	<0.001
HGB, median (IQR), g/dL	13.5 (12.4–14.5)	13.0 (11.9–14.4)	0.005
PLT, median (IQR), g/dL	243.0 (202.0–292.0)	300.0 (234.0–382.0)	<0.001
Albumin, median (IQR), g/dL	3.9 (3.6–4.1)	3.6 (3.1–3.9)	<0.001
Lactate, median (IQR), mg/dL	1.2 (0.9–1.6)	1.3 (1.1–2.1)	0.001
BUN, median (IQR), mg/dL	13.0 (10.0–17.0)	13.0 (10.0–18.0)	0.022
Cr, median (IQR), mg/dL	0.8 (0.7–1.0)	0.9 (0.7–1.2)	0.112
Na, median (IQR), mEq/L	139.0 (137.0–140.0)	137.0 (135.0–140.0)	<0.001
K, median (IQR), mEq/L	4.1 (3.8–4.4)	4.1 (3.7–4.4)	0.373
Cl, median (IQR), mEq/L	104.0 (102.0–106.0)	102.0 (100.0–104.0)	<0.001

Abbreviations: IQR—Interquartile range; ED—Emergency department; BLS—Basic life support; EMS—Emergency medical services; ESI—Emergency severity index; SBP—Systolic blood pressure; DBP—Diastolic blood pressure; BMI—Body mass index; CAD—Coronary artery disease; CHF—Congestive heart failure; DM—Diabetes mellitus; HTN—Hypertension; CKD—Chronic kidney disease; COPD—Chronic obstructive pulmonary disease; HGB—Hemoglobin; NEUT—Neutrophils; WBC—White blood cells; PLT—Platelets; CR—Creatinine; BUN—Blood Urea nitrogen; GLC—Glucose; NA—Sodium; K—Potassium; CL—Chloride; NYC—New York City.

Patients with complicated diverticulitis were more likely to be men, black, and arrive by basic life support ambulance or emergency medical services ambulance (Table 1).

Table 2 presents a single variable analysis of the laboratory variables associated with complicated diverticulitis in the entire cohort. Patients with complicated diverticulitis had higher absolute neutrophils (NEUT), white blood cells (WBC), platelets count (PLT), and lactate levels, and lower albumin, chloride (Cl), and sodium (Na) levels. NEUT had the highest AUC (0.73), followed by WBC (0.70).

Table 2. Areas under the receiver operating characteristic curves (AUC) of laboratory values for predicting worse outcome.

Laboratory Variable	AUC	Youden's Index
NEUT	0.73 (95% CI: 0.68–0.78)	10.5 × 10^3/μL
WBC	0.70 (95% CI: 0.65–0.76)	12.3 × 10^3/μL
Albumin	0.69 (95% CI: 0.63–0.74)	3.4 g/dL
PLT	0.68 (95% CI: 0.62–0.73)	312.0 × 10^3/μL
Cl	0.64 (95% CI: 0.59–0.69)	103.0 mEq/L
Lactate	0.61 (95% CI: 0.56–0.67)	0.9 mg/dL
Na	0.61 (95% CI: 0.56–0.66)	138.0 mEq/L
HGB	0.56 (95% CI: 0.50–0.61)	12.6 g/dL

Abbreviations: NEUT—Neutrophils; WBC—White blood cells; PLT—Platelets; Cl—Chloride; Na—Sodium; HGB—Hemoglobin.

Figure 2 presents the ten most common chief complaints in the cohort. Abdominal pain was by far the most common complaint, with 3299/4497 (73.4%) of the visits.

Machine Learning Models

Figure 2A,B presents the average AUCs of the recursive feature selection results. Both graphs show that the models improve up to about 7–8 features, then reach a plateau, with a slight gradual decline after 20 features. Both models peaked at an average AUC of 0.84–0.85 in the internal validation cohort.

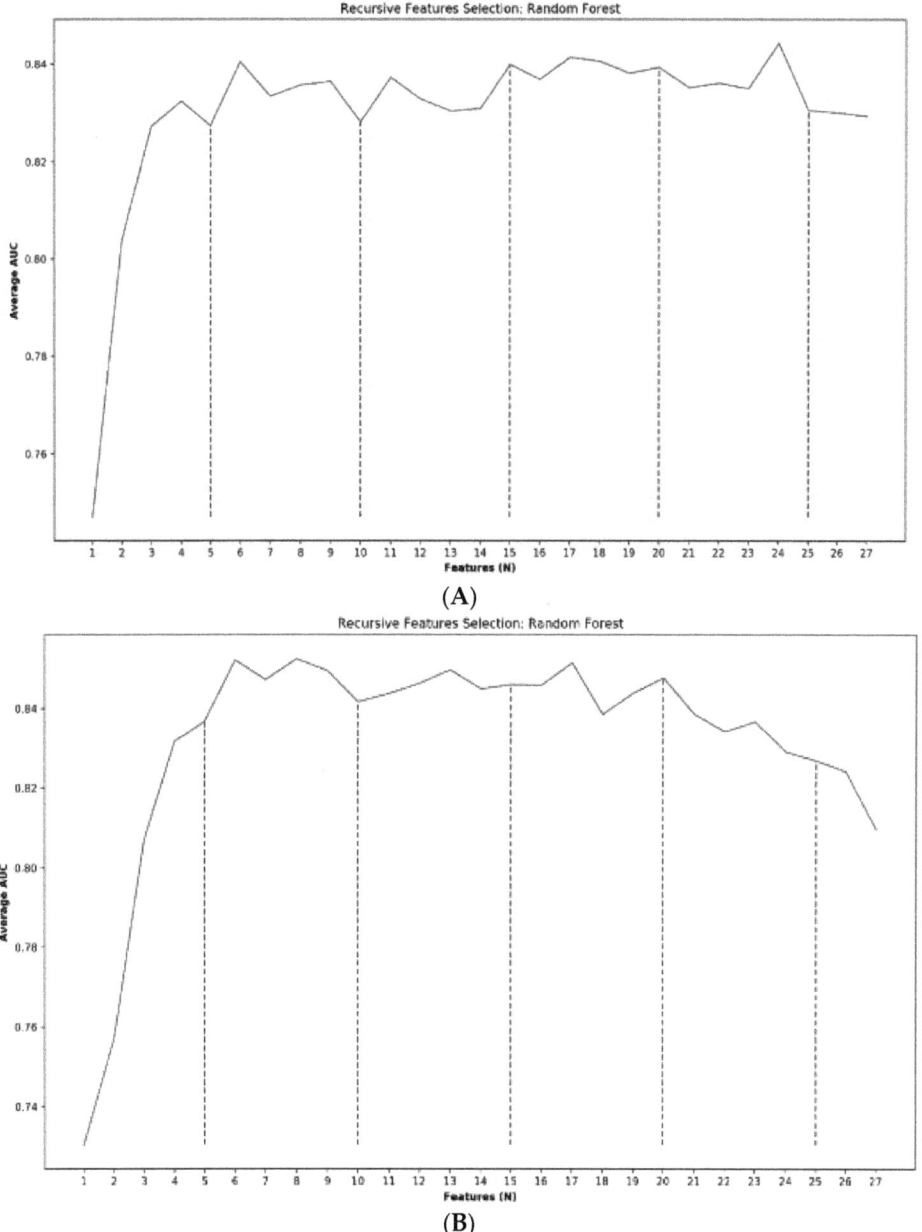

Figure 2. (**A,B**) Averaged areas under the receiver operating characteristic curves (AUC) of the recursive feature selection results. The models were trained and evaluated using 100 random splits of 90/10.

The models for evaluating the external validation cohort were built using the first 20 selected GB or RF features, respectively. GB slightly outperformed RF in the external validation cohort (GB AUC 0.85, 95% CI 0.78—0.91 vs. RF AUC 0.82, 95% CI 0.72—0.90). The SHAP explainability plots of the final GB and RF models are presented in Figure 3A,B.

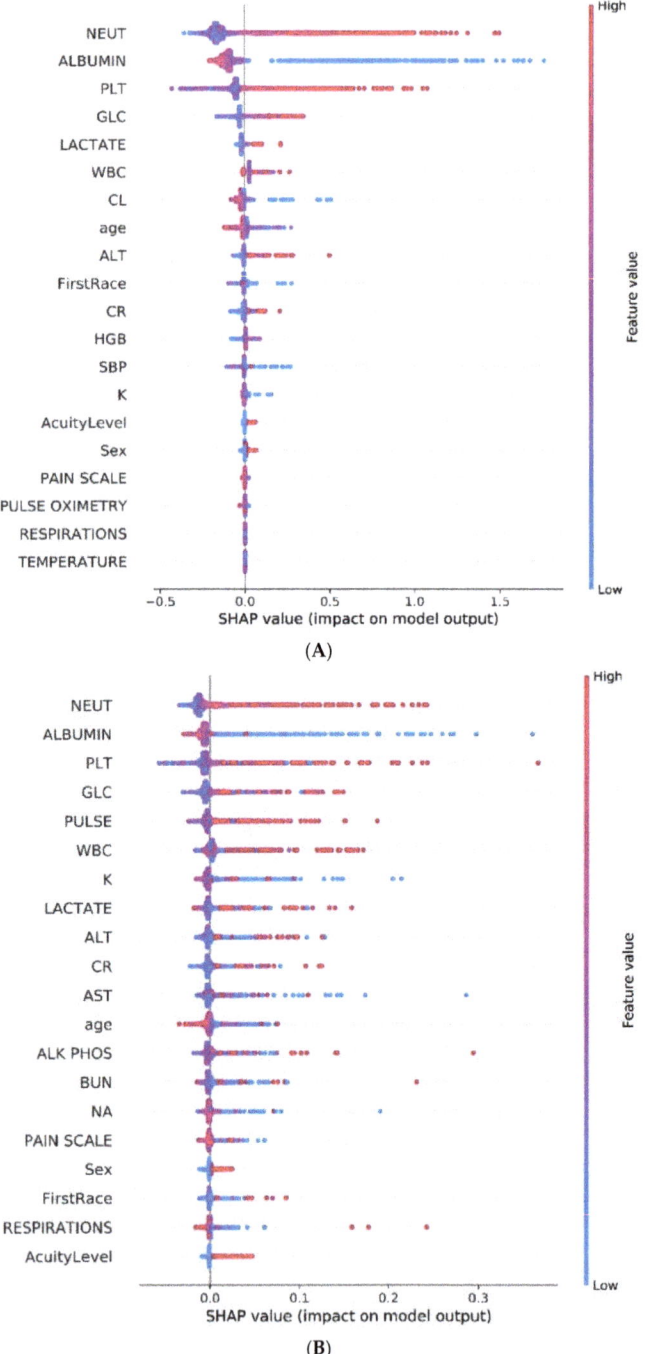

Figure 3. (**A**,**B**) SHAP explainability plots of the final gradient-boosting and random forest models.

For Youden's index, the final GB model showed a sensitivity of 88% with FPR 1:3.6 (Table 3).

Table 3. Metrics of the final gradient-boosting model.

Fixed Specificity	Sensitivity	Specificity	FPR	PPV	NPV	F1
Youden's index	0.88 (95% CI: 0.71–1.00)	0.72 (95% CI: 0.70–0.75)	1:3.6	0.05 (95% CI: 0.03–0.08)	0.99 (95% CI: 0.99–1.00)	0.10 (95% CI: 0.06–0.14)
90%	0.50 (95% CI: 0.30–0.70)	0.90	1:10	0.08 (95% CI: 0.04–0.13)	0.99 (95% CI: 0.98–1.00)	0.14 (95% CI: 0.07–0.22)
95%	0.38 (95% CI: 0.18–0.57)	0.95	1:20	0.12 (95% CI: 0.05–0.20)	0.99 (95% CI: 0.98–0.99)	0.18 (95% CI: 0.08–0.28)
99%	0.04 (95% CI: 0.00–0.14)	0.99	1:100	0.08 (95% CI: 0.00–0.25)	0.98 (95% CI: 0.98–0.99)	0.05 (95% CI: 0.00–0.16)

Abbreviations: FPR—False positive rate; PPV—Positive predictive value; NPV—Negative predictive value; F1—Harmonic mean of sensitivity and PPV.

4. Discussion

In recent years, there has been a clear rise in the incidence of hospitalizations for AD worldwide [8–10]. The rising numbers and the new therapeutic approach towards uncomplicated disease presentation, which supports outpatient conservative treatment [13,14], emphasize the need for effective risk stratification. While patients at risk of complications should be further evaluated, low-risk patients can be safely discharged from the ED for ambulatory treatment.

Herein, we present a gradient-boosting model derived from a large multi-site cohort including approximately 5000 ED visits that predicts the composite outcome of invasive intervention (either surgical or imaging-guided drainage) or in-hospital mortality. The model showed a sensitivity of 88%, FPR of 1:3.6, and NPV of 99%. Thus, it can help identify low-risk patients to be discharged from the ED with no need for further evaluation.

A recent study aimed at developing a diagnostic prediction model to differentiate complicated from uncomplicated AD [26]. This study included a single-center homogeneous group of 910 patients and used the surgical Hinchey classification for the definition of a complication [27]. Hinchey above 1A was classified as complicated. This classification included milder cases, and as a result 18% of patients were classified as complicated, while our study found 2.9% of patients with complicated diverticulitis. Since the classification of Hinchey class 1B as complicated is questionable, as patients at this stage have a favorable outcome in conservative treatment [28], we chose to only include patients treated with invasive interventions for a better disease stratification.

Similar to our results, the final validated diagnostic model included a high WBC as a prognostic factor. Other factors included in this model were CRP levels and abdominal guarding, which were not measured in our study.

Another recent study [29] developed a clinical score aiming at predicting complicated diverticular disease. This study was conducted on approximately 1000 patients, and the main complication presented by 67% of patients categorized as complicated was diverticular hemorrhage, which usually does not correlate with bowel inflammation and was not included in our study. The study used a multivariate logistic regression analysis and reached an AUC of 0.67.

To the best of our knowledge, our study is the largest ML-based multi-site study aimed at predicting the risk of complicated AD in the ED setting. The study inspects clinically relevant outcome measures and uses the composite outcome to assist in the triage of low-risk patients that can be managed safely in an ambulatory setting. Our patients' cohort is diverse in terms of ethnicity and socioeconomic status and comprises patients from five different hospitals. We assessed two types of models during data processing to compare their performance on this database in order to maximize the utility of the model in clinical practice.

Our model has reached a high accuracy in identifying low-risk patients, with a sensitivity of 88% for the prediction of high-risk patients. The FPR was 1:3.6 (Table 3), which indicates that one in four patients will be identified as at risk by mistake. Though not perfect, we believe that in the setting of finding a needle in a haystack and considering the risk of a missed complication, this is a reasonable trade-off.

Our study had several limitations. First, not all relevant laboratory results were available. Thus, though the CRP levels were shown in various studies [14,16–21,29] to correlate with the disease severity and prognosis, only 5% of our patients had this data, as CRP is not a routine laboratory examination in the ERs included in our study. Therefore, CRP levels were not included in the data analysis. Second, data were retrieved from electronic medical records and were retrospective. This might have caused some bias due to missing data. However, we believe that the large volume and patients' diversity can overcome this bias's impact.

Third, although patients were followed for recurrent ER visits, it is possible that a recurrent visit might have been missed if the patient chose to attend a different hospital. However, since data was collected from several hospitals covering a wide geographic distribution in New York City (NYC), it is very likely that a recurrent admission would have been registered.

In conclusion, an ML model trained on clinical measures provided a proof of concept performance in classifying low-risk patients presenting to the ED with AD.

Clinically, this implies that low-risk patients identified by our model may be discharged from the ED for further treatment under an ambulatory setting. Moreover, high-risk patients are identified by the model with a relatively high sensitivity, while only one out of four will be a false positive. We believe that ML can prevent unnecessary hospitalizations and assist in patients' risk stratification under clinical settings. Our results need to be validated in different geographic areas where there are populations of different ethnic origins, and more clinical studies are needed for further evaluations of the effect of ML models on clinical decision-making.

Author Contributions: Conceptualization, A.L. and E.K.; methodology, A.L. and E.K.; software, E.K. and Y.B.; validation, S.S., E.K. and Y.B.; formal analysis, E.K.; investigation, A.L.; resources, R.F. and M.A.L.; data curation E.K., M.A.L. and R.F.; writing—original draft preparation, A.L. and E.K.; writing—review and editing, A.L. and E.K.; All authors have read and agreed to the published version of the manuscript.

Funding: This research received no external funding.

Institutional Review Board Statement: The Mount Sinai Institutional Review Board (IRB) approved this study (Ethic code: STUDY-18-00573-MOD001).

Informed Consent Statement: The IRB committee waived informed consent.

Conflicts of Interest: The authors declare no conflict of interest.

References

1. Hughes, L.E. Postmortem survey of diverticular disease of the colon. *Gut* **1969**, *10*, 336–351. [CrossRef]
2. Garcia, G. Diverticulitis. In *Infecttions of the Gastrointestinal Tract*, 2nd ed.; Blaser, M.T., Smith, D.D., Ravdin, J.I., Greenberg, H.B., Guerrant, R.L., Eds.; Lippincott Williams & Wilkins: Philadelphia, PA, USA, 2002; pp. 306–316.
3. Parks, T.G. Natural History of Diverticular Disease of the Colon. *Clin. Gastroenterol.* **1975**, *4*, 53–69. [CrossRef]
4. Painter, N.S.; Burkitt, D.P. Diverticular disease of the colon, a 20th cencury problem. *Clin. Gastroenterol.* **1975**, *4*, 3–21. [CrossRef]
5. Farrell, R.J.; Farrell, J.J.; Morrin, M.M. Diverticular disease in the elderly. *Gastroenterol. Clic.* **2001**, *30*, 475–496. [CrossRef]
6. Wong, W.D.; Wexner, S.D.; Lowry, A.; Vernava, A., III; Burnstein, M.; Denstman, F.; Fazio, V.; Kerner, B.; Moore, R.; Oliver, G.; et al. Pratice parameters for the treatment of sigmoid diverticulitis-supporting documentation. *Dis. Colon. Rectum* **2000**, *43*, 289–297. [CrossRef] [PubMed]
7. Shahedi, K.; Fuller, G.; Bolus, R.; Cohen, E.; Vu, M.; Shah, R.; Agarwal, N.; Kaneshiro, M.; Atia, M.; Sheen, V.; et al. Long-term Risk of Acute Diverticulitis Among Patients With Incidental Diverticulosis Found During Colonoscopy. *Clin. Gastroenterol. Hepatol.* **2013**, *11*, 1609–1613. [CrossRef]
8. Peery, A.F.; Crockett, S.D.; Murphy, C.C.; Lund, J.L.; Dellon, E.S.; Williams, J.L.; Jensen, E.T.; Shaheen, N.J.; Barritt, A.S.; Lieber, S.R.; et al. Burden and Cost of Gastrointestinal, Liver, and Pancreatic Diseases in the United States: Update 2018. *Gastroenterology* **2019**, *156*, 254–272. [CrossRef] [PubMed]

9. Binda, G.A.; Mataloni, F.; Bruzzone, M.; Carabotti, M.; Cirocchi, R.; Nascimbeni, R.; Gambassi, G.; Amato, A.; Vettoretto, N.; Pinnarelli, L.; et al. Trends in hospital admission for acute diverticulitis in Italy from 2008 to 2015. *Tech. Coloproctol.* **2018**, *22*, 597–604. [CrossRef]
10. Jeyarajah, S.; Faiz, O.; Bottle, A.; Aylin, P.; Bjarnason, I.; Tekkis, P.P.; Papagrigoriadis, S. Diverticular disease hospital admissions are increasing, with poor outcomes in the elderly and emergency admissions. *Aliments Pharmacol. Ther.* **2009**, *30*, 1171–1182. [CrossRef] [PubMed]
11. Bharucha, A.E.; Parthasarathy, G.; Ditah, I.; Fletcher, J.G.; Ewelukwa, O.; Pendlimari, R.; Yawn, B.P.; Melton, J.L.; Schleck, C.; Zinsmeister, A.R. Temporal Trends in the Incidence and Natural History of Diverticulitis: A Population-Based Study. *Am. J. Gastroenterol.* **2015**, *110*, 1589–1596. [CrossRef] [PubMed]
12. Humes, D.J.; Solaymani–Dodaran, M.; Fleming, K.M.; Simpson, J.; Spiller, R.; West, J. A Population-Based Study of Perforated Diverticular Disease Incidence and Associated Mortality. *Gastroenterology* **2009**, *136*, 1198–1205. [CrossRef] [PubMed]
13. Bolkenstein, H.E.; Van De Wall, B.J.M.; Consten, E.C.J.; Broeders, I.; Draaisma, W.A. Risk factors for complicated diverticulitis: Systematic review and meta-analysis. *Int. J. Color. Dis.* **2017**, *32*, 1375–1383. [CrossRef] [PubMed]
14. Slim, K.; Joris, J.; Beyer-Berjot, L. The end of antibiotics in the management of uncomplicated acute diverticulitis. *J. Visc. Surg.* **2019**, *156*, 373–375. [CrossRef]
15. Strate, L.L.; Morris, A.M. Epidemiology, Pathophysiology, and Treatment of Diverticulitis. *Gastroenterology* **2019**, *156*, 1282–1298.e1. [CrossRef] [PubMed]
16. Mäkelä, J.T.; Klintrup, K.; Takala, H.; Rautio, T. The role of C-reactive protein in prediction of the severity of acute diverticulitis in an emergency unit. *Scand. J. Gastroenterol.* **2015**, *50*, 536–541. [CrossRef]
17. Nizri, E.; Spring, S.; Ben-Yehuda, A.; Khatib, M.; Klausner, J.; Greenberg, R. C-reactive protein as a marker of complicated diverticulitis in patients on anti-inflammatory medications. *Tech. Coloproctol.* **2014**, *18*, 145–149. [CrossRef]
18. Pisanu, A.; Vacca, V.; Reccia, I.; Podda, M.; Uccheddu, A. Acute Diverticulitis in the Young: The Same Disease in a Different Patient. *Gastroenterol. Res. Pr.* **2013**, *2013*, 867961. [CrossRef]
19. Tursi, A.; Brandimarte, G.; Giorgetti, G.; Elisei, W.; Maiorano, M.; Aiello, F. The Clinical Picture of Uncomplicated Versus Complicated Diverticulitis of the Colon. *Dig. Dis. Sci.* **2008**, *53*, 2474–2479. [CrossRef]
20. van de Wall, B.J.M.; Draaisma, W.A.; van der Kaaij, R.T.; Consten, E.C.J.; Wiezer, M.J.; Broeders, I.A.M.J. The value of inflammation markers and body temperature in acute diverticulitis. *Color. Dis.* **2013**, *15*, 621–626. [CrossRef]
21. Tan, J.P.; Barazanchi, A.W.; Singh, P.P.; Hill, A.G.; Maccormick, A.D. Predictors of acute diverticulitis severity: A systematic review. *Int. J. Surg.* **2016**, *26*, 43–52. [CrossRef]
22. Longstreth, G.F.; Iyer, R.L.; Chu, L.-H.X.; Chen, W.; Yen, L.S.; Hodgkins, P.; Kawatkar, A.A. Acute diverticulitis: Demographic, clinical and laboratory features associated with computed tomography findings in 741 patients. *Aliment. Pharmacol. Ther.* **2012**, *36*, 886–894. [CrossRef] [PubMed]
23. Cologne, K.G.; Skiada, D.; Beale, E.; Inaba, K.; Senagore, A.J.; Demetriades, D. Effects of diabetes mellitus in patients presenting with diverticulitis. *J. Trauma Acute Care Surg.* **2014**, *76*, 704–709. [CrossRef]
24. Barash, Y.; Soffer, S.; Grossman, E.; Tau, N.; Sorin, V.; Bendavid, E.; Irony, A.; Konen, E.; Zimlichman, E.; Klang, E. Alerting on mortality among patients discharged from the emergency department: A machine learning model. *Postgrad. Med. J.* **2020**. [CrossRef]
25. Soffer, S.; Klang, E.; Barash, Y.; Grossman, E.; Zimlichman, E. Predicting In-Hospital Mortality at Admission to the Medical Ward: A Big-Data Machine Learning Model. *Am. J. Med.* **2021**, *134*, 227–234.e4. [CrossRef]
26. Bolkenstein, H.E.; Van De Wall, B.J.; Consten, E.C.; van der Palen, J.; Broeders, I.A.; Draaisma, W.A. Development and validation of a diagnostic prediction model distinguishing complicated from uncomplicated diverticulitis. *Scand. J. Gastroenterol.* **2018**, *53*, 1291–1297. [CrossRef] [PubMed]
27. Hinchey, E.J.; Schaal, P.G.; Richards, G.K. Treatment of perforated diverticular disease of the colon. *Adv. Surg.* **1978**, *12*, 85–109.
28. Dharmarajan, S.; Hunt, S.R.; Birnbaum, E.H.; Fleshman, J.W.; Mutch, M.G. The efficacy of non-operative management of acute complicated diverticulitis. *Dis. Colon. Rectum* **2011**, *54*, 663–671. [CrossRef]
29. Covino, M.; Papa, V.; Tursi, A.; Simeoni, B.; Lopetuso, L.; Vetrone, L.; Franceschi, F.; Rapaccini, G.; Gasbarrini, A.; Papa, A. Development and Validation of Predictive Assessment of Complicated Diverticulitis Score. *J. Pers. Med.* **2021**, *11*, 80. [CrossRef] [PubMed]

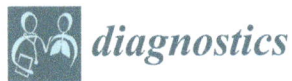

Article

Accuracy and Efficiency of Right-Lobe Graft Weight Estimation Using Deep-Learning-Assisted CT Volumetry for Living-Donor Liver Transplantation

Rohee Park [1], Seungsoo Lee [1,*], Yusub Sung [2], Jeeseok Yoon [3], Heung-Il Suk [3,4], Hyoungjung Kim [1] and Sanghyun Choi [1]

[1] Department of Radiology, Research Institute of Radiology, Asan Medical Center, University of Ulsan College of Medicine, Seoul 05505, Korea; bbakhyung91@gmail.com (R.P.); hjkim.radiology@gmail.com (H.K.); edwardchoi83@gmail.com (S.C.)
[2] Department of Convergence Medicine, Asan Medical Center, University of Ulsan College of Medicine, Seoul 05505, Korea; asmilez.sung@gmail.com
[3] Department of Brain and Cognitive Engineering, Korea University, Seoul 08308, Korea; wltjr1007@korea.ac.kr (J.Y.); hisuk@korea.ac.kr (H.-I.S.)
[4] Department of Artificial Intelligence, Korea University, Seoul 08308, Korea
* Correspondence: seungsoolee@amc.seoul.kr

Abstract: CT volumetry (CTV) has been widely used for pre-operative graft weight (GW) estimation in living-donor liver transplantation (LDLT), and the use of a deep-learning algorithm (DLA) may further improve its efficiency. However, its accuracy has not been well determined. To evaluate the efficiency and accuracy of DLA-assisted CTV in GW estimation, we performed a retrospective study including 581 consecutive LDLT donors who donated a right-lobe graft. Right-lobe graft volume (GV) was measured on CT using the software implemented with the DLA for automated liver segmentation. In the development group ($n = 207$), a volume-to-weight conversion formula was constructed by linear regression analysis between the CTV-measured GV and the intraoperative GW. In the validation group ($n = 374$), the agreement between the estimated and measured GWs was assessed using the Bland–Altman 95% limit-of-agreement (LOA). The mean process time for GV measurement was 1.8 ± 0.6 min (range, 1.3–8.0 min). In the validation group, the GW was estimated using the volume-to-weight conversion formula (estimated GW [g] = $206.3 + 0.653 \times$ CTV-measured GV [mL]), and the Bland–Altman 95% LOA between the estimated and measured GWs was $-1.7\% \pm 17.1\%$. The DLA-assisted CT volumetry allows for time-efficient and accurate estimation of GW in LDLT.

Keywords: deep learning; CT volumetry; segmentation; living right liver donors

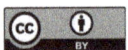

1. Introduction

Living-donor liver transplantation (LDLT) is an effective therapeutic option for patients with end-stage liver disease [1]. An adequate graft mass is a major component of a successful LDLT. The use of small-for-size grafts, with graft-to-recipient weight ratios of less than 0.8 to 1%, is associated with graft malfunction, while an insufficient remnant liver mass after harvesting a graft may threaten donor safety [2,3]. Therefore, the accurate preoperative estimation of graft weight is a prerequisite step in LDLT to ensure the safety of both recipients and donors.

CT volumetry has been widely used for preoperative graft volume measurement in LDLT [4–12]. Graft weight is usually estimated using CT-measured graft volume and a volume-to-weight conversion formula [10–15]. Although several studies have assessed the performance of CT volumetry in graft weight estimation [5,7,8,10–17], these studies had limitations. The volume-to-weight conversion formulae used in the previous studies were not reliable since they were derived from small study populations (i.e., ≤16 subjects) [10,11,14], pathologic liver conditions [10], or the assumption that the liver and water have the same density [12,13,15], which may have led to biased estimations of graft weight. Moreover, previous studies assessed the correlations or mean differences between the estimated and actual graft weights, but did not evaluate the measurement error of CT volumetric graft weight estimation [5–12], which is important to predict the range of actual graft weight in individual LDLT donors.

One obstacle that limits the clinical use of CT volumetry has been the time-consuming organ segmentation process. Recently, deep learning has emerged as a method for automated image analysis. Recent studies have demonstrated that a deep-learning algorithm (DLA) enables fully automated segmentation of the liver using CT images with high accuracy, allowing for automated liver volume measurement without user interaction [18]. Thus, the application of DLA for CT-based liver segmentation would dramatically improve the time efficiency of CT volumetry in estimating graft weight for LDLT.

Therefore, the purpose of our study was to construct a graft volume-to-weight conversion formula, and to evaluate the accuracy and time efficiency of DLA-assisted CT volumetry for estimating graft weight in a large cohort of living liver donors who donated right-lobe liver grafts.

2. Material and Method

This retrospective study was approved by our institutional review board, which waived the requirement for patients' informed consent.

2.1. Study Population

We retrospectively and consecutively enrolled living liver donors in our institution who donated right-lobe grafts from 2013 to 2015. Eligible donors were those who had undergone CT examinations within 3 months before liver donation and had data on intraoperative graft weight measurement. A total of 581 donors who satisfied the eligibility criteria comprised the study population (Figure 1). The study population was then divided into the development (liver donation in 2013, n = 207) and validation (liver donation from 2014 to 2015, n = 374) groups. A subset of 50 donors who were randomly selected from the validation group comprised the subgroup used to assess inter-reader agreement in graft volume measurement.

2.2. CT Examination

CT examinations were performed using various CT scanners and techniques (Supplementary Table S1). CT scans were obtained using 16-channel (Sensation 16, Simens Healthineers, Erlangen, Germany), 64-channel (Definition AS, Siemens Healthineers or Lightspeed VCT, GE Healthcare, Milwaukee, WI, USA), or 128-channel (Definition Flash, Siemens Healthineers) scanners. Portal venous phase images were obtained 76 s after intravenous contrast administration with tube voltages of 100 or 120 kVp, tube currents of 200–440 mA with automatic exposure control, matrix of 512 × 512, and section thicknesses of 3 or 5 mm with no gap. The total number of images ranged from 95 to 115 for the examinations with 5 mm slice thickness, and ranged from 155 to 188 for those with 3 mm slice thickness.

2.3. Graft Volume Measurement Using a Deep Learning Algorithm

The graft volume was measured by a reader who was a third-year radiology resident (P.R.) on portal venous phase CT images. The reader first analyzed CT data from the first 30 donors in the development group, together with an experienced radiologist (L.S.S, with 23 years of experience in abdominal imaging) for training purposes. The CT data were analyzed using the GoCDSS software (SmartCareworks Inc., Seoul, Korea), which applied a DLA for automated liver segmentation. The detailed information of the DLA was described previously [18], and its source code is provided at https://github.com/seungsoolee0007/liver_spleen_segmentation (accessed on 22 February 2022). Briefly, the algorithm performed whole-liver segmentation, excluding large hepatic vessels, with a dice similarity score of 97% in a computation time of 33 s for a typical abdominal CT examination [18]. Once the CT data were uploaded, the software automatically performed liver segmentation. Then, the reader reviewed CT images along with the deep-learning-generated liver segmentation results and corrected any segmentation errors. The liver volumes measured by automated segmentation by the deep learning algorithm and those measured after the reader's correction were recorded. The reader defined the resection plane for the right-lobe graft based on the Cantlie line by drawing two dividing lines (one along the main axis of the middle hepatic vein, superiorly, and the other along the imaginary line between the gallbladder and inferior vena cava, inferiorly) on the selected images (Figure 2). The software completed the resection plane by interpolation of the two dividing lines. The volumes of the whole liver and right-lobe liver graft were automatically calculated by summation of the area multiplied by the slice interval. The times required for reviewing CT images, correcting segmentation errors, and defining the resection plane were recorded. To assess inter-reader agreement, the second reader (L.S.S) independently measured graft volume in a subset of 50 donors from the validation group.

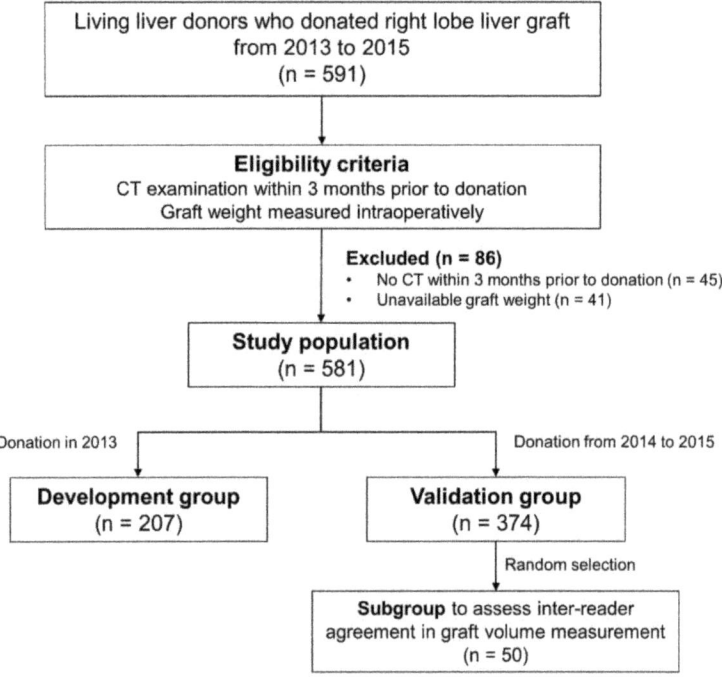

Figure 1. Flow diagram of the study population.

2.4. Clinical and Pathologic Data and Intraoperative Graft Weight Measurement

Clinical data including age, sex, height, weight, and body mass index (BMI) were obtained on the day of the CT examinations. The degree of hepatic steatosis (HS) was assessed by pathologic analysis of ultrasonography-guided percutaneous liver biopsy specimens, which was performed 1–78 days (median, 17 days) before liver donation as a part of donor workup. The degree of HS was graded as none (<5%), mild (5–33%), moderate (34–66%), or severe (>66%), as defined by the Non-alcoholic Steatohepatitis Clinical Research Network scoring system [19]. The graft weight was measured during the donor hepatectomy and served as the reference standard in our study. The donor hepatectomy was performed as described previously [5]. Briefly, the demarcation line of the right lobe was drawn based on the color change of the liver surface that occurred during temporary clamping of the right portal vein and right hepatic artery. Parenchymal dissection was performed with the middle hepatic vein as the anatomic landmark, i.e., along the right (graft without middle hepatic vein) or left (graft with middle hepatic vein) side of the middle hepatic vein. Dissection of the dorsal part of the liver was performed using a hanging maneuver that allowed transection of the liver parenchyma down to the inferior vena cava. After harvesting a right-lobe graft, the surgeons shook the excised graft to spill out the remaining blood, waited a few seconds for natural drainage, then measured the blood-free graft weight on an electronic laboratory scale (FD 110; Excel Precision, New Taipei City, Taiwan).

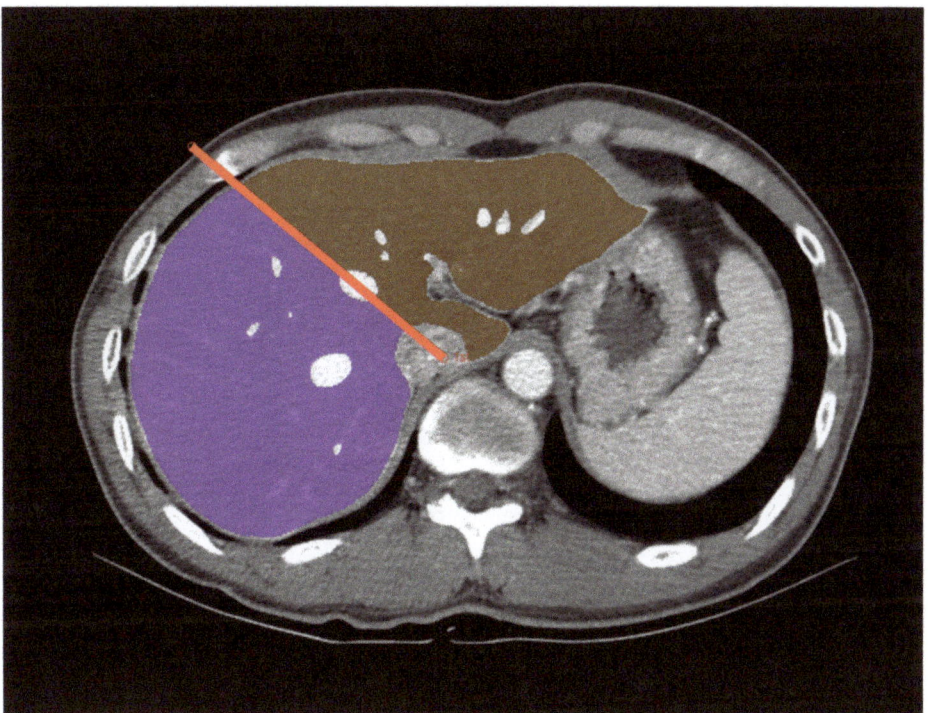

Figure 2. Measurement of the right-lobe graft volume using deep-learning-algorithm-assisted CT volumetry. An axial portal venous phase CT image in a 44-year-old male donor is overlaid with a right-lobe mask (purple), a left lobe mask (brown), and a dividing line (red line). CT image data were first processed by the deep learning algorithm for whole liver segmentation. The radiologist reviewed these results, corrected any segmentation errors, and defined the resection plane for the right-lobe graft by drawing the dividing lines.

2.5. Statistical Analysis

The characteristics of the development and validation groups were compared using independent t-tests or Fisher's exact tests. Agreements between the whole-liver volumes automatically measured by DLA and those measured after the radiologist's correction were evaluated using the Bland–Altman 95% limit of agreement (LOA). Bland–Altman 95% LOAs were expressed as percentages of the measured values and as the mean differences $\pm 1.96 \times$ standard deviation (SD) of the difference, where the mean difference represented systemic bias, and $1.96 \times$ SD of the difference represented the measurement error. In the developmental group, to evaluate the confounding effect of HS on the graft weight, multivariable linear regression analysis was performed by including the HS- and CT-measured graft volume as independent variables and graft weight as the dependent variable. Then, the formula to convert CT-measured graft volume to graft weight was built using univariable linear regression analysis. In the validation group, the graft weight was estimated using CT-measured graft volume, and the conversion formula derived from the development group. The agreement between the estimated and measured graft weights was then assessed using the concordance correlation coefficient (CCC) and Bland–Altman 95% LOA. In the subgroup including 50 donors in the validation group, the inter-reader agreement in the graft volumes between the two radiologists was assessed using the CCC and Bland–Altman 95% LOA. To assess the factors influencing the magnitude of error in graft weight estimation, multivariable linear regression analysis was performed in the validation cohort; this included the age, sex, BMI, HS, interval between CT scan and liver donation, and type of liver graft (right-lobe graft with or without middle hepatic vein) as independent variables; and the percentage difference between the estimated and measured graft weights, i.e., (estimated graft weight—measured graft weight)/measured graft weight, as the dependent variable. Statistical analyses were performed using IBM SPSS Statistics for Windows, version 21.0 (IBM Corp., Armonk, NY, USA) and MedCalc version 14.8.1 (MedCalc, Ostend, Belgium). p-values < 0.05 were considered to indicate significant differences.

3. Results

3.1. Characteristics of the Study Population

Table 1 summarizes the characteristics of the study population. The study population included 581 donors (413 men and 168 women; mean age, 27.7 years; age range, 17–54 years). Most donors had non-steatotic liver, and clinically relevant HS was present in 89 (15.3%) donors, with mild HS in 87 (15.0%) and moderate HS in two (0.3%) donors. The development and validation groups included 207 (132 men and 75 women; mean age, 27.6 years; age range, 18–54 years) and 374 (281 men and 93 women; mean age, 27.8 years; age range, 17–52 years) donors, respectively. The developmental and validation groups showed significant differences in sex ($p = 0.004$), BMI ($p = 0.015$), body weight ($p = 0.022$), and intraoperatively measured graft weight ($p = 0.004$).

Table 1. Characteristics of the study population.

KERRYPNX	Total	Developmental Group	Validation Group	p-Value *
Number of patients	581	207	374	
Age (years) [†]	27.7 ± 7.2	27.6 ± 6.9	27.8 ± 7.3	0.661
Sex				0.004
Male	413 (71.1)	132 (63.8)	282 (74.8)	
Hepatic steatosis				0.816
None	492 (84.7)	177 (85.5)	315 (84.2)	
Mild	87 (15.0)	29 (14.0)	58 (15.5)	
Moderate	2 (0.3)	1 (0.5)	1 (0.3)	
BMI (kg/m^2) [†]	22.9 ± 2.9	22.5 ± 2.9	23.1 ± 2.9	0.015
Height (cm) [†]	170.4 ± 8.1	169.9 ± 8.4	170.7 ± 7.9	0.268
Weight (kg) [†]	66.8 ± 11.4	65.4 ± 11.7	67.6 ± 11.1	0.022
Type of liver graft				0.151
RLG without MHV	559 (96.2)	196 (94.7)	363 (97.1)	
RLG with MHV	22 (3.8)	11 (5.3)	11 (2.9)	
Interval between CT and graft donation (days) [†]	30.6 ± 19.0	30.9 ± 18.8	30.4 ± 19.1	0.728
Graft weight (g) [†]	748.8 ± 129.3	728.1 ± 123.5	760.2 ± 131.2	0.004

Unless otherwise indicated, data are shown as the number of patients, with percentages in parentheses. RLG = right-lobe graft, MHV = middle hepatic vein. * p-values for comparisons between the development and validation groups; [†] Mean ± standard deviation.

3.2. Liver Segmentation and Graft Volume Estimation Using DLA

DLA-generated automated segmentation of the whole liver showed segmentation errors requiring radiologists' correction in 166 (28.6%) donors. Most segmentation errors were minor and were associated with a short correction time (the mean time required for the radiologists' correction ± standard deviation [SD], 12.8 ± 33.6 s) and a small change in volume (Bland–Altman 95% LOAs, 0.05% ± 3.0% of the measured liver volume). The mean process time, including the DLA-generated segmentation review, and correction and division of the segmented liver, was 1.8 ± 0.6 min (range, 1.3–8.0 min).

3.3. Construction of Graft Volume-to-Weight Conversion Formula in the Development Group

In the development group, the CT-measured graft volume and intraoperatively measured graft weight ranged from 454.9 mL to 1187.0 mL (mean ± SD, 1249.0 ± 237.9 mL) and from 420.0 g to 1025.0 g (mean ± SD, 728.1 ± 123.5 g), respectively. In multivariable linear regression analysis, HS did not have a significant effect on graft weight (coefficient, −0.34; $p = 0.667$) after accounting for the effect of graft volume on graft weight (coefficient, 0.655; $p < 0.001$). Therefore, we constructed the formula to convert CT-measured graft volume to graft weight in the entire development group, without excluding donors with HS (Figure 3). The conversion formula was as follows: estimated graft weight (g) = 206.3 + 0.653 × CT-measured graft volume (mL) ($r = 0.878$, $p < 0.001$).

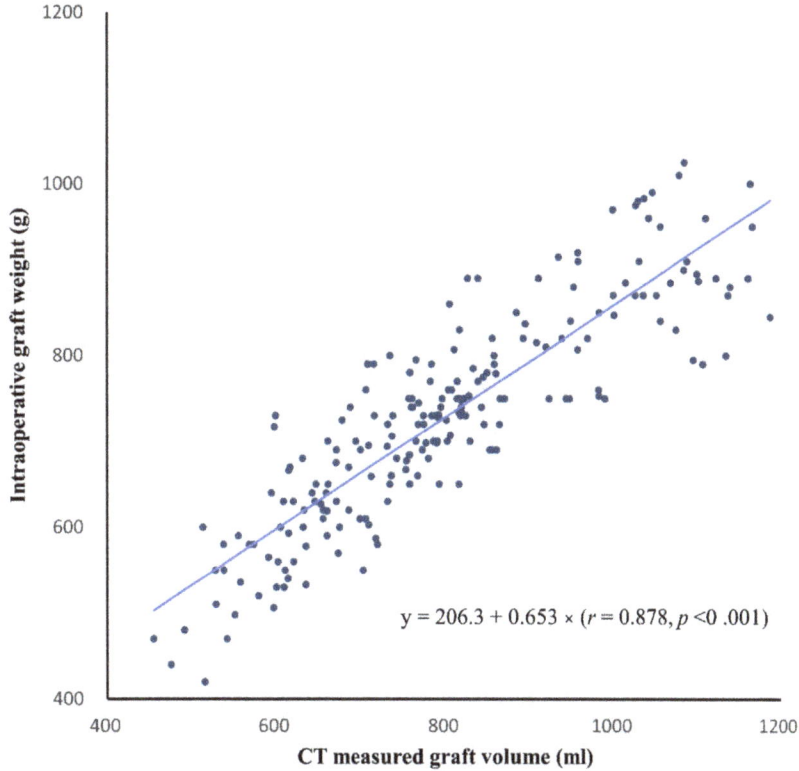

Figure 3. Scatter plot of the CT-measured graft volume versus intraoperative graft weight in the development group. The solid line indicates the best-fit regression line. The linear regression equation is also shown.

3.4. Agreement between the Estimated and Measured Graft Weights in the Validation Group

In the validation group, the CT-measured graft volume, estimated graft weight, and intraoperatively measured graft weight ranged from 722.9 mL to 2259.6 mL (mean ± SD, 1281.9 ± 233.4 mL), from 520.0 g to 1153.7 g (mean ± SD, 743.6 ± 104.0 g), and from 456.0 g to 1400.0 g (mean ± SD, 760.2 ± 131.2 g), respectively. The CCC for the agreement between the estimated and measured graft weights was 0.834 (95% confidence interval [CI], 0.804 to 0.860) (Figure 4). The Bland–Altman 95% LOA was −1.7% ± 17.1% ($p = 0.002$ for the difference of mean bias from zero), indicating a mean bias of −1.7% and measurement error of 17.1% of the graft weight (Figure 5).

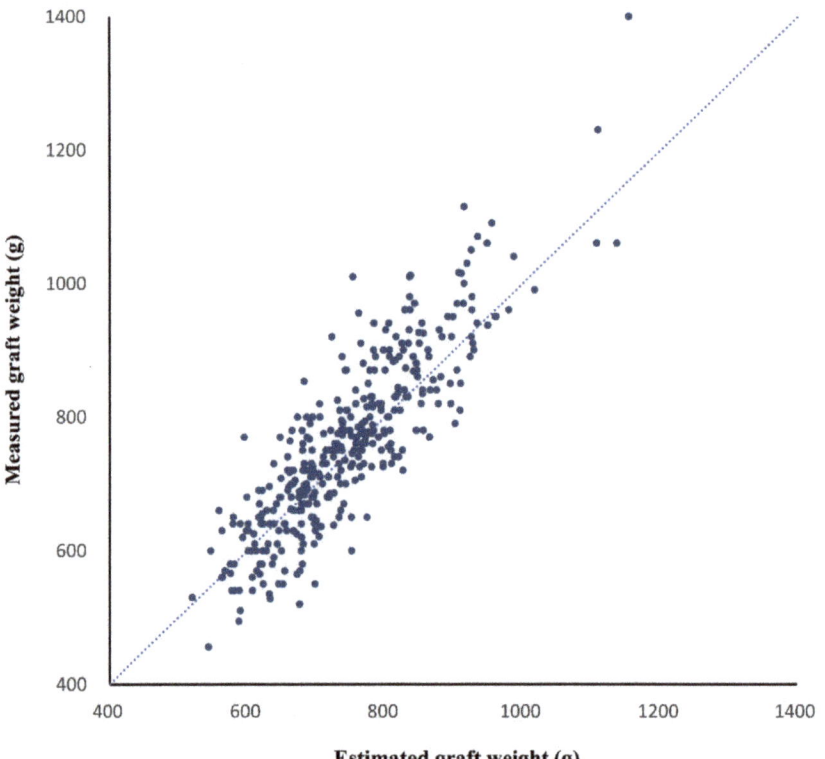

Figure 4. Scatter plot of the estimated and measured graft weights in the validation group. The dashed line is the reference line indicating complete agreement. The concordance correlation coefficient between the estimated and measured graft weights was 0.834 (95% confidence interval, 0.804 to 0.860), $p < 0.001$).

The inter-reader agreement for graft volume measurement was assessed in the subset of 50 donors in the validation cohort. The CCC for the agreement in the graft volume measurement between the two readers was 0.998 (95% CI, 0.996–0.999), and the Bland–Altman 95% LOA was 0.2% ± 1.8% ($p = 0.069$).

3.5. Factors Associated with Differences in Estimated and Measured Graft Weights

In the validation cohort, multivariable linear regression analysis revealed that sex (coefficient, −1.73; $p = 0.001$) and BMI (coefficient, −0.2; $p < 0.001$) showed significant independent associations with the percentage difference between the estimated and measured graft weights, while age ($p = 0.076$), HS degree ($p = 0.577$), interval between CT and liver donation ($p = 0.111$), and type of liver graft ($p = 0.279$) did not. The Bland–Altman 95% LOAs between the estimated and measured graft weights were −2.6% ± 16.8% ($p < 0.001$) and 0.9% ± 16.8% ($p = 0.306$) for men and women, respectively. When donors were sub-grouped according to BMI, the Bland–Altman 95% LOAs between the estimated and measured graft weights were −1.3% ± 16.2% ($p = 0.009$) and −4.2% ± 17.0% ($p < .001$) for donors with BMI <25 kg/m^2 and overweight or obese donors with BMI ≥25 kg/m^2, respectively.

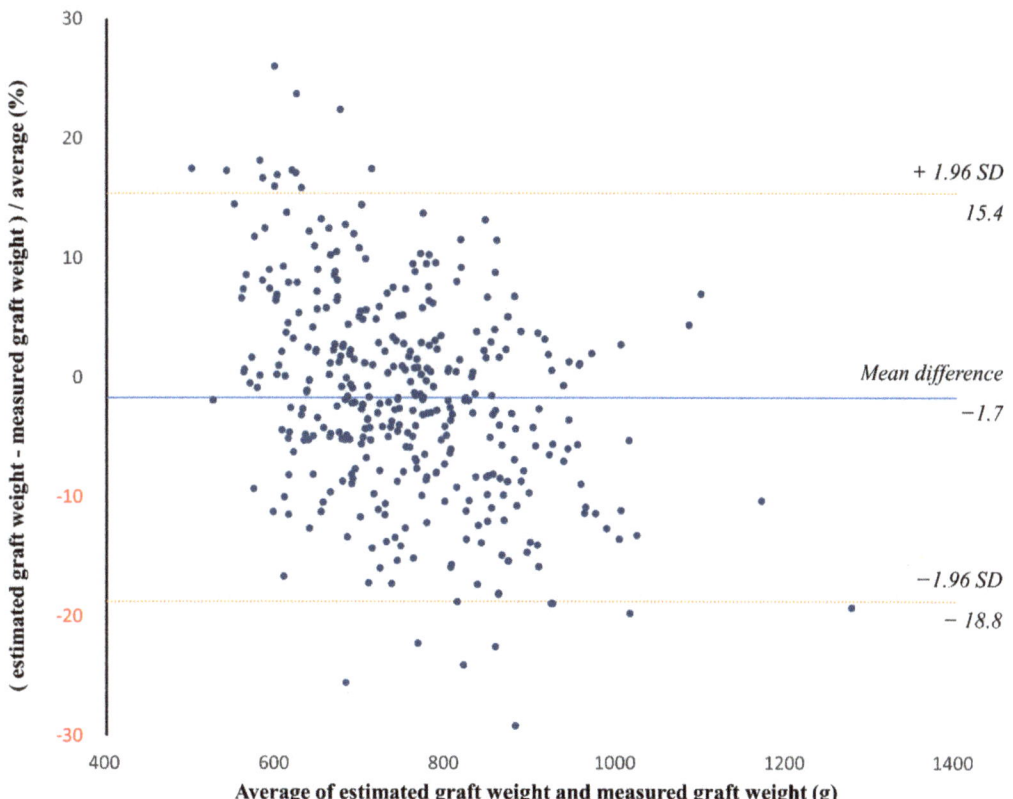

Figure 5. Bland–Altman plot of the agreement between the estimated and measured graft weights in the validation group. The solid line indicates the mean difference, while the dashed lines indicate the upper and lower limits of the 95% limits of agreement. The Bland–Altman 95% limit of agreement (LOA) was −1.7% ± 17.1% ($p = 0.002$ for the difference of mean bias from zero). SD = standard deviation.

4. Discussion

Our study evaluated the efficiency and accuracy of CT volumetry using a DLA for the preoperative estimation of right-lobe graft weight in LDLT. We found that the DLA allowed for a time-efficient measurement of graft volume on CT. The CT data analysis with the DLA was performed as a background process so that the reader reviewed CT images with DLA-generated liver segmentation results. The DLA enabled highly accurate segmentation of the liver. The DLA-generated liver segmentation results did not require additional correction in approximately 70% of donors; moreover, minor segmentation errors, which were rapidly corrected by the reviewing radiologist, were observed in only 30% of donors. As a result, CT volumetric assessment of right-lobe grafts was rapidly performed in an average process time of 1.8 min.

We developed the graft volume-to-weight conversion formula in a large number of donors (i.e., 207 donors) in the development group. In the validation group, graft weights that were estimated using the CT-measured graft volume and conversion formula showed an overall good agreement with the measured graft weights (CCC = 0.834). The Bland–Altman 95% LOA indicated a measurement error of graft weight of ±17.1%. Although this measurement error appears large, the range encompasses most (i.e., 95%) of the actual difference between the estimated and measured graft weights. Compared to our study, previous studies reported even greater differences between estimated and measured graft weights, ranging from −48.2% to 66.2% [5,8,12]. As suggested by previous studies, multiple factors may have contributed to the error in CT volumetric estimation of graft weight, including mismatches between expected and actual resection planes [6,12], graft dehydration [7,12], and variable amounts of blood remaining in the graft [8].

Our validation results showed a small but significant bias in the estimated graft weights, indicating that graft weight was underestimated by 1.7% in the validation group. The mean bias of 1.7% in our study was smaller than those reported previously (i.e., −9.8% to 2.4% of graft weight) [5,8], which may have been partly due to our use of a conversion formula developed in a larger study population. Though not yet fully understood, the bias in the estimated graft weights in the validation group may have been related to different characteristics between the development and validation groups. Our study showed that sex and BMI were significantly associated with the percentage difference between the estimated and measured graft weights. Graft weights tended to be underestimated in men (mean bias, −2.6%) and in donors with a higher BMI (mean bias, −4.2%). Thus, a significantly higher proportion of men and donors with a higher BMI in the validation group than in the development group may have led to a small underestimation of graft weight in the validation group.

We observed nearly perfect inter-reader agreement in graft volume measurement between the two readers (CCC = 0.998; Bland–Altman 95% LOA = −1.6% to 2.0% of the measured volume). This finding is noteworthy given the different level of experience between the two readers (i.e., third-year radiology resident vs. abdominal radiologist with 23 years of experience). The use of automated liver segmentation with the DLA may help to reduce inter-reader variability in liver segmentation, making CT-based graft volume measurement simple enough for a less experienced reader to learn after a short training session.

In our study, HS did not show a significant confounding effect on the association between graft volume and graft weight in the development cohort. In addition, the degree of HS was not a significant factor for the percentage difference between the estimated and measured graft weights. However, this finding should be interpreted with caution as most donors in our study population had no or mild HS. Despite some controversies, there have been a few prior reports suggesting the association of HS with increased liver volume [20–22]. Therefore, our results may not be directly generalizable to donors with moderate-to-severe HS.

Our study had several limitations. First, the retrospective design may be subject to selection bias and bias from missing data, despite our efforts to minimize such biases by enrolling consecutive donors. Second, we evaluated only right-lobe grafts since that is the preferred graft for LDLT to meet recipients' metabolic demands [23,24]. Thus, the measurement error range for CT volumetric graft weight estimation in our study may not be directly applicable to other types of liver graft. Finally, the development and validation groups in our study were enrolled in the same institution. External validation in a completely different population may have provided more conclusive validation results.

5. Conclusions

In conclusion, we proposed a graft volume-to-weight conversion formula for preoperative CT volumetric estimation of graft weight in LDLT. The DLA-assisted CT volumetry provided a time-efficient and accurate estimation of graft weight in LDLT. The measurement error of the CT volumetric estimation of right-lobe graft weight was approximately 17% of the graft weight.

Supplementary Materials: The following supporting information can be downloaded at: https://www.mdpi.com/article/10.3390/diagnostics12030590/s1, Table S1: CT imaging techniques used in the development and validation groups.

Author Contributions: Conceptualization, S.S.L.; data curation, R.P.; funding acquisition, S.L.; investigation, R.P., Y.S., J.Y., H.-I.S., H.K. and S.C.; project administration, S.L.; resources, Y.S. and J.Y.; software, H.-I.S.; writing—original draft, R.P.; writing—review & editing, H.K. and S.C. All authors have read and agreed to the published version of the manuscript.

Funding: This research was supported by a National Research Foundation of Korea (NRF) grant, funded by the Korean government (MSIT) (2020R1F1A1048826).

Institutional Review Board Statement: The Asan Medical Center Institutional Review Board approved this study (code 2021-0751) on 20 May 2021.

Informed Consent Statement: This retrospective study was approved by our institutional review board, which waived the requirement for patients' informed consent.

Conflicts of Interest: The authors declare no conflict of interest.

References

1. Hwang, S.; Lee, S.G.; Joh, J.W.; Suh, K.S.; Kim, D.G. Liver transplantation for adult patients with hepatocellular carcinoma in Korea: Comparison between cadaveric donor and living donor liver transplantations. *Liver Transpl.* **2005**, *11*, 1265–1272. [CrossRef] [PubMed]
2. Lee, S.G.; Hwang, S. How I do it: Assessment of hepatic functional reserve for indication of hepatic resection. *J. Hepato-Biliary-Pancreat. Surg.* **2005**, *12*, 38–43. [CrossRef] [PubMed]
3. Kiuchi, T.; Tanaka, K.; Ito, T.; Oike, F.; Ogura, Y.; Fujimoto, Y.; Ogawa, K. Small-for-size graft in living donor liver transplantation: How far should we go? *Liver Transpl.* **2003**, *9*, S29–S35. [CrossRef] [PubMed]
4. Lim, M.; Tan, C.; Cai, J.; Zheng, J.; Kow, A. CT volumetry of the liver: Where does it stand in clinical practice? *Clin. Radiol.* **2014**, *69*, 887–895. [CrossRef]
5. Kwon, H.J.; Kim, K.W.; Jang, J.K.; Lee, J.; Song, G.W.; Lee, S.G. Reproducibility and reliability of computed tomography volumetry in estimation of the right-lobe graft weight in adult-to-adult living donor liver transplantation: Cantlie's line vs portal vein territorialization. *J. Hepato-Biliary-Pancreat. Sci.* **2020**, *27*, 541–547. [CrossRef]
6. Jeong, W.K. Clinical implication of hepatic volumetry for living donor liver transplantation. *Clin. Mol. Hepatol.* **2018**, *24*, 51–53. [CrossRef]
7. Satou, S.; Sugawara, Y.; Tamura, S.; Yamashiki, N.; Kaneko, J.; Aoki, T.; Hasegawa, K.; Beck, Y.; Makuuchi, M.; Kokudo, N. Discrepancy between estimated and actual weight of partial liver graft from living donors. *J. Hepato-Biliary-Pancreat. Sci.* **2011**, *18*, 586–591. [CrossRef]
8. Kim, K.W.; Lee, J.; Lee, H.; Jeong, W.K.; Won, H.J.; Shin, Y.M.; Jung, D.-H.; Park, J.I.; Song, G.-W.; Ha, T.-Y. Right lobe estimated blood-free weight for living donor liver transplantation: Accuracy of automated blood-free CT volumetry—Preliminary results. *Radiology* **2010**, *256*, 433–440. [CrossRef]
9. Karlo, C.; Reiner, C.S.; Stolzmann, P.; Breitenstein, S.; Marincek, B.; Weishaupt, D.; Frauenfelder, T. CT- and MRI-based volumetry of resected liver specimen: Comparison to intraoperative volume and weight measurements and calculation of conversion factors. *Eur. J. Radiol.* **2010**, *75*, e107–e111. [CrossRef]
10. Nakayama, Y.; Li, Q.; Katsuragawa, S.; Ikeda, R.; Hiai, Y.; Awai, K.; Kusunoki, S.; Yamashita, Y.; Okajima, H.; Inomata, Y. Automated hepatic volumetry for living related liver transplantation at multisection CT. *Radiology* **2006**, *240*, 743–748. [CrossRef]
11. Lemke, A.-J.; Brinkmann, M.J.; Schott, T.; Niehues, S.M.; Settmacher, U.; Neuhaus, P.; Felix, R. Living donor right liver lobes: Preoperative CT volumetric measurement for calculation of intraoperative weight and volume. *Radiology* **2006**, *240*, 736–742. [CrossRef] [PubMed]
12. Hiroshige, S.; Shimada, M.; Harada, N.; Shiotani, S.; Ninomiya, M.; Minagawa, R.; Soejima, Y.; Suehiro, T.; Honda, H.; Hashizume, M.; et al. Accurate preoperative estimation of liver-graft volumetry using three-dimensional computed tomography. *Transplantation* **2003**, *75*, 1561–1564. [CrossRef] [PubMed]
13. Urata, K.; Kawasaki, S.; Matsunami, H.; Hashikura, Y.; Ikegami, T.; Ishizone, S.; Momose, Y.; Komiyama, A.; Makuuchi, M. Calculation of child and adult standard liver volume for liver transplantation. *Hepatology* **1995**, *21*, 1317–1321. [CrossRef]
14. Hwang, S.; Lee, S.; Kim, K.; Park, K.; Ahn, C. Correlation of blood-free graft weight and volumetric graft volume by an analysis of blood content in living donor liver grafts. *Transplant. Proc.* **2002**, *8*, 3293–3294. [CrossRef]
15. Hermoye, L.; Laamari-Azjal, I.; Cao, Z.; Annet, L.; Lerut, J.; Dawant, B.M.; Van Beers, B.E. Liver segmentation in living liver transplant donors: Comparison of semiautomatic and manual methods. *Radiology* **2005**, *234*, 171–178. [CrossRef] [PubMed]
16. Radtke, A.; Sotiropoulos, G.C.; Nadalin, S.; Molmenti, E.P.; Schroeder, T.; Lang, H.; Saner, F.; Valentin-Gamazo, C.; Frilling, A.; Schenk, A.; et al. Preoperative volume prediction in adult living donor liver transplantation: How much can we rely on it? *Am. J. Transplant.* **2007**, *7*, 672–679. [CrossRef]

17. Mokry, T.; Bellemann, N.; Muller, D.; Lorenzo Bermejo, J.; Klauss, M.; Stampfl, U.; Radeleff, B.; Schemmer, P.; Kauczor, H.U.; Sommer, C.M. Accuracy of estimation of graft size for living-related liver transplantation: First results of a semi-automated interactive software for CT-volumetry. *PLoS ONE* **2014**, *9*, e110201. [CrossRef]
18. Ahn, Y.; Yoon, J.S.; Lee, S.S.; Suk, H.I.; Son, J.H.; Sung, Y.S.; Lee, Y.; Kang, B.K.; Kim, H.S. Deep Learning Algorithm for Automated Segmentation and Volume Measurement of the Liver and Spleen Using Portal Venous Phase Computed Tomography Images. *Korean J. Radiol.* **2020**, *21*, 987–997. [CrossRef]
19. Kleiner, D.E.; Brunt, E.M.; Van Natta, M.; Behling, C.; Contos, M.J.; Cummings, O.W.; Ferrell, L.D.; Liu, Y.C.; Torbenson, M.S.; Unalp-Arida, A.; et al. Design and validation of a histological scoring system for nonalcoholic fatty liver disease. *Hepatology* **2005**, *41*, 1313–1321. [CrossRef]
20. Tang, A.; Chen, J.; Le, T.A.; Changchien, C.; Hamilton, G.; Middleton, M.S.; Loomba, R.; Sirlin, C.B. Cross-sectional and longitudinal evaluation of liver volume and total liver fat burden in adults with nonalcoholic steatohepatitis. *Abdom. Imaging* **2015**, *40*, 26–37. [CrossRef]
21. Bian, H.; Hakkarainen, A.; Zhou, Y.; Lundbom, N.; Olkkonen, V.M.; Yki-Järvinen, H. Impact of non-alcoholic fatty liver disease on liver volume in humans. *Hepatol. Res.* **2015**, *45*, 210–219. [CrossRef] [PubMed]
22. Siriwardana, R.C.; Chan, S.C.; Chok, K.S.; Lo, C.M.; Fan, S.T. Effects of the liver volume and donor steatosis on errors in the estimated standard liver volume. *Liver Transpl.* **2011**, *17*, 1437–1442. [CrossRef] [PubMed]
23. Miller, C.M.; Durand, F.; Heimbach, J.K.; Kim-Schluger, L.; Lee, S.G.; Lerut, J.; Lo, C.M.; Quintini, C.; Pomfret, E.A. The International Liver Transplant Society Guideline on Living Liver Donation. *Transplantation* **2016**, *100*, 1238–1243. [CrossRef] [PubMed]
24. Lee, S.; Park, K.; Hwang, S.; Lee, Y.; Kim, K.; Ahn, C.; Choi, D.; Joo, S.; Jeon, J.; Chu, C. Adult-to-adult living donor liver transplantation at the Asan Medical Center, Korea. *Asian J. Surg.* **2002**, *25*, 277–284. [CrossRef]

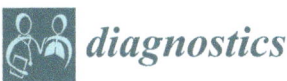

Article

Use of U-Net Convolutional Neural Networks for Automated Segmentation of Fecal Material for Objective Evaluation of Bowel Preparation Quality in Colonoscopy

Yen-Po Wang [1,2,3,4,†], Ying-Chun Jheng [1,4,5,†], Kuang-Yi Sung [1,2,4], Hung-En Lin [1,2,4], I-Fang Hsin [1,2,4], Ping-Hsien Chen [1,2,4], Yuan-Chia Chu [6,7,8], David Lu [1], Yuan-Jen Wang [4,9], Ming-Chih Hou [1,2,4], Fa-Yauh Lee [2,4] and Ching-Liang Lu [1,2,3,4,*]

1. Endoscopy Center for Diagnosis and Treatment, Department of Medicine, Taipei Veterans General Hospital, Taipei 112, Taiwan; ypwang@vghtpe.gov.tw (Y.-P.W.); cycom122@gmail.com (Y.-C.J.); ioudanny520@hotmail.com (K.-Y.S.); scottenx@gmail.com (H.-E.L.); ifhsin@gmail.com (I.-F.H.); u701117@gmail.com (P.-H.C.); david97lu@gmail.com (D.L.); mchou@vghtpe.gov.tw (M.-C.H.)
2. Division of Gastroenterology, Department of Medicine, Taipei Veterans General Hospital, Taipei 112, Taiwan; fylee@vghtpe.gov.tw
3. Institute of Brain Science, National Yang Ming Chiao Tung University School of Medicine, Taipei 112, Taiwan
4. Faculty of Medicine, National Yang Ming Chiao Tung University School of Medicine, Taipei 112, Taiwan; yjwang@vghtpe.gov.tw
5. Department of Medical Research, Taipei Veterans General Hospital, Taipei 112, Taiwan
6. Information Management Office, Taipei Veterans General Hospital, Taipei 112, Taiwan; xd.yuanchia@gmail.com
7. Big Data Center, Taipei Veterans General Hospital, Taipei 112, Taiwan
8. Department of Information Management, National Taipei University of Nursing and Health Sciences, Taipei 112, Taiwan
9. Healthcare and Management Center, Taipei Veterans General Hospital, Taipei 112, Taiwan
* Correspondence: cllu@vghtpe.gov.tw; Tel.: +886-2-2875-7272
† These authors contributed equally to this work.

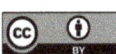

Abstract: Background: Adequate bowel cleansing is important for colonoscopy performance evaluation. Current bowel cleansing evaluation scales are subjective, with a wide variation in consistency among physicians and low reported rates of accuracy. We aim to use machine learning to develop a fully automatic segmentation method for the objective evaluation of the adequacy of colon preparation. Methods: Colonoscopy videos were retrieved from a video data cohort and transferred to qualified images, which were randomly divided into training, validation, and verification datasets. The fecal residue was manually segmented. A deep learning model based on the U-Net convolutional network architecture was developed to perform automatic segmentation. The performance of the automatic segmentation was evaluated on the overlap area with the manual segmentation. Results: A total of 10,118 qualified images from 119 videos were obtained. The model averaged 0.3634 s to segmentate one image automatically. The models produced a strong high-overlap area with manual segmentation, with 94.7% ± 0.67% of that area predicted by our AI model, which correlated well with the area measured manually (r = 0.915, $p < 0.001$). The AI system can be applied in real-time qualitatively and quantitatively. Conclusions: We established a fully automatic segmentation method to rapidly and accurately mark the fecal residue-coated mucosa for the objective evaluation of colon preparation.

Keywords: artificial intelligence; automated segmentation; U-NET; colonoscopy; colonoscopy preparation quality

1. Introduction

Colorectal cancer (CRC) is one of the main malignancies affecting humans, accounting for the second and third most common causes of cancer-related death, respectively, in males and females globally [1]. In the Asia–Pacific area, CRC incidence is also increasing rapidly, and CRC was ranked as the most common cancer over 10 years in Taiwan [1,2]. Colonoscopy is used to image the mucosa of the entire colon and is an effective method for reducing the CRC burden, since colonoscopy can detect CRC early and be used to remove adenomatous polyps, which can significantly improve CRC survival [3,4]. Despite this fact, interval cancer can sometimes be noted in patients who underwent a CRC surveillance program, which may stem from missed lesions due to an incomplete colonoscopy caused by inadequate bowel preparation [5–8].

Both the American and European Societies of Gastrointestinal Endoscopy have published guidelines on colon preparation to ensure the quality of bowel preparation during colonoscopy [9–11]. Inadequate bowel preparation may lead to repeated colonoscopies, prolonged prospective procedure time, increased operative risk, and rising medical costs [12]. Currently, there are three main validated bowel preparation scoring systems for evaluating the quality of colonoscopy preparation, including the Aronchick Scale, the Ottawa Bowel Preparation Scale (OBPS), and the Boston Bowel Preparation Score (BBPS) [13–15]. The Aronchick Scale and OBPS evaluate colon preparation before washing and suctioning, while the BBPS evaluates it afterwards [13–15]. OBPS also subjectively evaluates the amount of washing and suctioning required to achieve optimal visualization. In addition, the grading system, and the segments used to evaluate preparation (from the whole colon to five divided segments), are also different between the three systems [16,17]. The main concern with these scoring systems is that these scales depend on subjective evaluations to grade bowel cleanliness, which suffer from opinion-related bias [18,19]. That is to say, the inter-observer reliability, measured by intraclass correlations (ICC) or kappa coefficients, would be the major concern of these scales. For example, the Aronchick Scale showed a fair-to-substantial ICC of 0.31–0.76. The ICC of OBPS seems good at 0.94, but this was actually the result from a small-scale study on just a single gastroenterologist and a staff fellow for 97 colonoscopies. In addition, OBPS showed a fair agreement between nurses and physicians with a Pearson's $r = 0.60$ [20]. The reliability of BBPS is more frequently studied with a fair weighted kappa of 0.67 to 0.78. Among the three scales, the BBPS is the most thoroughly validated and is the most recommended one for use in a clinical setting [18]. Generally, the application of these three scales is time-consuming and requires detailed assessments and documentations. Therefore, in prospectively collected data from a large national endoscopic consortium, the proper application of these scales is rare; only about 11% of doctors in the United States thoroughly evaluate and document the suggested BBPS in clinical practice [21].

In recent years, with the application of artificial intelligence (AI), computer-aided detection and diagnosis software systems have been developed to help endoscopists enhance and characterize polyps during colonoscopy [22–25]. AI and machine learning techniques have also emerged to evaluate the quality of bowel preparation. Two previous studies explored the evaluation of bowel cleanliness in capsule endoscopy and colonoscopy [26,27]. These applied AI to classify bowel cleanliness based on experts' subjective grading. With this approach, human factors can still lead to potential bias in scoring due to the fair interobserver reliability of the grading scales used in these reports (capsule endoscopy, ICC = 0.37–0.66; colonoscopy, weighted kappa of 0.67–0.78 with BBPS). In our current study, we used a completely different approach by using a segmentation method to precisely label fecal material in the training dataset. With this method, we attempted to develop a fully automatic segmentation method through the application of convolutional neural networks (CNNs) to mark the mucosal area coated with fecal material using prospectively collected colonoscopy video imaging data. The proposed model can be a useful and novel tool for objectively evaluating the quality of colon preparation. To achieve this goal, we used U-Net, an AI architecture that focuses on biological images, as the backbone in the process [28]. The U-Net architecture won the 2015 International Symposium on Biomedical Imaging (ISBI) cell tracking challenge and is often used for brain tumor cutting [29], retinal image segmentation [30,31], endoscopy image segmentation [32,33], and other medical image segmentation tasks [34–36].

2. Materials and Methods

2.1. Data Collection

Endoscopy video and images from Jan 2019 to Feb 2020 were obtained from the Colonoscopy Video Database from the Endoscopy Center of Taipei Veterans General Hospital. The Colonoscopy Video Database was established by patients who were willing to contribute their colonoscopy video and related profiles for clinical study and consists of 520 videos as of February 2020. All the patients signed an informed consent form to contribute their colonoscopy video for clinical study, and a validated questionnaire for enquiring as to the possible factors contributing to the cleanliness of the bowel preparation was distributed to the participants. All patients received standardized bowel preparation with either 2 L of polyethylene glycol solution or BowKlean® powder (containing sodium picosulfate and magnesium oxite, Genovate Biotechnology, Taiwan) before the colonoscopy. Their endoscopy videos were prospectively obtained from the Colonoscopy Video Database from the Endoscopy Center. All colonoscopies were performed by using an Olympus Evis Lucera Elite CV-290 video processor and a high-definition colonoscope CF-HQ 290 or CF-H290 (Olympus Co., Ltd., Tokyo, Japan). The colonoscopy videos were recorded with a resolution of 1920 × 1080. The patients' individual information was de-identified and stored in the database. The study was approved by the Institutional Review Board of Taipei Veterans General Hospital.

2.2. Image Preprocessing

Initially, all videos were transformed into images according to their sampling rate in frames per second (FPS). Unqualified images were filtered out to ensure good image quality. The unqualified images were too blurred or murky to be recognized, low resolution, or in the improper format, or included frames without stool, or full of stool. Extranious information, such as the examination time, patient ID, name, and sex, were removed. These images were randomly divided into training (90% of the total images) and validation (10% of the total images). After establishing the final model, an independent verification dataset was collected from our center in different period to the time for training/validation [37]. The images used in the different datasets (training/validation/verification) were independent at patient level, indicating that the images from the same patients should be attributed to one particular dataset. The training and validation datasets were used to establish AI models, and the verification dataset served to verify the performance of established AI models. In this task, the data augmentation skill was applied to overcome the limitation of the data quantity and reinforce the performance of the AI model. It is worth mentioning that augmentation skill was only applied to the training dataset to enhance the variation in the training image, and measurement (augmentation) was not used in the validation and verification dataset. The augmentation methods included (1) random rotation (randomly rotated images with preservation), (2) random horizontal flip (horizontally flipped images with random radians), (3) random zoom in/out (zoomed in/out images at random scales), and (4) random Gaussian noise (randomly adding Gaussian noise to images).

2.3. Image Labeling

LabelMe (https://github.com/wkentaro/labelme, accessed on 1 October 2021), an annotation tool for executing image segmentation, is an open-source software and has been widely applied to perform image annotation tasks. The software was installed on a Windows system, and 3 senior endoscopic technicians were trained to perform endoscopy image segmentation labeling (Figure 1). The images show the areas where staining, residual stool, and/or opaque liquid, which influenced the visualization of mucosa, were marked for segmentation [14]. After the annotation, another senior technician rechecked the images to ensure labeling quality. When facing difficulty in image labeling, an experienced endoscopist (Wang YP) was consulted to make the final decision. All images with discernible information were removed and given a random serial number for subsequent model use.

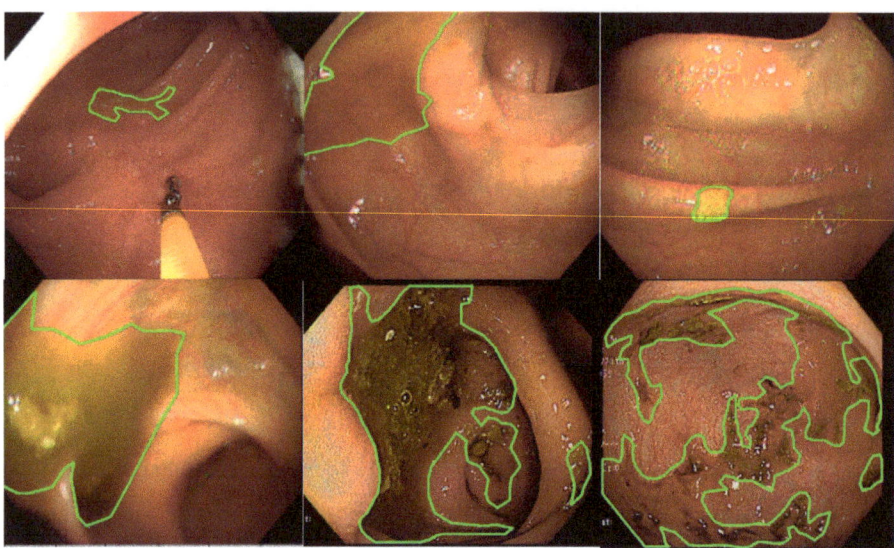

Figure 1. The manual segmentation samples. The figure represents the different types of fecal residues that were annotated and applied in this study.

2.4. Establishment and Validation of AI Models

U-Net was selected as the main architecture for developing our AI model since U-Net has been deemed valid for medical image recognition [28]. U-Net included 2 parts, the encoder and the decoder. The encoder extracted the important features of the images using the convolution method, and then the decoder applied these features to perform the segmentation task (Figure 2). Various encoders can be selected as the backbone in U-Net architecture for executing feature extraction, such as VGG19, ResNet34, InceptionV3, and EfficientNet-B5 [38]. EfficientNet-B5 was selected in our model because of its better accuracy and lower computational power (Table 1). One of the characteristics of U-Net was that it extracted features that can be transmitted and superimposed on subsequent layers to enhance the information and resolution of neural networks. The output result of U-Net was a probability map, and each pixel of an image had a binary value (0 or 1). The value of the pixels at the target location was segmented as 1, and the other pixel values were assigned to 0. Finally, the result of image segmentation was visualized based on each pixel value.

In U-Net, there still existed some hyperparameters that could be adjusted to enhance the AI performance, such as learning rate, number of epochs, and batch size. During the training process, the validation dataset was used to validate the performance in each trained model. Then, the model with the best performance was saved as the final model. The AI models were trained using Google cloud's platform with a two-core vCPU, 7.5 GB RAM, and an NVIDIA Tesla K80 GPU. Keras 2.2.4 and TensorFlow 1.6.0 running on CentOS 7 were used for training and validation.

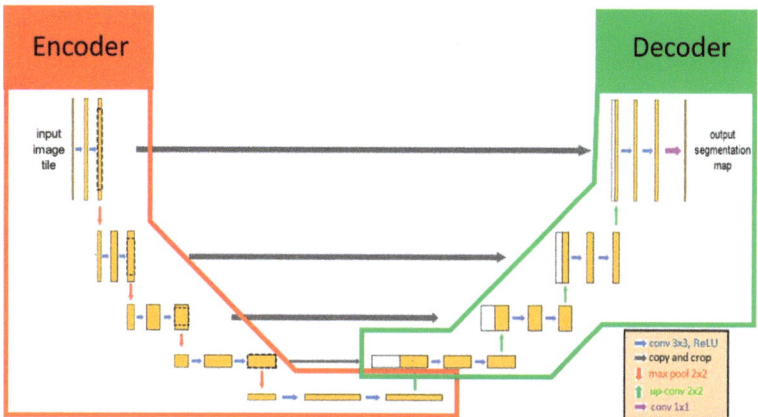

Figure 2. The architecture of U-Net. U-Net contained 2 parts: encoder and decoder. Initially, the input image included features extracted by the encoder, and those features were transmitted to the decoder as the important information for identifying whether each pixel was the target location. The red line and green line indicate the encoder and decoder, respectively, in the U-Net AI model.

Table 1. Comparison of accuracy using U-Net with different encoders.

Model	Top 1 Accuracy (%)	Top 5 Accuracy (%)	Parameters (M)
VGG19	71.1	89.8	143
Resnet34	73.31	91.4	26
ResNet50+SE	76.86	93.3	28
ResNeXt50	77.15	94.25	25
SENet-154	82.7	96.2	145.8
Inception V3	78	93.9	23.8
DenseNet121	74.5	91.8	8
MobileNet_v2	74.9	92.5	6
EfficientNet-B5	83.3	96.7	30

2.5. Verification of AI Models and Statistical Analysis

An independent dataset was selected for the verification of the best-established training model. The concept of a confusion matrix was applied to verify the performance of our trained AI model. In our image, the manually marked mucosal area coated by fecal residue was set as the ground truth, which was defined as the union area of false negative (FN) and true positive (TP) (Figure 3). The AI model-predicted area, i.e., the automated segmentation of fecal residue-covered mucosa, involved both the TP and false positive (FP). The intersection area of the ground truth and AI-predicted area was the TP. The area outside of the union of the ground truth and the AI-predicted area was defined as the true negative (TN). Accuracy was calculated as the addition of TP plus TN in proportion to the total mucosal area and was used to represent the performance of our AI model. The defined parameters are given in the following equations:

$$\text{Intersection over Union (IOU)} = TP/(TP + FP + FN)$$

$$\text{Accuracy (Acc)} = TP + TN/\text{total area}$$

$$\text{Predict} = (TP + FP)/\text{total area}$$

$$\text{GroundTruth} = (FN + TP)/\text{total area}$$

$$\text{Non\_union\_percent} = TN/\text{total area}$$

$$\text{Intersection\_percent} = TP/\text{total area}$$

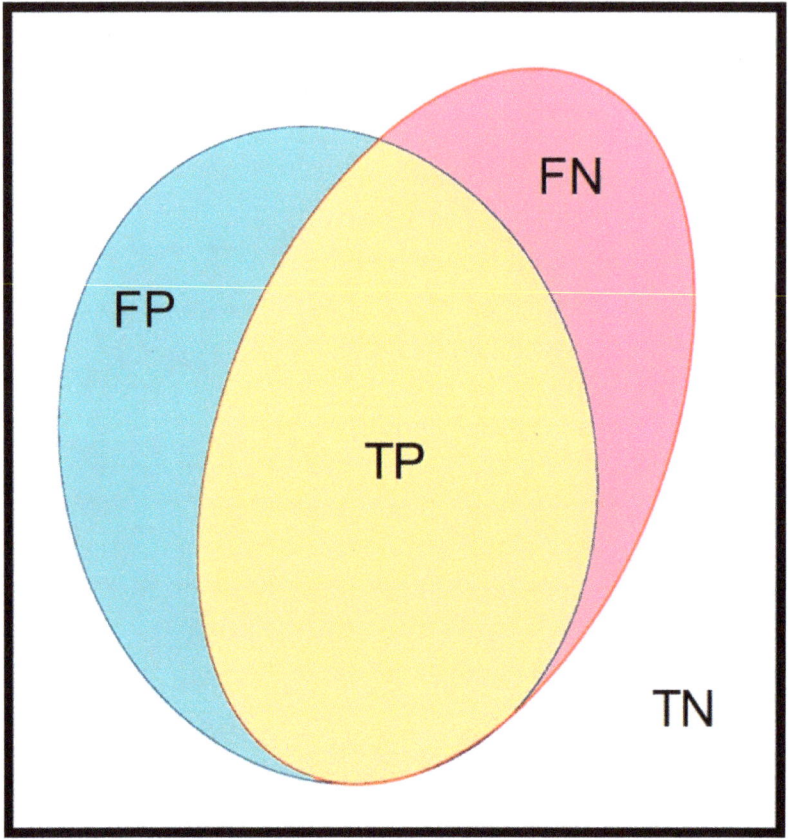

Figure 3. The major parameters in this study. The confusion matrix contained 4 parameters. The yellow area (true positive, TP) represents the intersection area of ground truth and the AI-predicted area. The union of red (false negative, FN) and yellow (true positive, TP) indicate the ground truth area. The blue area (false positive, FP) and yellow area (true positive, TP) indicate the AI-predicted area. The rest of the area out of the union of ground truth and the AI-predicted area was the true negative (TN).

The obtained area in pixels was measured, and all the data are presented as the mean ± S.E.M. The number of pixels in the AI-predicted surface area coated by fecal residue was computed. The proportion of AI-predicted surface area coated by fecal residue against total mucosa area as the octagonal area in the image was also computed and displayed in real time. Pearson correlation and a two-sided t-test were used to evaluate the association of the proportion of labelled areas against total area between automatic and manual segmentation. All statistical tests were performed at the $\alpha < 0.05$ level.

We also selected 3 short videos, each representing poor, good, and excellent preparation, for real-time verification. The final AI model was applied in the video to perform the auto-segmentation of mucosa covered by fecal residue in the video.

3. Results

3.1. Data Collection

A total of 119 endoscopy videos were collected from 119 patients (mean age: 53.13 years; male/female: 54/65). Successive image frames were then extracted from these videos. After image quality control, a total of 9066 images were selected and randomly divided into two groups, i.e., a training dataset with 8056 images (90% of all images) and a validation dataset with 1010 images (10% of all images). Another dataset for verification containing 1052 images was independently collected from those patients who underwent colonoscopy in a different time period from the training/validation datasets.

3.2. The Details of Model Establishment

U-Net, an AI architecture focused on biological image segmentation, was selected as the core architecture in this research. In the training stage, each image was resized to 288 × 288 pixels, the optimizer was set as Adam, the learning rate was set to 1e-4, and the loss function was set as binary cross-entropy. The total training epoch was set to 30, and the batch size was set to four (Table 2).

Table 2. The detailed parameters for training the models.

Model	U-Net
Backbone	EfficientNet-B5
Optimizer	Adam
Loss function	binary cross entropy
Learning rate	1e-4
Batch size	4
Total number of epochs run during training	30

3.3. The Performance of Automatic Segmentation (Results of Model Verification)

The average time required for the model to generate the automatic segmentation of each image was 0.3634 s. The accuracy of our AI model achieved 94.7 ± 0.67% with an IOU of 0.607 ± 0.17. The ground truth (technician-labelled) area of the total area was 14.8 ± 0.43%, while the AI-predicted area was 13.1 ± 0.38% of the total area. The intersection area of the ground truth and AI-predicted area was 11.3 ± 0.36% (fecal material detected by both technician and AI), and the area outside of the union of the ground truth and the AI-predicted area (nonunion area) was 83.4 ± 0.45% of the total measured area (Table 3).

Table 3. The detailed performance of the final trained models.

	Mean	S.E.M.
IOU	0.607	0.17
Accuracy	0.947	0.0067
Prediction	0.131	0.0038
Ground truth	0.148	0.0043
Intersection area	0.113	0.0036
Nonunion area	0.834	0.0045

IOU = Intersection over union.

Such results suggest that the AI-detected area is 3.5% less than the ground truth (technician-labelled area) (14.8% minus 11.3%), and the rate at which our model misdetected normal mucosa as fecal material is smaller at 1.8% (13.1% minus 11.3%). Example images of the best and worst results of our AI model are displayed in Figures 4 and 5.

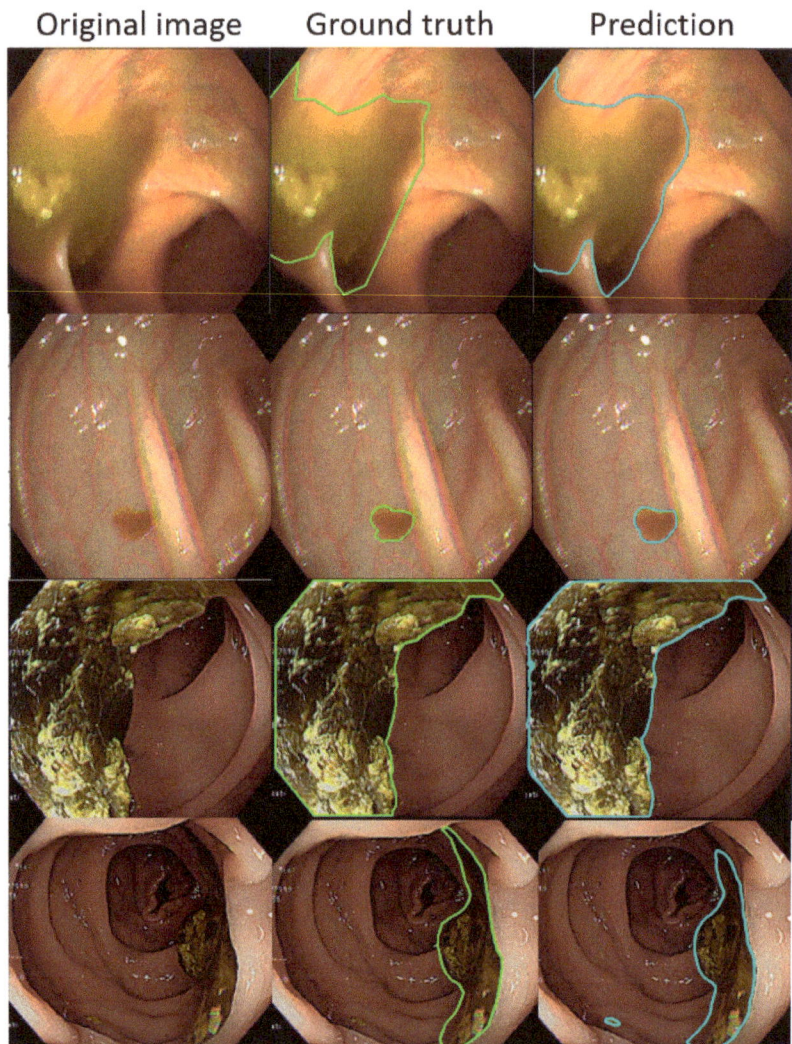

Figure 4. The better annotation example of AI model segmentation. The intersection over union (IOU) of those samples achieved approximately 0.90, meaning that the annotation result of the AI was similar to manual labeling. In those figures, the left, middle, and right columns represent the raw, manually annotated, and AI-annotated images, respectively. The green and blue lines indicate the segmentation labeled by endoscopy technicians and the trained AI model.

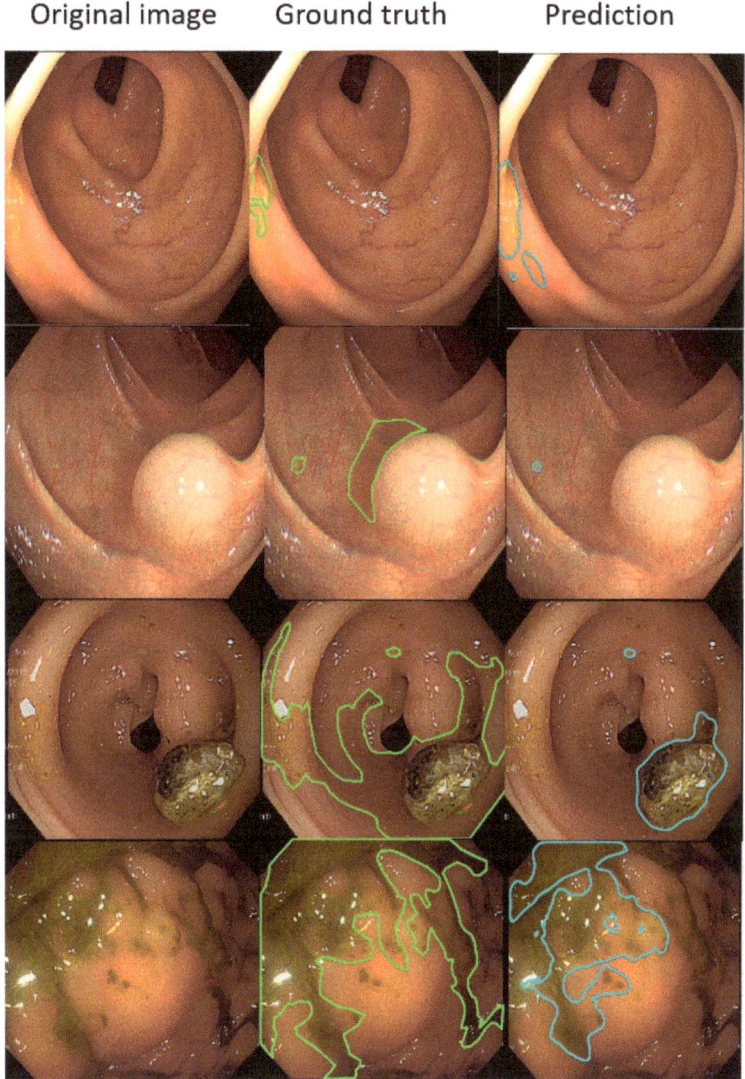

Figure 5. The worse annotation samples of the AI model segment. In each image, the left, middle, and right columns represent the raw, manually annotated, and AI-annotated images, respectively. The green and blue lines indicate the segmentation labeled by endoscopy technicians and the trained AI model. The IOU of these samples was less than 0.5.

In each visualized result, the left panel represents the raw image of the verification dataset. The green line in the middle panel indicates the ground truth annotated by endoscopic technicians, and the navy blue line in the right panel represents the result from the AI model prediction. The scatterplots in Figure 6 show that the area segmented manually was highly correlated to the area predicted by the AI ($r = 0.915$, $p < 0.001$), which suggested the independence of the accuracy with the bowel preparation adequacy. Our AI model was applied in real time in a colonoscopy video with a simultaneous display of the area of auto-segmentation and its percentage of AI-predicted fecal residue-covered mucosa. Example videos of poor, good, and excellent colon cleanliness are shown in Supplementary Videos S1–S3.

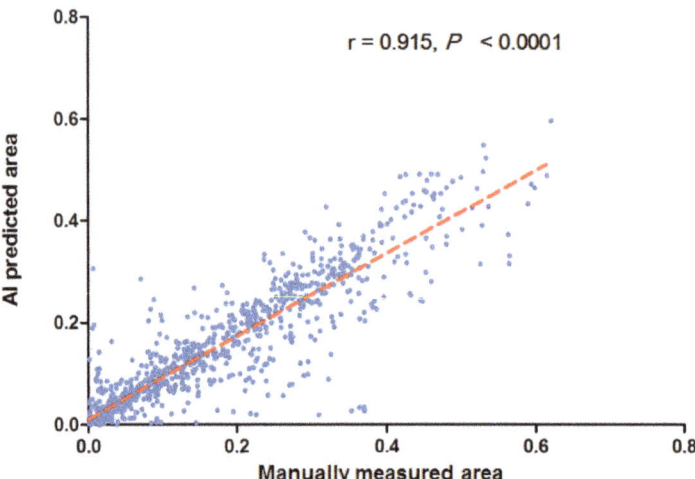

Figure 6. Scatterplots show a comparison of the area produced from manual and automatic segmentation methods.

4. Discussion

In the current study, we used machine learning to evaluate colon preparation using automated segmentation of the mucosal area covered by fecal residue. We demonstrated that this automated segmentation displayed comparable results and high accuracy when compared with manual annotation. To the best of our knowledge, our current article may present the first examples of deep CNN being used for automatically segmenting in the evaluation of the quality of bowel preparation during colonoscopy.

Proper reporting of the preparation quality after colonoscopy is extremely important. Inadequate bowel preparation in colonoscopy will lead to an increased risk of missed lesions, increased procedural time, increased costs, and potentially increased adverse events [21,37]. Furthermore, good preparation scored by the validated bowel preparation scale is associated with an increased polyp detection rate [18]. Currently, there are three main validated bowel preparation scoring systems for evaluating the quality of colonoscopy preparation, including the Aronchick Scale, the OBPS, and the BBPS [13–15]. It has been reported that reliability varies between studies and between scales [18,19]. All these scoring systems depend on the endoscopists' subjective evaluations and are dependent on the raters' interpretation of visual descriptions. The potential subjective opinion-related bias may lead to a wide difference in grading the adequacy of bowel preparation among physicians, especially in patients with moderate preparation quality that may lead to poor scoring and to a repeat colonoscopy [19]. In this study, we first established an objective evaluation system for bowel preparation by measuring the area of clearly visible mucosa and colon mucosa not clearly visualized due to staining, residual stool, and/or opaque liquid. This machine learning-based scoring system can shift the subjective grading into objectively obtained mucosal areas. The accuracy of this CNN-based model is highly comparable to the manually marked measurement. With this objective measurement system, we may evaluate colon preparation more precisely compared with the subjective grading system. Future studies are mandatory to apply the current AI model to real-world practice and set up an objective threshold for adequate bowel preparation.

Most of the past studies on AI for medical image recognition used retrospectively collected images or video frames to develop their AI models [38–40]. In our study, however, we only used video frames to develop our model, which will experience more difficulty achieving a satisfactory result than studies using images or images combined with video frames. This is because video frames are more easily influenced by focus distance, lighting, and vibrations. Therefore, the quality of the frame will often be much lower than that of still images. In some studies, the video verification dataset was significantly lower than the image verification dataset [41–43]. Nevertheless, our current model, developed from video frames, displayed satisfactory performance with high auto-segmentation accuracy. Furthermore, after the establishment of our AI model, we verified our model using a dataset that was independent from the dataset used to develop the model. This approach was used to avoid overlap of the training and validation datasets [43].

As shown in the Introduction, we chose U-Net as the core architecture because of its good performance. It may be argued that other architectures may perform better. For example, DeepLab achieved a higher IOU than U-Net in other reports [44–48]. In the decode part, DeepLab would directly quadruple the encoder features as the output result [49], while U-Net obtained the output result by repeating the up-sampling process four times [28]. Hence, U-Net can preserve more low-level features in the final output result. In our case, the fecal material in the image may be relatively small when compared to the entire image. Therefore, we suggest that U-Net may be able to detect more fecal materials, at greater detail, which is more suitable for our purpose. Recent research does suggest that there may be new lightweight encoder networks that may be able to achieve performance on par with the current available encoder with fewer samples while having faster image processing [50]. Future investigations comparing different backbones, especially the lightweight ones, may be necessary to further improve the accuracy and efficiency in AI-assisted fecal material detection during colonoscopy.

Limitations are present in this study. The accuracy of our model when detecting material is high (94%), while the IOU is relatively low (0.61). This may be due to the relatively small annotated area when compared to the entire image, contributing to a high TN in the current model. In addition, our data showed that the area between our model and the ground truth sat in the best line below 0.4 (40% of total area), and it seemed to become more disparate after 0.4 on the scatterplot. Such a result suggests that the current AI model can be less predictive upon poor bowel preparation (images with fecal material more than 40% of total area). The disparate results may be due to the relatively small amount of fecal material in most images used for training. By including more images of poor bowel preparation containing more fecal material during training, we may be able to increase the IOU and improve the accuracy. Concerns may also be raised regarding the accuracy of the manual segmentation as the ground truth, since there are multiple potential variabilities during human annotation. In addition, the cut-off value used to represent the adequacy of bowel preparation and its comparability with the currently validated scoring system are unknown. Additionally, severe bowel inflammation, ulcerations or bleeding may mimic poor colon preparation that influence the evaluation accuracy. Furthermore, we treated the current model as a proof of concept, so the model was established with relatively few images in the validation dataset and lacks the application of k-fold cross-validation. Future studies are mandatory to see whether there are differences among endoscopic technicians on the same images and whether our model falls into the same percentage of errors and deviations in future confirmatory clinical trials.

5. Conclusions

In conclusion, we used deep CNN to establish a fully automatic segmentation method to rapidly and accurately mark the mucosal area coated with fecal residue during colonoscopy for the objective evaluation of colon preparation. It is important to evaluate the clinical impact by comparing the application of this novel AI system with the currently available bowel preparation scales.

Supplementary Materials: The following supporting information can be downloaded at: https://www.mdpi.com/article/10.3390/diagnostics12030613/s1, Video S1: Example video of poor colon cleanliness, Video S2: Example video of good colon cleanliness, Video S3: Example video of excellent colon cleanliness.

Author Contributions: Conceptualization, Y.-P.W., Y.-C.J. and C.-L.L.; methodology, Y.-P.W., Y.-C.J., P.-H.C., I.-F.H., M.-C.H., F.-Y.L. and C.-L.L.; software, Y.-C.J., Y.-C.C. and D.L.; validation, Y.-P.W., Y.-C.J., Y.-C.C. and D.L.; formal analysis, Y.-P.W., Y.-C.J., Y.-C.C. and D.L.; investigation, Y.-P.W., Y.-C.J., K.-Y.S., H.-E.L., Y.-J.W. and C.-L.L.; resources, M.-C.H., F.-Y.L., Y.-J.W. and C.-L.L.; writing—original draft preparation, Y.-P.W., Y.-C.J., P.-H.C., I.-F.H. and C.-L.L.; writing—review and editing, M.-C.H., F.-Y.L., Y.-J.W. and C.-L.L.; visualization, Y.-C.J., D.L., Y.-C.C., K.-Y.S. and H.-E.L.; supervision, M.-C.H., F.-Y.L., Y.-J.W. and C.-L.L.; project administration, Y.-J.W. and C.-L.L.; funding acquisition, Y.-J.W. and C.-L.L. All authors have read and agreed to the published version of the manuscript.

Funding: This research was funded by Taipei Veterans General Hospital, grant number V108B-020, V109B-041, V1083-004-4, V109E-002-5, V110E-002-3. The funders had no role in the design of the study; in the collection, analyses, or interpretation of data; in the writing of the manuscript, or in the decision to publish the results.

Institutional Review Board Statement: The study was conducted in accordance with the Declaration of Helsinki, and approved by the Institutional Review Board of Taipei Veterans General Hospital (protocol code 2018-11-011CC, date of approval on 25 October 2018).

Informed Consent Statement: Informed consent was obtained from all subjects involved in the study.

Data Availability Statement: The data presented in this study are available on request from the corresponding author. The data are not publicly available due to Institutional Review Board's regulation.

Conflicts of Interest: All authors report no financial relationships with commercial interest and no competing interest.

References

1. Sung, J.J.; Lau, J.Y.; Goh, K.L.; Leung, W.K.; Asia Pacific Working Group on Colorectal Cancer. Increasing incidence of colorectal cancer in Asia: Implications for screening. *Lancet Oncol.* **2005**, *6*, 871–876. [CrossRef]
2. Chiang, C.J.; Lo, W.C.; Yang, Y.W.; You, S.L.; Chen, C.J.; Lai, M.S. Incidence and survival of adult cancer patients in Taiwan, 2002–2012. *J. Med. Assoc.* **2016**, *115*, 1076–1088. [CrossRef] [PubMed]
3. Shaukat, A.; Mongin, S.J.; Geisser, M.S.; Lederle, F.A.; Bond, J.H.; Mandel, J.S.; Church, T.R. Long-term mortality after screening for colorectal cancer. *N. Engl. J. Med.* **2013**, *369*, 1106–1114. [CrossRef] [PubMed]
4. Loberg, M.; Kalager, M.; Holme, O.; Hoff, G.; Adami, H.O.; Bretthauer, M. Long-term colorectal-cancer mortality after adenoma removal. *N. Engl. J. Med.* **2014**, *371*, 799–807. [CrossRef] [PubMed]
5. Sanduleanu, S.; Le Clercq, C.M.; Dekker, E.; Meijer, G.A.; Rabeneck, L.; Rutter, M.D.; Valori, R.; Young, G.P.; Schoen, R.E. Definition and taxonomy of interval colorectal cancers: A proposal for standardising nomenclature. *Gut* **2015**, *64*, 1257–1267. [CrossRef]
6. Patel, S.G.; Ahnen, D.J. Prevention of interval colorectal cancers: What every clinician needs to know. *Clin. Gastroenterol. Hepatol.* **2014**, *12*, 7–15. [CrossRef]
7. Mitchell, R.M.; McCallion, K.; Gardiner, K.R.; Watson, R.G.; Collins, J.S. Successful colonoscopy; completion rates and reasons for incompletion. *Ulst. Med. J.* **2002**, *71*, 34–37.
8. Shah, H.A.; Paszat, L.F.; Saskin, R.; Stukel, T.A.; Rabeneck, L. Factors associated with incomplete colonoscopy: A population-based study. *Gastroenterology* **2007**, *132*, 2297–2303. [CrossRef]
9. Hassan, C.; Bretthauer, M.; Kaminski, M.F.; Polkowski, M.; Rembacken, B.; Saunders, B.; Benamouzig, R.; Holme, O.; Green, S.; Kuiper, T.; et al. Bowel preparation for colonoscopy: European Society of Gastrointestinal Endoscopy (ESGE) guideline. *Endoscopy* **2013**, *45*, 142–150. [CrossRef]
10. ASGE Standards of Practice Committee; Saltzman, J.R.; Cash, B.D.; Pasha, S.F.; Early, D.S.; Muthusamy, V.R.; Khashab, M.A.; Chathadi, K.V.; Fanelli, R.D.; Chandrasekhara, V.; et al. Bowel preparation before colonoscopy. *Gastrointest. Endosc.* **2015**, *81*, 781–794. [CrossRef]
11. Rex, D.K.; Schoenfeld, P.S.; Cohen, J.; Pike, I.M.; Adler, D.G.; Fennerty, M.B.; Lieb, J.G., 2nd; Park, W.G.; Rizk, M.K.; Sawhney, M.S.; et al. Quality indicators for colonoscopy. *Gastrointest. Endosc.* **2015**, *81*, 31–53. [CrossRef] [PubMed]
12. Lieberman, D.A.; Rex, D.K.; Winawer, S.J.; Giardiello, F.M.; Johnson, D.A.; Levin, T.R. Guidelines for colonoscopy surveillance after screening and polypectomy: A consensus update by the US Multi-Society Task Force on Colorectal Cancer. *Gastroenterology* **2012**, *143*, 844–857. [CrossRef] [PubMed]
13. Aronchick, C.A.; Lipshutz, W.H.; Wright, S.H.; DuFrayne, F.; Bergman, G. Validation of an instrument to assess colon cleansing. *Am. J. Gastroenterol.* **1999**, *9*, 2667.
14. Lai, E.J.; Calderwood, A.H.; Doros, G.; Fix, O.K.; Jacobson, B.C. The Boston bowel preparation scale: A valid and reliable instrument for colonoscopy-oriented research. *Gastrointest. Endosc.* **2009**, *69*, 620–625. [CrossRef]
15. Calderwood, A.H.; Jacobson, B.C. Comprehensive validation of the Boston Bowel Preparation Scale. *Gastrointest. Endosc.* **2010**, *72*, 686–692. [CrossRef] [PubMed]

16. Johnson, D.A.; Barkun, A.N.; Cohen, L.B.; Dominitz, J.A.; Kaltenbach, T.; Martel, M.; Robertson, D.J.; Boland, C.R.; Giardello, F.M.; Lieberman, D.A.; et al. Optimizing adequacy of bowel cleansing for colonoscopy: Recommendations from the US multi-society task force on colorectal cancer. *Gastroenterology* **2014**, *147*, 903–924. [CrossRef]
17. Kastenberg, D.; Bertiger, G.; Brogadir, S. Bowel preparation quality scales for colonoscopy. *World J. Gastroenterol.* **2018**, *24*, 2833–2843. [CrossRef]
18. Parmar, R.; Martel, M.; Rostom, A.; Barkun, A.N. Validated Scales for Colon Cleansing: A Systematic Review. *Am. J. Gastroenterol.* **2016**, *111*, 197–204, quiz 205. [CrossRef]
19. Heron, V.; Martel, M.; Bessissow, T.; Chen, Y.I.; Desilets, E.; Dube, C.; Lu, Y.; Menard, C.; McNabb-Baltar, J.; Parmar, R.; et al. Comparison of the Boston Bowel Preparation Scale with an Auditable Application of the US Multi-Society Task Force Guidelines. *J. Can. Assoc. Gastroenterol.* **2019**, *2*, 57–62. [CrossRef]
20. Martinato, M.; Krankovic, I.; Caccaro, R.; Scacchi, M.; Cesaro, R.; Marzari, F.; Colombara, F.; Compagno, D.; Judet, S.; Sturniolo, G. P.15.8 Assessment of boewel preparation for colonoscopy: Comparison between different tools and different healthcare professionals. *Dig. Liver Dis.* **2013**, *45*, S195–S196. [CrossRef]
21. Kluge, M.A.; Williams, J.L.; Wu, C.K.; Jacobson, B.C.; Schroy, P.C., 3rd; Lieberman, D.A.; Calderwood, A.H. Inadequate Boston Bowel Preparation Scale scores predict the risk of missed neoplasia on the next colonoscopy. *Gastrointest. Endosc.* **2018**, *87*, 744–751. [CrossRef] [PubMed]
22. Kudo, S.E.; Misawa, M.; Mori, Y.; Hotta, K.; Ohtsuka, K.; Ikematsu, H.; Saito, Y.; Takeda, K.; Nakamura, H.; Ichimasa, K.; et al. Artificial Intelligence-assisted System Improves Endoscopic Identification of Colorectal Neoplasms. *Clin. Gastroenterol. Hepatol.* **2019**, *18*, 1874–1881. [CrossRef]
23. Gong, D.; Wu, L.; Zhang, J.; Mu, G.; Shen, L.; Liu, J.; Wang, Z.; Zhou, W.; An, P.; Huang, X.; et al. Detection of colorectal adenomas with a real-time computer-aided system (ENDOANGEL): A randomised controlled study. *Lancet Gastroenterol. Hepatol.* **2020**, *5*, 352–361. [CrossRef]
24. Chen, P.J.; Lin, M.C.; Lai, M.J.; Lin, J.C.; Lu, H.H.; Tseng, V.S. Accurate Classification of Diminutive Colorectal Polyps Using Computer-Aided Analysis. *Gastroenterology* **2018**, *154*, 568–575. [CrossRef] [PubMed]
25. Byrne, M.F.; Chapados, N.; Soudan, F.; Oertel, C.; Linares Perez, M.; Kelly, R.; Iqbal, N.; Chandelier, F.; Rex, D.K. Real-time differentiation of adenomatous and hyperplastic diminutive colorectal polyps during analysis of unaltered videos of standard colonoscopy using a deep learning model. *Gut* **2019**, *68*, 94–100. [CrossRef]
26. Buijs, M.M.; Ramezani, M.H.; Herp, J.; Kroijer, R.; Kobaek-Larsen, M.; Baatrup, G.; Nadimi, E.S. Assessment of bowel cleansing quality in colon capsule endoscopy using machine learning: A pilot study. *Endosc. Int. Open* **2018**, *6*, E1044–E1050. [CrossRef]
27. Zhou, J.; Wu, L.; Wan, X.; Shen, L.; Liu, J.; Zhang, J.; Jiang, X.; Wang, Z.; Yu, S.; Kang, J.; et al. A novel artificial intelligence system for the assessment of bowel preparation (with video). *Gastrointest. Endosc.* **2020**, *91*, 428–435.e2. [CrossRef]
28. Ronneberger, O.; Fischer, P.; Brox, T. *U-Net: Convolutional Networks for Biomedical Image Segmentation*; Springer: Cham, Switzerland, 2015; pp. 234–241.
29. Dong, H.; Yang, G.; Liu, F.; Mo, Y.; Guo, Y. Automatic Brain Tumor Detection and Segmentation Using U-Net Based Fully Convolutional Networks. In *Medical Image Understanding and Analysis*; Springer: Cham, Switzerland, 2017; pp. 506–517.
30. De Fauw, J.; Ledsam, J.R.; Romera-Paredes, B.; Nikolov, S.; Tomasev, N.; Blackwell, S.; Askham, H.; Glorot, X.; O'Donoghue, B.; Visentin, D.; et al. Clinically applicable deep learning for diagnosis and referral in retinal disease. *Nat. Med.* **2018**, *24*, 1342–1350. [CrossRef]
31. Chiu, S.J.; Li, X.T.; Nicholas, P.; Toth, C.A.; Izatt, J.A.; Farsiu, S. Automatic segmentation of seven retinal layers in SDOCT images congruent with expert manual segmentation. *Opt. Express* **2010**, *18*, 19413–19428. [CrossRef]
32. Laves, M.-H.; Bicker, J.; Kahrs, L.A.; Ortmaier, T. A dataset of laryngeal endoscopic images with comparative study on convolution neural network-based semantic segmentation. *Int. J. Comput. Assist. Radiol. Surg.* **2019**, *14*, 483–492. [CrossRef]
33. De Groof, A.J.; Struyvenberg, M.R.; van der Putten, J.; van der Sommen, F.; Fockens, K.N.; Curvers, W.L.; Zinger, S.; Pouw, R.E.; Coron, E.; Baldaque-Silva, F.; et al. Deep-Learning System Detects Neoplasia in Patients with Barrett's Esophagus with Higher Accuracy than Endoscopists in a Multistep Training and Validation Study with Benchmarking. *Gastroenterology* **2020**, *158*, 915–929.e4. [CrossRef] [PubMed]
34. Zafar, K.; Gilani, S.O.; Waris, A.; Ahmed, A.; Jamil, M.; Khan, M.N.; Sohail Kashif, A. Skin Lesion Segmentation from Dermoscopic Images Using Convolutional Neural Network. *Sensors* **2020**, *20*, 1601. [CrossRef] [PubMed]
35. Bui, T.D.; Wang, L.; Chen, J.; Lin, W.; Li, G.; Shen, D. Multi-task Learning for Neonatal Brain Segmentation Using 3D Dense-Unet with Dense Attention Guided by Geodesic Distance. In *Domain Adaptation and Representation Transfer and Medical Image Learning with Less Labels and Imperfect Data: First MICCAI Workshop, DART 2019, and first International Work*; Springer: Cham, Switzerland, 2019; Volume 11795, pp. 243–251. [CrossRef]
36. Gadosey, P.K.; Li, Y.; Adjei Agyekum, E.; Zhang, T.; Liu, Z.; Yamak, P.T.; Essaf, F. SD-UNet: Stripping Down U-Net for Segmentation of Biomedical Images on Platforms with Low Computational Budgets. *Diagnostics* **2020**, *10*, 110. [CrossRef] [PubMed]
37. Clark, B.T.; Protiva, P.; Nagar, A.; Imaeda, A.; Ciarleglio, M.M.; Deng, Y.; Laine, L. Quantification of Adequate Bowel Preparation for Screening or Surveillance Colonoscopy in Men. *Gastroenterology* **2016**, *150*, 396–405. [CrossRef]

38. Gulshan, V.; Peng, L.; Coram, M.; Stumpe, M.C.; Wu, D.; Narayanaswamy, A.; Venugopalan, S.; Widner, K.; Madams, T.; Cuadros, J.; et al. Development and Validation of a Deep Learning Algorithm for Detection of Diabetic Retinopathy in Retinal Fundus Photographs. *JAMA* **2016**, *316*, 2402–2410. [CrossRef] [PubMed]
39. Misawa, M.; Kudo, S.E.; Mori, Y.; Cho, T.; Kataoka, S.; Yamauchi, A.; Ogawa, Y.; Maeda, Y.; Takeda, K.; Ichimasa, K.; et al. Artificial Intelligence-Assisted Polyp Detection for Colonoscopy: Initial Experience. *Gastroenterology* **2018**, *154*, 2027–2029.e3. [CrossRef]
40. Hwang, D.-K.; Hsu, C.-C.; Chang, K.-J.; Chao, D.; Sun, C.-H.; Jheng, Y.-C.; Yarmishyn, A.A.; Wu, J.-C.; Tsai, C.-Y.; Wang, M.-L.; et al. Artificial intelligence-based decision-making for age-related macular degeneration. *Theranostics* **2019**, *9*, 232–245. [CrossRef]
41. Fernandez-Esparrach, G.; Bernal, J.; Lopez-Ceron, M.; Cordova, H.; Sanchez-Montes, C.; Rodriguez de Miguel, C.; Sanchez, F.J. Exploring the clinical potential of an automatic colonic polyp detection method based on the creation of energy maps. *Endoscopy* **2016**, *48*, 837–842. [CrossRef]
42. Wang, Y.; Tavanapong, W.; Wong, J.; Oh, J.H.; de Groen, P.C. Polyp-Alert: Near real-time feedback during colonoscopy. *Comput. Methods Programs Biomed.* **2015**, *120*, 164–179. [CrossRef]
43. Wang, P.; Xiao, X.; Glissen Brown, J.R.; Berzin, T.M.; Tu, M.; Xiong, F.; Hu, X.; Liu, P.; Song, Y.; Zhang, D.; et al. Development and validation of a deep-learning algorithm for the detection of polyps during colonoscopy. *Nat. Biomed. Eng.* **2018**, *2*, 741–748. [CrossRef]
44. Jiang, Y.; Xiao, C.; Li, L.; Chen, X.; Shen, L.; Han, H. An Effective Encoder-Decoder Network for Neural Cell Bodies and Cell Nucleus Segmentation of EM Images. In Proceedings of the 41st Annual International Conference of the IEEE Engineering in Medicine and Biology Society (EMBC), Berlin, Germany, 23–27 July 2019; pp. 6302–6305.
45. El-Bana, S.; Al-Kabbany, A.; Sharkas, M. A Two-Stage Framework for Automated Malignant Pulmonary Nodule Detection in CT Scans. *Diagnostics* **2020**, *10*, 131. [CrossRef] [PubMed]
46. Yao, X.; Yang, H.; Wu, Y.; Wu, P.; Wang, B.; Zhou, X.; Wang, S. Land Use Classification of the Deep Convolutional Neural Network Method Reducing the Loss of Spatial Features. *Sensors* **2019**, *19*, 2792. [CrossRef]
47. Dozen, A.; Komatsu, M.; Sakai, A.; Komatsu, R.; Shozu, K.; Machino, H.; Yasutomi, S.; Arakaki, T.; Asada, K.; Kaneko, S.; et al. Image Segmentation of the Ventricular Septum in Fetal Cardiac Ultrasound Videos Based on Deep Learning Using Time-Series Information. *Biomolecules* **2020**, *10*, 1526. [CrossRef] [PubMed]
48. Zhang, Z.; Gao, S.; Huang, Z. An Automatic Glioma Segmentation System Using a Multilevel Attention Pyramid Scene Parsing Network. *Curr. Med. Imaging* **2021**, *17*, 751–761. [CrossRef] [PubMed]
49. Chen, L.-C.; Zhu, Y.; Papandreou, G.; Schroff, F.; Adam, H. Encoder-Decoder with Atrous Separable Convolution for Semantic Image Segmentation. In Proceedings of the Computer Vision—ECCV 2018, Munich, Germany, 8–14 September 2018; pp. 833–851.
50. Jeon, Y.; Watanabe, A.; Hagiwara, S.; Yoshino, K.; Yoshioka, H.; Quek, S.T.; Feng, M. Interpretable and Lightweight 3-D Deep Learning Model For Automated ACL Diagnosis. *IEEE J. Biomed. Health Inform.* **2021**, *25*, 2388–2397. [CrossRef]

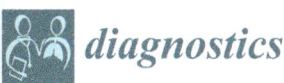

Review

Artificial Intelligence and Machine Learning in the Diagnosis and Management of Gastroenteropancreatic Neuroendocrine Neoplasms—A Scoping Review

Athanasios G. Pantelis [1,*], Panagiota A. Panagopoulou [2] and Dimitris P. Lapatsanis [1]

[1] 4th Department of Surgery, Evaggelismos General Hospital of Athens, 10676 Athens, Greece; dimitrislapatsanis@gmail.com
[2] Protypo Dialysis Center of Piraeus, 18233 Piraeus, Greece; giota81@gmail.com
* Correspondence: ath.pantelis@gmail.com

Abstract: Neuroendocrine neoplasms (NENs) and tumors (NETs) are rare neoplasms that may affect any part of the gastrointestinal system. In this scoping review, we attempt to map existing evidence on the role of artificial intelligence, machine learning and deep learning in the diagnosis and management of NENs of the gastrointestinal system. After implementation of inclusion and exclusion criteria, we retrieved 44 studies with 53 outcome analyses. We then classified the papers according to the type of studied NET (26 Pan-NETs, 59.1%; 3 metastatic liver NETs (6.8%), 2 small intestinal NETs, 4.5%; colorectal, rectal, non-specified gastroenteropancreatic and non-specified gastrointestinal NETs had from 1 study each, 2.3%). The most frequently used AI algorithms were Supporting Vector Classification/Machine (14 analyses, 29.8%), Convolutional Neural Network and Random Forest (10 analyses each, 21.3%), Random Forest (9 analyses, 19.1%), Logistic Regression (8 analyses, 17.0%), and Decision Tree (6 analyses, 12.8%). There was high heterogeneity on the description of the prediction model, structure of datasets, and performance metrics, whereas the majority of studies did not report any external validation set. Future studies should aim at incorporating a uniform structure in accordance with existing guidelines for purposes of reproducibility and research quality, which are prerequisites for integration into clinical practice.

Keywords: neuroendocrine tumors; neuroendocrine neoplasms; carcinoid; gastroenteropancreatic; GEP-NETs; Pan-NENs; SI-NETs; artificial intelligence; machine learning; deep learning

1. Introduction

Neuroendocrine neoplasms (NENs) of the gastrointestinal tract and the pancreas are rare tumors that tend to be diagnosed incidentally but with an increasing frequency [1,2]. GEP-NENs arise from the neural crest and may be located in the stomach, the small intestine, the appendix, the colon, the rectum, the pancreas, the ampulla of Vater, and the extrahepatic bile ducts, as well as the liver in the form of metastases. For the purposes of this review, we will focus on the former group of organs. For purposes of systematization, NENs can be divided into well differentiated neuroendocrine tumors (NETs) and poorly differentiated neuroendocrine carcinomas (NECs), the latter representing 10–20% of NENs [3]. This classification is not arbitrary, as NETs and NECs represent two genetically and biologically separate entities. NETs may be further classified into NETs arising from the gastrointestinal tract (GI-NETs, also known as carcinoids; ~50% of GEP-NETs) and ones affecting the pancreas (Pan-NENs; ~30% of GEP-NETs). NENs may or may not be functional. Nonfunctioning NENs are usually asymptomatic (especially early-stage ones), but may cause gastrointestinal bleeding and anemia, as well as obstructive effects which may present as jaundice, small bowel obstruction, intussusception, appendicitis and palpable abdominal mass depending on their anatomic location. Functioning GI-NENs may cause flushing, diarrhea, endocardial fibrosis and wheezing, owing to the synergistic effect of secreted vasoactive substances such as prostaglandins, kinins, serotonin and histamine. These symptoms signal the so-called carcinoid syndrome and usually herald liver metastases, because normally the liver inactivates products secreted into the portal circulation [4]. On the other hand, functioning Pan-NENs cause distinctive syndromes depending on the secreted product (i.e., gastrinoma–Zollinger-Ellison syndrome (ZES), insulinoma–Whipple's triad, glucagonoma–necrolytic erythema and hyperglycemia, VIPoma–watery diarrhea-hypokalemia-achlorhydria syndrome, somatostatinoma–diabetes, gallstone formation and steatorrhea etc) [1,2]. Gastric NETs merit special mention, as they may manifest with atypical symptoms that are not related to hormone secretion [1]. Type 1 gastric NETs (70–80% of gastric NETs) are related to atrophic gastritis that leads to secondary hypergastrinemia, which in turn causes hyperplasia of the enterochromaffin-like (ECL) cells. With continuous stimulation, ECLs give rise to aggregates which constitute foci of NETs. Type 2 gastric NETs (approximately 30%) are associated with ZES and multiple endocrine neoplasia type 1 (MEN-1). Type 3 gastric NETs are not related to other syndromes, are sporadic and are the most aggressive, as they tend to metastasize in 50–100% of the cases. Finally, type 4 gastric NETs are poorly differentiated and typically non-amenable to surgical manipulations.

Various biomarkers (mainly in immunohistochemistry) serve different purposes in the spectrum of NENs: Ki-67 is the most well-known among them, it has a prognostic relevance and is an essential component of the WHO grading of NENs [5]; SSTR-2/5 are useful for the detection of somatostatin receptors when functional imaging (with ^{68}Ga-DOTATATE PET/CT) is not possible; DAXX/ATRX has a prognostic relevance for Pan-NETs and is useful for distinguishing between NETs and NECs; p53/pRb are used for the classification of poorly differentiated NECs and the distinction from G3 NETs; and MGMT has a predictive response for the chemotherapeutic temozolomide [3]. Chromogranin A (CgA) is a useful circulating biomarker, especially for the diagnosis of asymptomatic NETs [1]. The NETest is a multigene mRNA assay that provides a broad molecular characterization GEP-NENs with high sensitivity and specificity and better diagnostic accuracy when compared to isolated biomarkers such as CgA [2]. Functional imaging with ^{68}Ga-DOTATATE, which binds to somatostatin receptors (SSRTs), is the cornerstone of diagnosis (and particularly localization and staging) of NETs, especially in the cases of small intestinal NETs (SI-NETs), large NETs and metastatic NETs [1].

Artificial intelligence (AI) is the process of simulating human learning by a machine, in the context of which large quantities of digitized data (input) are fed to a computer, the computer processes them with the aid of AI algorithms, and it ultimately reaches conclusions, makes decisions, or adjusts its function (output). Input data may derive from electronic health records (EHRs) and large databases, such as the Surveillance, Epidemiology, and End-Results Program (SEER) registry, digitized histology samples and whole slide images (WSIs), digital imaging studies (computed tomography—CT, magnetic resonance imaging—MRI, endoscopic ultrasonography—EUS, positron emission tomography—PET etc.), endoscopic study videos and so forth. AI is an umbrella term and includes supervised machine learning (ML), unsupervised machine learning, deep learning (DL) and reinforcement learning [6]. Each discipline differs from the preceding one in that it entails a greater degree of autonomy from the operator's supervision. AI with its subcategories is gradually entering healthcare and pertinent studies have had an exponential publication rate over the last five years, with various applications being integrated into clinical practice [7]. For the non-familiar clinician, AI should not be deemed as a substitute to their pivotal role in the patient care continuum or as an incomprehensible field belonging exclusively to computer experts but should rather be approached as a valuable tool in the process of decision-making, as well as a novel statistical method which, unlike traditional ones, may reveal hidden relationships between causes of disease and diagnosis, management and potentially cure.

With the present study we attempt to map the current status of AI and its applications in the diagnosis and management of gastroenteropancreatic NENs (GEP-NENs). Given on the one hand that NENs are relatively rare entities and on the other hand that AI, ML and DL are novel in the field of Medicine, we deemed it a rather uncharted area of interest and opted for a scoping review.

2. Materials and Methods

This review was performed according to the PRISMA extension for scoping reviews [8]. We performed literature search using the PubMed database in January 2021. The combined search terms were [artificial intelligence; machine learning; deep learning] AND [neuroendocrine; NET; NEN; carcinoid; insulinoma; glucagonoma; gastrinoma; VIPoma] AND [gastrointest*; GI; small intest*; appendi*; colon*; rect*; colorect *; stomach; gastric; duoden*; pancrea*; biliary; bile duct; Vater; ampulla; liver; hepa*]. There was no chronological restriction. Included articles had to have study populations with diagnosed NEN or NEN should be included in the differential diagnosis. They should also have at least 1 ML/DL algorithm for the process of their data, irrespective of the study design. The presence of a comparison group (external validation) was desired but not mandatory. Similarly, the report of at least one benchmarking metric, among accuracy, F1-score, area under receiver operator characteristic curve (AUROC) or area under precision-recall curve (AUPRC) were desired but not mandatory. Table 1 summarizes eligibility criteria. Only full-text publications were considered. Articles not in English language or not providing full text were excluded.

Table 1. Inclusion criteria.

Parameter	Inclusion Criteria
Population	Diagnosed cases with NEN (NET/NEC) or NEN included in the differential diagnosis.
Intervention	Analysis with a ML/DL algorithm.
Comparison	External validation desired but not mandatory.
Outcome	Report of accuracy, F1-score, AUROC or AUPRC desired but not mandatory.
Study design	Any. Abstract-only studies were excluded

NEN: neuroendocrine neoplasm; NET: neuroendocrine tumor; NEC: neuroendocrine carcinoma; ML: machine learning; DL: deep learning; AUROC: area under receiver operator characteristic (ROC) curve; AUPRC: area under precision-recall (PR) curve.

Data extraction was performed by two independent researchers (A.G.P., P.A.P.) using a predefined template with the eligibility and exclusion criteria. In case of disagreement, a third researcher (D.P.L.) made the decision whether to include the article or not. For the collection of relevant data we consulted the Guidelines for Developing and Reporting Machine Learning Predictive Models in Biomedical Research [9]. We collected data on year of publication, country of origin, DOI number, study design (prospective vs. retrospective), classification vs. regression, NEN type studied, dataset (number of patients or samples), input (predictors), output (outcomes), tested AI algorithm(s), training set, test set, internal and external validation sets, cross-validation method, accuracy, F1-score, AUROC (with 95% CI, if available) and AUPRC (with 95% CI, if available).

Numerical variables are presented as mean ± standard deviation (SD). Categorical variables are presented using frequencies and percentages. Calculations and statistical analysis were carried out using the online tool Prism®, GraphPad Software, San Diego, CA, USA.

3. Results

Literature search across PubMed yielded 1327 articles. In addition, 9 articles were retrieved through other sources (Google® search, screening through articles' literature). After screening of titles and abstracts, removal of duplicates, and implementation of eligibility criteria, 44 unique articles were included in the final analysis (Figure 1) [10–53].

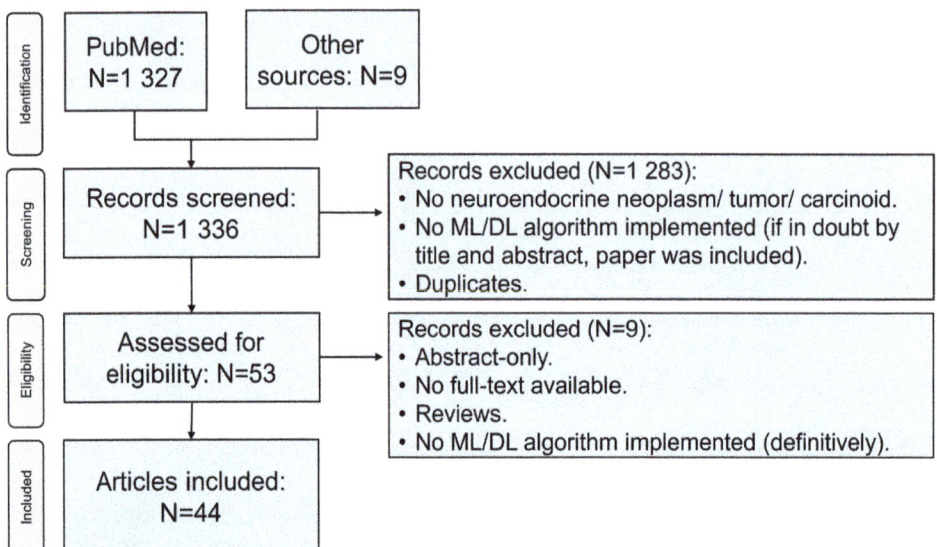

Figure 1. Flowchart depicting the selection process of sources of evidence. ML: machine learning; DL: deep learning.

Regarding geographical distribution (Figure 2), the included studies originated from 12 different countries, with major contributors being the USA (22 studies, 50%), China (12 studies, 27.3%) and Italy (3 studies, 6.8%). Among them, there were 4 coalitions of countries. The studies spanned a 13-year period (2007–2021), with a significant rise over time (Figure 3). Notably, 2/3 of studies were published over 2019–2021, which follows the general increase of publications regarding AI [54].

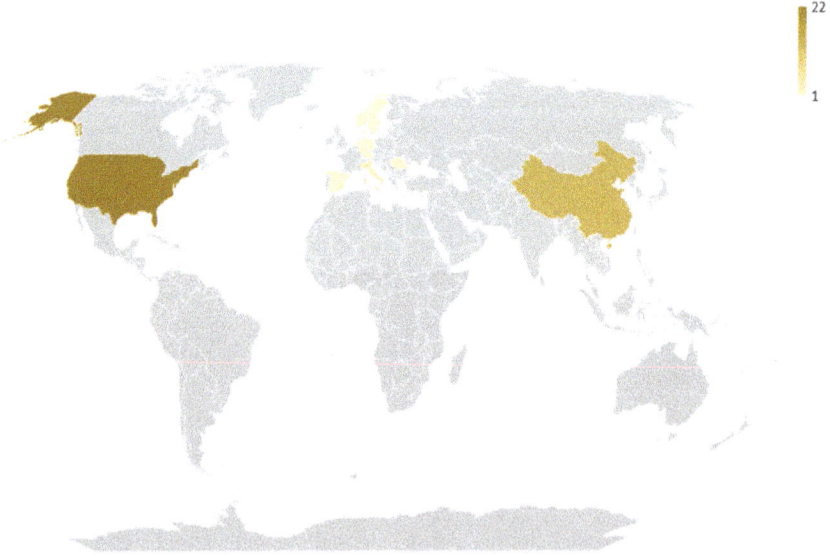

Figure 2. Geographic distribution of the studies included in the review. The darker the hue, the larger the number of studies coming from this particular country.

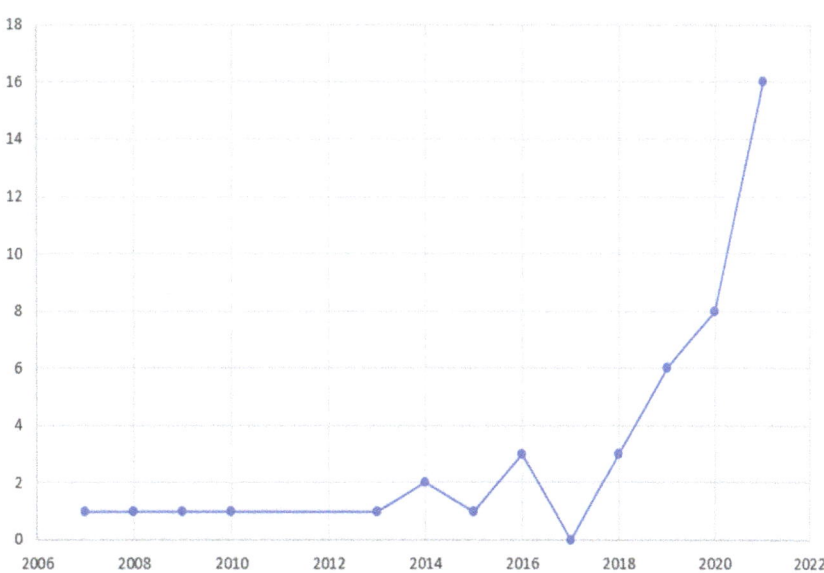

Figure 3. Temporal distribution of the studies included in the review according to year of publication.

In order to identify the prediction problem of each study, we collected data on study design, nature of the prediction, and continuity of the target variable, as per Luo et al. [9]. Consequently, there were 19 prospective (42.2%) and 26 retrospective (57.8%) analyses. Notably, one study had 2 stages, one prospective and one retrospective [13], hence the discrepancy between the total number of studies (44) and the sum of analysis based on prospective-retrospective study design (45). Regarding the nature of the prediction, we dichotomized the studies into diagnostic vs. prognostic, depending on whether the prediction referred to healthy subjects or subjects with already diagnosed NET, respectively [55]. The analysis yielded 24 diagnostic (54.5%) and 20 prognostic (45.5%) studies. Finally, all studies but one [24] had to do with classification. The prediction characteristics of each study are summarized in Table 2.

We then classified the papers according to the type of studied NET. Twenty-six studies were about Pan-NETs (59.1%) [10,11,15–20,24,25,27,28,30,31,34,38,41–43,45–47,49,51–53], 3 studies had to do with (metastatic) liver NETs (6.8%) [36,37,44], 2 studies analyzed SI-NETs (4.5%) [14,35], whereas colon and rectum [12], rectum [22], non-specified GEP [39], and non-specified GI NETs [50] had from 1 study each (2.3%). There were 4 studies with multiple types of NETs with separate data for each one of them provided (9.1%) [21,23,29,33], and another 2 studies with non-specified multiple types of NETs (4.5%) [13,48]. Figure 4 shows the relevant distribution of studies by NET type.

Regarding the source of data, there were 15 studies with histology-based analyses [10,15,20,23,24,33,38–43,45,47,50] and another 15 studies with imaging-based analyses (34.1% each). Six studies were structured based on patient databases (16.7%) [13,22,27,29,32,48], 5 on genetic assays (11.4%) [18,21,30,35,36], and 3 on plasma/serum (6.8%) [12,14,26]. Imaging-based studies were further distinguished in CT-based (6/15, 40%) [17,28,34,46,51,53], EUS-based (4/15, 26.7%) [11,19,25,31], MRI-based (3/15, 20%) [44,49,52], and PET/CT (2/15, 13.3%) [16,37]. Genetic assays included gene expression assays [35,36] and miRNA analyses [18,21] (2 studies each), as well as 1 genome-wide association study (GWAS) [30]. Figure 5 shows the relevant distribution of studies by source of data.

Table 2. Collective representation of the studies included in the present review, with respective prediction characteristics, technical characteristics, datasets and benchmarking. For reasons of conciseness, we have included only AUC of all the mentioned benchmarking measurements.

Study ID				Prediction Characteristics			Technical Characteristics				Datasets & Benchmarking			
First Author	Year of Publication	DOI	Ref. No.	Study Design	Nature of Prediction	Continuity of Output	NET Type	Source of Data	Tested AI Algorithm(s)	Training	AUC-Training	Cross-Validation	Test	AUC-Test	Ext. Validation	AUC
Bevilacqua A	2021	10.3390/diagnostics11050670	[10]	Prospective	Prognostic	Classification	Pancreas	Histology	LDA-model A	Y	0.870–0.940	3-fold x100	Y	0.870–0.900	N	
Chen K	2018	10.1016/S1470-2045(20)30323-5	[11]	Retrospective	Prognostic	Classification	Pancreas	Imaging (EUS)	DT, LR, NN, RF, SVM	N		N	Y	0.879–0.997	N	
Cheng X	2021	10.3389/fsurg.2021.745220	[22]	Retrospective	Prognostic	Classification	Rectum	Database	Adaboost, NB, Nu-SVC, SVC, RF, XGB	Y	0.780–0.850	10-fold	Y	0.890	Y	0.830–0.890
Drozdov I	2009	10.1002/cncr.24180	[33]	Prospective	Diagnostic	Classification	Primary small intestine; metastatic liver	Histology	DT, SVM	Y		10-fold	Y		N	
Drozdov I	2009	10.1002/cncr.24180	[33]	Prospective	Prognostic	Classification	Primary small intestine; metastatic liver	Histology	Perceptron	Y		N	N		N	
Feherenbach U	2021	10.3390/cancers13112726	[44]	Prospective	Prognostic	Classification	Liver	Imaging (MRI)	Not specified	Y	0.908–1.000	N	Y		N	
Gao X	2019	10.1007/s11548-019-02070-5	[49]	Prospective	Prognostic	Classification	Pancreas	Imaging (MRI)	CNN	Y	0.915 *	5-fold	Y	0.893 *	N	
Govind D	2020	10.1038/s41598-020-67880-z	[50]	Prospective	Prognostic	Classification	GI	Histology	deep-SKIE, SKIE (GAN-based), deep-SKIE (GAN-based)	Y		N	Y		N	
Han X	2021	10.3389/fonc.2021.606677	[51]	Retrospective	Diagnostic	Classification	Pancreas	Imaging (CT)	Adaboost, DT, GBDT, GNB, KNN, LDA, LR, SVM, RF	Y		10-fold x1000	Y	0.946–0.997 *	N	
Huang B	2021	10.1109/JBHI.2020.3043236	[52]	Retrospective	Prognostic	Classification	Pancreas	Imaging (MRI)	DFSR	N		N	Y	0.919	Y	0.688–0.840
Huang B	2021	10.1109/JBHI.2021.3070708	[53]	Retrospective	Prognostic	Classification	Pancreas	Imaging (CT)	GBDT, LR, RF, SVM	Y	0.660–0.760	N	Y	0.700–0.870	Y	0.710–0.830
Ito H	2020	10.4251/wjgo.v12.i11.1311	[12]	Retrospective	Diagnostic	Classification	Colon & rectum	Serum	BT	Y		N	N		N	
Kidd M	2021	10.1159/000508573	[13]	Retrospective	Prognostic	Classification	Multiple	Database	DT	N		N	N		N	
Kidd M	2021	10.1159/000508573	[13]	Prospective	Prognostic	Classification	Multiple	Database	DT	N		N	Y		N	
Kjelman	2021	10.1159/000510483; 10.1159/000510483	[14]	Prospective	Diagnostic	Classification	Small intestine	Serum	RF	Y	0.970–0.990	5-fold	N		N	
Klimov S	2021	10.3389/fonc.2020.593211	[15]	Retrospective	Prognostic	Classification	Pancreas	Histology	CNN	Y		5-fold	Y		N	
Klimov S	2021	10.3389/fonc.2020.593211	[15]	Retrospective	Prognostic	Classification	Pancreas	Histology	CNN, ML, "zoo" (18 different models)	Y		5-fold, leave-one-out	N		N	
Liu Y	2014	10.1016/j.media.2014.02.005.	[16]	Prospective	Prognostic	Classification	Pancreas	Imaging (PET/CT)	RDM	N		N	N		N	
Luo Y	2019	10.1159/000503291	[17]	Retrospective	Prognostic	Classification	Pancreas	Imaging (CT)	CNN, LR, RF, SVM	Y	0.570–0.810	8-fold	Y	0.820	N	
Nanayakkara J	2020	10.1093/narcan/zcaa009	[18]	Retrospective	Diagnostic	Classification	Pancreas	miRNA	data mining	N		N	Y		N	
Nguyen VX	2010	10.7863/jum.2010.29.9.1345	[19]	Retrospective	Diagnostic	Classification	Pancreas	Imaging (EUS)	ANN	Y		N	Y	0.890	N	
Niazi MKK	2018	10.1371/journal.pone.0195621	[20]	Retrospective	Diagnostic	Classification	Pancreas	Histology	Inception v3-C1 (type of CNN), Bootstrapped Inception v3-C1	N		N	Y	0.922–0.973	N	
Panarelli N	2019	10.1530/ERC-18-0244	[21]	Retrospective	Diagnostic	Classification	Appendix, GEP, ileum, pancreas, rectum	miRNA	SVM	Y		10-fold	Y		N	
Redemann J	2020	10.4103/jpi.jpi_37_20	[23]	Retrospective	Diagnostic	Classification	Appendix, colon & rectum, duodenum, pancreas, small intestine, stomach, total (icl. lung)	Histology	CNN	Y		N	Y		N	

Table 2. Cont.

Study ID			Prediction Characteristics			Technical Characteristics				Datasets & Benchmarking				
First Author	Year of Publication	DOI	Ref. No.	Study Design	Nature of Prediction	Continuity of Output	NET Type	Source of Data	Tested AI Algorithm(s)	Training	AUC-Training	Cross-Validation	Test	AUC-Test	Ext. Validation	AUC
Saccomandi P	2016	10.1007/s10103-016-1948-1	[24]	Retrospective	Prognostic	Regression	Pancreas	Histology	Inverse Monte Carlo	N		N	N		N	
Saffioti A	2008	10.1016/j.gie.2008.04.031	[25]	Prospective	Diagnostic	Classification	Pancreas	Imaging (EUS)	MLP	Y	0.779–0.982	10-fold	Y		N	
Soldevilla B	2021	10.3390/cancers13112634	[26]	Prospective	Diagnostic	Classification	Not specified	Plasma	OPLS-DA supervised model	Y		N	N		N	
Song Y	2018	10.7150/jca.26649	[27]	Retrospective	Prognostic	Classification	Pancreas	Database	DL, LR, SVM, RF	Y		10-fold	Y	0.870 (DL)	N	
Song C	2021	10.21037/atm-21-25	[28]	Retrospective	Prognostic	Classification	Pancreas	Imaging (CT)	SVM (various models)	Y	0.580–0.830	10-fold	Y	0.480–0.770	Y	0.520–0.560
Tchelebi JH	2021	10.3390/diagnostics11050804	[29]	Retrospective	Prognostic	Classification	GI; pancreas	Database	DT, GB GNB, KNN, MLP, MNB, LR, RF, SVC, XT	Y		10-fold	Y		N	
Tiresh A	2019	10.1002/cncr.31930	[30]	Prospective	Diagnostic	Classification	Pancreas	GWAS	Unsupervised clustering analysis	N		N	N		N	
Udristoiu AL	2021	10.1371/journal.pone.0251701	[31]	Prospective	Diagnostic	Classification	Pancreas	Imaging (EUS)	CNN-LSTM (different models)	Y		N	Y	0.970–0.990	N	
van Gerven MAJ	2007	10.1016/j.artmed.2006.09.003	[32]	Retrospective	Prognostic	Classification	Not specified	Database	NTC	Y		leave-one-out	N		N	
Wan Y	2021	10.1002/mp.15199	[34]	Retrospective	Prognostic	Classification	Pancreas	Imaging (CT)	SAE, hybrid (SAE+handcrafted)	Y	0.766–0.934	5-fold	Y	0.759	N	
Wang Q	2020	10.1042/BSR20193860	[35]	Prospective	Diagnostic	Classification	Small intestine	Gene expression assay	ANN	N		N	N		N	
Wang Q	2021	10.3389/fonc.2021.725988	[36]	Retrospective	Diagnostic	Classification	Liver	Gene expression assay	SVM	N		N	Y	0.945–1.000	N	
Wehrend J	2021	10.1186/s13550-021-00859-x	[37]	Retrospective	Diagnostic	Classification	Liver	Imaging (PET/CT)	CNN	Y		5-fold	Y	0.700–0.730 **	N	
Xing F	2013	10.1007/978-3-642-40811-3_55	[38]	Prospective	Diagnostic	Classification	Pancreas	Histology	SVM	N		N	Y		N	
Xing F	2014	10.1109/TBME.2013.2291703	[39]	Prospective	Diagnostic	Classification	GEP	Histology	SVM	N		3-fold	N		N	
Xing F	2015	10.1007/978-3-319-24574-4_40	[40]	Prospective	Diagnostic	Classification	Not specified	Histology	CNN	N		N	Y		N	
Xing F	2016	10.1007/978-3-319-46726-9_22	[41]	Prospective	Diagnostic	Classification	Pancreas	Histology	CNN	Y		N	Y		N	
Xing F	2016	10.1109/TMI.2015.2461436	[42]	Prospective	Diagnostic	Classification	Pancreas	Histology	CNN	Y		N	Y		N	
Xing F	2019	10.1109/TBME.2019.2900378	[43]	Prospective	Diagnostic	Classification	Pancreas	Histology	FCN-8s, FGRNA, FGRNB, FRCN, KiNet, SFCNOPI, U-Net	Y		N	Y	0.525–0.724	N	
Zhang X	2020	10.1200/CCI.19.00108	[45]	Retrospective	Diagnostic	Classification	Pancreas	Histology	GADA	Y	0.627–0.857	2-fold	Y	0.462–0.775	N	
Zhang T	2021	10.3389/fonc.2020.521831	[46]	Retrospective	Prognostic	Classification	Pancreas	Imaging (CT)	DC + Adaboost, DC + GBDT, XGB + RF	Y		N	Y	0.570–0.860	N	
Zhou RQ	2019	10.12998/wjcc.v7.i13.1611	[47]	Retrospective	Prognostic	Classification	Pancreas	Histology	LDA, LR, MLP, SVM	N		leave-one-out	Y		N	
Zimmerman NM	2021	10.2217/fon-2020-1254	[48]	Retrospective	Prognostic	Classification	Multiple	Database	DT	N		N	N		N	

* Only the algorithm with the best performance is mentioned. ** AUPRC (instead of AUROC).

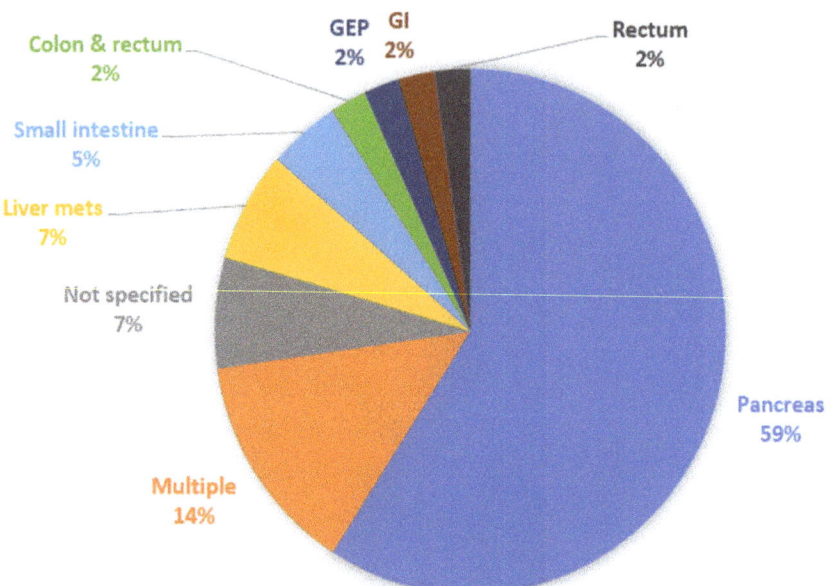

Figure 4. Distribution of studies by type of NET analyzed. GEP: gastroenteropancreatic; GI: gastrointestinal.

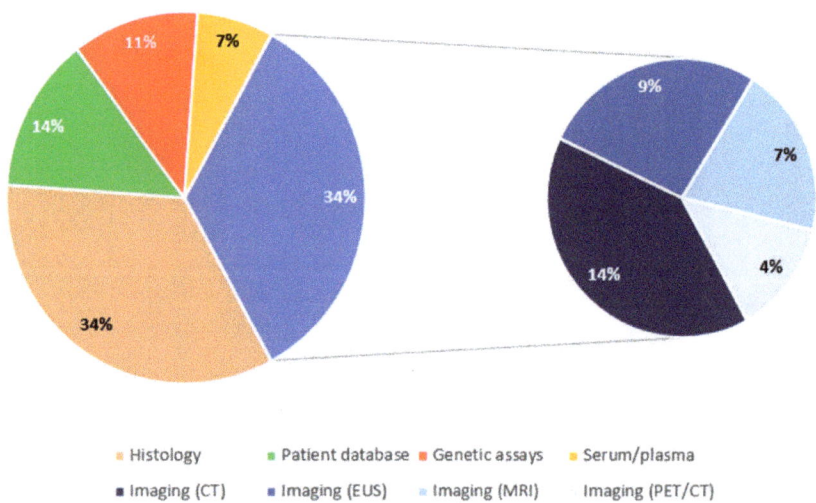

- Histology
- Patient database
- Genetic assays
- Serum/plasma
- Imaging (CT)
- Imaging (EUS)
- Imaging (MRI)
- Imaging (PET/CT)

Figure 5. Distribution of studies by source of data. CT: computed tomography; EUS: endoscopic ultrasound; MRI: magnetic resonance imaging; PET: positron emission tomography.

In the set of 44 studies, there were 53 outcome analyses, i.e., 7 studies with more than 1 outcome (5 with two outcomes [13,38,43,45,53], and 2 with three outcomes [15,33]). The most popular outcome analyses were tumor type identification and tumor grade (10 analyses each, 18.9%), tumor detection (5 analyses, 9.4%), and 5-year survival, cell segmentation, disease progression, disease recurrence and Ki-67 scoring (2 analyses each, 3.8%). Table 3 summarizes these outcome analyses, along with the references to relevant studies.

Table 3. Most popular outcome analyses within the included studies.

Outcome	Number of Studies (%)	Reference No.
Tumor type identification	10 (18.9)	[12,18,19,21,23,25,31,36,37,51]
Tumor grade	10 (18.9)	[10,11,17,34,46,47,49,50,52,53]
Tumor detection	5 (9.4)	[14,20,26,33,43]
5-year survival	2 (3.8)	[22,27]
Cell segmentation	2 (3.8)	[40,42]
Disease progression	2 (3.8)	[13,29]
Disease recurrence	2 (3.8)	[28,53]
Ki-67 scoring	2 (3.8)	[38,39]

The next analysis we performed was on the number of AI algorithms mentioned within the included studies. As it is expected, a number of studies included more than one AI algorithms, either in an attempt to find the most accurate among them or in the form of comparison of a novel AI model against established ones. In total, we identified 47 different models, with 10 among them being the most utilized ones (Figure 6), i.e., Supporting Vector Classification/Machine (14 analyses, 29.8%) [11,17,21,22,27–29,33,36,38,39,47,51,53], Convolutional Neural Network (10 analyses, 21.3%) [15,17,20,23,31,37,40–42,49], Random Forest (9 analyses, 19.1%) [11,14,17,22,27,29,46,51,53], Logistic Regression (8 analyses, 17.0%) [11,17,27,29,32,47,51,53], Decision Tree (6 analyses, 12.8%) [11,13,29,33,48,51], Gradient Boosting Decision Tree [29,46,51,53], Multi-Layer Perceptron [25,29,33,47], and (Gaussian) Naïve Bayes [22,29,32,51] (4 analyses each; 8.5%), and AdaBoost [22,46,51], and Linear Discriminant Analysis [10,47,51] with 3 analyses each (6.4%).

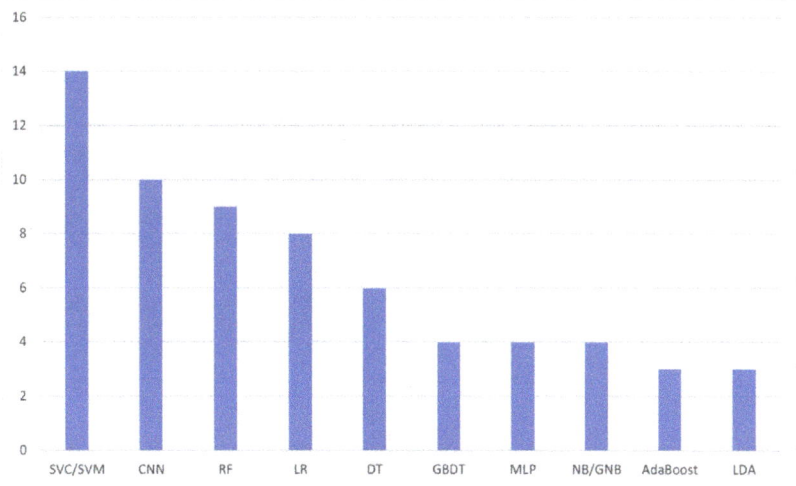

Figure 6. The most frequently appearing artificial intelligence algorithms within the included studies. SVC: Supporting Vector Classification; SVM: Supporting Vector Machine; CNN: Convolutional Neural Network; RF: Random Forest; LR: Logistic Regression; DT: Decision Tree; GBDT: Gradient Boosting Decision Tree; MLP: Multi-Layer Perceptron; NB/GNB: (Gaussian) Naïve Bayes; LDA: Linear Discriminant Analysis.

We then proceeded with the potential of quantitative assessment of the included studies. Again, we utilized the seminal study of Luo et al. [9] and evaluated the included studies for reporting their training sets, testing sets, cross-validation method and external validation sets. As surrogate metrics of performance for the studied AI algorithms, we considered Accuracy, F1-score, AUROC (95% CI) and AUPRC (95% CI). Only 33 studies out of the included 44 (75%) reported clearly on their training set [10,12,14–17,19,21–23,25–

34,37,39,41–47,49–51,53], 19 mentioned a cross-validation method (43.2%) [10,14,15,17,21,22, 25,27–29,32–34,37,39,45,47,49,51], 36 reported their test set (81.8%) [10,11,13,15,17–23,25,27– 29,31,33,34,36–53], and only 4 had an external validation set (9.1%) [22,28,42,53]. Thirty-five studies (79.5%) reported at least 1 performance metric in at least 1 dataset (training or test). However, this feature was very heterogenous and non-consistent and we decided not to proceed with further analysis (Supplemental Table S1). Regarding training sets, the highest reported Accuracy value was 1.000 (SVM, MLP) [21,33] and the lowest was 0.540 (noisy threshold classifier) [32], the highest reported F1-score was 0.876 (SVC) [29] and the lowest was 0.578 (FCRNA) [43], and the highest reported AUROC was 1.000 (algorithm not specified) [44], while the lowest one was 0.570 (CNN) [17]. With respect to test sets, the highest reported Accuracy value was 1.000 (SVM) [21] and the lowest was 0.310 (CNN) [23], the highest reported F1-score was 0.989 (Decision Tree, Random Forest) [51] and the lowest was 0.578 (FCRNA) [43], and the highest reported AUROC was 1.000 (SVM) [35], whilst the lowest one was 0.462 (Generative Adversarial Domain Adaptation) [45]. Table 2 summarizes the prediction characteristics, the source of data, the implemented AI algorithm(s), and the datasets for each of study included in our scoping review.

4. Discussion

This scoping review deals with the current applications of artificial intelligence in the diagnosis and management of gastrointestinal and pancreatic neuroendocrine neoplasms (GEP-NENs). GEP-NENs are inherently rare neoplasms, as such an empirical approach to their management would be unreliable. One of the advantages of AI and its application through machine learning and deep learning is that it can integrate a vast amount of data collected anywhere in the world (big data) and then render them applicable into clinical practice in an individualized manner.

Despite the rarity of NENs, our research yielded a total of 44 relevant studies, the vast majority of which have been published over the last three years. On the one hand, this harmonizes with the general tendency of incremental accumulation of pertinent evidence in Medicine [54,56], on the other hand it may reflect an increasing diagnosis rate of NENs, as it has been documented by the SEER registry [2]. In any case, this establishment may pave the way for future research.

Nevertheless, available studies have several limitations. First, a major restriction are the small datasets of the majority of the studies. There were only 3 among them which used data from large databases with populations of 13,830 [48], 10,580 [22] and 9,663,315 [27] patients, whereas the rest of the studies had populations of 50–361 individuals. Another serious point is that most of the studies did not provide clear information on the structure of the prediction problem (i.e., study design, prognostic vs. diagnostic, classification vs. regression), as such these pieces of information were derived after strenuous digest through the text. Most importantly, there is a non-negligible number of studies with poorly defined training and test sets. Another area of confusion is the lack of universal nomenclature regarding the discrete data sets (i.e., training, validation and test). Some studies use the terms "test set" and "validation set" interchangeably, whereas others are structured based on all three datasets. Future studies should also present their findings on AI algorithm performance in a robust way, including accuracy, F1-score, AUROC and AUPRC, because each one measures different performance aspects and may be a better predictor than the other ones under certain circumstances [57]. Also, such quantification will pave the way for meta-analyses. Furthermore, the ultimate goal of AI is the implementation of the findings of relevant studies into clinical practice. This can be achieved only if the performance of AI algorithms is benchmarked against established tests. Given the small number of studies with an external validation dataset, there is plenty of room for improvement in the field. As mentioned earlier, future endeavors in the field should follow a universal structure as per the existing guidelines, for purposes of both reproducibility and quality [9,58].

As one proceeds from the structure to the content of relevant studies, as we documented, the most popular topics are tumor type identification and grade, tumor detection, 5-year survival, cell segmentation, disease progression, disease recurrence and Ki-67 scoring. In a recent review, Yang et al. showed similar applications of AI with satisfactory prediction accuracy in the diagnosis, risk stratification and prognosis of small intestinal tumors [59]. Interestingly, this review shares 3 studies with the review in hand [14,21,33], which is not surprising given the rarity of small intestinal tumors and the major share of NENs among them. Kim et al. performed a similar analysis of the usefulness of AI in gastric neoplasms [60].

The combination of radiomics, i.e., the multitude of features and technical parameters that can be extracted from imaging studies, with the capability of big data processing offered by AI has opened new frontiers and has led to an exponential burst of pertinent literature. The fundamentals of the process of transforming an imaging study into data that can be processed by an AI algorithm are image acquisition, segmentation (i.e., selection of a region of interest in two dimensions), preprocessing (which allows data homogenization), data extraction, data selection and modelization. Given the routine performance of a constellation of imaging studies in clinical practice, this concept could contribute to the prompt diagnosis of NENs even at a preclinical stage. Promising evidence from imaging of pancreatic tumors with CT and MRI shows that this technology could find more widespread application in the field of NENs [61]. Partouche et al. performed a systematic review and meta-analysis of 161 studies on AI and imaging for Pan-NETs [62]. In accordance with our review, they documented wide heterogeneity of practices, poor procedural compliance with international guidelines, and poor reporting of clinical protocols. They reach the conclusion that standardization and homogenization is the key to future research if AI has the aspiration to enter clinical practice as a standard of care. In an another recent review on the role of radiomics in Pan-NETs, Bezzi et al. also acknowledge the need for further validations before widespread clinical adoption, nevertheless this discipline has great potential in decision-making regarding diagnosis and management [63].

In a process similar to data extraction from imaging studies, histology images can be utilized for processing with the aid of AI algorithms, following a pipeline from whole slide images (WSIs), segmentation into tiles, biomarker visualization and classification. Kuntz et al. recently published a review of 16 studies that used CNN in order to analyze gastrointestinal cancer histology images and showed good performance metrics with external validation, but none of them had clinical implementation for the time being [64].

The main limitation of the review in hand is the heterogeneity of the included studies, on grounds of methodology, dataset allocation and performance benchmarking, which did not allow for a meta-analysis. Structured publications are consequently mandatory in order to facilitate reproducible evidence of high quality. Another predicament for our study is set by the heterogeneity of NENs itself, which may raise methodological limitations. Nevertheless, given the probing nature of our research, an inclusive search strategy was inevitable. Future reviews could focus on specific histologic neuroendocrine types or disease stages.

5. Conclusions

To our knowledge, this is the first attempt to systematize existing evidence on the applications of AI in the field of NENs. Published studies focus mostly on diagnosis (tumor detection, tumor identification and tumor grading) rather than management and decision-making, mainly with the use of imaging studies and histology samples. Future directions should take into serious consideration the reporting and quality prerequisites set by already existing guidelines.

Supplementary Materials: The following supporting information can be downloaded at: https://www.mdpi.com/article/10.3390/diagnostics12040874/s1, Table S1: Raw data.

Author Contributions: Conceptualization, A.G.P. and P.A.P.; methodology, A.G.P.; validation, A.G.P., P.A.P. and D.P.L.; formal analysis, A.G.P.; investigation, A.G.P.; resources, A.G.P.; data curation, A.G.P.; writing—original draft preparation, A.G.P.; writing—review and editing, P.A.P.; visualization, A.G.P.; supervision, D.P.L.; project administration, A.G.P. All authors have read and agreed to the published version of the manuscript.

Funding: This research received no external funding.

Institutional Review Board Statement: Not applicable.

Informed Consent Statement: Not applicable.

Data Availability Statement: Not applicable.

Conflicts of Interest: The authors declare no conflict of interest.

References

1. Bonds, M.; Rocha, F.G. Neuroendocrine Tumors of the Pancreatobiliary and Gastrointestinal Tracts. *Surg. Clin.* **2020**, *100*, 635–648. [CrossRef] [PubMed]
2. Clift, A.K.; Kidd, M.; Bodei, L.; Toumpanakis, C.; Baum, R.P.; Oberg, K.; Modlin, I.M.; Frilling, A. Neuroendocrine Neoplasms of the Small Bowel and Pancreas. *Neuroendocrinology* **2020**, *110*, 444–476. [CrossRef] [PubMed]
3. Pavel, M.; Öberg, K.; Falconi, M.; Krenning, E.P.; Sundin, A.; Perren, A.; Berruti, A. Gastroenteropancreatic neuroendocrine neoplasms: ESMO Clinical Practice Guidelines for diagnosis, treatment and follow-up. *Ann. Oncol.* **2020**, *31*, 844–860. [CrossRef]
4. Modlin, I.M.; Kidd, M.; Latich, I.; Zikusoka, M.N.; Shapiro, M.D. Current Status of Gastrointestinal Carcinoids. *Gastroenterology* **2005**, *128*, 1717–1751. [CrossRef] [PubMed]
5. IARC Publications Website—Digestive System Tumours. Available online: https://publications.iarc.fr/579 (accessed on 26 February 2022).
6. Loftus, T.J.; Tighe, P.J.; Filiberto, A.C.; Efron, P.A.; Brakenridge, S.C.; Mohr, A.M.; Rashidi, P.; Upchurch, G.R., Jr.; Bihorac, A. Artificial Intelligence and Surgical Decision-Making. *JAMA Surg.* **2020**, *155*, 148–158. Available online: https://jamanetwork.com/journals/jamasurgery/fullarticle/2756311 (accessed on 18 December 2019). [CrossRef] [PubMed]
7. Yu, K.H.; Beam, A.L.; Kohane, I.S. Artificial intelligence in healthcare. *Nat. Biomed. Eng.* **2018**, *2*, 719–731. [CrossRef]
8. Tricco, A.C.; Lillie, E.; Zarin, W.; O'Brien, K.K.; Colquhoun, H.; Levac, D.; Moher, D.; Peters, M.D.J.; Horsley, T.; Weeks, L.; et al. PRISMA extension for scoping reviews (PRISMA-ScR): Checklist and explanation. *Ann. Intern. Med.* **2018**, *169*, 467–473. [CrossRef]
9. Luo, W.; Phung, Q.-D.; Tran, T.; Gupta, S.; Rana, S.; Karmakar, C.; Shilton, A.; Yearwood, J.L.; Dimitrova, N.; Ho, T.B.; et al. Guidelines for Developing and Reporting Machine Learning Predictive Models in Biomedical Research: A Multidisciplinary View. *J. Med. Internet Res.* **2016**, *18*, e323. [CrossRef]
10. Bevilacqua, A.; Calabrò, D.; Malavasi, S.; Ricci, C.; Casadei, R.; Campana, D.; Baiocco, S.; Fanti, S.; Ambrosini, V. A [68Ga] Ga-DOTANOC PET/CT Radiomic Model for Non-Invasive Prediction of Tumour Grade in Pancreatic Neuroendocrine Tumours. *Diagnostics* **2021**, *11*, 870. [CrossRef]
11. Chen, K.; Zhang, W.; Zhang, Z.; He, Y.; Liu, Y.; Yang, X. Simple Vascular Architecture Classification in Predicting Pancreatic Neuroendocrine Tumor Grade and Prognosis. *Am. J. Dig. Dis.* **2018**, *63*, 3147–3152. [CrossRef]
12. Ito, H.; Uragami, N.; Miyazaki, T.; Yang, W.; Issha, K.; Matsuo, K.; Kimura, S.; Arai, Y.; Tokunaga, H.; Okada, S.; et al. Highly accurate colorectal cancer prediction model based on Raman spectroscopy using patient serum. *World J. Gastrointest. Oncol.* **2020**, *12*, 1311–1324. [CrossRef] [PubMed]
13. Kidd, M.; Kitz, A.; Drozdov, I.A.; Modlin, I.M. Neuroendocrine Tumor Omic Gene Cluster Analysis Amplifies the Prognostic Accuracy of the NETest. *Neuroendocrinology* **2021**, *111*, 490–504. [CrossRef] [PubMed]
14. Kjellman, M.; Knigge, U.; Welin, S.; Thiis-Evensen, E.; Gronbaek, H.; Schalin-Jäntti, C.; Sorbye, H.; Joergensen, M.T.; Johanson, V.; Metso, S.; et al. A Plasma Protein Biomarker Strategy for Detection of Small Intestinal Neuroendocrine Tumors. *Neuroendocrinology* **2021**, *111*, 840–849. [CrossRef] [PubMed]
15. Klimov, S.; Xue, Y.; Gertych, A.; Graham, R.P.; Jiang, Y.; Bhattarai, S.; Pandol, S.J.; Rakha, E.A.; Reid, M.D.; Aneja, R. Predicting Metastasis Risk in Pancreatic Neuroendocrine Tumors Using Deep Learning Image Analysis. *Front. Oncol.* **2021**, *10*, 593211. [CrossRef]
16. Liu, Y.; Sadowski, S.M.; Weisbrod, A.B.; Kebebew, E.; Summers, R.M.; Yao, J. Patient specific tumor growth prediction using multimodal images. *Med. Image Anal.* **2014**, *18*, 555–566. [CrossRef]
17. Luo, Y.; Chen, X.; Chen, J.; Song, C.; Shen, J.; Xiao, H.; Chen, M.; Li, Z.-P.; Huang, B.; Feng, S.-T. Preoperative Prediction of Pancreatic Neuroendocrine Neoplasms Grading Based on Enhanced Computed Tomography Imaging: Validation of Deep Learning with a Convolutional Neural Network. *Neuroendocrinology* **2020**, *110*, 338–350. [CrossRef]
18. Nanayakkara, J.; Tyryshkin, K.; Yang, X.; Wong, J.J.M.; Vanderbeck, K.; Ginter, P.S.; Scognamiglio, T.; Chen, Y.-T.; Panarelli, N.; Cheung, N.-K.; et al. Characterizing and classifying neuroendocrine neoplasms through microRNA sequencing and data mining. *NAR Cancer* **2020**, *2*, zcaa009. [CrossRef]

19. Nguyen, V.X.; Nguyen, C.C.; Li, B.; Das, A. Digital image analysis is a useful adjunct to endoscopic ultrasonographic diagnosis of subepithelial lesions of the gastrointestinal tract. *J. Ultrasound Med.* **2010**, *29*, 1345–1351. [CrossRef]
20. Niazi, M.K.K.; Tavolara, T.E.; Arole, V.; Hartman, U.J.; Pantanowitz, L.; Gurcan, M.N. Identifying tumor in pancreatic neuroendocrine neoplasms from Ki67 images using transfer learning. *PLoS ONE* **2018**, *13*, e0195621. [CrossRef]
21. Panarelli, N.; Tyryshkin, K.; Wong, J.; Majewski, A.; Yang, X.; Scognamiglio, T.; Kim, M.K.; Bogardus, K.; Tuschl, T.; Chen, Y.-T.; et al. Evaluating gastroenteropancreatic neuroendocrine tumors through microRNA sequencing. *Endocr. Relat. Cancer* **2019**, *26*, 47–57. [CrossRef]
22. Cheng, X.; Li, J.; Xu, T.; Li, K.; Li, J. Predicting Survival of Patients With Rectal Neuroendocrine Tumors Using Machine Learning: A SEER-Based Population Study. *Front. Surg.* **2021**, *8*, 745220. [CrossRef] [PubMed]
23. Hanson, J.A.; Redemann, J.; Schultz, F.A.; Martinez, C.; Harrell, M.; Clark, D.P.; Martin, D.R. Comparing deep learning and immunohistochemistry in determining the site of origin for well-differentiated neuroendocrine tumors. *J. Pathol. Inform.* **2020**, *11*, 32. [CrossRef] [PubMed]
24. Saccomandi, P.; Larocca, E.S.; Rendina, V.; Schena, E.; D'Ambrosio, R.; Crescenzi, A.; Di Matteo, F.M.; Silvestri, S. Estimation of optical properties of neuroendocrine pancreas tumor with double-integrating-sphere system and inverse Monte Carlo model. *Lasers Med. Sci.* **2016**, *31*, 1041–1050. [CrossRef] [PubMed]
25. Săftoiu, A.; Vilmann, P.; Gorunescu, F.; Gheonea, D.I.; Gorunescu, M.; Ciurea, T.; Popescu, G.L.; Iordache, A.; Hassan, H.; Iordache, S. Neural network analysis of dynamic sequences of EUS elastography used for the differential diagnosis of chronic pancreatitis and pancreatic cancer. *Gastrointest. Endosc.* **2008**, *68*, 1086–1094. [CrossRef] [PubMed]
26. Soldevilla, B.; López-López, A.; Lens-Pardo, A.; Carretero-Puche, C.; Lopez-Gonzalvez, A.; La Salvia, A.; Gil-Calderon, B.; Riesco-Martinez, M.; Espinosa-Olarte, P.; Sarmentero, J.; et al. Comprehensive Plasma Metabolomic Profile of Patients with Advanced Neuroendocrine Tumors (NETs). Diagnostic and Biological Relevance. *Cancers* **2021**, *13*, 2634. [CrossRef]
27. Song, Y.; Gao, S.; Tan, W.; Qiu, Z.; Zhou, H.; Zhao, Y. Multiple Machine Learnings Revealed Similar Predictive Accuracy for Prognosis of PNETs from the Surveillance, Epidemiology, and End Result Database. *J. Cancer* **2018**, *9*, 3971–3978. [CrossRef]
28. Song, C.; Wang, M.; Luo, Y.; Chen, J.; Peng, Z.; Wang, Y.; Zhang, H.; Li, Z.-P.; Shen, J.; Huang, B.; et al. Predicting the recurrence risk of pancreatic neuroendocrine neoplasms after radical resection using deep learning radiomics with preoperative computed tomography images. *Ann. Transl. Med.* **2021**, *9*, 833. [CrossRef]
29. Telalovic, J.H.; Pillozzi, S.; Fabbri, R.; Laffi, A.; Lavacchi, D.; Rossi, V.; Dreoni, L.; Spada, F.; Fazio, N.; Amedei, A.; et al. A Machine Learning Decision Support System (DSS) for Neuroendocrine Tumor Patients Treated with Somatostatin Analog (SSA) Therapy. *Diagnostics* **2021**, *11*, 804. [CrossRef]
30. Tirosh, A.; Mukherjee, S.; Lack, J.; Gara, S.K.; Wang, S.; Quezado, M.M.; Keutgen, X.M.; Wu, X.; Cam, M.; Kumar, S.; et al. Distinct genome-wide methylation patterns in sporadic and hereditary nonfunctioning pancreatic neuroendocrine tumors. *Cancer* **2019**, *125*, 1247–1257. [CrossRef]
31. Udriștoiu, A.L.; Cazacu, I.M.; Gruionu, L.G.; Gruionu, G.; Iacob, A.V.; Burtea, D.E.; Ungureanu, B.S.; Costache, M.I.; Constantin, A.; Popescu, C.F.; et al. Real-time computer-aided diagnosis of focal pancreatic masses from endoscopic ultrasound imaging based on a hybrid convolutional and long short-term memory neural network model. *PLoS ONE* **2021**, *16*, e0251701. [CrossRef]
32. van Gerven, M.A.; Jurgelenaite, R.; Taal, B.G.; Heskes, T.; Lucas, P.J. Predicting carcinoid heart disease with the noisy-threshold classifier. *Artif. Intell. Med.* **2007**, *40*, 45–55. [CrossRef] [PubMed]
33. Drozdov, I.; Kidd, M.; Nadler, B.; Camp, R.L.; Mane, S.M.; Hauso, O.; Gustafsson, B.I.; Modlin, I.M. Predicting neuroendocrine tumor (carcinoid) neoplasia using gene expression profiling and supervised machine learning. *Cancer* **2009**, *115*, 1638–1650. [CrossRef] [PubMed]
34. Wan, Y.; Yang, P.; Xu, L.; Yang, J.; Luo, C.; Wang, J.; Chen, F.; Wu, Y.; Lu, Y.; Ruan, D.; et al. Radiomics analysis combining unsupervised learning and handcrafted features: A multiple-disease study. *Med. Phys.* **2021**, *48*, 7003–7015. [CrossRef] [PubMed]
35. Wang, Q.; Yu, C. Expression profiling of small intestinal neuroendocrine tumors identified pathways and gene networks linked to tumorigenesis and metastasis. *Biosci. Rep.* **2020**, *40*, BSR20193860. [CrossRef] [PubMed]
36. Wang, Q.; Li, F.; Jiang, Q.; Sun, Y.; Liao, Q.; An, H.; Li, Y.; Li, Z.; Fan, L.; Guo, F.; et al. Gene Expression Profiling for Differential Diagnosis of Liver Metastases: A Multicenter, Retrospective Cohort Study. *Front. Oncol.* **2021**, *11*, 725988. [CrossRef] [PubMed]
37. Wehrend, J.; Silosky, M.; Xing, F.; Chin, B.B. Automated liver lesion detection in 68Ga DOTATATE PET/CT using a deep fully convolutional neural network. *EJNMMI Res.* **2021**, *11*, 98. [CrossRef]
38. Xing, F.; Su, H.; Yang, L. An Integrated Framework for Automatic Ki-67 Scoring in Pancreatic Neuroendocrine Tumor. *Med. Image Comput. Comput. Assist. Interv.* **2013**, *16*, 436–443. [CrossRef]
39. Xing, F.; Su, H.; Neltner, J.; Yang, L. Automatic Ki-67 Counting Using Robust Cell Detection and Online Dictionary Learning. *IEEE Trans. Biomed. Eng.* **2014**, *61*, 859–870. [CrossRef]
40. Xing, F.; Yang, L. Fast Cell Segmentation Using Scalable Sparse Manifold Learning and Affine Transform-Approximated Active Contour. *Med. Image Comput. Comput. Assist. Interv.* **2015**, *9351*, 332–339. [CrossRef]
41. Xing, F.; Shi, X.; Zhang, Z.; Cai, J.; Xie, Y.; Yang, L. Transfer Shape Modeling Towards High-Throughput Microscopy Image Segmentation. *Med. Image Comput. Comput. Assist. Interv.* **2016**, *9902*, 183–190. [CrossRef]
42. Xing, F.; Xie, Y.; Yang, L. An Automatic Learning-Based Framework for Robust Nucleus Segmentation. *IEEE Trans. Med. Imaging* **2016**, *35*, 550–566. [CrossRef] [PubMed]

43. Xing, F.; Cornish, T.C.; Bennett, T.; Ghosh, D.; Yang, L. Pixel-to-Pixel Learning With Weak Supervision for Single-Stage Nucleus Recognition in Ki67 Images. *IEEE Trans. Biomed. Eng.* **2019**, *66*, 3088–3097. [CrossRef] [PubMed]
44. Fehrenbach, U.; Xin, S.; Hartenstein, A.; Auer, T.; Dräger, F.; Froböse, K.; Jann, H.; Mogl, M.; Amthauer, H.; Geisel, D.; et al. Automatized Hepatic Tumor Volume Analysis of Neuroendocrine Liver Metastases by Gd-EOB MRI—A Deep-Learning Model to Support Multidisciplinary Cancer Conference Decision-Making. *Cancers* **2021**, *13*, 2726. [CrossRef] [PubMed]
45. Zhang, X.; Cornish, T.C.; Yang, L.; Bennett, T.D.; Ghosh, D.; Xing, F. Generative Adversarial Domain Adaptation for Nucleus Quantification in Images of Tissue Immunohistochemically Stained for Ki-67. *JCO Clin. Cancer Inform.* **2020**, *4*, 666–679. [CrossRef] [PubMed]
46. Zhang, T.; Zhang, Y.; Liu, X.; Xu, H.; Chen, C.; Zhou, X.; Liu, Y.; Ma, X. Application of Radiomics Analysis Based on CT Combined With Machine Learning in Diagnostic of Pancreatic Neuroendocrine Tumors Patient's Pathological Grades. *Front. Oncol.* **2021**, *10*, 521831. [CrossRef]
47. Zhou, R.-Q.; Ji, H.-C.; Liu, Q.; Zhu, C.-Y.; Liu, R. Leveraging machine learning techniques for predicting pancreatic neuroendocrine tumor grades using biochemical and tumor markers. *World J. Clin. Cases* **2019**, *7*, 1611–1622. [CrossRef]
48. Zimmerman, N.M.; Ray, D.; Princic, N.; Moynihan, M.; Clarke, C.; Phan, A. Exploration of machine learning techniques to examine the journey to neuroendocrine tumor diagnosis with real-world data. *Futur. Oncol.* **2021**, *17*, 3217–3230. [CrossRef]
49. Gao, X.; Wang, X. Deep learning for World Health Organization grades of pancreatic neuroendocrine tumors on contrast-enhanced magnetic resonance images: A preliminary study. *Int. J. Comput. Assist. Radiol. Surg.* **2019**, *14*, 1981–1991. [CrossRef]
50. Govind, D.; Jen, K.-Y.; Matsukuma, K.; Gao, G.; Olson, K.A.; Gui, D.; Wilding, G.E.; Border, S.P.; Sarder, P. Improving the accuracy of gastrointestinal neuroendocrine tumor grading with deep learning. *Sci. Rep.* **2020**, *10*, 11064. [CrossRef]
51. Han, X.; Yang, J.; Luo, J.; Chen, P.; Zhang, Z.; Alu, A.; Xiao, Y.; Ma, X. Application of CT-Based Radiomics in Discriminating Pancreatic Cystadenomas From Pancreatic Neuroendocrine Tumors Using Machine Learning Methods. *Front. Oncol.* **2021**, *11*, 606677. [CrossRef]
52. Huang, B.; Tian, J.; Zhang, H.; Luo, Z.; Qin, J.; Huang, C.; He, X.; Luo, Y.; Zhou, Y.; Dan, G.; et al. Deep Semantic Segmentation Feature-Based Radiomics for the Classification Tasks in Medical Image Analysis. *IEEE J. Biomed. Health Inform.* **2021**, *25*, 2655–2664. [CrossRef] [PubMed]
53. Huang, B.; Lin, X.; Shen, J.; Chen, X.; Chen, J.; Li, Z.-P.; Wang, M.; Yuan, C.; Diao, X.-F.; Luo, Y.; et al. Accurate and Feasible Deep Learning Based Semi-Automatic Segmentation in CT for Radiomics Analysis in Pancreatic Neuroendocrine Neoplasms. *IEEE J. Biomed. Health Inform.* **2021**, *25*, 3498–3506. [CrossRef] [PubMed]
54. Kulkarni, S.; Seneviratne, N.; Baig, M.S.; Khan, A.H.A. Artificial Intelligence in Medicine: Where Are We Now? *Acad. Radiol.* **2020**, *27*, 62–70. [CrossRef] [PubMed]
55. Collins, G.S.; Reitsma, J.B.; Altman, D.G.; Moons, K.G.M. Transparent reporting of a multivariable prediction model for individual prognosis or diagnosis (TRIPOD): The TRIPOD statement. *Eur. J. Clin. Investig.* **2015**, *45*, 204–214. [CrossRef]
56. Schaefer, J.; Lehne, M.; Schepers, J.; Prasser, F.; Thun, S. The use of machine learning in rare diseases: A scoping review. *Orphanet J. Rare Dis.* **2020**, *15*, 145. [CrossRef]
57. F1 Score vs ROC AUC vs Accuracy vs PR AUC: Which Evaluation Metric Should You Choose?—Neptune.ai. Available online: https://neptune.ai/blog/f1-score-accuracy-roc-auc-pr-auc (accessed on 27 February 2022).
58. de Hond, A.A.H.; Leeuwenberg, A.M.; Hooft, L.; Kant, I.M.J.; Nijman, S.W.J.; van Os, H.J.A.; Aardoom, J.J.; Debray, T.P.A.; Schuit, E.; van Smeden, M.; et al. Guidelines and quality criteria for artificial intelligence-based prediction models in healthcare: A scoping review. *Npj Digit. Med.* **2022**, *5*, 2. [CrossRef]
59. Yang, Y.; Li, Y.-X.; Yao, R.-Q.; Du, X.-H.; Ren, C. Artificial intelligence in small intestinal diseases: Application and prospects. *World J. Gastroenterol.* **2021**, *27*, 3734–3747. [CrossRef]
60. Kim, J.H.; Nam, S.-J.; Park, S.C. Usefulness of artificial intelligence in gastric neoplasms. *World J. Gastroenterol.* **2021**, *27*, 3543–3555. [CrossRef]
61. Bartoli, M.; Barat, M.; Dohan, A.; Gaujoux, S.; Coriat, R.; Hoeffel, C.; Cassinotto, C.; Chassagnon, G.; Soyer, P. INVITED REVIEW CT and MRI of pancreatic tumors: An update in the era of radiomics. *Jpn. J. Radiol.* **2020**, *38*, 1111–1124. [CrossRef]
62. Partouche, E.; Yeh, R.; Eche, T.; Rozenblum, L.; Carrere, N.; Guimbaud, R.; Dierickx, L.O.; Rousseau, H.; Dercle, L.; Mokrane, F.-Z. Updated Trends in Imaging Practices for Pancreatic Neuroendocrine Tumors (PNETs): A Systematic Review and Meta-Analysis to Pave the Way for Standardization in the New Era of Big Data and Artificial Intelligence. *Front. Oncol.* **2021**, *11*, 628408. [CrossRef]
63. Bezzi, C.; Mapelli, P.; Presotto, L.; Neri, I.; Scifo, P.; Savi, A.; Bettinardi, V.; Partelli, S.; Gianolli, L.; Falconi, M.; et al. Radiomics in pancreatic neuroendocrine tumors: Methodological issues and clinical significance. *Eur. J. Pediatr.* **2021**, *48*, 4002–4015. [CrossRef] [PubMed]
64. Kuntz, S.; Krieghoff-Henning, E.; Kather, J.N.; Jutzi, T.; Höhn, J.; Kiehl, L.; Hekler, A.; Alwers, E.; von Kalle, C.; Fröhling, S.; et al. Gastrointestinal cancer classification and prognostication from histology using deep learning: Systematic review. *Eur. J. Cancer* **2021**, *155*, 200–215. [CrossRef] [PubMed]

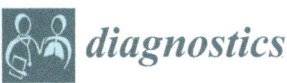

Article

Performance of Convolutional Neural Networks for Polyp Localization on Public Colonoscopy Image Datasets

Alba Nogueira-Rodríguez [1,2], Miguel Reboiro-Jato [1,2], Daniel Glez-Peña [1,2] and Hugo López-Fernández [1,2,*]

1. CINBIO, Department of Computer Science, ESEI-Escuela Superior de Ingeniería Informática, Universidade de Vigo, 32004 Ourense, Spain; alnogueira@uvigo.es (A.N.-R.); mrjato@uvigo.es (M.R.-J.); dgpena@uvigo.es (D.G.-P.)
2. SING Research Group, Galicia Sur Health Research Institute (IIS Galicia Sur), SERGAS-UVIGO, 36213 Vigo, Spain
* Correspondence: hlfernandez@uvigo.es; Tel.: +34-988387027

Abstract: Colorectal cancer is one of the most frequent malignancies. Colonoscopy is the de facto standard for precancerous lesion detection in the colon, i.e., polyps, during screening studies or after facultative recommendation. In recent years, artificial intelligence, and especially deep learning techniques such as convolutional neural networks, have been applied to polyp detection and localization in order to develop real-time CADe systems. However, the performance of machine learning models is very sensitive to changes in the nature of the testing instances, especially when trying to reproduce results for totally different datasets to those used for model development, i.e., inter-dataset testing. Here, we report the results of testing of our previously published polyp detection model using ten public colonoscopy image datasets and analyze them in the context of the results of other 20 state-of-the-art publications using the same datasets. The F1-score of our recently published model was 0.88 when evaluated on a private test partition, i.e., intra-dataset testing, but it decayed, on average, by 13.65% when tested on ten public datasets. In the published research, the average intra-dataset F1-score is 0.91, and we observed that it also decays in the inter-dataset setting to an average F1-score of 0.83.

Keywords: colorectal cancer; deep learning; convolutional neural network (CNN); polyp detection; polyp localization

Citation: Nogueira-Rodríguez, A.; Reboiro-Jato, M.; Glez-Peña, D.; López-Fernández, H. Performance of Convolutional Neural Networks for Polyp Localization on Public Colonoscopy Image Datasets. *Diagnostics* 2022, 12, 898. https://doi.org/10.3390/diagnostics12040898

Academic Editors: Eun-Sun Kim and Kwang-Sig Lee

Received: 23 February 2022
Accepted: 1 April 2022
Published: 4 April 2022

Publisher's Note: MDPI stays neutral with regard to jurisdictional claims in published maps and institutional affiliations.

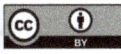

Copyright: © 2022 by the authors. Licensee MDPI, Basel, Switzerland. This article is an open access article distributed under the terms and conditions of the Creative Commons Attribution (CC BY) license (https://creativecommons.org/licenses/by/4.0/).

1. Introduction

In the last few years, significant research has been published on the application of deep learning (DL) for colorectal polyp detection and characterization in colonoscopy images, as demonstrated by the growing number of reviews on the topic [1–4]. Polyp detection is way more advanced than characterization, and several randomized control trials (RCT) have already been conducted [5–10], some of which are associated with the development of commercial systems [3].

This difference is also reflected in the availability of public colonoscopy image datasets. In the case of polyp detection, one of the most relevant events in this field was the celebration of the MICCAI 2015 conference [11], since it hosted a sub-challenge on automatic polyp detection for which the first and most well-known public colonoscopy datasets were published. These are the CVC-ClinicDB [12], ETIS-Larib [13], and ASU-Mayo Clinic Colonoscopy Video [14] datasets. Since then, several new datasets have been released, significantly increasing the number publicly available data. In addition, in the particular case of the CVC-ClinicDB dataset, its creators have extended it with three more public datasets: CVC-ColonDB [15,16], CVC-PolypHD [15,16], and CVC-ClinicVideoDB [17,18]. The growth in the volume of public data has seen a remarkable increase in recent years with the release of PICCOLO [19], Kvasir-SEG [20], LDPolypVideo [21], SUN [22], and

KUMC [23], each including several thousands of polyp images, with the latter three exceeding the total volume of images published so far. All these datasets include annotations of the polyp locations as either bounding boxes or binary masks and, therefore, are suitable for polyp localization. In contrast, there are only three public datasets suitable for polyp characterization. The first dataset was published by Mesejo et al. [24] in 2016 and, since then, only the PICCOLO [19] and KUMC [23] datasets have included the necessary annotations for this task.

In our previous review [1], we collected the most relevant studies applying DL for polyp detection and characterization in colonoscopy and analyzed them from a technical point of view, focusing on the low-level details for the implementation of the DL models. Together with the review, we created a GitHub repository (https://github.com/sing-group/deep-learning-colonoscopy (accessed on 22 February 2022)) containing the most relevant information, especially the performance metrics reported by each study and the test datasets used. Since then, we have been continuously updating the repository to add new works and datasets as they were published. As a result of carrying out the work presented here, we improved the repository by adding information about the train datasets used in each analysis and by detailing the type of evaluation carried out in polyp detection. It is important to note that we do not consider preprints for inclusion in the repository due to the high activity in the field and the fact that we are not able to track and curate all of them in an appropriate and sustainable way. Nevertheless, there are some recent preprints, such as the work of Ali et al., 2021, presenting the PolypGen [25] dataset, that will be included as soon they are published in a peer-reviewed journal.

Despite this, comparing the models developed in different works is not straightforward, since they use different ways of assessing their performance. Most of them use private datasets for model development and testing, hindering the reproducibility. Other works use only public datasets for both model development and testing. Finally, there are hybrid works where the performance of a model developed with a private dataset is evaluated on a public dataset.

In a recent work, we published a real-time polyp detection model based on a YOLOv3 [26] pretrained with PASCAL VOC datasets [27] that we fine-tuned using a private dataset (28,576 annotated images from 941 different polyps). This model achieved an F1-score of 0.88 (recall = 0.87, precision = 0.89) in a bounding-box-based evaluation using still images (a test partition of our private dataset).

Nevertheless, the performance of ML models is very sensitive to changes in the nature of the testing instances when compared to those instances used for developing them, especially when trying to reproduce results on completely different datasets to those used for model development (inter-dataset testing). Aiming at gaining insights for taking further steps for improving our model following a data-centric approach, in this work, we systematically evaluate the performance of our published model, without retrain, on ten public datasets. This is, to the best of our knowledge, the first time that such extensive evaluation has been carried out. In addition, we also include a comparison of published research on polyp localization, including the best performances reported by each study on public datasets. In this regard, there is interest in comparing intra-dataset performances (i.e., a performance evaluation on a test split of the dataset used for model development, either private or public) versus inter-dataset performances (i.e., a performance evaluation on a dataset different than the one used for model development).

2. Materials and Methods

2.1. Our Polyp Localization Network

In a previous work [26], we reported the results of training and evaluating a real-time automatic polyp detection system based on YOLOv3. For this purpose, in the context of the PolyDeep project (http://polydeep.org (accessed on 22 February 2022)), we created a private dataset containing 28,576 polyp images from 941 different polyps, out of which 21 046 were acquired under white light (WL) and 7530 under narrow-band imaging (NBI) light. The images were manually annotated by expert endoscopists to specify the polyp locations as bounding boxes. This image dataset is part of a larger collection of annotated polyp videos and images, named PIBAdb, which is already available through the IISGS BioBank (https://www.iisgaliciasur.es/home/biobanco/cohorte-pibadb (accessed on 22 February 2022)).

For model development, we set aside a test partition containing 30% of the polyps (283; 8658 images) to perform a bounding-box-based evaluation. The remaining 70% was, in turn, split into train (70%; 460 polyps; 13,873 images) and validation (30%; 198 polyps; 6045 images) partitions. It is important to note that this image dataset only includes polyp images with exactly one polyp.

The YOLOv3 model used as a basis was the Apache MxNet [28] implementation that the GluonCV toolkit [29] provides pre-trained with the PASCAL VOC 2007 and 2012 challenges' [27] train and validation datasets. This base model was fine-tuned using the train partition of our dataset, achieving an F1-score of 0.88 (recall = 0.87, precision = 0.89) and an average precision (AP) of 0.87 in a bounding-box-based evaluation using the test partition. The results are on par with other state-of-the-art models, and the model was able to process frames at a rate of 0.041 s/frame, thus being able to operate in real time.

This model was used, without retrain, to carry out the experiments described in Section 2.4 in order to evaluate its performance on different public datasets. Although the dataset used to develop the model does not include images with multiple polyps or images without polyps, given the nature of YOLOv3, the model is able to predict multiple polyps when necessary, as it will be shown.

2.2. Public Colonoscopy Image Datasets and Polyp Localization Studies Selection

Figure 1 shows the criteria for selecting public colonoscopy image datasets and polyp localization studies. This selection started with the 44 studies and 13 public datasets collected as of February 2022 in the GitHub repository associated with our review on DL for polyp detection and classification in colonoscopy, mentioned above.

Since one of our objectives is to draw a comparison of published research that reports performance metrics of public datasets, 17 studies were excluded in the first place because they only evaluated the models on private datasets. In addition, two datasets were also excluded for different reasons: (*i*) the CP-CHILD dataset [30] was also excluded since it only provides frames labeled as "polyp" and "non-polyp" and not a suitable ground truth including the polyp localizations; and (*ii*) the ASU-Mayo Clinic Colonoscopy Video dataset [14] was excluded since we were not able to access the dataset after repeated attempts to contact the authors without obtaining a response. Because of the exclusion of the ASU-Mayo Clinic Colonoscopy dataset, three studies that used it were also discarded.

From the remaining 23 studies, the following three were excluded: (*i*) the study by Misawa et al., 2021 [22] was excluded since they evaluate the detection performance instead of the localization performance, despite the fact they were using an object detection network architecture (YOLOv3); and (*ii*) the studies from Tashk et al., 2019 [31] and Sánchez-Peralta et al., 2020 [19] were excluded since they performed polyp segmentation and, therefore, provide pixel-based performance metrics, which are not comparable with the bounding-box-based performance metrics of the polyp localization studies. This latter cause of exclusion also motivated the discard of the CVC-EndoSceneStill dataset.

So, after applying the selection criteria seen in Figure 1, 20 studies and 10 public datasets were selected for evaluating the performance of our polyp localization model.

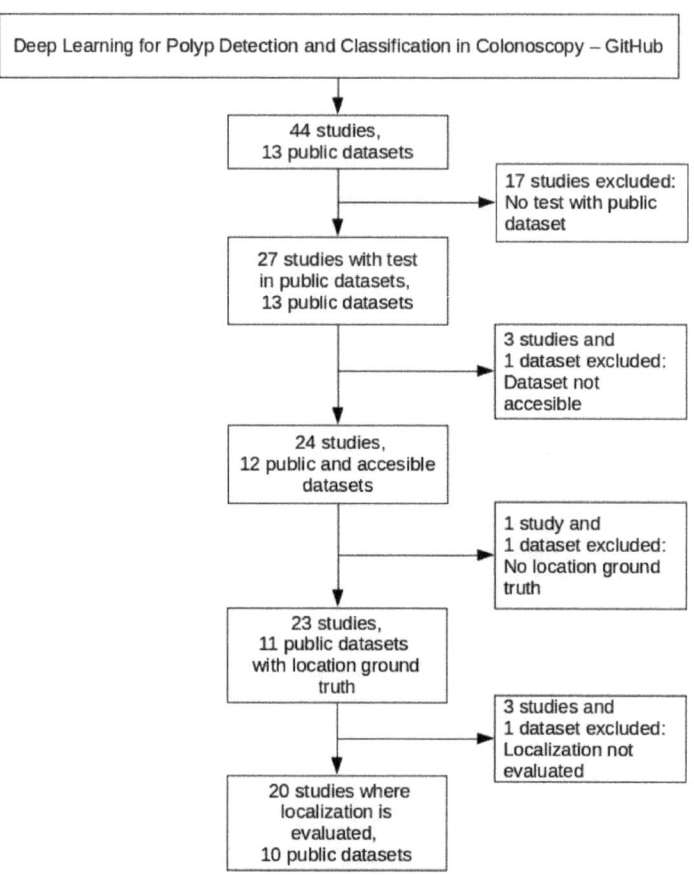

Figure 1. Criteria for selecting polyp localization studies and public colonoscopy image datasets.

2.3. Public Colonoscopy Image Datasets Description and Preprocessing

Table 1 shows the most relevant details of the ten public colonoscopy image datasets selected for the analysis. Regarding the type of ground truth provided, seven of them provide polyps annotated with binary masks, namely CVC-ClinicDB [12], CVC-ColonDB [15,16], CVC-PolypHD [15,16], ETIS-Larib [13], CVC-ClinicVideoDB [17,18], and PICCOLO [19]. In these cases, we converted the binary masks into bounding boxes to be able to analyze them with our model (the procedure is described below in this section). Three of them provide polyp locations as bounding boxes, namely the KUMC [23], SUN [22], and LDPolypVideo [21] datasets. Finally, Kvasir-SEG [20] provides both segmentation and localization information.

The public datasets show a lot of variability in terms of number of images, number of polyps, image resolution, capturing device, etc., as shown in Table 1. The trend in the most recent datasets is to include non-polyp images. In addition, as can be seen in Figure 2, which shows one random image of each dataset included, the variability in the appearance of the images themselves and the polyps contained in them is also high (e.g., Kvasir-SEG contains images with superimposed text and/or the presence of instruments, etc.).

As explained before, almost all datasets provide polyp locations as binary masks, and thus are suitable for object segmentation models. Since our model works with bounding boxes information, the binary masks were converted into this representation using the scikit-image Python library. Figure 3 shows an example of this conversion procedure, where it can be seen that the scikit-image functions allow obtaining the minimum bounding boxes that cover the original binary masks. In addition, the organization of the images and annotations in the datasets was also adapted to the PASCAL VOC dataset format that our evaluation pipeline uses as input. This adaptation process usually required three steps: (*i*) folder reorganization, in which all original and mask images are moved into two separate folders if necessary; (*ii*) format conversion, to covert the original images to the JPG format if necessary; and (*iii*) conversion to PASCAL VOC dataset format, in which the dataset is adapted to this format, including the transformation of binary masks into bounding boxes when needed.

Table 1. Descriptions of the ten public colonoscopy image datasets for polyp localization.

Dataset	Paper Publication Year	Description	Resolution	Ground Truth	Presence of Multiple Polyp Images	Presence of Non-Polyp Images
CVC-ClinicDB [12]	2015	612 sequential WL images with polyps extracted from 31 sequences (23 patients) with 31 different polyps	384 × 288	Binary mask to locate the polyp	yes	no
CVC-ColonDB [15,16]	2012	300 sequential WL images with polyps extracted from 13 sequences (13 patients)	574 × 500	Binary mask to locate the polyp	no	no
CVC-PolypHD [15,16]	2018	56 WL images	1920 × 1080	Binary mask to locate the polyp	yes	no
ETIS-Larib [13]	2014	196 WL images with polyps extracted from 34 sequences with 44 different polyps	1225 × 966	Binary mask to locate the polyp	yes	no
Kvasir-SEG [20]	2020	1000 polyp images	332 × 487 1920 × 1072	Binary mask and bounding box to locate the polyp	yes	no
CVC-ClinicVideoDB [17,18]	2017	11,954 images in total with 10,025 images of polyps	384 × 288	Binary mask to locate the polyp	no	yes
PICCOLO [19]	2020	3433 images (2131 WL and 1302 NBI) from 76 lesions from 40 patients	854 × 480 1920 × 1080	Binary mask to locate the polyp	yes	yes
KUMC dataset [23]	2021	37,899 images in total, including the CVC-ColonDB, ASU-Mayo Clinic Colonoscopy Video, and Colonoscopic Dataset datasets	Various resolutions	Bounding box to locate the polyp	no	yes
SUN [22]	2021	49,136 images with polyps. The polyp samples of 100 cases	1240 × 1080	Bounding box to locate the polyp	no	no *
LDPolypVideo [21]	2021	160 videos (40,187 frames: 33,876 polyp images and 6311 non-polyp images) with 200 labeled polyps.	560 × 480	Bounding box to locate the polyp	yes	yes

* The SUN dataset contains 109,554 non-polyp frames that were not downloaded for our experiments.

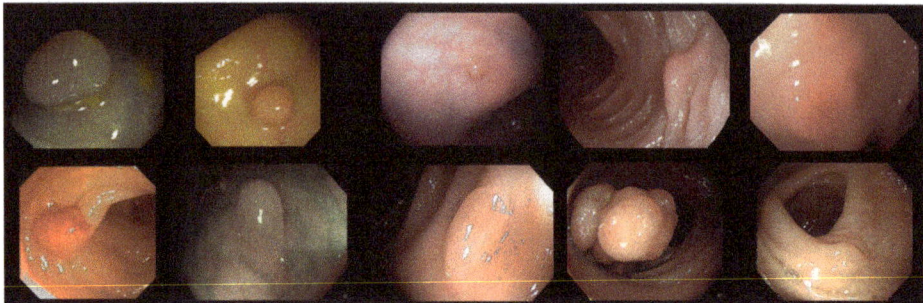

Figure 2. Examples of polyp images from the included datasets. Upper row (left to right): CVC-ClinicDB, CVC-ColonDB, CVC-PolypHD, ETIS-Larib, and Kvasir-SEG. Bottom row (left to right): CVC-ClinicVideoDB, PICCOLO, KUMC, SUN, and LDPolypVideo.

The scripts to make such conversions were published in the following GitHub repository: https://github.com/sing-group/public-datasets-to-voc (accessed on 22 February 2022). The specific process of converting each of the datasets to this common format is discussed below. In Supplementary Table S1, we summarize the most relevant information regarding the datasets structure (number and image formats, scripts used to process them, etc.). This table also shows the number of bounding boxes obtained for each dataset along with the average relative bounding box size with respect to the whole image.

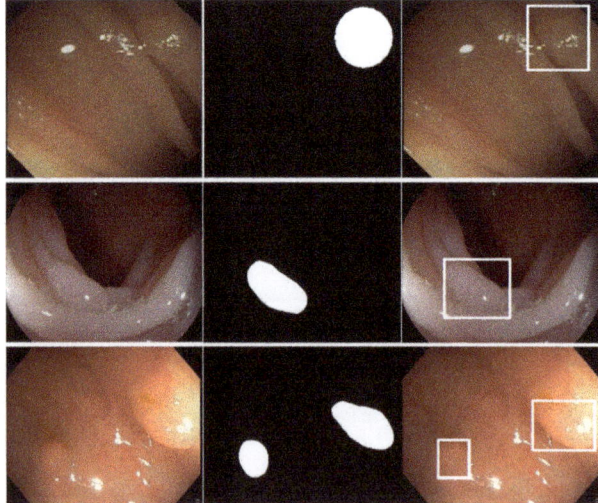

Figure 3. Conversion from binary mask annotations to bounding boxes. First column: original polyp images. Second column: binary mask annotations. Third column: obtained bounding box annotations over the original polyp images.

The CVC-ColonDB and CVC-ClinicDB datasets share the same folder structure and include several mask types for each image. The original polyp images are provided in their own folder, while the images of each mask type are placed in separate folders. All the images are provided in a BMP format, except for the "gtpolyp" mask images in CVC-ClinicDB, which are provided in a TIFF format. For our experiment, the "gtpolyp" mask images were used. The original polyp images were first converted to JPG using the convert_format.sh script. Finally, the dataset was converted into the PASCAL VOC dataset format using the CVC-ToVOC.py script.

The CVC-ClinicVideoDB dataset is structured as two folders, containing development (train and validation) and test partitions, and provides original polyp and mask images in a PNG format. Because the test partition does not include annotations, its images were discarded, and therefore only the images from the development partition were used. In this partition, original polyp and mask images are stored in separate folders by polyp. The original polyp and mask images were first separated into two different folders using the separate_folder_ClinicVideo.sh script, and then the original polyp images were converted into a JPG format using the convert_format.sh script. Finally, the dataset was converted into the PASCAL VOC dataset format using the ClinicVideoToVOC.py script.

The CVC-PolypHD dataset provides a single folder containing both the original polyp and mask images in BMP and TIFF formats, respectively. The original polyp and mask images were first separated into two different folders using the separate_folder_PolypHD.sh script, and then the original polyp images were converted into a JPG format using the convert_format.sh script. Finally, the dataset was converted into the PASCAL VOC dataset format using the PolypHDToVOC.py script.

The ETIS-Larib dataset is structured as two folders containing the original polyp and binary mask images in a TIFF format. The original polyp images were first converted into a JPG format using the convert_format.sh script, and then the dataset was converted into the PASCAL VOC dataset format using the ETIS-LaribToVOC.py script.

The Kvasir-SEG dataset is structured as two folders containing the original polyp and binary mask images in a JPG format and a JSON file that contains the bounding box locations of each image. The conversion of this dataset to the PASCAL VOC dataset format was carried out using the KvasirToVOC.py script.

The PICCOLO dataset is structured as three folders, containing the train, validation, and test partitions, and provides original polyp and mask images in PNG and TIFF formats, respectively. In this case, the original polyp and binary mask images were moved into two single separate folders using the merge_PICCOLO.sh script in order to get rid of the partitions and be able to use the whole dataset as a test set. Then, the original polyp images were converted into a JPG format using the convert_format.sh script, and the dataset was converted into the PASCAL VOC dataset format using the PICCOLOToVOC.py script.

The KUMC dataset is structured as three folders, containing the train, validation, and test partitions, respectively, which are already in the PASCAL VOC dataset format. In this case, we grouped the images into a single folder (i.e., merge train, validation, and test partitions) in order to be able to use the entire dataset as a test set. It is important to note that this dataset includes some annotations that do not have an image associated and, therefore, we excluded those annotations to create a usable version of this dataset. Also, this dataset includes labels for "adenomatous" and "hyperplastic" polyps, which were also merged into a single "polyp" annotation to be able to use them with our model (trained to locate images of class "polyp"). The whole conversion process of this dataset was carried out using the KUMCToVOC.sh script.

The SUN dataset provides one folder for each polyp, containing one or more images of the polyp in a JPG format and a text file with the bounding box location and the class (polyp vs. non-polyp) of each image. In this case, we grouped the images into a single folder in order to be able to use the entire dataset as a test set, using the merge_SUN.sh script. Finally, the dataset was converted into the PASCAL VOC dataset format using the SUNToVOC.sh script.

Finally, the LDPolypVideo dataset is structured as two folders, containing the development (train and validation) and test partitions, and provides original polyp images in a JPG format and a text file with the bounding box location of each image. In this case, we grouped the images into a single folder in order to be able to use the entire dataset as a test set, using the merge_and_rename_LDPolypVideo.sh script, which also renames the original image names to avoid duplicates when all images are put in the same folder. Finally, the dataset was converted into the PASCAL VOC dataset format using the LDPolypVideoToVOC.py script.

2.4. Experiments

The experiments consisted in evaluating the performance of our model (presented in Section 2.1) in the ten public colonoscopy image datasets selected, without retrain. The model was developed using a set of Compi pipelines [32,33] available at this GitHub repository: https://github.com/sing-group/polydeep-object-detection (accessed on 22 February 2022). In order to carry out the experiments presented in this work, the test pipeline (test.xml) was used to load the trained model and analyze the performance on the ten public datasets after converting them to the PASCAL VOC format (as described in Section 2.3). This allowed us to obtain the performance results presented in Section 3.

2.5. Performance of Studies on Public Colonoscopy Image Datasets

Table 2 includes all published studies reporting bounding-box-based performance metrics (i.e., comparing predicted bounding boxes against the true bounding boxes of the ground truth) in at least one of the selected public colonoscopy image datasets, as resulted from the selection process explained in Section 2.2. These data were used then to analyze the performance of various models on the public datasets included in this study and compare our detection model with them. It is important to note that some studies evaluate the performance of several models and, in this case, we selected only the metrics of the best performing ones to perform our analyses and compare them.

The table includes one row for each study experiment with the following information: training set, testing set, recall, precision, F1-score, and F2-score. It is important to note that: (*i*) we only included the performance metrics for the selected public datasets, although some works reported performances with other datasets (e.g., Shin Y. et al., 2018 [34] reports the performance for the ASU-Mayo Clinic Colonoscopy Video, but it is not included, as we could not access the dataset); (*ii*) we included the performance metrics for private dataset partitions (Wang et al., 2018 [35], Wittenberg et al., 2019 [36], and Young Lee J. et al., 2020 [37]) since they able to compare those studies against us.

Each row of Table 2 (i.e., experiment performance) can be categorized as: (*i*) intra-dataset performance, when the evaluation was carried out on a test split of the dataset used for model development; or (*ii*) inter-dataset performance, when the performance evaluation was carried out on a dataset different than the one used for model development. From the 20 studies, there are 10 that only show their performance results for evaluating one public dataset, 8 that use at least two public datasets, 2 that use three datasets, and 1 that uses four public datasets.

Table 2. Performance results of studies evaluating DL models for polyp localization in at least one of the selected public colonoscopy image datasets.

Paper	Train	Test	Results			
			Recall	Precision	F1-Score	F2-Score
Brandao et al., 2018 [38]	CVC-ClinicDB + ASU-Mayo	ETIS-Larib	0.90	0.73	0.81	0.86
		CVC-ColonDB	0.90	0.80	0.85	0.88
Zheng Y. et al., 2018 [39]	CVC-ClinicDB + CVC-ColonDB	ETIS-Larib	0.74	0.77	0.76	0.75
Shin Y. et al., 2018 [34]	CVC-ClinicDB	ETIS-Larib	0.80	0.87	0.83	0.82
		CVC-Clinic VideoDB	0.84	0.90	0.87	0.85
Wang et al., 2018 [35]	Private	CVC-ClinicDB	0.88	0.93	0.91	0.89
		Private *	0.94	0.96	0.95	0.95
Qadir et al., 2019 [40]	CVC-ClinicDB	CVC-ClinicVideoDB	0.84	0.90	0.87	0.85
Tian Y. et al., 2019 [41]	Private	ETIS-Larib	0.64	0.74	0.69	0.66
Ahmad et al., 2019 [42]	Private	ETIS-Larib	0.92	0.75	0.83	0.88
Sornapudi et al., 2019 [43]	CVC-ClinicDB	ETIS-Larib	0.80	0.73	0.76	0.79
		CVC-ColonDB	0.92	0.90	0.91	0.91
		CVC-PolypHD	0.78	0.83	0.81	0.79

Table 2. Cont.

Paper	Train	Test	Results			
			Recall	Precision	F1-Score	F2-Score
Wittenberg et al., 2019 [36]	Private	ETIS-Larib	0.83	0.74	0.79	0.81
		CVC-ClinicDB	0.86	0.80	0.82	0.85
		Private	0.93	0.86	0.89	0.92
Jia X. et al., 2020 [44]	CVC-ColonDB	CVC-ClinicDB	0.92	0.85	0.88	0.91
	CVC-ClinicDB	ETIS-Larib	0.82	0.64	0.72	0.77
Ma Y. et al., 2020 [45]	CVC-ClinicDB	CVC-ClinicVideoDB	0.92	0.88	0.90	0.91
Young Lee J. et al., 2020 [37]	Private	CVC-ClinicDB	0.90	0.98	0.94	0.96
		Private	0.97	0.97	0.97	0.97
Podlasek J. et al., 2020 [46]	Private	ETIS-Larib	0.67	0.79	0.73	0.69
		CVC-ClinicDB	0.91	0.97	0.94	0.92
		CVC-ColonDB	0.74	0.92	0.82	0.77
		Hyper-Kvasir	0.88	0.98	0.93	0.90
Qadir et al., 2021 [47]	CVC-ClinicDB	ETIS-Larib	0.87	0.86	0.86	0.86
		CVC-ColonDB	0.91	0.88	0.90	0.90
Xu J. et al., 2021 [48]	CVC-ClinicDB	ETIS-Larib	0.72	0.83	0.77	0.74
		CVC-ClinicVideoDB	0.66	0.89	0.76	0.70
Pacal et al., 2021 [49]	CVC-ClinicDB	ETIS-Larib	0.83	0.92	0.87	0.84
		CVC-ColonDB	0.97	0.96	0.96	0.97
Liu et al., 2021 [50]	CVC-ClinicDB	ETIS-Larib	0.88	0.78	0.82	0.85
Li K. et al., 2021 [23]	KUMC	KUMC-Test **	0.86	0.91	0.89	0.87
Ma Y. et al., 2021 [21]	CVC-ClinicDB	CVC-ClinicVideoDB	0.64	0.85	0.73	0.67
		LDPolypVideo	0.47	0.65	0.55	0.50
Pacal et al., 2022 [51]	SUN + PICCOLO + CVC-ClinicDB	ETIS-Larib	0.91	0.91	0.91	0.91
	SUN	SUN ***	0.86	0.96	0.91	0.88
	PICCOLO	PICCOLO	0.80	0.93	0.86	0.82

* Wang et al., 2018 evaluated the test performance using a different private dataset from the one used for model training. However, we consider this as an intra-dataset experiment since the private dataset for model development was collected in the Endoscopy Center of Sichuan Provincial People's Hospital between January 2007 and December 2015 and the private test dataset was collected in the same center using the same devices between January and December 2016, and we understand that the distribution should be very similar.
** Li K. et al., 2021 used a partition of the KUMC dataset as testing set in their experiments (KUMC-Test in the table).
*** Pacal et al., 2022 used a partition of the SUN dataset that includes "non-polyp" images and, therefore, it is not comparable to our performance with the SUN dataset, which includes all polyp images.

Among the public datasets, as Figure 4 shows, the ETIS-Larib dataset was the most widely used for testing the detection models (14 out of 20 studies), probably due to the fact that it was one of the test datasets for the automatic polyp detection subchallenge at MICCAI 2015 [11]. The highest F1-score in this dataset was achieved by Pacal et al., 2022 [51] (0.91). The next datasets used by the greatest number of studies (5 out of 20) were CVC-ColonDB, for which the highest F1 (0.96) was achieved by Pacal et al., 2021 [49], CVC-ClinicDB, for which both Young Lee J. et al., 2020 [37] and Podlasek J. et al., 2020 [46] achieved an F1 of 0.94, and CVC-ClinicVideoDB, for which Ma Y. et al., 2020 [45] achieved the top F1-score of 0.90.

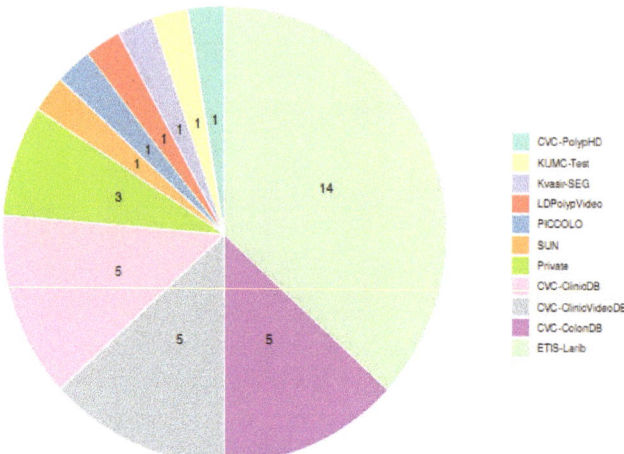

Figure 4. Usage of datasets for model evaluation among studies in Table 2. Each study using several datasets contributes one point for each testing dataset used.

3. Results and Discussion

Table 3 shows the performance results of our model when evaluated on the ten selected public colonoscopy image datasets. As shown in Figure 5, the F1-score of our model decayed in all public datasets with respect to the performance in our private test partition (F1 = 0.88, recall = 0.87, precision = 0.89). The average F1 decay was 13.65%, reaching its maximum with the whole LDPolypVideo dataset (F1 = 0.52), for which we also had the lowest recall (0.49).

Table 3. Performance results of our model when evaluated on the ten selected public colonoscopy image datasets.

Dataset	Number of Images for Test	Results				
		Recall	Precision	F1-Score	F2-Score	AP
CVC-ClinicDB	612	0.82	0.87	0.85	0.83	0.82
CVC-ColonDB	300	0.84	0.81	0.83	0.83	0.85
CVC-PolypHD	56	0.75	0.86	0.80	0.77	0.79
ETIS-Larib	196	0.72	0.71	0.72	0.72	0.69
Kvasir-SEG	1000	0.78	0.84	0.81	0.82	0.79
PICCOLO	3433	0.60	0.76	0.67	0.62	0.63
CVC-ClinicVideoDB	11,954	0.80	0.75	0.77	0.79	0.77
KUMC dataset	37,899	0.81	0.83	0.82	0.81	0.83
KUMC dataset–Test	4872	0.76	0.81	0.78	0.77	0.79
SUN	49,136	0.78	0.83	0.81	0.79	0.81
LDPolypVideo	40,186	0.49	0.56	0.52	0.50	0.44

The three datasets in which our model decayed the most were LDPolypVideo (−40.75%), PICCOLO (−24.27%), and ETIS-Larib (−18.54%). These datasets share two characteristics that the private dataset used to develop and test our model does not have: (*i*) the presence of non-polyp images (LDPolypVideo and PICCOLO), which may decrease our precision as we are showing more test images without polyps and our model has more chances to emit false positives; and (*ii*) the presence of images with multiple-polyp images (LDPolypVideo, PICCOLO, and ETIS-Larib), which may decrease our recall even though our model is able to locate multiple polyps (e.g., PICCOLO contains almost 10% of images annotated with multiple polyps, and our recall in this dataset (0.60) was significantly lower than in others).

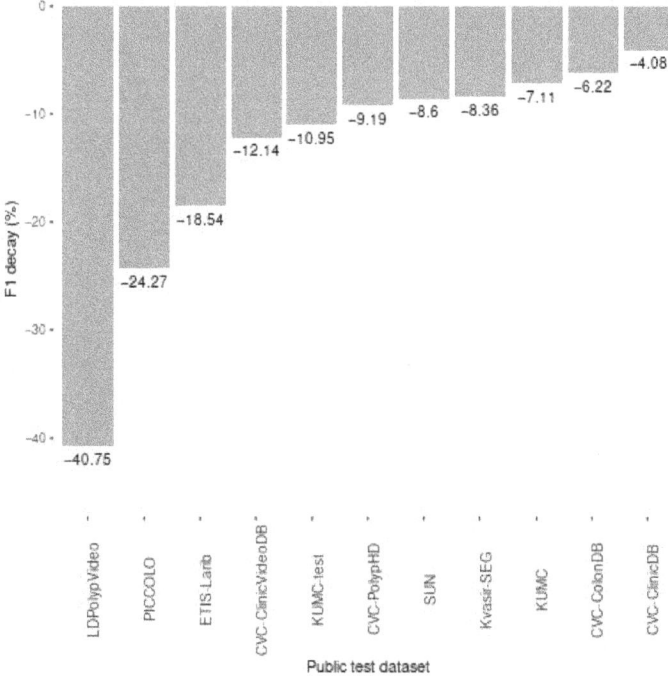

Figure 5. F1 decay (%) in public colonoscopy image datasets compared to the performance of our model in our private dataset reported in Nogueira-Rodríguez et al., 2021 (0.88) [26].

The low performance in the LDPolypVideo dataset is not surprising, as authors state in their publication that the dataset contains images selected to include a high degree of diversity in polyp morphology, multiple polyps, motion blur, and specular reflections, in order to create a challenging dataset [21]. In fact, they fine-tuned several state-of-the-art object detection models (including YOLOv3, the same as us) using the CVC-ClinicDB dataset and evaluated their performance using the CVC-ClinicVideoDB dataset and their new LDPolypVideo dataset, obtaining a significantly lower performance in the LDPolypVideo dataset evaluation with all models. Their best F1-score (0.55) in the LDPolypVideo dataset was obtained using RetinaNet, while their YOLOv3 model obtained an F1-score of 0.41 (compared to our F1-score of 0.52).

Intrigued by the low F1-score in the whole PICCOLO dataset, we analyzed the performance of our model in the three original partitions of the dataset separately, obtaining an F1-score 0.71 in the train partition (recall = 0.63, precision = 0.80, 2203 images), an F1-score 0.53 in the validation partition (recall = 0.49, precision = 0.61, 897 images), and an F1-score 0.74 in the test partition (recall = 0.69, precision = 0.80, 333 images). As can be seen, the performance in the validation partition was significantly worse than in the other two partitions, which we believe to be the main cause of the performance decrease when testing with the whole dataset. Figure 6 shows several incorrect predictions of our model against the ground truth in the train, validation, and tests splits of the PICCOLO dataset. We noted that the validation split contains many big bounding boxes as ground truth, and we computed the average relative size of the bounding boxes with respect to the whole image in the three partitions, obtaining 0.20 in train, 0.33 in validation, and 0.16 in test. Thus, bounding boxes in the validation set are clearly bigger than in the other two partitions. We also observed the majority of polyps in the validation partition look like the three images shown in the middle column of Figure 6, while polyps in our dataset look like the three images taken from the PICCOLO training set in the first column. We understand that polyp images in the validation set, where our model decayed the most, follow a different distribution than the ones in our private training set. Nevertheless, some of these errors (seen in the bottom-left or upper-right images in Figure 6) are caused because the intersection between the predicted and the actual bounding boxes is below the threshold, but in practical terms, an endoscopist would be able to localize the polyp in real-time when using the model.

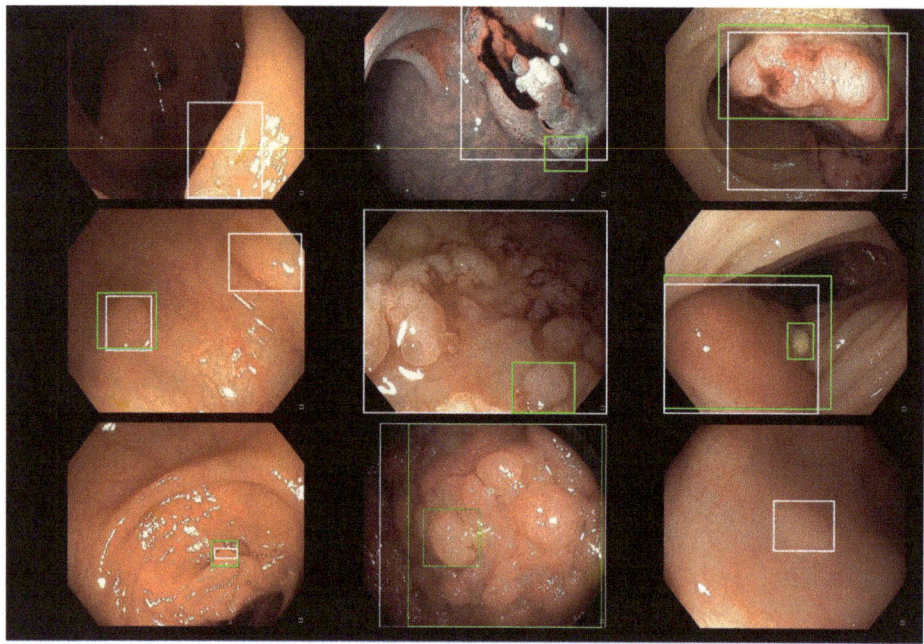

Figure 6. Incorrect prediction examples of our detection model over the different splits of the PICCOLO dataset. From left to right, there are three examples taken from the train, validation, and test splits. Predicted boxes are depicted in green, whereas ground truth boxes are in white.

Only 3 out of the 20 studies had the same exact setup that we had: training the model with a private dataset, testing it with a test partition of the private dataset (intra-dataset performance), and finally testing it using one or more public datasets (inter-dataset performance estimation). As shown in Figure 7, the F1-score also decayed in those studies when analyzing the public datasets with respect to the private test set. In the case of the CVC-ClinicDB dataset, used by the four studies, the average decay was about 5%. In the ETIS-Larib dataset, the Wittenberg et al., 2019 [36] study decayed by 11.24%, compared to our 18.54% decrease.

With the aim of further exploring the intra-to-inter performance decay in other studies, we analyzed the evaluations on public datasets collected in Section 2.5. Such evaluations are heterogeneous regarding the datasets used for training and testing, the models used, and other similar factors. Thus, we compared the intra-dataset performances (i.e., a performance evaluation on a test split of the dataset used for model development, either private or public) against the inter-dataset performances (i.e., a performance evaluation on a dataset different than the one used for model development). As Figure 8A shows, the intra-dataset performances were usually higher than the inter-dataset performances. Figure 8B shows the inter-dataset distribution disaggregated by the public dataset on which the evaluation was carried out. It is important to note that three public datasets (PICCOLO, KUMC, and SUN) are under the intra-dataset performance box, as they are only used in intra-dataset setups. These results are in line with the results obtained in our experiment that show a decay in the F1-score when the evaluation was carried out on a different test dataset.

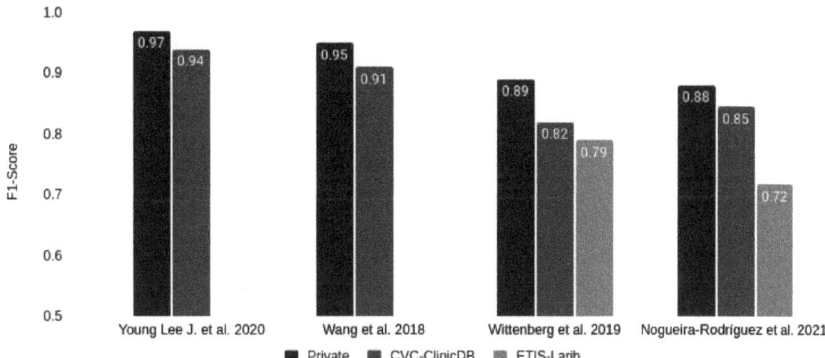

Figure 7. Comparison of F1-score decay on public colonoscopy image datasets of those studies reporting their performance for the private test set partition.

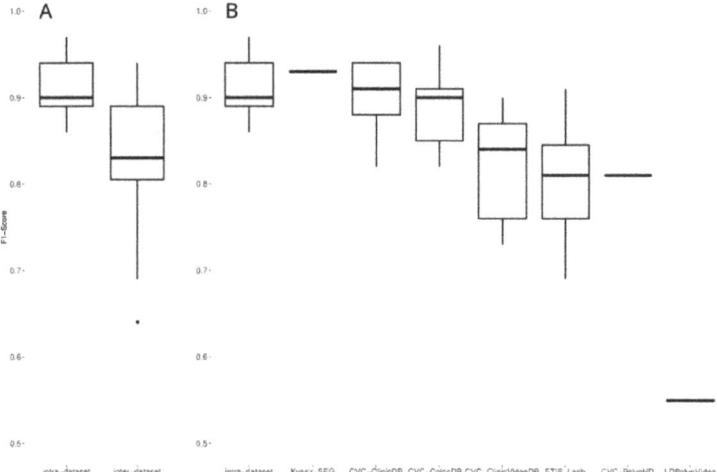

Figure 8. (**A**) Comparison of intra-dataset and inter-dataset performances of the 20 selected studies. (**B**) Same as A, with the inter-dataset performances disaggregated by dataset.

Interestingly, the two datasets in which the decay of our model was lower (CVC-ClinicDB and CVC-ColonDB) are also two of the three datasets in which the published studies obtained performances closer to the intra-dataset ones; also, two of the three datasets in which the performance was worse in the published studies (ETIS-Larib and LDPolypVideo) were two of the most challenging for our model. In the light of these observations, we correlated our performance in the seven datasets shown in Figure 8B with the median inter-dataset performances of the published studies. Figure 9 allows us to observe that such correlation exists (p-value < 0.001), showing that our exhaustive testing reveals the inherent degree of difficulty of the public datasets; a single model (ours) showed the same behavior as the aggregation of the published research, taking into account that studies are heterogeneous (different models and different training datasets) and that we picked the highest F1-scores of those performing several analyses.

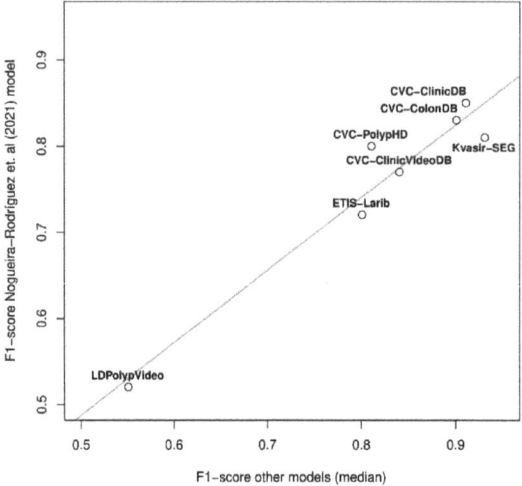

Figure 9. Correlation between the median inter-dataset F1-score of published studies and ours in seven public colonoscopy image datasets.

4. Conclusions

In this work, we performed the biggest systematic evaluation of a polyp localization model trained using a private dataset and tested it on ten public colonoscopy image datasets, including the most recent PICCOLO, SUN, and KUMC datasets. The biggest evaluation to date was carried out by Podlasek J. et al., 2020 [46], who tested their model with four datasets. As a result of performing such an evaluation, we have published a set of scripts for converting the public datasets into the PASCAL VOC format for polyp localization, providing a valuable resource for other researchers aiming to perform similar analyses.

Our experiments and the analysis of the published research allowed us to observe that there is a performance decay when performing an inter-dataset evaluation. The F1-score of our model was 0.88 when evaluated on a private test partition and decayed, on average, 13.65% when tested on the ten public datasets selected. In the published research, the average F1-score was 0.91 when the evaluation was performed on a test split of the dataset used for mode development, compared to the 0.83 average F1 obtained when such models were tested with external datasets, keeping in mind that these F1-scores are the best ones among the reported performances. This confirms our initial hypothesis that models developed using one dataset are sensitive to changes in the nature of the testing instances. Also, we observed that this decay is associated with the test dataset; while studies on datasets such as CVC-ClinicDB and CVC-ColonDB obtain F1-scores closer to their development performances, other datasets such as ETIS-Larib and LDPolypVideo, are more challenging.

In light of these findings, our future work to keep improving our model will be data-centric. In the first place, we will use an updated version of our dataset (now available through the IISGS BioBank: https://www.iisgaliciasur.es/home/biobanco/cohorte-pibadb (accessed on 22 February 2022)) that includes more annotated images for polyp localization. In this updated version, we have also included annotated non-polyp images, which some studies also used during training to improve the performance of the model [22]. Finally, we will also evaluate the possibility of augmenting our training data with public datasets, as some studies have attempted [51], giving priority to those datasets where our model decays the most, such as ETIS-Larib, PICCOLO, or LDPolypVideo. Doing this would also allow us to train our model using images annotated with multiple polyps.

Supplementary Materials: The following supporting information can be downloaded at: https://www.mdpi.com/article/10.3390/diagnostics12040898/s1. Supplementary Table S1: Summary of datasets' structure and conversion process statistics.

Author Contributions: Conceptualization, A.N.-R., D.G.-P. and H.L.-F.; Data curation, A.N.-R. and H.L.-F.; Funding acquisition, M.R.-J. and D.G.-P.; Investigation, A.N.-R., D.G.-P. and H.L.-F.; Methodology, A.N.-R., D.G.-P. and H.L.-F.; Project administration, M.R.-J. and D.G.-P.; Software, A.N.-R.; Supervision, D.G.-P. and H.L.-F.; Writing—original draft, A.N.-R. and H.L.-F.; Writing—review and editing, A.N.-R., M.R.-J., D.G.-P. and H.L.-F. All authors have read and agreed to the published version of the manuscript.

Funding: This work was partially supported by: (*i*) grant PolyDeep (DPI2017-87494-R) funded by MEIC/AEI/10.13039/501100011033 and by ERDF A way of making Europe; (*ii*) grant PolyDeepAdvance (PDC2021-121644-I00) funded by MCIN/AEI/10.13039/501100011033 and by the European Union NextGenerationEU/PRTR; (*iii*) by Consellería de Educación, Universidades e Formación Profesional (Xunta de Galicia) under the scope of the strategic funding ED431C2018/55-GRC Competitive Reference Group; and (*iv*) by National Funds through Fundação para a Ciência e a Tecnologia (FCT) through the individual scientific employment program contract with Hugo López-Fernández (2020.00515.CEECIND). A. Nogueira-Rodríguez is supported by a pre-doctoral contract from Xunta de Galicia (ED481A-2019/299). H. López-Fernández is supported by a "María Zambrano" post-doctoral contract from Ministerio de Universidades (Gobierno de España).

Data Availability Statement: Publicly available datasets were analyzed in this study. The CVC-ClinicDB, CVC-ColonDB, CVC-ClinicVideoDB, and CVC-PolypHD datasets are publicly available here: https://giana.grand-challenge.org. The ETIS-Larib dataset is publicly available here: https://polyp.grand-challenge.org/EtisLarib. The Kvasir-SEG dataset is publicly available here: https://datasets.simula.no/kvasir-seg. The PICCOLO dataset is publicly available here: https://www.biobancovasco.org/en/Sample-and-data-catalog/Databases/PD178-PICCOLO-EN.html. The KUMC dataset is publicly available here: https://dataverse.harvard.edu/dataset.xhtml?persistentId=doi:10.7910/DVN/FCBUOR. The SUN dataset is publicly available here: http://amed8k.sundatabase.org/. The LDPolypVideo dataset is publicly available here: https://github.com/dashishi/LDPolypVideo-Benchmark (accessed on 22 February 2022).

Acknowledgments: We want to acknowledge Jorge Bernal for the support in accessing the CVC datasets and Heyato Itoh for giving us access to the SUN dataset. The PICCOLO dataset included in this study was provided by the Basque Biobank (http://www.biobancovasco.org (accessed on 22 February 2022)). The SING group thanks the CITI (Centro de Investigación, Transferencia e Innovación) from the University of Vigo for hosting its IT infrastructure.

Conflicts of Interest: The authors declare no conflict of interest.

References

1. Nogueira-Rodríguez, A.; Domínguez-Carbajales, R.; López-Fernández, H.; Iglesias, A.; Cubiella, J.; Fdez-Riverola, F.; Reboiro-Jato, M.; Glez-Peña, D. Deep Neural Networks approaches for detecting and classifying colorectal polyps. *Neurocomputing* **2020**, *423*, 721–734. [CrossRef]
2. Viscaino, M.; Bustos, J.T.; Muñoz, P.; Cheein, C.A.; Cheein, F.A. Artificial intelligence for the early detection of colorectal cancer: A comprehensive review of its advantages and misconceptions. *World J. Gastroenterol.* **2021**, *27*, 6399–6414. [CrossRef] [PubMed]
3. Hann, A.; Troya, J.; Fitting, D. Current status and limitations of artificial intelligence in colonoscopy. *United Eur. Gastroenterol. J.* **2021**, *9*, 527–533. [CrossRef] [PubMed]
4. Ashat, M.; Klair, J.S.; Singh, D.; Murali, A.R.; Krishnamoorthi, R. Impact of real-time use of artificial intelligence in improving adenoma detection during colonoscopy: A systematic review and meta-analysis. *Endosc. Int. Open* **2021**, *9*, E513–E521. [CrossRef]
5. Wang, P.; Berzin, T.M.; Brown, J.R.G.; Bharadwaj, S.; Becq, A.; Xiao, X.; Liu, P.; Li, L.; Song, Y.; Zhang, D.; et al. Real-time automatic detection system increases colonoscopic polyp and adenoma detection rates: A prospective randomised controlled study. *Gut* **2019**, *68*, 1813–1819. [CrossRef]
6. Gong, D.; Wu, L.; Zhang, J.; Mu, G.; Shen, L.; Liu, J.; Wang, Z.; Zhou, W.; An, P.; Huang, X.; et al. Detection of colorectal adenomas with a real-time computer-aided system (ENDOANGEL): A randomised controlled study. *Lancet Gastroenterol. Hepatol.* **2020**, *5*, 352–361. [CrossRef]
7. Wang, P.; Liu, X.; Berzin, T.M.; Brown, J.R.G.; Liu, P.; Zhou, C.; Lei, L.; Li, L.; Guo, Z.; Lei, S.; et al. Effect of a deep-learning computer-aided detection system on adenoma detection during colonoscopy (CADe-DB trial): A double-blind randomised study. *Lancet Gastroenterol. Hepatol.* **2020**, *5*, 343–351. [CrossRef]

8. Huang, J.; Liu, W.-N.; Zhang, Y.-Y.; Bian, X.-Q.; Wang, L.-J.; Yang, Q.; Zhang, X.-D. Study on detection rate of polyps and adenomas in artificial-intelligence-aided colonoscopy. *Saudi J. Gastroenterol.* **2020**, *26*, 13–19. [CrossRef]
9. Su, J.-R.; Li, Z.; Shao, X.-J.; Ji, C.-R.; Ji, R.; Zhou, R.-C.; Li, G.-C.; Liu, G.-Q.; He, Y.-S.; Zuo, X.-L.; et al. Impact of a real-time automatic quality control system on colorectal polyp and adenoma detection: A prospective randomized controlled study (with videos). *Gastrointest. Endosc.* **2019**, *91*, 415–424.e4. [CrossRef]
10. Repici, A.; Badalamenti, M.; Maselli, R.; Correale, L.; Radaelli, F.; Rondonotti, E.; Ferrara, E.; Spadaccini, M.; Alkandari, A.; Fugazza, A.; et al. Efficacy of Real-Time Computer-Aided Detection of Colorectal Neoplasia in a Randomized Trial. *Gastroenterology* **2020**, *159*, 512–520.e7. [CrossRef]
11. Bernal, J.; Tajkbaksh, N.; Sánchez, F.J.; Matuszewski, B.J.; Chen, H.; Yu, L.; Angermann, Q.; Romain, O.; Rustad, B.; Balasingham, I.; et al. Comparative Validation of Polyp Detection Methods in Video Colonoscopy: Results from the MICCAI 2015 Endoscopic Vision Challenge. *IEEE Trans. Med. Imaging* **2017**, *36*, 1231–1249. [CrossRef] [PubMed]
12. Bernal, J.; Sánchez, F.J.; Fernández-Esparrach, M.G.; Gil, D.; Rodríguez, C.; Vilariño, F. WM-DOVA maps for accurate polyp highlighting in colonoscopy: Validation vs. saliency maps from physicians. *Comput. Med. Imaging Graph.* **2015**, *43*, 99–111. [CrossRef] [PubMed]
13. Silva, J.S.; Histace, A.; Romain, O.; Dray, X.; Granado, B. Toward embedded detection of polyps in WCE images for early diagnosis of colorectal cancer. *Int. J. Comput. Assist. Radiol. Surg.* **2013**, *9*, 283–293. [CrossRef] [PubMed]
14. Tajbakhsh, N.; Gurudu, S.R.; Liang, J. Automated Polyp Detection in Colonoscopy Videos Using Shape and Context Information. *IEEE Trans. Med. Imaging* **2015**, *35*, 630–644. [CrossRef] [PubMed]
15. Bernal, J.; Sánchez, J.; Vilariño, F. Towards automatic polyp detection with a polyp appearance model. *Pattern Recognit.* **2012**, *45*, 3166–3182. [CrossRef]
16. Vázquez, D.; Bernal, J.; Sánchez, F.J.; Fernández-Esparrach, M.G.; López, A.M.; Romero, A.; Drozdzal, M.; Courville, A. A Benchmark for Endoluminal Scene Segmentation of Colonoscopy Images. *J. Health Eng.* **2017**, *2017*, 1–9. [CrossRef]
17. Angermann, Q.; Bernal, J.; Sánchez-Montes, C.; Hammami, M.; Fernández-Esparrach, G.; Dray, X.; Romain, O.; Sánchez, F.J.; Histace, A. Towards Real-Time Polyp Detection in Colonoscopy Videos: Adapting Still Frame-Based Methodologies for Video Sequences Analysis. In *Computer Assisted and Robotic Endoscopy and Clinical Image-Based Procedures*; Cardoso, M.J., Arbel, T., Luo, X., Wesarg, S., Reichl, T., González Ballester, M.Á., McLeod, J., Drechsler, K., Peters, T., Erdt, M., et al., Eds.; Springer International Publishing: Cham, Switzerland, 2017; pp. 29–41. [CrossRef]
18. Bernal, J.J.; Histace, A.; Masana, M.; Angermann, Q.; Sánchez-Montes, C.; Rodriguez, C.; Hammami, M.; Garcia-Rodriguez, A.; Córdova, H.; Romain, O.; et al. Polyp Detection Benchmark in Colonoscopy Videos using GTCreator: A Novel Fully Configurable Tool for Easy and Fast Annotation of Image Databases. In Proceedings of the 32nd CARS Conference, Berlin, Germany, 22–23 June 2018.
19. Sánchez-Peralta, L.F.; Pagador, J.B.; Picón, A.; Calderón, Á.J.; Polo, F.; Andraka, N.; Bilbao, R.; Glover, B.; Saratxaga, C.L.; Sánchez-Margallo, F.M. PICCOLO White-Light and Narrow-Band Imaging Colonoscopic Dataset: A Performance Comparative of Models and Datasets. *Appl. Sci.* **2020**, *10*, 8501. [CrossRef]
20. Jha, D.; Smedsrud, P.H.; Riegler, M.A.; Halvorsen, P.; de Lange, T.; Johansen, D.; Johansen, H.D. Kvasir-SEG: A Segmented Polyp Dataset. *Int. Conf. Multimed. Model.* **2019**, *11962*, 451–462. [CrossRef]
21. Ma, Y.; Chen, X.; Cheng, K.; Li, Y.; Sun, B. LDPolypVideo Benchmark: A Large-Scale Colonoscopy Video Dataset of Diverse Polyps. *Int. Conf. Med. Image Comput. Comput.-Assist. Interv.* **2021**, *12905*, 387–396. [CrossRef]
22. Misawa, M.; Kudo, S.-E.; Mori, Y.; Hotta, K.; Ohtsuka, K.; Matsuda, T.; Saito, S.; Kudo, T.; Baba, T.; Ishida, F.; et al. Development of a computer-aided detection system for colonoscopy and a publicly accessible large colonoscopy video database (with video). *Gastrointest. Endosc.* **2020**, *93*, 960–967.e3. [CrossRef]
23. Li, K.; Fathan, M.I.; Patel, K.; Zhang, T.; Zhong, C.; Bansal, A.; Rastogi, A.; Wang, J.S.; Wang, G. Colonoscopy polyp detection and classification: Dataset creation and comparative evaluations. *PLoS ONE* **2021**, *16*, e0255809. [CrossRef]
24. Mesejo, P.; Pizarro, D.; Abergel, A.; Rouquette, O.; Beorchia, S.; Poincloux, L.; Bartoli, A. Computer-Aided Classification of Gastrointestinal Lesions in Regular Colonoscopy. *IEEE Trans. Med Imaging* **2016**, *35*, 2051–2063. [CrossRef] [PubMed]
25. Ali, S.; Jha, D.; Ghatwary, N.; Realdon, S.; Cannizzaro, R.; Salem, O.E.; Lamarque, D.; Daul, C.; Riegler, M.A.; Anonsen, K.V.; et al. PolypGen: A multi-center polyp detection and segmentation dataset for generalisability assessment. *arXiv* **2021**, arXiv:2106.04463. [CrossRef]
26. Nogueira-Rodríguez, A.; Domínguez-Carbajales, R.; Campos-Tato, F.; Herrero, J.; Puga, M.; Remedios, D.; Rivas, L.; Sánchez, E.; Iglesias, A.; Cubiella, J.; et al. Real-time polyp detection model using convolutional neural networks. *Neural Comput. Appl.* **2021**, 1–22. [CrossRef]
27. Everingham, M.; Van Gool, L.; Williams, C.K.I.; Winn, J.; Zisserman, A. The Pascal Visual Object Classes (VOC) Challenge. *Int. J. Comput. Vis.* **2009**, *88*, 303–338. [CrossRef]
28. Chen, T.; Li, M.; Li, Y.; Lin, M.; Wang, N.; Wang, M.; Xiao, T.; Xu, B.; Zhang, C.; Zhang, Z. MXNet: A Flexible and Efficient Machine Learning Library for Heterogeneous Distributed Systems. *arXiv* **2015**, arXiv:1512.01274.
29. Guo, J.; He, H.; He, T.; Lausen, L.; Li, M.; Lin, H.; Shi, X.; Wang, C.; Xie, J.; Zha, S.; et al. GluonCV and GluonNLP: Deep Learning in Computer Vision and Natural Language Processing. *J. Mach. Learn. Res.* **2020**, *21*, 1–7.
30. Wang, W.; Tian, J.; Zhang, C.; Luo, Y.; Wang, X.; Li, J. An improved deep learning approach and its applications on colonic polyp images detection. *BMC Med. Imaging* **2020**, *20*, 83. [CrossRef]

31. Tashk, A.; Herp, J.; Nadimi, E. Fully Automatic Polyp Detection Based on a Novel U-Net Architecture and Morphological Post-Process. In Proceedings of the 2019 International Conference on Control, Artificial Intelligence, Robotics & Optimization (ICCAIRO), Athens, Greece, 8–10 December 2019; pp. 37–41. [CrossRef]
32. López-Fernández, H.; Graña-Castro, O.; Nogueira-Rodríguez, A.; Reboiro-Jato, M.; Glez-Peña, D. Compi: A framework for portable and reproducible pipelines. *PeerJ Comput. Sci.* **2021**, *7*, e593. [CrossRef] [PubMed]
33. Nogueira-Rodríguez, A.; López-Fernández, H.; Graña-Castro, O.; Reboiro-Jato, M.; Glez-Peña, D. Compi Hub: A Public Repository for Sharing and Discovering Compi Pipelines. In *Practical Applications of Computational Biology & Bioinformatics, 14th International Conference (PACBB 2020)*; Panuccio, G., Rocha, M., Fdez-Riverola, F., Mohamad, M.S., Casado-Vara, R., Eds.; Springer International Publishing: Cham, Switzerland, 2021; pp. 51–59. [CrossRef]
34. Shin, Y.; Qadir, H.A.; Aabakken, L.; Bergsland, J.; Balasingham, I. Automatic Colon Polyp Detection Using Region Based Deep CNN and Post Learning Approaches. *IEEE Access* **2018**, *6*, 40950–40962. [CrossRef]
35. Wang, P.; Xiao, X.; Brown, J.R.G.; Berzin, T.M.; Tu, M.; Xiong, F.; Hu, X.; Liu, P.; Song, Y.; Zhang, D.; et al. Development and validation of a deep-learning algorithm for the detection of polyps during colonoscopy. *Nat. Biomed. Eng.* **2018**, *2*, 741–748. [CrossRef] [PubMed]
36. Wittenberg, T.; Zobel, P.; Rathke, M.; Mühldorfer, S. Computer Aided Detection of Polyps in Whitelight- Colonoscopy Images using Deep Neural Networks. *Curr. Dir. Biomed. Eng.* **2019**, *5*, 231–234. [CrossRef]
37. Lee, J.Y.; Jeong, J.; Song, E.M.; Ha, C.; Lee, H.J.; Koo, J.E.; Yang, D.-H.; Kim, N.; Byeon, J.-S. Real-time detection of colon polyps during colonoscopy using deep learning: Systematic validation with four independent datasets. *Sci. Rep.* **2020**, *10*, 8379. [CrossRef] [PubMed]
38. Brandao, P.; Zisimopoulos, O.; Mazomenos, E.; Ciuti, G.; Bernal, J.; Visentini-Scarzanella, M.; Menciassi, A.; Dario, P.; Koulaouzidis, A.; Arezzo, A.; et al. Towards a Computed-Aided Diagnosis System in Colonoscopy: Automatic Polyp Segmentation Using Convolution Neural Networks. *J. Med Robot. Res.* **2018**, *3*, 1840002. [CrossRef]
39. Zheng, Y.; Zhang, R.; Yu, R.; Jiang, Y.; Mak, T.W.C.; Wong, S.H.; Lau, J.Y.W.; Poon, C.C.Y. Localisation of Colorectal Polyps by Convolutional Neural Network Features Learnt from White Light and Narrow Band Endoscopic Images of Multiple Databases. In Proceedings of the 2018 40th Annual International Conference of the IEEE Engineering in Medicine and Biology Society (EMBC), Honolulu, HI, USA, 18–21 July 2018; pp. 4142–4145. [CrossRef]
40. Qadir, H.A.; Balasingham, I.; Solhusvik, J.; Bergsland, J.; Aabakken, L.; Shin, Y. Improving Automatic Polyp Detection Using CNN by Exploiting Temporal Dependency in Colonoscopy Video. *IEEE J. Biomed. Health Inform.* **2019**, *24*, 180–193. [CrossRef]
41. Tian, Y.; Pu, L.Z.; Singh, R.; Burt, A.D.; Carneiro, G. One-Stage Five-Class Polyp Detection and Classification. In Proceedings of the 2019 IEEE 16th International Symposium on Biomedical Imaging (ISBI 2019), Venice, Italy, 8–11 April 2019; pp. 70–73. [CrossRef]
42. Ahmad, O.F.; Brandao, P.; Sami, S.S.; Mazomenos, E.; Rau, A.; Haidry, R.; Vega, R.; Seward, E.; Vercauteren, T.K.; Stoyanov, D.; et al. Tu1991 Artificial intelligence for real-time polyp localisation in colonoscopy withdrawal videos. *Gastrointest. Endosc.* **2019**, *89*, AB647. [CrossRef]
43. Sornapudi, S.; Meng, F.; Yi, S. Region-Based Automated Localization of Colonoscopy and Wireless Capsule Endoscopy Polyps. *Appl. Sci.* **2019**, *9*, 2404. [CrossRef]
44. Jia, Y.; Mai, X.; Cui, Y.; Yuan, Y.; Xing, X.; Seo, H.; Xing, L.; Meng, M.Q.-H. Automatic Polyp Recognition in Colonoscopy Images Using Deep Learning and Two-Stage Pyramidal Feature Prediction. *IEEE Trans. Autom. Sci. Eng.* **2020**, *17*, 1570–1584. [CrossRef]
45. Ma, Y.; Chen, X.; Sun, B. Polyp Detection in Colonoscopy Videos by Bootstrapping Via Temporal Consistency. In Proceedings of the 2020 IEEE 17th International Symposium on Biomedical Imaging (ISBI), Iowa City, IA, USA, 3–7 April 2020; pp. 1360–1363. [CrossRef]
46. Podlasek, J.; Heesch, M.; Podlasek, R.; Kilisiński, W.; Filip, R. Real-time deep learning-based colorectal polyp localization on clinical video footage achievable with a wide array of hardware configurations. *Endosc. Int. Open* **2021**, *09*, E741–E748. [CrossRef]
47. Qadir, H.A.; Shin, Y.; Solhusvik, J.; Bergsland, J.; Aabakken, L.; Balasingham, I. Toward real-time polyp detection using fully CNNs for 2D Gaussian shapes prediction. *Med. Image Anal.* **2020**, *68*, 101897. [CrossRef]
48. Xu, J.; Zhao, R.; Yu, Y.; Zhang, Q.; Bian, X.; Wang, J.; Ge, Z.; Qian, D. Real-time automatic polyp detection in colonoscopy using feature enhancement module and spatiotemporal similarity correlation unit. *Biomed. Signal. Process. Control.* **2021**, *66*, 102503. [CrossRef]
49. Pacal, I.; Karaboga, D. A robust real-time deep learning based automatic polyp detection system. *Comput. Biol. Med.* **2021**, *134*, 104519. [CrossRef]
50. Liu, X.; Guo, X.; Liu, Y.; Yuan, Y. Consolidated domain adaptive detection and localization framework for cross-device colonoscopic images. *Med. Image Anal.* **2021**, *71*, 102052. [CrossRef] [PubMed]
51. Pacal, I.; Karaman, A.; Karaboga, D.; Akay, B.; Basturk, A.; Nalbantoglu, U.; Coskun, S. An efficient real-time colonic polyp detection with YOLO algorithms trained by using negative samples and large datasets. *Comput. Biol. Med.* **2021**, *141*, 105031. [CrossRef] [PubMed]

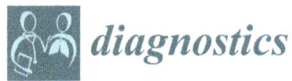

Article

Computer-Aided Image Enhanced Endoscopy Automated System to Boost Polyp and Adenoma Detection Accuracy

Chia-Pei Tang [1,2], Chen-Hung Hsieh [3] and Tu-Liang Lin [3,*]

1. Division of Gastroenterology, Department of Internal Medicine, Dalin Tzu Chi Hospital, Buddhist Tzu Chi Medical Foundation, Chiayi City 62224, Taiwan; franktg@hotmail.com
2. School of Medicine, Tzu Chi University, Hualien City 97004, Taiwan
3. Department of Management Information System, National Chiayi University, Chiayi City 600023, Taiwan; a0903355322@gmail.com
* Correspondence: tuliang@mail.ncyu.edu.tw

Abstract: Colonoscopy is the gold standard to detect colon polyps prematurely. Early detection, characterization and resection of polyps decrease colon cancer incidence. Colon polyp missing rate remains high despite novel methods development. Narrowed-band imaging (NBI) is one of the image enhance techniques used to boost polyp detection and characterization, which uses special filters to enhance the contrast of the mucosa surface and vascular pattern of the polyp. However, the single-button-activated system is not convenient for a full-time colonoscopy operation. We selected three methods to simulate the NBI system: Color Transfer with Mean Shift (CTMS), Multi-scale Retinex with Color Restoration (MSRCR), and Gamma and Sigmoid Conversions (GSC). The results show that the classification accuracy using the original images is the lowest. All color transfer methods outperform the original images approach. Our results verified that the color transfer has a positive impact on the polyp identification and classification task. Combined analysis results of the mAP and the accuracy show an excellent performance of the MSRCR method.

Keywords: colonoscopy; narrow-band image; colon polyp; Retinex; gamma and sigmoid conversion; YOLO

1. Introduction

Colonoscopy is considered as the standard method for the diagnosis and surveillance of colon polyps. Subsequent polypectomy after colonoscopy is the most effective colorectal cancer (CRC) prevention [1]. Early colonoscopy detection and removal of polyps reduces the incidence of colorectal cancer (CRC) by 76% [2]. The most common polyps are hyperplastic and adenomatous. According to the American Society for Gastrointestinal Endoscopy, the "resect and discard" and "diagnose and leave" strategies propose that the hyperplastic polyp need not to be removed. Since hyperplastic polyps are most diminutive and non-malignant, these strategies save a great deal of resection time and pathologic analysis cost [3,4]. The traditional white light (WL) colonoscopy yields an adenoma miss rate of 26%, especially for those <5 mm in size [5,6]. Adenomatous polyps are the primary lesion which evolve to CRC and develop to an interval cancer missed in an initial colonoscopy. The identification and resection of adenomatous polyp is essential to prevent CRC [7]. Innovative methods have been introduced to decrease polyp and adenoma miss rate [8,9].

As the field of colonoscopy technology thrives, new diagnostic modalities have been introduced to improve polyp detection. Image-enhanced endoscopy (IEE) is one of the state-of-the-art tools. Digital IEE includes Olympus narrowed-band imaging (NBI), PENTAX i-scan, and FUJI linked-color imaging (LCI), which improves the diagnostic ability by enhancing polyp mucosa microstructure and microvasculature. The Olympus NBI filters the specific wavelengths to enhance mucosa and vascular pattern. PENTAX i-scan is a real time post-image software-driven modification of contrast, hue and sharpness to enhance polyp mucosa. The NBI remains the most adopted and widely used method at present [10].

NBI incorporated Olympus colonoscopy has a superb ability to detect and identify hyperplastic and adenomatous polyps. This one-button-activated electrical system is an innovative image technology and aids endoscopists to better detect and characterize polyps [11]. NBI technology allows only blue and green lights to pass through a filter placed in the colonoscope light source. The NBI wavelength of the trichromatic optical filters is between 415 and 540 nm with a bandwidth of 30 nm, which has a shallow penetration depth [12]. Two peaks of tissue hemoglobin are absorbed with the wavelength at 415 nm (blue light) and 540 nm (green light) [13]. The narrowed spectrum light highlights the mucosa surface microvasculature pattern to differentiate non-neoplastic (hyperplastic) from neoplastic (adenoma) polyp [14,15] (Figure 1). However, the bowel content of fecal material, debris or filthy water appears bright red color in contrast to the deep dark brown normal mucosa in the NBI environment, which is a visual irritant. The full-time activated NBI system might trigger visual fatigue and discomfort owing to the high color contrast image. Studies indicate that NBI increases polyp and adenoma detection rate with the full-time activated system [12,16–18]. In the real world, endoscopists only activate the NBI system in the circumstances of analyzing the type and margin of the polyp. Switching between WL and NBI back and forth during the withdrawal phase in a colonoscopy is time consuming and not cost-effective. As a consequence, endoscopists leave the system off in most of the colonoscopy observation period. The polyp and adenoma detection rates are not increased with the NBI system in daily clinical practice. In the era of artificial intelligence, we can overcome this issue with a tailor-made image enhancement CNN model to boost the polyp detection and classification without affecting an endoscopist's routine performance.

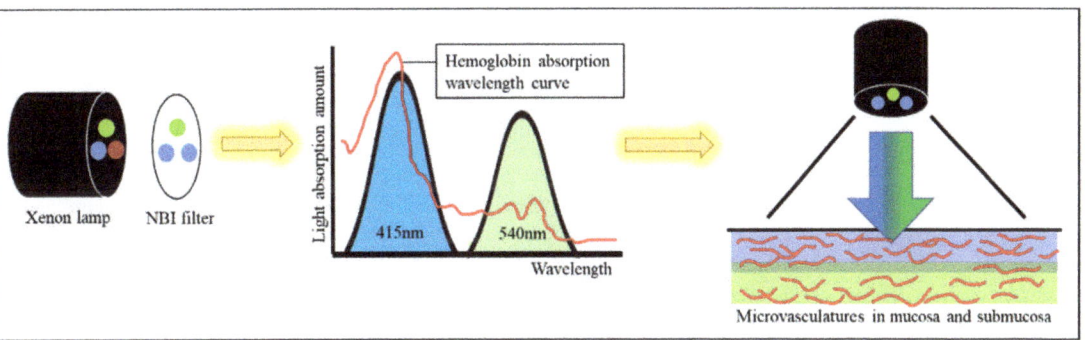

Figure 1. Physics of the NBI endoscopy system. The optical filter on the xenon lamp filters the red light to enhance the vascular and mucosa surface pattern.

The output connection of the Olympus NBI system from the colonoscopy equipment to an external computer is not feasible. We need to convert the original WL image from the colonoscopy source to an NBI simulated CNN-based model on the background and show the WL image with the bounding box in the monitor (Figure 2). We selected three methods to simulate the NBI system for image enhancement: Color Transfer with Mean Shift (CTMS), Multi-scale Retinex (MSR), and gamma and sigmoid conversions. We also compared the selected methods with two conventional image enhancement methods, Histogram Equalization (HE) [19,20] and Contrast Limited Adaptive Histogram Equalization (CLAHE) [21].

The CTMS conversion process is inspired by the work of Xiao et al. [22], who transferred the insufficient training dataset images from the RGB color space to the CIE-LAB color space using a U-Net architecture, to generate the data augmented images.

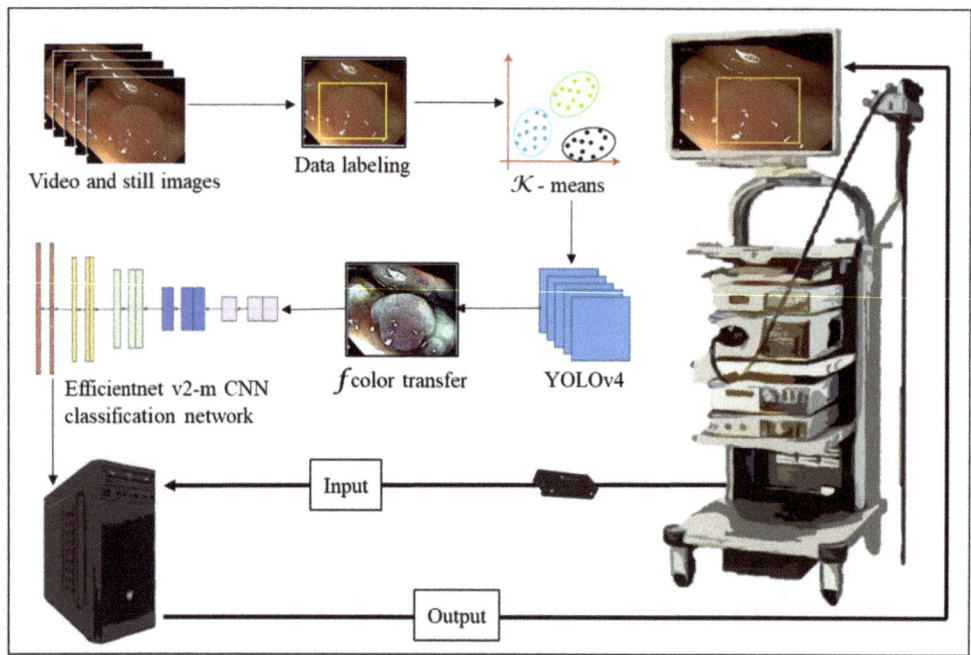

Figure 2. NBI simulated image enhancement system workflow. The polyp images are labeled and trained with YOLOv4 before color transfer to boost detection and classification accuracy.

MSR algorithm is an image enhancement method mimicking human visual perception which provides dynamic range compression, tonal rendition and color constancy [23–26]. Our eyes perceive colors by the light reflection back from an object with a certain wavelength. The human visual system captures colors irrespective of the illumination source under different spectral lighting conditions from a scene. The MSR algorithm separates the original image into a base and a detailed layer, which are processed to improve nonuniform illumination [27]. It has been used for various issues as image dehazing [28], image enhancement and defogging [29] and color constancy computation [30]. In real-world colonoscopy images, the illumination varies with uneven darkness and brightness owing to the light source on the tip of the colonoscope [31]. Luo et al. [32] used a modified MSR with detailed layer to solve the nonuniform and directional illumination on the surgical endoscopy field. Their combined visibility was improved from 0.81 to 1.06 and outperformed existent Retinex methods. Wang et al. [33] corrected color images based on a MSR with a nonlinear functional transformation. They improved the overall brightness and contrast of an image and preserved the image details. Vani et al. [31] discussed the use of MSR and Adaptive Histogram Equalization to suppress noise and improve visibility in wireless capsule endoscopy. Deeba et al. [34] proposed a two-stage automated algorithm with Retinex and saliency region detection algorithm. They achieved a sensitivity of 97.33% and specificity of 79%. MSR provides superb endoscopy image enhancement with balanced brightness and contrast to detect subtle lesions in colonoscopy.

The sigmoidal-remapping function is accomplished by enhancing the image contrast in the limited dynamic range. That is, the lightness between the highlight and shadow in an image can be controlled with the lightness and darkness of the contrast in the sigmoid function [35]. The sigmoidal-remapping function is a continuous nonlinear activation curve [36]. Deeba et al. [37] used a sigmoidal remapping curve to enhance the blue and green light channels in the endoscopy image combined with saliency map formation and histogram of gradient for feature extraction. They achieved a recall and F2 score of 86.33% and 75.51%, respectively.

In this study, we aim to establish a NBI simulated image enhancement technique combined with the computer-aided system to boost polyp detection and classification. We chose three different methods and compared them to each other for their effectiveness in endoscopy image enhancement.

2. Materials and Methods

2.1. Materials

The colonoscopy images were taken from colonoscopies performed with high-definition colonoscopes (CF-H290I, Olympus, Tokyo, Japan) in Dalin Tzu Chi hospital, a teaching hospital in Taiwan, from December 2021 to March 2022, with the approval of the Institutional Review Board (B11004010).

2.1.1. Dataset

The polyp dataset for the training of the deep learning network model was divided into two parts according to the obtaining method. The first part was the static colonoscopy images that were manually selected and captured. Most of the manually selected polyp images were clear compared with those captured from colonoscopy videos. The manual selection process ensured the better image quality and avoided the similarity of polyp images. There were a total of 3796 images, of which 3693 images had more than one polyp. The remaining 103 images were background images which did not contain polyp. The second part of the dataset was extracted from 25 recorded colonoscopy videos performed by senior endoscopists. The total duration of the 25 videos was about 3.1 h (around 336,780 frames), and the number of detected polyps in each video varied. There were 3 complete colonoscopy inspection videos, and the remaining 22 were the segments of detected polyp videos. After deleting the unrecognizable images, 2719 images were included in this study and 1347 images were without polyps. The images were stored with a resolution of 1920 × 1080.

The dataset was divided into three categories according to the types of polyp, i.e., hyperplastic polyp (HP), tubular adenomatous polyp (TA), and sessile serrated adenoma (SSA). The TA and SSA polyps require resection and the HP polyps are considered to not need resection during colonoscopy. There were 1486 images of HP, 2687 images of TA, and 892 images of SSA polyps. Table 1 shows the statistics of the images.

Table 1. The number of images in each polyp category of the dataset.

	TA	SSA	HP	Background
Number of images	2687	892	1486	1450

2.1.2. Data Labeling

Polyps were labeled using the LabelImg image label tool in this study. The labeled images in this study were divided into three categories. The first step was to label all polyps in the dataset, which was to identify the presence of polyp in the image. The identified polyps were divided into three types: TA, HP, and SSA.

2.1.3. Data Augmentation

Data augmentation is a common technique in object recognition. By scaling, cropping, and rotating, the amount of training data for the model training increases to improve the accuracy of the model. In Yolo v4 network training, the image is randomly rotated by plus or minus 180 degrees. The hue and saturation are adjusted. The images are randomly scaled, cropped, and collaged with Mosaic's data augmentation method for training.

2.2. Methods

2.2.1. Color Transfer with Mean Shift

Xiao et al. proposed a novel Color Transfer with Mean Shift method, a data augmentation technique to improve the performance of the deep learning network model for small data. Xiao et al. transferred the training data from the RGB color space to the CIE-LAB color space, a color space defined by the International Commission on Illumination (CIE), through a matrix. The method proposed by Xiao et al. selected a target image and calculated the color mean value of the target image; the mean value is imposed on the original image to generate a new image. The process is formulated as Equation (1). $C_{transferred}$ represents the converted value, $C_{original}$ represents the value of the image to be converted, $\overline{C}_{original}$ represents the mean value of channel C calculated from the main coloring area of the original image, and $\overline{C}_{target}$ represents the mean value of channel C in the transferred area of the target image.

$$C_{transferred} = C_{original} - \overline{C}_{original} + \overline{C}_{target} \tag{1}$$

Their study proved that the proposed data augmentation method had better performance than the traditional geometric data augmentation methods (scaling and rotation). The network model trained with this data augmentation method generalized better [22].

We applied the Color Transfer with Mean Shift to the polyp detection. For mimicking the features of NBI colonoscopy image using WL images, we converted the channels A* and B* using Equation (2). The C is the converted channel value, C_{WL} represents the channel value of WL colonoscopy images, $\overline{C}_{WL}$ represents the mean value of WL colonoscopy image channels, $\overline{C}_{NBI}$ represents the mean value of channels in NBI colonoscopy image, x is the coefficient to adjust the NBI image value of the channel, and y is the constant to fine-tune the color tone.

$$C_{transferred} = C_{WL} - \overline{C}_{WL} + x * \overline{C}_{NBI} + y \tag{2}$$

Figures 3 and 4 are the color transfer examples of two types of polyps, adenomatous and hyperplastic polyps. Figures 3 and 4 show the images of TA and HP polyps after Color Transfer with Mean Shift.

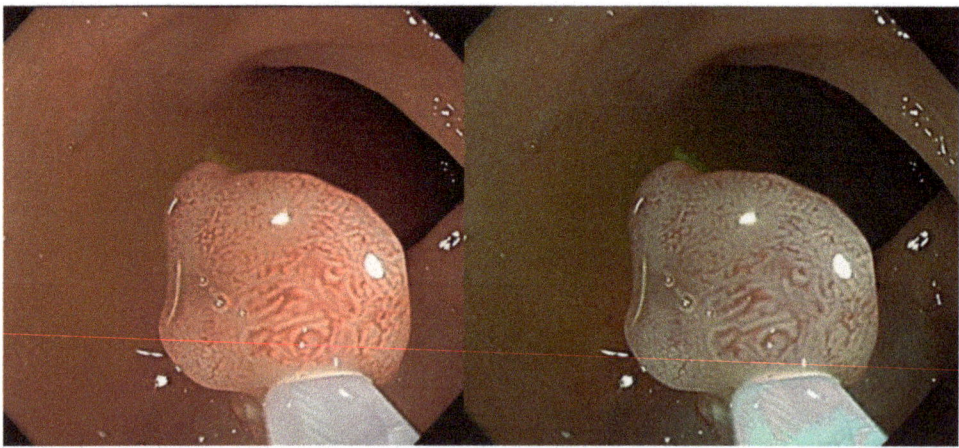

Figure 3. Images of TA polyps after Color Transfer with Mean Shift. (**Left**): Original WL, (**Right**): Color Transferred).

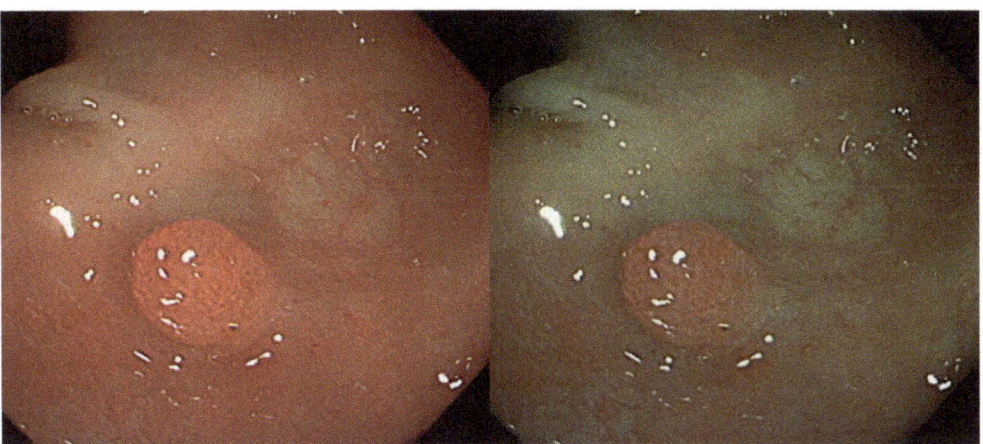

Figure 4. Images of HP polyps after Color Transfer with Mean Shift. ((**Left**): Original WL, (**Right**): Color Transferred).

2.2.2. Retinex

Retinex is a common method for image enhancement, a term combining retina and cortex. Retinex minimizes the effect of a light source on the image to achieve color constancy. Retinex has three steps to maintain the color constancy. First, the image is dynamically compressed to preserve the details of the original image. The second step is to isolate the color from the spectrum of the scene's light source. Finally, the color of the object in the image is restored and reproduced.

We formulate the above mentioned three steps into the following mathematic expressions. Each pixel in the image is expressed as the product of the light source intensity and the reflection intensity as Equation (3), where S is the pixel value of coordinate (x, y) in the image, R is the reflection expression, and L is the intensity of the light source.

$$S(x,y) = R(x,y) * L(x,y) \tag{3}$$

Dynamic range compression is used to compress the original signal into a smaller range. In the digital image, the signal is compressed into the range of the according signal. To obtain the details in the image, Retinex dynamically compresses the image logarithmically as Equation (4).

$$\log(R(x,y)) = \log(S(x,y)) - \log(L(x,y)) \tag{4}$$

The natural color is independent of the spectrum of the light source. The goal of Retinex is to eliminate the influence of a different light source intensity. The elimination is expressed as Equation (5), where R_i is the result of the output on channel I, I_i is the pixel value of channel i in the image. F is the Gaussian Surround Function that simulates the illumination of light sources in nature, as Equation (6); c is the Gaussian surround space constant.

$$R_i(x, y) = \log[I_i(x,y)] - \log[F(x,y) * I_i(x,y)] \tag{5}$$

$$F(x, y) = e^{-r^2/c^2} \tag{6}$$

When the Gaussian surrounding space constant is small ($c < 20$), it has an improved dynamic range compression effect and retains more image details. When the constant is increased ($c > 200$), better color restoration is achieved [38]. The Gaussian surrounding space constant is used only once in the Single Scale Retinex (SSR); trade-off is made between the two. Therefore, Multi-Scale Retinex (MSR) was developed, which uses multiple

Gaussian surrounding space constants in the image to gain the advantages of different scales simultaneously, as in Equation (7).

$$R_{MSR_i} = \sum_{n=1}^{N} w_n R_{ni} \tag{7}$$

$$F_n(x,y) = ke^{-r^2/c_n^2} \tag{8}$$

R_{MSR_i} in Equation (7) is the output of the ith channel of MSR, w_n is the weight, R_{ni} is the result of SSR output using c_n as the Gaussian surrounding space constant, and Equation (8) is the Gaussian surrounding function in MSR. In several experiments, it is shown that three scales are sufficient for MSR, a small scale ($c_n < 20$), a large scale ($c_n > 200$), and an intermediate scale. The weights were assigned equally for the 3 scales, i.e., 1/3 of each scale [23].

Originally, the Retinex algorithm was based on the Gray-World Assumption. As the reflectance of the image is the same in all three primary color channels, it meets the Gray-World Assumption. This assumption is violated when the image is not colorful or has a large number of single blocks of color, which results in Retinex being grayed out or having severely reduced saturation. Therefore, D. J. Jobson proposed that adding a color restoration function to the MSR and converting it to the Multi-Scale Retinex with Color Restoration (MSRCR) as in Equations (9) and (10), where β = 46, α = 125, b = -30, and G = 192 [38].

$$R_{MSRCR_i}(x,y) = G[C_i(x,y)R_{MSR_i}(x,y) + b] \tag{9}$$

$$C_i(x,y) = \beta \log[\alpha I'_i(x,y)] = \beta \log[\alpha I_i(x,y)] - \beta \log[\sum_{i=1}^{S} I_i(x,y)] \tag{10}$$

Parthasarathy and Sankaran improved MSRCR by proposing an automated multiscale Retinex for color restoration, adding a hue conversion function to the MSRCR output. They used a histogram to calculate color pixel thresholds, limiting all to two thresholds [39].

Figures 5–7 are the Retinex examples of three polyp types, TA, HP, and SSA.

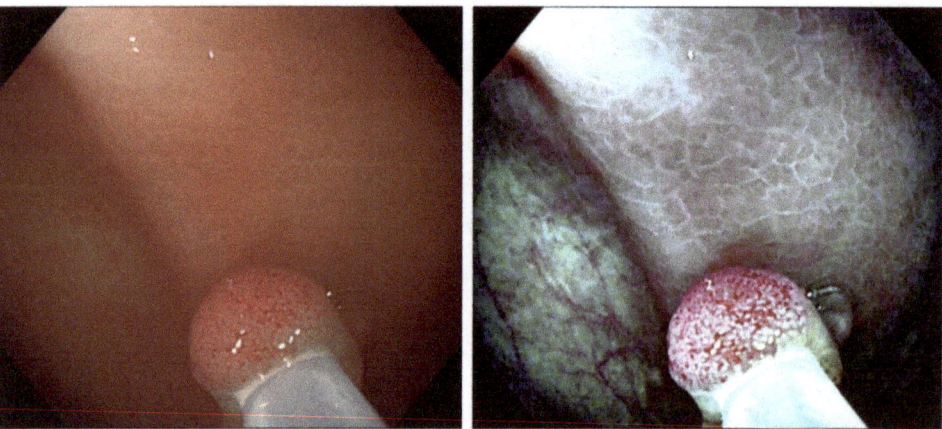

Figure 5. Images of TA polyp after Retinex. ((**Left**): Original WL, (**Right**): Retinex).

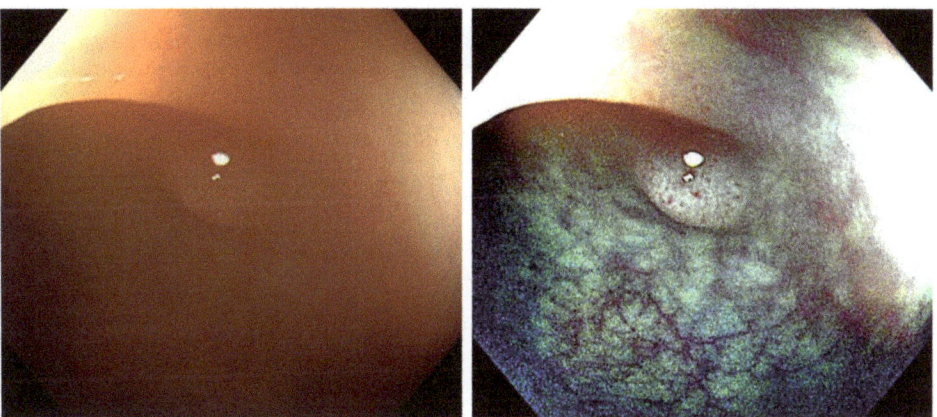

Figure 6. Images of HP polyp after Retinex ((**Left**): Original WL, (**Right**): Retinex).

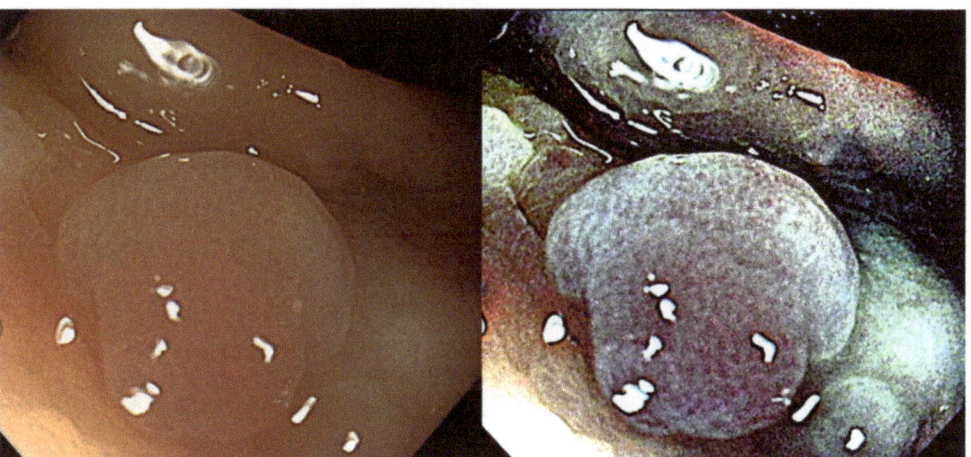

Figure 7. Images of SSA polyp after Retinex. ((**Left**): Original WL, (**Right**): Retinex).

2.2.3. Gamma and Sigmoid Conversions

Deeba et al. proposed a computer-aided polyp detection algorithm for wireless capsule endoscopy [37]. Their proposed method is divided into three steps. The image is enhanced, followed by the generation of salient graphics to highlight the location of possible polyps, and finally the histogram of gradient values (HOG) is calculated for feature extraction. Deeba et al. enhanced the blue and green light channels by using the sigmoid curve in the image, as in Equation (11).

$$I_s = I_{MAX} * \frac{1}{1 + e^{-a(I-c)}} \tag{11}$$

The values at both ends of the sigmoid curve are compressed, and the values in the middle are stretched between 0 and 1. The I_s is the result of sigmoid calculation, I_{MAX} is the maximum pixel value in a single channel, a and c are constants, the size of the constant is adjusted according to the image, and the red channel is suppressed using the Transform-based Gamma Correction (TGC) curve in Equation (12).

$$I_G = (I_{MAX} - S) * (I/I_{MAX})^r \tag{12}$$

The I_G is the calculated result of the gamma curve and S is a constant that controls the effect of curve suppression [37]. Figure 8 shows the gamma and sigmoid conversion of RGB channels. Figure 9 shows the images after adjusting the parameters of the sigmoid curve and gamma correction curve using colonoscopy images.

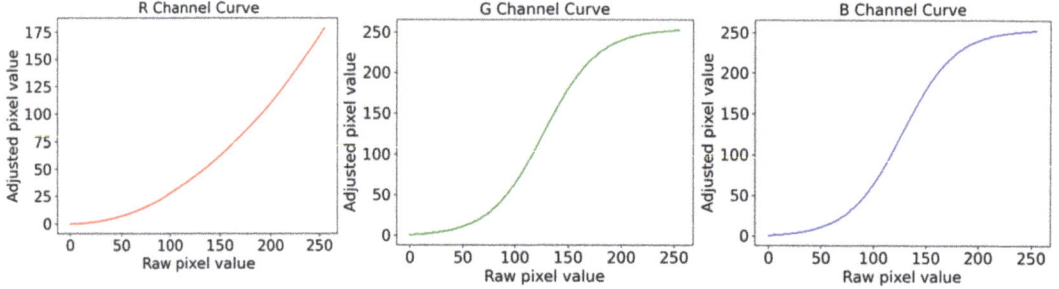

Figure 8. Conversion diagram of RGB in gamma and sigmoid conversion.

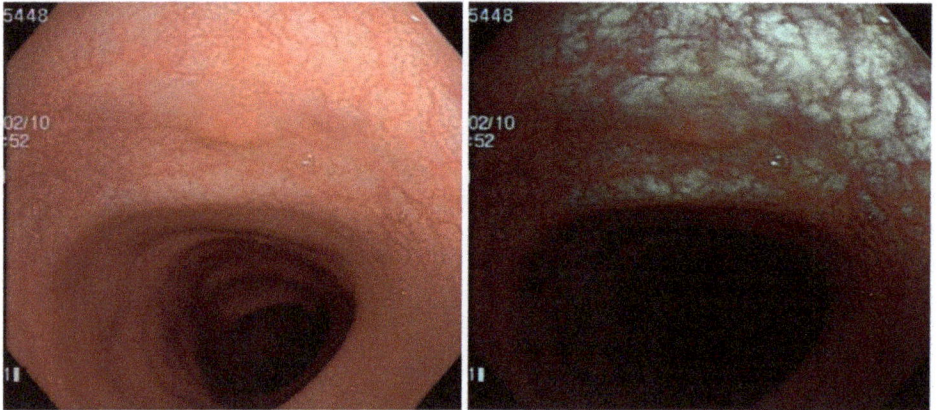

Figure 9. Image of SSA polyp after gamma and sigmoid conversion. ((**Left**): Original WL, (**Right**): Gamma and Sigmoid Conversion).

2.2.4. YOLOv4

YOLOv4 is a one-stage object recognition method proposed by Alexey Bochkovskiy et al. in 2020 [40]. Based on Yolov3 [41], YOLOv4 has made improvements in various areas. YOLOv4 has improved both the speed and accuracy of recognition compared with previous versions. The recognition AP of MS COCO dataset on Tesla V100 GPU reaches 43.5%, and the recognition speed is about 65FPS. The network model of object recognition is divided into four parts according to their different functions, which are the input layer responsible for image input, the backbone of the main body of the object recognition network, the neck connecting the backbone and the head, and the layer responsible for classification and bounding boxes. The head of YOLOv4 follows the original YOLOv3, the trunk uses CSPDarknet53 previously developed by the author, and the neck uses Spatial Pyramid Pooling (SPP) and Path Aggregation Network (PANet).

YOLOv4 refers to several of the latest object recognition methods mentioned on the Browse State-of-the-Art website in the field of object recognition, which are applied to various parts of the network to evaluate their quality. YOLOv4 selects the best performance method and was further improved. The author conducted experiments and improvements on six parts, including data amplification, activation function, bounding box regression loss, normalization, normalization of network activation through mean and variance, and skip-connections. After experiments and comparisons, YOLOv4 finally added CutMix, Mosaic data amplification, Class Label Smoothing, DropBlock, Mish activation function, Cross-stage partial connections and Multi-input weighted residual connections to the backbone part; and CIoU loss, CmBN, DropBlock, Mosaic data augmentation, Self-Adversarial Training, Eliminate grid sensitivity, Cosine annealing scheduler, Optimal hyperparameters, Mish activation function, SPP, SAM, PANet, and DIoU to the head section—technologies such as NMS.

In addition to the improvement in accuracy and speed, YOLOv4 proves that complete training on a general consumer-grade graphic card is possible, making the YOLOv4 algorithm more widely adopted [40].

2.2.5. Research Design

In this research, the colorectal polyp identification is performed using two experimental designs. In the first experimental design (Figure 10), the color transfer is performed on the entire colonoscopy image. In the implementation, we found that when the color transfer is performed on the entire high-resolution image, it takes some extra time to convert every pixel of the entire image. However, in the actual diagnosis process, it is expected that the system can generate instant results. Therefore, in order to improve this immediacy problem, this study further proposes a second experimental design (Figure 11). First, the WL endoscopic image is used to identify the polyp and performs color transfer in the identified polyp areas. The entire process takes less time and enhances its immediacy due to a smaller area for color transfer.

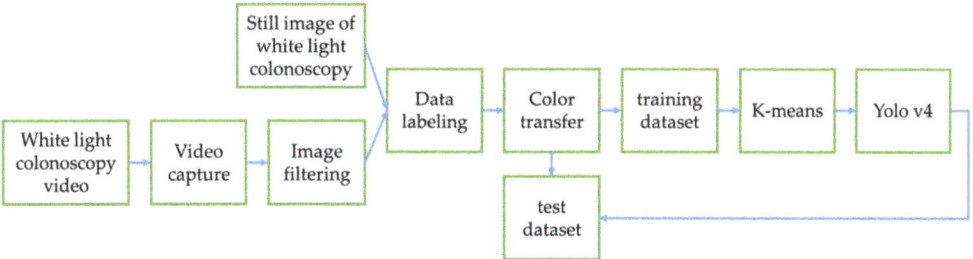

Figure 10. Experimental Design 1.

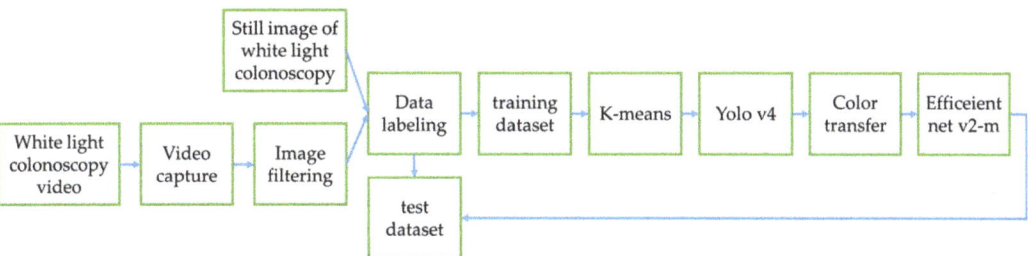

Figure 11. Experimental Design 2.

Figure 10 is the structure diagram of the first experimental design. The first step is the collection and arrangement of the dataset. The video of the colonoscopy is captured into static images. Poor quality images are filtered out. They are merged with the static images of the colonoscopy. The LabelImg tool is adopted to label the location and type of polyps. The second step is pre-processing, converting the labeled data using the color transfer function, then randomly splitting the data into a training dataset and a testing dataset in a ratio of 8 to 2, and using K-means to convert the object frames into groups. The third step is to add the data into the deep learning network for training and evaluate the network model with the test dataset.

The second experiment design is to add an image classification network of Efficientnet v2-m after obtaining the polyp identification results from the first experiment as shown in Figure 11. In the first experiment design, we collected 11,957 images with polyps and 9369 images without polyps and trained a polyp recognition model using Yolov4 to detect polyps in images. The final mAP of the model was 92.4%. After the recognition results of Yolov4, we performed color transfer on the object frame output by the network and trained the types of polyps using the Efficientnet v2-m network. Because the color transfer is only performed on the object frames rather than the entire image, we reduced the time complexity, making polyp image recognition quicker than the first experiment.

This study attempts to remove unimportant information in colonoscopy images using a special color transfer processing method to preserve or highlight the details of polyps. Three different color transfer methods are used, Color Transfer with Mean Shift, automatic multi-scale Retinex for color restoration, and gamma and sigmoid conversion. In this study, it is believed that Color Transfer with Mean Shift and NBI have similar concepts in reducing original data, and the gamma and sigmoid conversion simulate the same pattern as NBI suppresses red light. Since the colonoscopy is illuminated by a direct single light source, the bright area is interspersed with uneven dark shadows owing to folds or fecal debris. In this study, the color and detail contours which disappeared in the image are restored using the automatic MSR algorithm.

2.2.6. Model Training

This research uses YOLOv4 to train the model. First, the dataset is grouped into 9 scales that conform to the ground truth of the dataset using k-means. The model uses the calculated 9 scales as the anchor boxes size in the final output layer of the network. In the model training, the loss graph of the model is monitored until the loss becomes flat, and the training stops, that is, the model has converged.

2.2.7. Evaluation Metrics

This research adopts the mean Average Precision (mAP) to measure the accuracy of the model. The calculation of mAP is an AP calculation for all categories which takes the average. mAP is used as a metric for object detection. Intersection over union (IoU) is also added to measure the correctness of the target position marked by the model. The IoU is the intersection of the model-predicted box and the ground truth divided by the union of the two boxes as in Equation (13). The calculation of AP is as in Equation (14). In short, the AP is the average precision of one category and mAP is the mean average precision of all categories. The higher the mAP value, the higher the accuracy of the search results.

$$\text{IoU}(A, B) = |\frac{A \cap B}{A \cup B}| \tag{13}$$

$$AP = \frac{1}{11} \sum_{r \in \{0, 0.1..., 1\} f} P_{interp}(r) \tag{14}$$

In the calculation of mAP, an IoU is usually set as the critical value (usually set to 0.5). When the IoU is greater than the preset critical value, it is classified as True Positive (TP); otherwise, it is classified as a false positive (FP). The real object is not predicted by the model classified as false negatives (FN), and the false object is not predicted as true negatives (TN). AP is calculated according to these values and estimates the area under the PR curve (Precision-Recall) (AUC). In machine learning, there are two methods to measure the model: Precision as Equation (14) and Recall as Equation (15).

$$\text{Precision} = \frac{TP}{TP + FP} \tag{15}$$

$$\text{Recall} = \frac{TP}{TP + FN} \tag{16}$$

In the PASCAL VOC challenge, Equation (14) is used to calculate the AP average of 11 Recall interpolation points as the AP of the object. Finally, the AP of all objects in the model is averaged to gain the mAP. The mAP in this research is calculated using the program on Yolo v4-AlexeyAB GitHub.

In the Efficientnet v2-m classification network, the accuracy is used as the evaluation standard. If the quasi-class predicted by the model is the same as the real situation, it belongs to TP or TN, and if the predicted result does not match the real situation, it belongs to FP or FN. Finally, the accuracy is calculated using the four values of the confusion matrix. As in Equation (17), the accuracy is the percentage of correct predicted results in the total sample.

$$\text{Accuracy} = \frac{TP + TN}{TP + FP + FN + TN} \tag{17}$$

3. Results

In this study, different color transfer methods were trained using deep learning networks and were compared with the model trained on the original images to evaluate the effect of color transfer methods on polyp identification and classification. The data are divided into three datasets according to different classification methods. The first dataset is divided into three types of polyps (TA, HP and SSA). The second dataset divides polyps into neoplastic (TA and SSA) and non-neoplastic (HP). The third dataset excludes the SSA due to them being scarce in number.

3.1. YOLOv4 Training Results in Experimental Design 1

In this section, the three datasets use MSRCR, gamma and sigmoid conversion, Color Transfer with Mean Shift, and original images to train the model with Yolov4 network, and we compare the model results. The neoplastic polyps, TA and SSA, are grouped into the same category for color transfer comparison. We use the MSRCR to compare with other color transfer methods and it shows the highest value at 77.6162 in mAP. The results of the conventional HE and CLAHE are also included to benchmark with the selected color transfer methods. The images are first transferred from the RGB color space to LAB color space and the HE and CLAHE are performed on the lightness L channel. There are two main operational parameters, tile size and clip limit, in the CLAHE image enhancement process. The tile size is the number of the non-overlapping tiles to which the original image is partitioned and is set to 8 × 8 in the experiments. The clip limit is the threshold that will be used to trim the histograms of the pixel distribution and is set to 2 in the experiments. The MSRCR performs best in the two groups of polyps (Table 2). Therefore, MSRCR is the most suitable color transfer method to use in two classes.

Table 2. mAP results of 3 color transfer methods in HP vs. combination of TA and SSA.

Method	HP	TA+SSA	mAP
Original Image	76.18	76.08	76.1296
HE	73.86	75.89	74.8799
CLAHE	75.31	75.92	75.615
Multi-scale Retinex with Color Restoration	**78.53**	**76.70**	**77.6162**
Gamma and Sigmoid Conversions	76.54	76.38	76.4582
Color Transfer with Mean Shift	78.30	76.40	77.3478

HE: Histogram Equalization, CLAHE: Contrast Limited Adaptive Histogram Equalization.

Then, the dataset is divided into three categories according to different types of polyps for further comparison of color transfer methods. The gamma and sigmoid conversion mAP have the highest value of 72.1863 (Table 3). Therefore, gamma and sigmoid conversion are suitable for color transfer in terms of the three polyp classes.

Table 3. mAP results of 3 color transfer methods in 3 polyp classes.

Method	HP	TA	SSA	mAP
Original Image	74.80	84.09	46.17	68.3590
HE	73.42	84.4	55.24	71.0244
CLAHE	73.6	85.5	55.37	71.4944
Multi-scale Retinex with Color Restoration	75.40	86.16	48.08	69.8782
Gamma and Sigmoid Conversions	**75.69**	**87.85**	53.02	**72.1863**
Color Transfer with Mean Shift	75.19	84.44	45.88	68.1714

HE: Histogram Equalization, CLAHE: Contrast Limited Adaptive Histogram Equalization.

Since the SSA is a rare polyp with insufficient data, it affects the accuracy of the identification result. We exclude the SSA category and compared the mAP results of the two categories of HP and TA for color transfer. The mAP demonstrates that the MSRCR is the most suitable color transfer method, and its mAP value is 86.8422 (Table 4).

Table 4. mAP results of 3 color transfer methods in 2 polyp classes, HP and TA.

Method	HP	TA	mAP
Original Image	80.40	86.15	83.2753
HE	79.48	87.23	83.3543
CLAHE	80.56	86.24	83.3963
Multi-scale Retinex with Color Restoration	**84.43**	**89.35**	**86.8422**
Gamma and Sigmoid conversions	79.83	87.30	83.5650
Color Transfer with Mean Shift	81.71	88.07	84.8913

HE: Histogram Equalization, CLAHE: Contrast Limited Adaptive Histogram Equalization.

Comparing the results of the three color transfer methods, the MSRCR has the best mAP result in two polyp classes. Although gamma and sigmoid conversion has a better result in three polyp classes analysis, we need to consider the low probability in the SSA group owing to scarce data. By excluding the SSA, the mAP of MSRCR color transfer is higher than using gamma and sigmoid conversion with TA and SSA combined. We speculate that the higher accuracy of gamma and sigmoid conversion on SSA results in better mAP than the MSRCR in three polyp classes. After considering the distribution of the dataset and the mAP results, this study selects MSRCR as the color transfer method.

3.2. Classifier Training Results in Experimental Design 2

In this section, the MSRCR, gamma and sigmoid conversion, Color Transfer with Mean Shift and original image dataset are adopted to train the model using Efficientnet v2-m network in three datasets. The polyps are automatically cropped from images and the classification task is performed based on the cropped polyp images. The accuracy is used as the criteria for polyp classification evaluation. The classification is correct if the type of polyp identified by the model matches the ground truth.

The results in the case of HP vs. combination of TA and SSA polyps can be seen from the above table (Table 5). The result shows the best accuracy of MSRCR with 0.8643. Therefore, the MSRCR is the most accurate method for color transfer classification.

Table 5. Accuracy of 3 color transfer methods in HP vs. combination of TA and SSA.

Method	Accuracy
Original Image	0.8377
HE	0.8394
CLAHE	0.8377
Multi-scale Retinex with Color Restoration	**0.8643**
Gamma and Sigmoid Conversions	0.8533
Color Transfer with Mean Shift	0.8502

HE: Histogram Equalization, CLAHE: Contrast Limited Adaptive Histogram Equalization.

Then, the classification was performed in three polyp classes. The gamma and sigmoid conversion show the best accuracy of 0.7517, and the accuracy of MSRCR is 0.7491 (Table 6). The values are similar. In this classification analysis, both methods are suitable for the task.

Table 6. Accuracy of 3 color transfer methods in 3 polyp classes.

Method	Accuracy
Original Image	0.7257
HE	0.7474
CLAHE	0.7487
Multi-scale Retinex with Color Restoration	0.7491
Gamma and Sigmoid Conversions	**0.7517**
Color Transfer with Mean Shift	0.7474

HE: Histogram Equalization, CLAHE: Contrast Limited Adaptive Histogram Equalization.

For the results after excluding SSA polyps, the MSRCR accuracy is the highest with a value of 0.8428 (Table 7). Under this classification task, the most suitable color transfer method is MSRCR.

Table 7. Accuracy of the 3 color transfer methods in 2 polyp classes, HP and TA.

Method	Accuracy
Original Image	0.8017
HE	0.8200
CLAHE	0.8384
Multi-scale Retinex with Color Restoration	**0.8428**
Gamma and Sigmoid Conversions	0.8394
Color Transfer with Mean Shift	0.8308

HE: Histogram Equalization, CLAHE: Contrast Limited Adaptive Histogram Equalization.

From the accuracy comparison of the different methods in several classes, the classification accuracy of the original image is the lowest. All color transfer methods using datasets other than the original image perform better. The results demonstrated that the color transfer has a positive impact on the polyp identification. Combining the mAP results from the previous section and the accuracy results in this section, we concluded that the Retinex has an excellent outcome and is the best choice for color transfer.

4. Discussion

We aim to demonstrate that color transfer is useful for the correct identification of polyps. We developed a deep learning network to predict the test dataset; three color transfer methods are compared with the base prediction of the original image dataset for the optimal identification model selection. Several image results were selected for comparison. The detected image result of MSRCR vs. Original Image are shown in Figures 12–14. In the original image models of Figures 12–14, the polyps were undetected or misclassified.

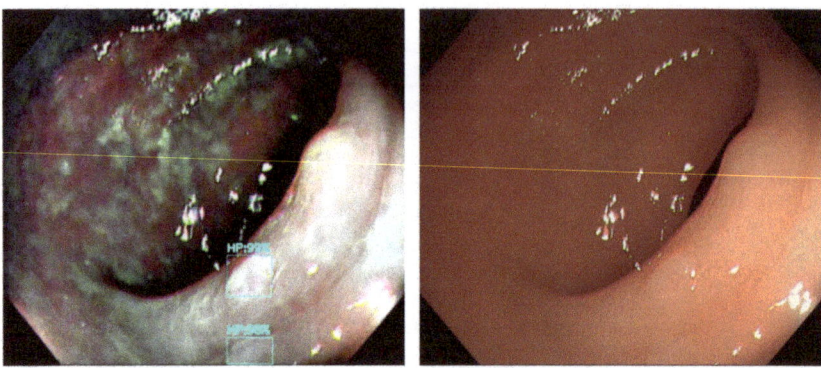

Figure 12. The correct results of MSRCR vs. the undetected polyp in original image. ((**Left**): MSRCR, (**Right**): Original).

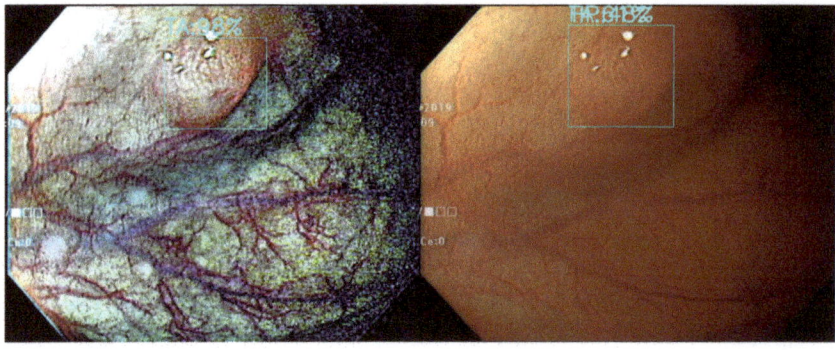

Figure 13. The correct results of MSRCR vs. the misclassified polyp of original image. ((**Left**): MSRCR, (**Right**): Original).

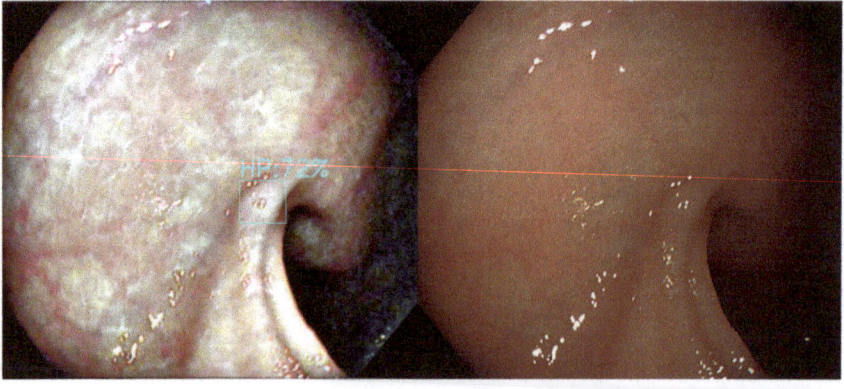

Figure 14. The correct results of MSRCR vs. the undetected polyp of original image. ((**Left**): MSRCR, (**Right**): Original).

5. Conclusions

In this study, color transfer methods were successfully applied to polyp identification. The colon polyp detection accuracy and classification increased. From different experimental settings in this study, the comparison of the three color transfer methods showed that the MSRCR method outperforms others. The scarce SSA polyp images led to suboptimal results. The dataset ought to increase for the accuracy improvement of SSA detection.

We developed two research designs in this study. The first design converts each pixel of the image individually because of the nature of the color transfer. We concluded that the computation time was reduced to improve the response time. The second research design was proposed to identify the position of polyps, perform the color transfer, and classify them according to the conversion results. This ensures immediacy by reducing the area of conversion to increase the speed of the entire process.

Author Contributions: Conceptualization, T.-L.L.; Data curation, C.-P.T. and C.-H.H.; Formal analysis, C.-P.T.; Methodology, T.-L.L.; Software, C.-H.H.; Writing—original draft, C.-P.T.; Writing—review & editing, T.-L.L. All authors have read and agreed to the published version of the manuscript.

Funding: This research was funded by Dalin Tzu Chi Hospital, Buddhist Tzu Chi Medical Foundation, grant number DTCRD 111-I-14.

Institutional Review Board Statement: The study was conducted in accordance with the Declaration of Helsinki, and approved by the Institutional Review Board of Dalin Tzu Chi Hospital (protocol code B11004010 approved on 24 November 2021).

Informed Consent Statement: Not applicable.

Conflicts of Interest: The authors declare no conflict of interest.

References

1. Zauber, A.G.; Winawer, S.J.; O'Brien, M.J.; Lansdorp-Vogelaar, I.; van Ballegooijen, M.; Hankey, B.F.; Shi, W.; Bond, J.H.; Schapiro, M.; Panish, J.F. Colonoscopic polypectomy and long-term prevention of colorectal-cancer deaths. *N. Engl. J. Med.* **2012**, *366*, 687–696. [CrossRef] [PubMed]
2. Winawer, S.J.; Zauber, A.G.; Ho, M.N.; O'brien, M.J.; Gottlieb, L.S.; Sternberg, S.S.; Waye, J.D.; Schapiro, M.; Bond, J.H.; Panish, J.F. Prevention of colorectal cancer by colonoscopic polypectomy. *N. Engl. J. Med.* **1993**, *329*, 1977–1981. [CrossRef] [PubMed]
3. Duong, A.; Pohl, H.; Djinbachian, R.; Deshêtres, A.; Barkun, A.N.; Marques, P.N.; Bouin, M.; Deslandres, E.; Aguilera-Fish, A.; Leduc, R. Evaluation of the polyp-based resect and discard strategy: A retrospective study. *Endoscopy* **2022**, *54*, 128–135. [CrossRef] [PubMed]
4. Zachariah, R.; Samarasena, J.; Luba, D.; Duh, E.; Dao, T.; Requa, J.; Ninh, A.; Karnes, W. Prediction of Polyp Pathology Using Convolutional Neural Networks Achieves 'Resect and Discard' Thresholds. *Am. J. Gastroenterol.* **2020**, *115*, 138. [CrossRef]
5. Rex, D.K.; Cutler, C.S.; Lemmel, G.T.; Rahmani, E.Y.; Clark, D.W.; Helper, D.J.; Lehman, G.A.; Mark, D.G. Colonoscopic miss rates of adenomas determined by back-to-back colonoscopies. *Gastroenterology* **1997**, *112*, 24–28. [CrossRef]
6. Van Rijn, J.C.; Reitsma, J.B.; Stoker, J.; Bossuyt, P.M.; Van Deventer, S.J.; Dekker, E. Polyp miss rate determined by tandem colonoscopy: A systematic review. *Off. J. Am. Coll. Gastroenterol. ACG* **2006**, *101*, 343–350. [CrossRef]
7. Zhang, R.; Zheng, Y.; Mak, T.W.C.; Yu, R.; Wong, S.H.; Lau, J.Y.; Poon, C.C. Automatic detection and classification of colorectal polyps by transferring low-level CNN features from nonmedical domain. *IEEE J. Biomed. Health Inform.* **2016**, *21*, 41–47. [CrossRef]
8. Tang, C.-P.; Chen, K.-H.; Lin, T.-L. Computer-Aided Colon Polyp Detection on High Resolution Colonoscopy Using Transfer Learning Techniques. *Sensors* **2021**, *21*, 5315. [CrossRef]
9. Tang, C.-P.; Shao, P.P.; Hsieh, Y.-H.; Leung, F.W. A review of water exchange and artificial intelligence in improving adenoma detection. *Tzu-Chi Med. J.* **2021**, *33*, 108.
10. Alharbi, O.R.; Alballa, N.S.; AlRajeh, A.S.; Alturki, L.S.; Alfuraih, I.M.; Jamalaldeen, M.R.; Almadi, M.A. Use of image-enhanced endoscopy in the characterization of colorectal polyps: Still some ways to go. *Saudi J. Gastroenterol. Off. J. Saudi Gastroenterol. Assoc.* **2019**, *25*, 89.
11. Gupta, N.; Bansal, A.; Rao, D.; Early, D.S.; Jonnalagadda, S.; Edmundowicz, S.A.; Sharma, P.; Rastogi, A. Accuracy of in vivo optical diagnosis of colon polyp histology by narrow-band imaging in predicting colonoscopy surveillance intervals. *Gastrointest. Endosc.* **2012**, *75*, 494–502. [CrossRef]
12. Ikematsu, H.; Saito, Y.; Tanaka, S.; Uraoka, T.; Sano, Y.; Horimatsu, T.; Matsuda, T.; Oka, S.; Higashi, R.; Ishikawa, H. The impact of narrow band imaging for colon polyp detection: A multicenter randomized controlled trial by tandem colonoscopy. *J. Gastroenterol.* **2012**, *47*, 1099–1107. [CrossRef]

13. Vișovan, I.I.; Tanțău, M.; Pascu, O.; Ciobanu, L.; Tanțău, A. The role of narrow band imaging in colorectal polyp detection. *Bosn. J. Basic Med. Sci.* **2017**, *17*, 152. [CrossRef]
14. East, J.E.; Suzuki, N.; Saunders, B.P. Comparison of magnified pit pattern interpretation with narrow band imaging versus chromoendoscopy for diminutive colonic polyps: A pilot study. *Gastrointest. Endosc.* **2007**, *66*, 310–316. [CrossRef]
15. Machida, H.; Sano, Y.; Hamamoto, Y.; Muto, M.; Kozu, T.; Tajiri, H.; Yoshida, S. Narrow-band imaging in the diagnosis of colorectal mucosal lesions: A pilot study. *Endoscopy* **2004**, *36*, 1094–1098. [CrossRef]
16. Ogiso, K.; Yoshida, N.; Siah, K.T.H.; Kitae, H.; Murakami, T.; Hirose, R.; Inada, Y.; Dohi, O.; Okayama, T.; Kamada, K. New-generation narrow band imaging improves visibility of polyps: A colonoscopy video evaluation study. *J. Gastroenterol.* **2016**, *51*, 883–890. [CrossRef]
17. Horimatsu, T.; Sano, Y.; Tanaka, S.; Kawamura, T.; Saito, S.; Iwatate, M.; Oka, S.; Uno, K.; Yoshimura, K.; Ishikawa, H. Next-generation narrow band imaging system for colonic polyp detection: A prospective multicenter randomized trial. *Int. J. Colorectal Dis.* **2015**, *30*, 947–954. [CrossRef]
18. Ng, S.C.; Lau, J.Y. Narrow-band imaging in the colon: Limitations and potentials. *J. Gastroenterol. Hepatol.* **2011**, *26*, 1589–1596. [CrossRef]
19. Pizer, S.M.; Amburn, E.P.; Austin, J.D.; Cromartie, R.; Geselowitz, A.; Greer, T.; ter Haar Romeny, B.; Zimmerman, J.B.; Zuiderveld, K. Adaptive histogram equalization and its variations. *Comput. Vis. Graph. Image Process.* **1987**, *39*, 355–368. [CrossRef]
20. Stark, J.A. Adaptive image contrast enhancement using generalizations of histogram equalization. *IEEE Trans. Image Process.* **2000**, *9*, 889–896. [CrossRef]
21. Reza, A.M. Realization of the contrast limited adaptive histogram equalization (CLAHE) for real-time image enhancement. *J. VLSI Signal Process. Syst. Signal. Image Video Technol.* **2004**, *38*, 35–44. [CrossRef]
22. Xiao, Y.; Decencière, E.; Velasco-Forero, S.; Burdin, H.; Bornschlögl, T.; Bernerd, F.; Warrick, E.; Baldeweck, T. A new color augmentation method for deep learning segmentation of histological images. In Proceedings of the 2019 IEEE 16th International Symposium on Biomedical Imaging (ISBI 2019), Venice, Italy, 8–11 April 2019; pp. 886–890.
23. Rahman, Z.-U.; Jobson, D.J.; Woodell, G.A. Multi-scale retinex for color image enhancement. In Proceedings of the 3rd IEEE International Conference on Image Processing, Lausanne, Switzerland, 19 September 1996; pp. 1003–1006.
24. Wang, L.; Xiao, L.; Liu, H.; Wei, Z. Variational Bayesian method for retinex. *IEEE Trans. Image Process.* **2014**, *23*, 3381–3396. [CrossRef]
25. Ng, M.K.; Wang, W. A total variation model for Retinex. *SIAM J. Imaging Sci.* **2011**, *4*, 345–365. [CrossRef]
26. Provenzi, E.; Fierro, M.; Rizzi, A.; De Carli, L.; Gadia, D.; Marini, D. Random spray Retinex: A new Retinex implementation to investigate the local properties of the model. *IEEE Trans. Image Process.* **2006**, *16*, 162–171. [CrossRef]
27. Sato, T. TXI: Texture and color enhancement imaging for endoscopic image enhancement. *J. Healthc. Eng.* **2021**, *2021*, 5518948. [CrossRef]
28. Galdran, A.; Alvarez-Gila, A.; Bria, A.; Vazquez-Corral, J.; Bertalmío, M. On the duality between retinex and image dehazing. In Proceedings of the IEEE Conference on Computer Vision and Pattern Recognition, Salt Lake City, UT, USA, 18–23 June 2018; pp. 8212–8221.
29. Luo, X.; McLeod, A.J.; Pautler, S.E.; Schlachta, C.M.; Peters, T.M. Vision-based surgical field defogging. *IEEE Trans. Med. Imaging* **2017**, *36*, 2021–2030. [CrossRef]
30. McCann, J.J. Retinex at 50: Color theory and spatial algorithms, a review. *J. Electron. Imaging* **2017**, *26*, 031204. [CrossRef]
31. Vani, V.; Prashanth, K.M. Color image enhancement techniques in Wireless Capsule Endoscopy. In Proceedings of the 2015 International Conference on Trends in Automation, Communications and Computing Technology (I-TACT-15), Bangalore, India, 21–22 December 2015; pp. 1–6.
32. Luo, X.; Zeng, H.-Q.; Wan, Y.; Zhang, X.-B.; Du, Y.-P.; Peters, T.M. Endoscopic vision augmentation using multiscale bilateral-weighted retinex for robotic surgery. *IEEE Trans. Med. Imaging* **2019**, *38*, 2863–2874. [CrossRef]
33. Wang, W.; Chen, Z.; Yuan, X.; Wu, X. Adaptive image enhancement method for correcting low-illumination images. *Inf. Sci.* **2019**, *496*, 25–41. [CrossRef]
34. Deeba, F.; Mohammed, S.K.; Bui, F.M.; Wahid, K.A. Unsupervised abnormality detection using saliency and retinex based color enhancement. In Proceedings of the 2016 38th Annual International Conference of the IEEE Engineering in Medicine and Biology Society (EMBC), Orlando, FL, USA, 16–20 August 2016; pp. 3871–3874.
35. Braun, G.J.; Fairchild, M.D. Image lightness rescaling using sigmoidal contrast enhancement functions. *J. Electron. Imaging* **1999**, *8*, 380–393. [CrossRef]
36. Nguyen-Thi, K.-N.; Che-Ngoc, H.; Pham-Chau, A.-T. An efficient image contrast enhancement method using sigmoid function and differential evolution. *J. Adv. Eng. Comput.* **2020**, *4*, 162–172. [CrossRef]
37. Deeba, F.; Bui, F.M.; Wahid, K.A. Computer-aided polyp detection based on image enhancement and saliency-based selection. *Biomed. Signal Process. Control.* **2020**, *55*, 101530. [CrossRef]
38. Jobson, D.J.; Rahman, Z.-u.; Woodell, G.A. A multiscale retinex for bridging the gap between color images and the human observation of scenes. *IEEE Trans. Image Process.* **1997**, *6*, 965–976. [CrossRef] [PubMed]
39. Parthasarathy, S.; Sankaran, P. An automated multi scale retinex with color restoration for image enhancement. In Proceedings of the 2012 National Conference on Communications (NCC), Kharagpur, India, 3–5 February 2012; pp. 1–5.
40. Bochkovskiy, A.; Wang, C.-Y.; Liao, H.-Y.M. Yolov4: Optimal speed and accuracy of object detection. *arXiv* **2020**, arXiv:2004.10934.
41. Redmon, J.; Farhadi, A. Yolov3: An incremental improvement. *arXiv* **2018**, arXiv:1804.02767.

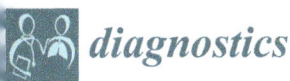

Article

Performance of a Deep Learning System for Automatic Diagnosis of Protruding Lesions in Colon Capsule Endoscopy

Miguel Mascarenhas [1,2,3,*,†], João Afonso [1,2,†], Tiago Ribeiro [1,2], Hélder Cardoso [1,2,3], Patrícia Andrade [1,2,3], João P. S. Ferreira [4,5], Miguel Mascarenhas Saraiva [6] and Guilherme Macedo [1,2,3]

1. Department of Gastroenterology, São João University Hospital, Alameda Professor Hernâni Monteiro, 4200-427 Porto, Portugal; joaoafonso28@gmail.com (J.A.); tiagofcribeiro@outlook.pt (T.R.); hc@sapo.pt (H.C.); anapatriciarandrade@gmail.com (P.A.); guilhermemacedo59@gmail.com (G.M.)
2. WGO Gastroenterology and Hepatology Training Center, 4200-427 Porto, Portugal
3. Faculty of Medicine of the University of Porto, Alameda Professor Hernâni Monteiro, 4200-427 Porto, Portugal
4. Department of Mechanical Engineering, Faculty of Engineering of the University of Porto, Rua Dr. Roberto Frias, 4200-465 Porto, Portugal; j.ferreira@fe.up.pt
5. INEGI—Institute of Science and Innovation in Mechanical and Industrial Engineering, Rua Dr. Roberto Frias, 4200-465 Porto, Portugal
6. ManopH Gastroenterology Clinic, Rua Sá da Bandeira 752, 4000-432 Porto, Portugal; miguelms.manoph@gmail.com
* Correspondence: miguelmascarenhassaraiva@gmail.com
† These authors contributed equally to this work.

Abstract: Background: Colon capsule endoscopy (CCE) is an alternative for patients unwilling or with contraindications for conventional colonoscopy. Colorectal cancer screening may benefit greatly from widespread acceptance of a non-invasive tool such as CCE. However, reviewing CCE exams is a time-consuming process, with risk of overlooking important lesions. We aimed to develop an artificial intelligence (AI) algorithm using a convolutional neural network (CNN) architecture for automatic detection of colonic protruding lesions in CCE images. An anonymized database of CCE images collected from a total of 124 patients was used. This database included images of patients with colonic protruding lesions or patients with normal colonic mucosa or with other pathologic findings. A total of 5715 images were extracted for CNN development. Two image datasets were created and used for training and validation of the CNN. The AUROC for detection of protruding lesions was 0.99. The sensitivity, specificity, PPV and NPV were 90.0%, 99.1%, 98.6% and 93.2%, respectively. The overall accuracy of the network was 95.3%. The developed deep learning algorithm accurately detected protruding lesions in CCE images. The introduction of AI technology to CCE may increase its diagnostic accuracy and acceptance for screening of colorectal neoplasia.

Keywords: colon capsule endoscopy; artificial intelligence; convolutional neural network; colorectal neoplasia

1. Introduction

Capsule endoscopy (CE) is a primary diagnostic tool for the investigation of patients with suspected small bowel disease. Colon capsule endoscopy has been recently introduced as a minimally invasive alternative to conventional colonoscopy for evaluation of the colonic mucosa [1,2]. This system allows overcoming some of the drawbacks associated with conventional colonoscopy, including the potential for pain, use of sedation, and the risk of adverse events, including bleeding and perforation [3]. The clinical application of this tool has been most extensively studied in the setting of colorectal cancer screening, particularly for patients with previous incomplete colonoscopy, or for whom the latter exam is contraindicated, unfeasible or unwanted [4,5]. The role of CCE as an alternative to conventional colonoscopy in the setting of colorectal cancer screening is growing. A recent meta-analysis by Vuik and coworkers reported similar performance levels for conventional colonoscopy and CCE as well as the superiority of CCE compared to computed tomography colonography (virtual colonoscopy) [6]. Moreover, a single full-length CCE video may produce over 50,000 images, and reviewing these images is a monotonous and time-consuming task, requiring approximately 50 min for completion [2]. Furthermore, any given frame may capture only a fragment of a mucosal abnormality and lesions may be depicted in a very small number of frames. Therefore, the risk of overlooking important lesions is not insignificant [2].

The combination of enhanced computational power with large clinical datasets has potentiated the research and development of AI tools for clinical implementation. The application of automated algorithms to diverse medical fields has provided promising results regarding disease identification and classification [7–9]. Convolutional neural networks (CNN) are a type of multi-layered deep learning algorithm tailored for image analysis. The application of these technological solutions to small bowel CE has provided promising results in the detection of several types of lesions [10–13]. The introduction of AI tools for real-time detection of colorectal neoplasia in conventional colonoscopy has suggested a high diagnostic yield for CNN-based algorithms [14]. The impact of AI algorithms for detection of colorectal neoplasia in CCE images has been scarcely evaluated. Enhanced reading of CCE images through the application of these tools may improve the diagnostic accuracy of CCE for colorectal neoplasia, which is currently unsatisfactory [2]. Importantly, the implementation of automated algorithms may help to reduce the time required for reading a single CCE exam. The aim of this study was to develop and validate a CNN-based algorithm for the automatic detection of colonic protruding lesions using CCE images.

2. Materials and Methods

2.1. Study Design

A multicenter study was performed for development and validation of a CNN for automatic detection of colonic protruding lesions. CCE images were retrospectively collected from two different institutions: São João University Hospital (Porto, Portugal) and ManopH Gastroenterology Clinic (Porto, Portugal). One hundred and twenty-four CCE exams (124 patients, 24 from São João University Hospital and 100 from ManopH Gastroenterology Clinic), performed between 2010 and 2020, were included. The full-length video of all participants was reviewed, and a total of 5715 frames of the colonic mucosa were ultimately extracted. Significant frames were included regardless of image quality and bowel cleansing quality. Inclusion and classification of frames were performed by three gastroenterologists with experience in CCE (Miguel Mascarenhas, Hélder Cardoso and Miguel Mascarenhas Saraiva), each with an experience of >1500 CE previous to this study. A final decision on frame labelling required the agreement of at least two of the three researchers.

This study was approved by the ethics committee of São João University Hospital (No. CE 407/2020). The study protocol was conducted respecting the original and subsequent revisions of the declaration of Helsinki. This study is retrospective and of non-interventional nature. Thus, the output provided by the CNN had no influence on the clinical management of each included patient. Any information susceptible to identify the included patients was omitted, and each patient was assigned a random number in order to guarantee effective data anonymization for researchers involved in CNN development. A team with Data Protection Officer (DPO) certification (Maastricht University) confirmed the non-traceability of data and conformity with the general data protection regulation (GDPR).

2.1.1. Colon Capsule Endoscopy Procedure

For all patients, CCE procedures were conducted using the *PillCam*™ COLON 2 system (Medtronic, Minneapolis, MN, USA). This system consists of three major components: the endoscopic capsule, an array of sensors connected to a data recorder, and a software for frame revision. The capsule measures 32.3 mm in length and 11.6 mm in width. It has

2 high-resolution cameras, each with a 172° angle of view. The system frame rate varied automatically between 4 and 35 frames per second, depending on bowel motility. Each frame had a resolution of 512 × 512 pixels. The battery of the endoscopic capsule has an estimated life of ≥10 h [2]. This system was launched in 2009 and was not submitted to hardware updates since then. Thus, no significant changes in image quality were evident during this period. The images were reviewed using *PillCam*™ software version 9.0 (Medtronic, Minneapolis, MN, USA). Each frame was processed in order to remove information allowing patient identification (name, operating number, date of procedure).

Each patient received bowel preparation according to previously published guidelines [15]. Summarily, patients initiated a clear liquid diet in the day preceding capsule ingestion, with fasting in the night before examination. A solution consisting of polyethylene glycol was used in split-dosage (2 L in the evening and 2 L in the morning of capsule ingestion). Prokinetic therapy (10 mg domperidone) was used if the capsule remained in the stomach 1 h after ingestion, upon real-time image review on the recorder. Two boosters consisting of a sodium phosphate solution were applied after the capsule has entered the small bowel and with a 3 h interval. Only complete CCE exams were included. A complete exam was considered if the capsule was excreted.

2.1.2. Development of the Convolutional Neural Network

A deep learning CNN was developed for automatic detection of colonic protruding lesions. Protruding lesions included all polyps, epithelial tumors, and subepithelial lesions. From the collected pool of images (n = 5715), 2410 showed protruding lesions and 3305 displayed normal mucosa or other mucosal lesions (ulcers, erosions, red spots, angiectasia, varices and lymphangiectasia). This pool of images was split for constitution of training and validation image datasets. The training dataset was composed by 80% of the consecutively extracted images (n = 4572). The remaining 20% were used as the validation dataset (n = 1143). The validation dataset was used for assessing the performance of the CNN (Figure 1).

To create the CNN, we modified the *Xception* model with its weights trained on *ImageNet* (a large-scale image dataset aimed for use in development of object recognition software). To transfer this learning to our data, we kept the convolutional layers of the model. We replaced the last fully connected layers with 2 dense layers of size 2048 and 1024, respectively, and then attached a fully connected layer based on the number of classes we used to classify our endoscopic images. To avoid overfitting, a dropout layer of 0.3 drop rate was added between convolutional and classification components of the network. We applied gradient-weighted class activation mapping on the last convolutional layer [16], in order to highlight important features for predicting protruding lesions. The size of each image was set for 300 pixels of height and width. The learning rate of 0.0001, batch size of 128 and the number of epochs of 30 was set by trial and error. We used Tensorflow 2.3 and Keras libraries to prepare the data and run the model. The analyses were performed with a computer equipped with a 2.1 GHz Intel® Xeon® Gold 6130 processor (Intel, Santa Clara, CA, USA) and a double NVIDIA Quadro® RTX™ 8000 graphic processing unit (NVIDIA Corporate, Santa Clara, CA, USA).

2.1.3. Model Performance and Statistical Analysis

The primary outcome measures included sensitivity, specificity, positive and negative predictive values, and accuracy. Moreover, we used receiver operating characteristic (ROC) curve analysis and area under the ROC curve (AUROC) to measure the performance of our model in the distinction between the categories. For each image, the trained CNN calculated the probability for each of the categories (protruding lesions vs. normal colonic mucosa or other findings). A higher probability value translated in a greater confidence in the CNN prediction. The software generated heatmaps that localized features that predicted a class probability (Figure 2A). The category with the highest probability score was outputted as the CNN's predicted classification (Figure 2B). The output provided by the network was compared to the specialists' classification (*gold standard*). We performed a 3-fold cross validation. Therefore, the entire dataset was split into 3 even-sized image groups. Training and validation datasets were created for each of the five groups, at a proportion of 80% and 20% for training and validation datasets, respectively. Sensitivities, specificities, positive and negative predictive values are presented as means ± standard deviations (SD). Additionally, the image processing performance of the network was determined by calculating the time required for the CNN to provide output for all images in the validation image dataset. Sensitivities, specificities, positive and negative predictive values were obtained using one iteration and are presented as percentages. Statistical analysis was performed using Sci-Kit learn v0.22.2 [17].

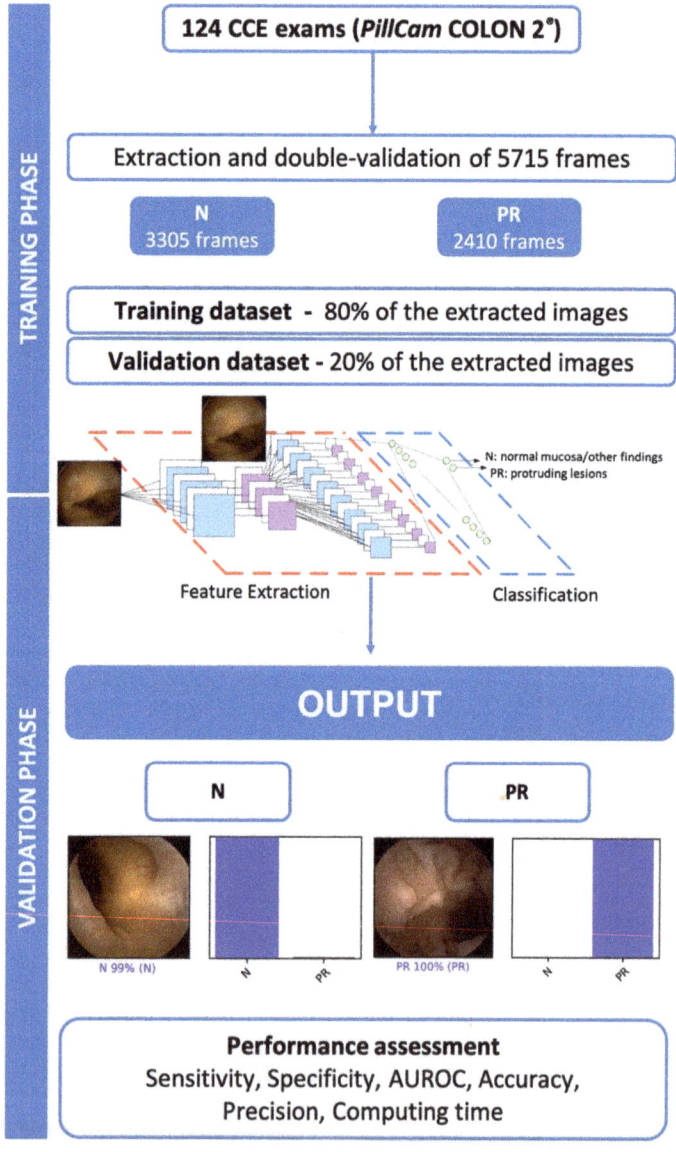

Figure 1. Summary of study design for the training and validation phases. PR—protruding lesion; N—normal mucosa or other findings.

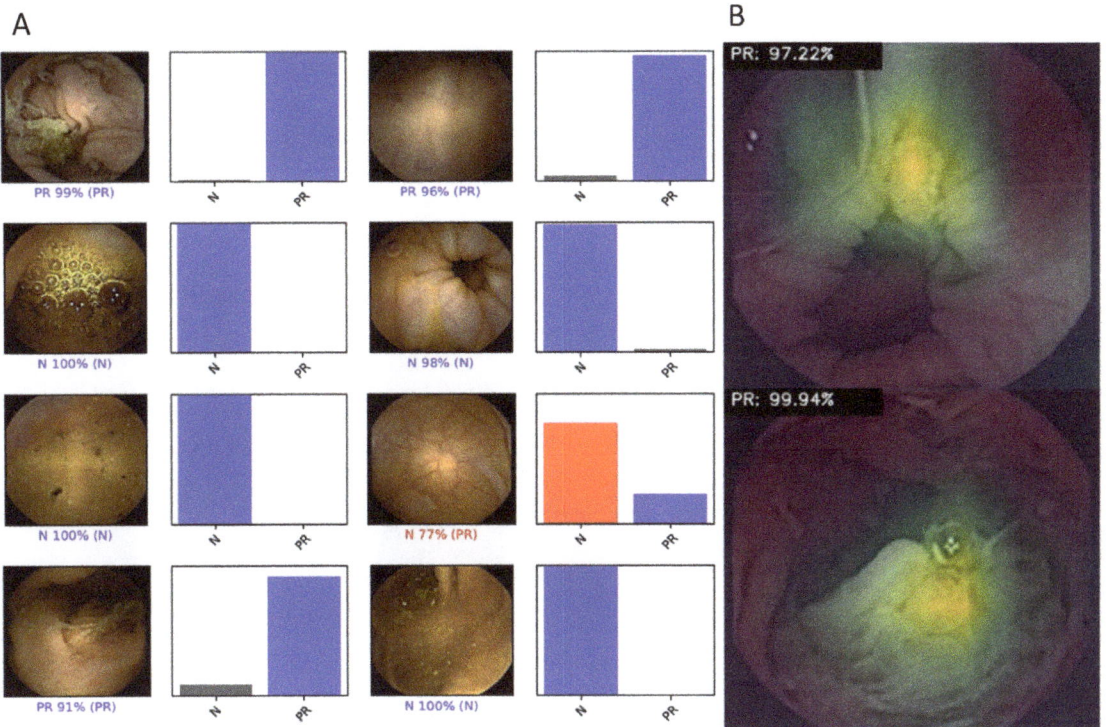

Figure 2. Heatmaps (**A**) and output (**B**) obtained from the application of the convolutional neural network. (**A**) Examples of heatmaps showing CCE features of protruding lesions as identified by the CNN. (**B**) The bars represent the probability estimated by the network.

3. Results

3.1. Construction of the Network

One hundred and twenty-four patients were submitted to CCE and enrolled in this study. A total of 5715 frames were extracted, 2410 showing protruding lesions (2303 polyps, 8 subepithelial lesions and 99 epithelial tumors) and 3305 showing normal colonic mucosa or other findings. The training dataset was constituted by 80% of the total image pool. The remaining 20% of frames (n = 1143) were used for testing the model. This validation dataset was composed by 482 (42.2%) images with evidence of protruding lesions and 661 (57.8%) images with normal colonic mucosa/other findings. The CNN evaluated each image and predicted a classification (protruding lesions vs. normal mucosa/other lesions), which was compared with the classification provided by gastroenterologists. Repeated inputs of data to the CNN resulted in the improvement of its accuracy (Figure 3).

3.2. Overall Performance of the Network

The confusion matrix between the trained CNN and expert classifications is shown in Table 1. Overall, the developed model had a sensitivity and specificity for the detection of protruding lesions of 90.0% and 99.1%, respectively. The positive and negative predictive values were, respectively, 98.6% and 93.2%. The overall accuracy of the network was 95.3% (Table 1). The AUROC for detection of protruding lesions was 0.99 (Figure 4).

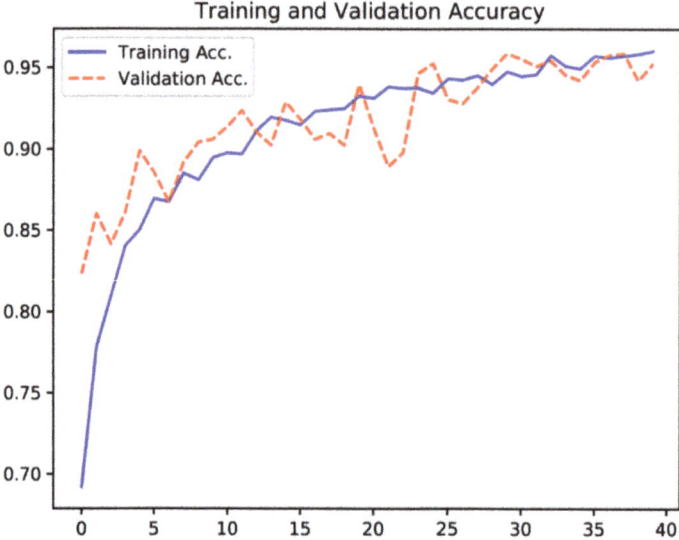

Figure 3. Evolution of the accuracy of the convolutional neural network during training and validation phases, as the training and validation datasets were repeatedly inputted in the neural network.

Table 1. Confusion matrix and performance marks.

			Expert Classification	
			Protruding Lesion	Normal Mucosa
CNN classification		Protruding lesion	434	6
		Normal mucosa	48	655
		Sensitivity	90.0%	
		Specificity	99.1%	
		PPV	98.6%	
		NPV	93.2%	
		Accuracy	95.3%	

Abbreviations: CNN—convolutional neural network; PPV—positive predictive value; NPV—negative predictive value.

We performed a 3-fold cross validation, where the entire dataset was randomized and split in 3 equivalent parts. The performance results for the three experiments are shown in Table 2. Overall, the estimated model accuracy was 95.6 ± 1.1%. The mean sensitivity and specificity of the model were 87.4 ± 4.6% and 96.1 ± 1.4%. The algorithm had a mean AUC of 0.976 ± 0.006.

3.3. Computational Performance of the CNN

The CNN completed the reading of the testing dataset in 17.5 s (approximately 15.4 ms/frame). This translates into an approximated reading rate of 65 frames per second. At this rate, the CNN would complete the revision of a full-length CCE video containing an estimate of 50,000 frames in approximately 13 min.

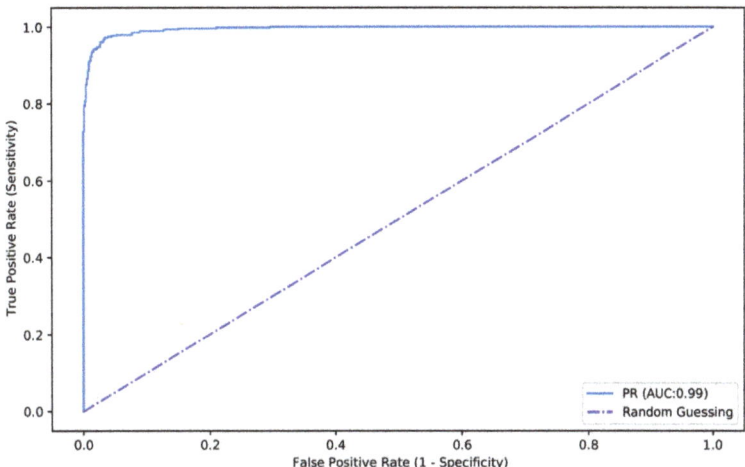

Figure 4. ROC analyses of the network's performance in the detection of protruding lesions vs. normal colonic mucosa/other findings. ROC—receiver operator characteristics. PR—protruding lesion.

Table 2. Three-fold cross validation.

	Sensitivity (%)	Specificity (%)	PPV (%)	NPV (%)	Accuracy (%)	AUC
Fold 1	82.8	97.5	62.6	99.1	96.9	0.980
Fold 2	87.4	95.9	57.1	99.2	95.4	0.970
Fold 3	92.1	94.7	48.4	99.6	94.6	0.980
Overall, mean (±SD)	87.4 ± 4.6	96.1 ± 1.4	56.0 ± 7.1	99.3 ± 0.2	95.6 ± 1.1	0.976 ± 0.006

Abbreviations: ±SD—±standard deviation; PPV—positive predictive value; NPV—negative predictive value; AUC—area under the receiving operator characteristics curve.

4. Discussion

The exploration of AI algorithms for application to conventional endoscopic techniques for automatic detection of colorectal neoplasia has been producing promising results over the last decade. The development and implementation of these systems has been recently endorsed (although with limitations) by the European Society of Gastrointestinal Endoscopy [18]. Furthermore, a recent meta-analysis has suggested that the application of AI models for adenoma and polyp's identification may substantially increase the adenoma detection rate and the number of adenomas detected per colonoscopy [19]. These improvements in commonly used performance metrics have shown not to be affected by factors known to influence detection by the human eye, including the size and morphology of the lesions [19]. Artificial intelligence is expected to play a major role in improving the acceptability and the diagnostic yield of CCE [20]. These systems may help in several steps of the CCE process, from predicting the quality of colon cleanliness, lesion detection and the distinction of colorectal lesions [20–22].

In our study, we have developed a deep learning tool based on a CNN architecture for automatic detection of protruding lesions in the colonic lumen using CCE images. This study has several highlights. First, our model demonstrated high levels of performance, with a sensitivity of 90.0%, a specificity of 99.1, an accuracy of 95.3% and an AUROC of 0.99. Obtaining fairly high levels of sensitivity and negative predictive value is paramount for CNN-assisted reading systems, which are designed to lessen the probability of missing lesions, while maintaining a high specificity. Third, our network had a remarkable image processing performance, being capable of reading 65 images per second.

The precise role of CCE in everyday clinical practice is yet to be defined. Thus far, most studies highlight its potential when applied in the setting of colorectal cancer screening. Although colonoscopy remains the undisputed *gold standard*, studies have suggested that CCE could be viewed as a non-invasive complement, rather than substitutive of conventional colonoscopy, particularly in the setting of a previous incomplete colonoscopy [23]. Current guidelines on colorectal cancer screening list CCE as a valid alternative to colonoscopy for the screening of an average-risk population [15]. Studies comparing the diagnostic yield of CCE with another non-invasive screening test, CT colonography, have shown the superiority of CCE [24]. Moreover, when following a first positive fecal-immunological test, CCE may reduce the need for more invasive conventional colonoscopy [25]. Although conflicting evidence exist, some studies have shown that adoption of CCE as a screening method may lead to a higher uptake rate compared to conventional colonoscopy [26]. Moreover, CCE may not only be seen as an alternative to conventional colonoscopy but rather as a complementary solution in programmed screening settings. Indeed, CCE may help to shorten waiting lists, decrease hospital appointments and make screening available to remote areas [27]. In this setting, the cost-effectiveness of CCE appears to be greater when the prevalence of colorectal cancer is lower and the uptake rate is superior to that of conventional colonoscopy [28]. However, the use of CCE is hampered by its purely diagnostic character, the need for a rigorous bowel cleansing protocol, as well as the time required for reading each CCE exam.

The development of AI tools for detection of colorectal neoplasia in CCE images has been poorly explored. Automatic detection of these lesions is limited by the poor resolution of CCE images combined with their variable morphology, size and color. To our knowledge, only two other studies have assessed the potential of the application of CNN models to CCE images. Yamada et al. was the first to explore the implementation of AI algorithms for the identification of colorectal neoplasia in frames extracted from CCE exams. Their network was developed using a relatively large pool of CCE images (17,783 frames from 178 patients). Overall, their algorithm achieved a good performance (AUROC of 0.90) [29]. However, the sensitivity of their model was modest (79%) compared to that of our network. Blanes-Vidal et al. adapted a preexisting CNN (*AlexNet*) and trained it for the detection of colorectal polyps. The sensitivity, specificity and accuracy expressed in their paper were 97%, 93% and 96%, respectively. In our perspective, the development of these technologies should aim to support a clinical decision rather than substitute the role of the clinician. Therefore, these systems must remain highly sensitive in order to minimize the risk of missing lesions.

Our network demonstrated a high image processing performance (65 frames/second). To date, no value for comparison exists regarding CCE. Nevertheless, these performance marks exceed those published for CNNs applied to other CE systems [11,30]. The development of highly efficient networks may, in the near future, translate into shorter reading times, thus overcoming one of the main drawbacks of CCE. Further well-designed studies are required to assess if a high image processing capacity in experimental settings can be reproduced as an enhanced time efficiency regarding reading times of CCE exams comparing to conventional reading. The combination of enhanced diagnostic accuracy and time efficiency may have a pivotal role in widening the indications for CCE and its acceptance as a valid screening and diagnostic tool.

This study has several limitations. First, it is a retrospective study. Therefore, further prospective multicentric studies in a real-life setting are desirable to confirm the clinical value of our results. Second, although we included a large number of patients from two distinct medical centers, the number of extracted images is small. This limited number of extracted images was mainly dictated by the low number of frames showing protruding lesions. In order to produce a balanced dataset while minimizing the risk of missing lesions, an equilibrium between the number of images showing protruding lesions and normal mucosa was fostered. This may partially explain the suboptimal sensitivity. We are currently expanding our image pool in order to increase the robustness of our model, thus contributing to decrease the rate of false negative CE exams, which should be one of the main endpoints in developing these algorithms. The multicentric nature of our work reinforces the validity of our results. Nevertheless, multicentric studies including larger populations are required to ensure the clinical significance of our findings. Moreover, future studies for clinical validation of these tools must contemplate the comparison of performance between AI software and conventional colonoscopy, the *gold standard* technique for the detection and characterization of these lesions.

In conclusion, we developed a highly sensitive and specific CNN-based model for detection of protruding lesions in CCE images. We believe that the implementation of AI tools to clinical practice will be a crucial step for wider acceptance of CCE for non-invasive screening and diagnosis of colorectal neoplasia. Future studies should assess the impact of AI algorithms in mitigating the limitations of CCE in a real-life clinical setting, particularly the time required for reviewing each exam, as well as evaluate the potential benefits in terms of diagnostic yield.

Author Contributions: M.M.—study design, revision of videos, image extraction and labelling and construction and development of the Convolutional Neural Network (CNN), data interpretation. J.A.—study design, organization of patient database, image extraction, organization of the dataset, construction and development of the Convolutional Neural Network (CNN), data interpretation and drafting of the manuscript. T.R.—study design, construction and development of the CNN, bibliographic review, drafting of the manuscript. H.C.—study design, revision of videos, image extraction and labelling, data interpretation. P.A.—study design, data interpretation, drafting of the manuscript. J.P.S.F.—study design, construction and development of the CNN, statistical analysis. M.M.S.—study design, revision of scientific content of the manuscript. G.M.—study design, revision of scientific content of the manuscript. All authors have read and agreed to the published version of the manuscript.

Funding: The authors acknowledge Fundação para a Ciência e Tecnologia (FCT) for supporting the computational costs related to this study through CPCA/A0/7363/2020 grant. This entity had no role in study design, data collection, data analysis, preparation of the manuscript and publishing decision.

Institutional Review Board Statement: The study was conducted in accordance with the Declaration of Helsinki, and approved by the Ethics Committee of São João University Hospital (No. CE 407/2020).

Informed Consent Statement: Informed consent was obtained from all subjects involved in the study.

Conflicts of Interest: The authors declare no conflict of interest.

References

1. Eliakim, R.; Fireman, Z.; Gralnek, I.M.; Yassin, K.; Waterman, M.; Kopelman, Y.; Lachter, J.; Koslowsky, B.; Adler, S.N. Evaluation of the PillCam Colon capsule in the detection of colonic pathology: Results of the first multicenter, prospective, comparative study. *Endoscopy* **2006**, *38*, 963–970. [CrossRef] [PubMed]
2. Eliakim, R.; Yassin, K.; Niv, Y.; Metzger, Y.; Lachter, J.; Gal, E.; Sapoznikov, B.; Konikoff, F.; Leichtmann, G.; Fireman, Z.; et al. Prospective multicenter performance evaluation of the second-generation colon capsule compared with colonoscopy. *Endoscopy* **2009**, *41*, 1026–1031. [CrossRef] [PubMed]
3. Niikura, R.; Yasunaga, H.; Yamada, A.; Matsui, H.; Fushimi, K.; Hirata, Y.; Koike, K. Factors predicting adverse events associated with therapeutic colonoscopy for colorectal neoplasia: A retrospective nationwide study in Japan. *Gastrointest. Endosc.* **2016**, *84*, 971–982.e976. [CrossRef] [PubMed]
4. Spada, C.; Hassan, C.; Bellini, D.; Burling, D.; Cappello, G.; Carretero, C.; Dekker, E.; Eliakim, R.; de Haan, M.; Kaminski, M.F.; et al. Imaging alternatives to colonoscopy: CT colonography and colon capsule. European Society of Gastrointestinal Endoscopy (ESGE) and European Society of Gastrointestinal and Abdominal Radiology (ESGAR) Guideline—Update 2020. *Endoscopy* **2020**, *52*, 1127–1141. [CrossRef]
5. Milluzzo, S.M.; Bizzotto, A.; Cesaro, P.; Spada, C. Colon capsule endoscopy and its effectiveness in the diagnosis and management of colorectal neoplastic lesions. *Exp. Rev. Anticancer Ther.* **2019**, *19*, 71–80. [CrossRef]
6. Vuik, F.E.R.; Nieuwenburg, S.A.V.; Moen, S.; Spada, C.; Senore, C.; Hassan, C.; Pennazio, M.; Rondonotti, E.; Pecere, S.; Kuipers, E.J.; et al. Colon capsule endoscopy in colorectal cancer screening: A systematic review. *Endoscopy* **2021**, *53*, 815–824. [CrossRef]
7. Yasaka, K.; Akai, H.; Abe, O.; Kiryu, S. Deep Learning with Convolutional Neural Network for Differentiation of Liver Masses at Dynamic Contrast-enhanced CT: A Preliminary Study. *Radiology* **2018**, *286*, 887–896. [CrossRef]

8. Esteva, A.; Kuprel, B.; Novoa, R.A.; Ko, J.; Swetter, S.M.; Blau, H.M.; Thrun, S. Dermatologist-level classification of skin cancer with deep neural networks. *Nature* **2017**, *542*, 115–118. [CrossRef]
9. Gargeya, R.; Leng, T. Automated Identification of Diabetic Retinopathy Using Deep Learning. *Ophthalmology* **2017**, *124*, 962–969. [CrossRef]
10. Aoki, T.; Yamada, A.; Aoyama, K.; Saito, H.; Tsuboi, A.; Nakada, A.; Niikura, R.; Fujishiro, M.; Oka, S.; Ishihara, S.; et al. Automatic detection of erosions and ulcerations in wireless capsule endoscopy images based on a deep convolutional neural network. *Gastrointest. Endosc.* **2019**, *89*, 357–363.e352. [CrossRef]
11. Aoki, T.; Yamada, A.; Kato, Y.; Saito, H.; Tsuboi, A.; Nakada, A.; Niikura, R.; Fujishiro, M.; Oka, S.; Ishihara, S.; et al. Automatic detection of blood content in capsule endoscopy images based on a deep convolutional neural network. *J. Gastroenterol. Hepatol.* **2020**, *35*, 1196–1200. [CrossRef] [PubMed]
12. Ding, Z.; Shi, H.; Zhang, H.; Meng, L.; Fan, M.; Han, C.; Zhang, K.; Ming, F.; Xie, X.; Liu, H.; et al. Gastroenterologist-Level Identification of Small-Bowel Diseases and Normal Variants by Capsule Endoscopy Using a Deep-Learning Model. *Gastroenterology* **2019**, *157*, 1044–1054.e1045. [CrossRef] [PubMed]
13. Tsuboi, A.; Oka, S.; Aoyama, K.; Saito, H.; Aoki, T.; Yamada, A.; Matsuda, T.; Fujishiro, M.; Ishihara, S.; Nakahori, M.; et al. Artificial intelligence using a convolutional neural network for automatic detection of small-bowel angioectasia in capsule endoscopy images. *Dig. Endosc.* **2020**, *32*, 382–390. [CrossRef] [PubMed]
14. Repici, A.; Badalamenti, M.; Maselli, R.; Correale, L.; Radaelli, F.; Rondonotti, E.; Ferrara, E.; Spadaccini, M.; Alkandari, A.; Fugazza, A.; et al. Efficacy of Real-Time Computer-Aided Detection of Colorectal Neoplasia in a Randomized Trial. *Gastroenterology* **2020**, *159*, 512–520.e517. [CrossRef]
15. Spada, C.; Hassan, C.; Galmiche, J.P.; Neuhaus, H.; Dumonceau, J.M.; Adler, S.; Epstein, O.; Gay, G.; Pennazio, M.; Rex, D.K.; et al. Colon capsule endoscopy: European Society of Gastrointestinal Endoscopy (ESGE) Guideline. *Endoscopy* **2012**, *44*, 527–536. [CrossRef]
16. Selvaraju, R.R.; Cogswell, M.; Das, A.; Vedantam, R.; Parikh, D.; Batra, D. Grad-cam: Visual explanations from deep networks via gradient-based localization. In Proceedings of the IEEE International Conference on Computer Vision, Venice, Italy, 22–29 October 2017; pp. 618–626.
17. Pedregosa, F.; Varoquaux, G.; Gramfort, A.; Michel, V.; Thirion, B.; Grisel, O.; Blondel, M.; Prettenhofer, P.; Weiss, R.; Dubourg, V.; et al. Scikit-learn: Machine Learning in Python. *J. Mach. Learn. Res.* **2011**, *12*, 2825–2830.
18. Bisschops, R.; East, J.E.; Hassan, C.; Hazewinkel, Y.; Kamiński, M.F.; Neumann, H.; Pellisé, M.; Antonelli, G.; Bustamante Balen, M.; Coron, E.; et al. Advanced imaging for detection and differentiation of colorectal neoplasia: European Society of Gastrointestinal Endoscopy (ESGE) Guideline—Update 2019. *Endoscopy* **2019**, *51*, 1155–1179. [CrossRef]
19. Hassan, C.; Spadaccini, M.; Iannone, A.; Maselli, R.; Jovani, M.; Chandrasekar, V.T.; Antonelli, G.; Yu, H.; Areia, M.; Dinis-Ribeiro, M.; et al. Performance of artificial intelligence in colonoscopy for adenoma and polyp detection: A systematic review and meta-analysis. *Gastrointest. Endosc.* **2021**, *93*, 77–85.e76. [CrossRef]
20. Bjørsum-Meyer, T.; Koulaouzidis, A.; Baatrup, G. Comment on "Artificial intelligence in gastroenterology: A state-of-the-art review". *World J. Gastroenterol.* **2022**, *28*, 1722–1724. [CrossRef]
21. Nakazawa, K.; Nouda, S.; Kakimoto, K.; Kinoshita, N.; Tanaka, Y.; Tawa, H.; Koshiba, R.; Naka, Y.; Hirata, Y.; Ota, K.; et al. The Differential Diagnosis of Colorectal Polyps Using Colon Capsule Endoscopy. *Intern. Med.* **2021**, *60*, 1805–1812. [CrossRef]
22. Yamada, K.; Nakamura, M.; Yamamura, T.; Maeda, K.; Sawada, T.; Mizutani, Y.; Ishikawa, E.; Ishikawa, T.; Kakushima, N.; Furukawa, K.; et al. Diagnostic yield of colon capsule endoscopy for Crohn's disease lesions in the whole gastrointestinal tract. *BMC Gastroenterol.* **2021**, *21*, 75. [CrossRef]
23. Spada, C.; Barbaro, F.; Andrisani, G.; Minelli Grazioli, L.; Hassan, C.; Costamagna, I.; Campanale, M.; Costamagna, G. Colon capsule endoscopy: What we know and what we would like to know. *World J. Gastroenterol.* **2014**, *20*, 16948–16955. [CrossRef] [PubMed]
24. Cash, B.D.; Fleisher, M.R.; Fern, S.; Rajan, E.; Haithcock, R.; Kastenberg, D.M.; Pound, D.; Papageorgiou, N.P.; Fernández-Urién, I.; Schmelkin, I.J.; et al. Multicentre, prospective, randomised study comparing the diagnostic yield of colon capsule endoscopy versus CT colonography in a screening population (the TOPAZ study). *Gut* **2020**, *70*, 2115–2122. [CrossRef] [PubMed]
25. Holleran, G.; Leen, R.; O'Morain, C.; McNamara, D. Colon capsule endoscopy as possible filter test for colonoscopy selection in a screening population with positive fecal immunology. *Endoscopy* **2014**, *46*, 473–478. [CrossRef] [PubMed]
26. Groth, S.; Krause, H.; Behrendt, R.; Hill, H.; Börner, M.; Bastürk, M.; Plathner, N.; Schütte, F.; Gauger, U.; Riemann, J.F.; et al. Capsule colonoscopy increases uptake of colorectal cancer screening. *BMC Gastroenterol.* **2012**, *12*, 80. [CrossRef]
27. Bjoersum-Meyer, T.; Spada, C.; Watson, A.; Eliakim, R.; Baatrup, G.; Toth, E.; Koulaouzidis, A. What holds back colon capsule endoscopy from being the main diagnostic test for the large bowel in cancer screening? *Gastrointest. Endosc.* **2021**, *95*, 168–170. [CrossRef]
28. Hassan, C.; Zullo, A.; Winn, S.; Morini, S. Cost-effectiveness of capsule endoscopy in screening for colorectal cancer. *Endoscopy* **2008**, *40*, 414–421. [CrossRef]

29. Yamada, A.; Niikura, R.; Otani, K.; Aoki, T.; Koike, K. Automatic detection of colorectal neoplasia in wireless colon capsule endoscopic images using a deep convolutional neural network. *Endoscopy* **2020**, *53*, 832–836. [CrossRef]
30. Saito, H.; Aoki, T.; Aoyama, K.; Kato, Y.; Tsuboi, A.; Yamada, A.; Fujishiro, M.; Oka, S.; Ishihara, S.; Matsuda, T.; et al. Automatic detection and classification of protruding lesions in wireless capsule endoscopy images based on a deep convolutional neural network. *Gastrointest. Endosc.* **2020**, *92*, 144–151.e141. [CrossRef]

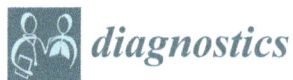 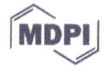

Systematic Review

Artificial Intelligence in Colon Capsule Endoscopy—A Systematic Review

Sarah Moen, Fanny E. R. Vuik, Ernst J. Kuipers and Manon C. W. Spaander *

Department of Gastroenterology and Hepatology, Erasmus MC University Medical Center, 3015 CE Rotterdam, The Netherlands
* Correspondence: v.spaander@erasmusmc.nl; Tel.: +31-(0)-10-7035643; Fax: +31-(0)-10-7035172

Abstract: Background and aims: The applicability of colon capsule endoscopy in daily practice is limited by the accompanying labor-intensive reviewing time and the risk of inter-observer variability. Automated reviewing of colon capsule endoscopy images using artificial intelligence could be timesaving while providing an objective and reproducible outcome. This systematic review aims to provide an overview of the available literature on artificial intelligence for reviewing colonic mucosa by colon capsule endoscopy and to assess the necessary action points for its use in clinical practice. **Methods**: A systematic literature search of literature published up to January 2022 was conducted using Embase, Web of Science, OVID MEDLINE and Cochrane CENTRAL. Studies reporting on the use of artificial intelligence to review second-generation colon capsule endoscopy colonic images were included. **Results**: 1017 studies were evaluated for eligibility, of which nine were included. Two studies reported on computed bowel cleansing assessment, five studies reported on computed polyp or colorectal neoplasia detection and two studies reported on other implications. Overall, the sensitivity of the proposed artificial intelligence models were 86.5–95.5% for bowel cleansing and 47.4–98.1% for the detection of polyps and colorectal neoplasia. Two studies performed per-lesion analysis, in addition to per-frame analysis, which improved the sensitivity of polyp or colorectal neoplasia detection to 81.3–98.1%. By applying a convolutional neural network, the highest sensitivity of 98.1% for polyp detection was found. **Conclusion**: The use of artificial intelligence for reviewing second-generation colon capsule endoscopy images is promising. The highest sensitivity of 98.1% for polyp detection was achieved by deep learning with a convolutional neural network. Convolutional neural network algorithms should be optimized and tested with more data, possibly requiring the set-up of a large international colon capsule endoscopy database. Finally, the accuracy of the optimized convolutional neural network models need to be confirmed in a prospective setting.

Keywords: colon capsule endoscopy; artificial intelligence; polyp detection; bowel cleansing

1. Introduction

Colon Capsule Endoscopy (CCE) provides a promising non-invasive alternative to colonoscopy for exploration of the colonic mucosa [1,2]. It uses an ingestible, wireless, disposable capsule to explore the colon without the need for sedation or gas insufflation. The first generation CCE was introduced in 2006 and a second generation CCE was developed in 2009 (PillCam Colon 2, Medtronic, Minneapolis, MN, USA) [3]. The second generation colon capsule endoscopy (CCE-2) has a high diagnostic accuracy for the detection of colorectal polyps, with a sensitivity of 85% and specificity of 85% for polyps of any size, sensitivity of 87% and specificity of 88% for polyps ≥ 6mm, and a sensitivity of 87% and specificity of 95% for polyps ≥ 10 mm [4].

An important limitation of the applicability of CCE in daily practice is the accompanying labor-intensive reviewing time for the CCE images. A recent study showed a median reading time of 70 min for the entire gastrointestinal tract and 55 min for review of the colon alone [5]. On top of that, agreement in and between different readers may also be

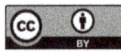

a topic of concern. Literature regarding intra- and inter-observer variability in reviewing CCE images is scarce, but one study demonstrated a poor level of agreement among both expert and beginner readers in determining the indication for follow-up colonoscopy based on the number and size of detected polyps [6]. There was also a poor level of agreement in determining the bowel cleansing quality.

Automated reviewing of CCE images using artificial intelligence (AI) could be timesaving for clinicians while providing an objective and reproducible outcome. AI is a very broad term that describes a computerized approach that includes machine and deep learning methods for interpreting data that normally requires human intelligence [7,8]. Basic AI methods can classify images by computing scores based on features such as texture and color. Machine learning based on pre-defined features is a another AI method used to classify images, where a classifying algorithm is created based on feature classification by experts. An important example of this method is the support vector machine (SVM). Deep learning is a sub-class of machine learning where features do not have to be pre-defined. It is based on a neural network structure that can learn discriminative features from data automatically, giving them the ability to solve very complex problems. Convolutional neural network (CNN) is the most common deep learning algorithm for classifying images. It uses many images to develop and train a classification model by learning rich features and repeating patterns from these images [9].

In colonoscopy, research investigating the use of AI as an aid for the detection of colorectal lesions is already rapidly evolving [10,11]. However, blindly applying the same automated methods to CCE would be blunt due to the differences in the images provided by CCE and colonoscopy. For example, localizing polyps and determining their exact number is more difficult using CCE since the capsule spins around and moves back and forth while the lack of air insufflation causes the intestinal wall to protrude into the lumen, sometimes mimicking polyps. Therefore, a reliable AI method specifically developed for reviewing CCE images is warranted. Some literature is available regarding automated methods for reviewing small bowel capsule endoscopy (SBCE) [7], but literature on AI using CCE is scarce. This systematic review aims to give an overview of the available literature on AI methods for reviewing the colonic mucosa by CCE and assess the necessary action points to evolve AI technology for the use of CCE in daily clinical practice.

2. Methods

A systematic search aiming to retrieve published trials and abstracts reporting on AI using CCE was conducted following the guidelines of the Preferred Reporting Items for Systematic Review and Meta-Analyses (PRISMA) [12]. A systematic search was conducted on literature databases from inception until the 4th of January 2022. Embase, Web of Science, OVID MEDLINE and Cochrane CENTRAL were used as potential sources. The search was conducted using controlled vocabulary supplemented with several key words (Table 1).

In 2006, the first-generation colon capsule (CCE-1) was developed, and in 2011, the second-generation colon capsule (CCE-2) came to the market. New technology was implemented in the second-generation colon capsule: the capsule frame rate increased from 4 to 35 images per second; the angle of view increased from 156° to 172° for each lens and the data recorder was improved. The CCE-2 achieved a substantially higher sensitivity and specificity to detect polyps compared to the first-generation colon capsule [3]. Therefore, studies using CCE-1 were excluded. Two independent reviewers (S.M. and F.E.R.V.) first screened the selected studies by title and abstract. Studies reporting on AI for reviewing CCE-2 colonic images were selected. Included studies could report on the use of AI for the detection of abnormalities, determining the location of the capsule in the colon and assessing bowel cleansing quality. A full-text examination of the selected publications was performed by the same reviewers independently. Reference lists of the included studies were hand-searched to identify potentially relevant studies that were not retrieved in the original search.

Table 1. Systematic literature search. * = *symbol that broadens a search by finding words that start with the same letters.*

Embase.com (1971-)
('capsule endoscopy'/exp OR 'capsule endoscope'/de OR ((capsule * OR videocapsule *) NEAR/3 (endoscop * OR colonoscop *)):ab,ti) AND ('large intestine'/exp OR 'large intestine disease'/exp OR 'large intestine tumor'/exp OR colonoscopy/exp OR (colon * OR colorectal * OR rectal OR rectum OR large-intestin *):ab,ti) AND ('artificial intelligence'/exp OR 'machine learning'/exp OR 'software'/exp OR 'algorithm'/exp OR automation/de OR 'computer analysis'/de OR 'computer assisted diagnosis'/de OR 'image processing'/de OR ((artificial * NEAR/3 intelligen *) OR (machine NEAR/3 learning) OR (compute * NEAR/3 (aided OR assist * OR technique *)) OR software * OR algorithm * OR automat * OR (image NEAR/3 (processing OR matching OR analy *)) OR support-vector * OR svm OR hybrid * OR neural-network * OR autonom * OR (unsupervis * NEAR/3 (learn * OR classif *))):Ab,ti) NOT ([animals]/lim NOT [humans]/lim)
Medline ALL Ovid (1946-)
(Capsule Endoscopy/OR Capsule Endoscopes/OR ((capsule * OR videocapsule *) ADJ3 (endoscop * OR colonoscop *)).ab,ti.) AND (Intestine, Large/OR Colorectal Neoplasms/OR exp Colonoscopy/OR (colon * OR colorectal * OR rectal OR rectum OR large-intestin *).ab,ti.) AND (exp Artificial Intelligence/OR exp Machine Learning/OR Software/OR Algorithms/OR Automation/OR Diagnosis, Computer-Assisted/OR Image Processing, Computer-Assisted/OR ((artificial * ADJ3 intelligen *) OR (machine ADJ3 learning) OR (compute * ADJ3 (aided OR assist * OR technique *)) OR software * OR algorithm * OR automat * OR (image ADJ3 (processing OR matching OR analy *)) OR support-vector * OR svm OR hybrid * OR neural-network * OR autonom * OR (unsupervis * ADJ3 (learn * OR classif *))).ab,ti.) NOT (exp animals/ NOT humans/)
Web of Science Core Collection (1975-)
TS=((((capsule * OR videocapsule *) NEAR/2 (endoscop * OR colonoscop *))) AND ((colon * OR colorectal * OR rectal OR rectum OR large-intestin *)) AND (((artificial * NEAR/2 intelligen *) OR (machine NEAR/2 learning) OR (compute * NEAR/2 (aided OR assist * OR technique *)) OR software * OR algorithm * OR automat * OR (image NEAR/2 (processing OR matching OR analy *)) OR support-vector * OR svm OR hybrid * OR neural-network * OR autonom * OR (unsupervis * NEAR/2 (learn * OR classif *)))))
Cochrane CENTRAL register of Trials (1992-)
((((capsule * OR videocapsule *) NEAR/3 (endoscop * OR colonoscop *)):ab,ti) AND ((colon * OR colorectal * OR rectal OR rectum OR large-intestin *):ab,ti) AND (((artificial * NEAR/3 intelligen *) OR (machine NEAR/3 learning) OR (compute * NEAR/3 (aided OR assist * OR technique *)) OR software * OR algorithm * OR automat * OR (image NEAR/3 (processing OR matching OR analy *)) OR support-vector * OR svm OR hybrid * OR neural-network * OR autonom * OR (unsupervis * NEAR/3 (learn * OR classif *)))):Ab,ti)
Google scholar
"capsule I videocapsule endoscopy I colonoscopy" colon I colonoscopy I colorectal "artificial intelligence" I "machine learning" I "computer aided I assisted" I software I algorithm I automated I "image processing I matching I analysis" I "support vector" I "neural network"

Details regarding the development of the proposed AI models and numbers on the performance of these models were extracted from the final set of included studies. A meta-analysis could not be performed due to the heterogeneity of the study designs.

Quality Assessment of the Included Studies

The quality of the included studies in terms of risk of bias and concerns regarding applicability were independently assessed by two reviewers (S.M. and F.E.R.V.) using the Quality Assessment of Diagnostic Accuracy Studies (QUADAS) -2 assessment tool [13].

3. Results

3.1. Literature Search

After removal of duplicates, retrieved articles were screened for eligibility based on their title and/or abstract (Figure 1). A total of 1017 articles were evaluated for eligibility, after which 903 were excluded. The remaining 114 studies underwent full-text review, after which 105 were excluded for various reasons. No additional studies were retrieved by hand-search. A total of nine studies were included in the final review.

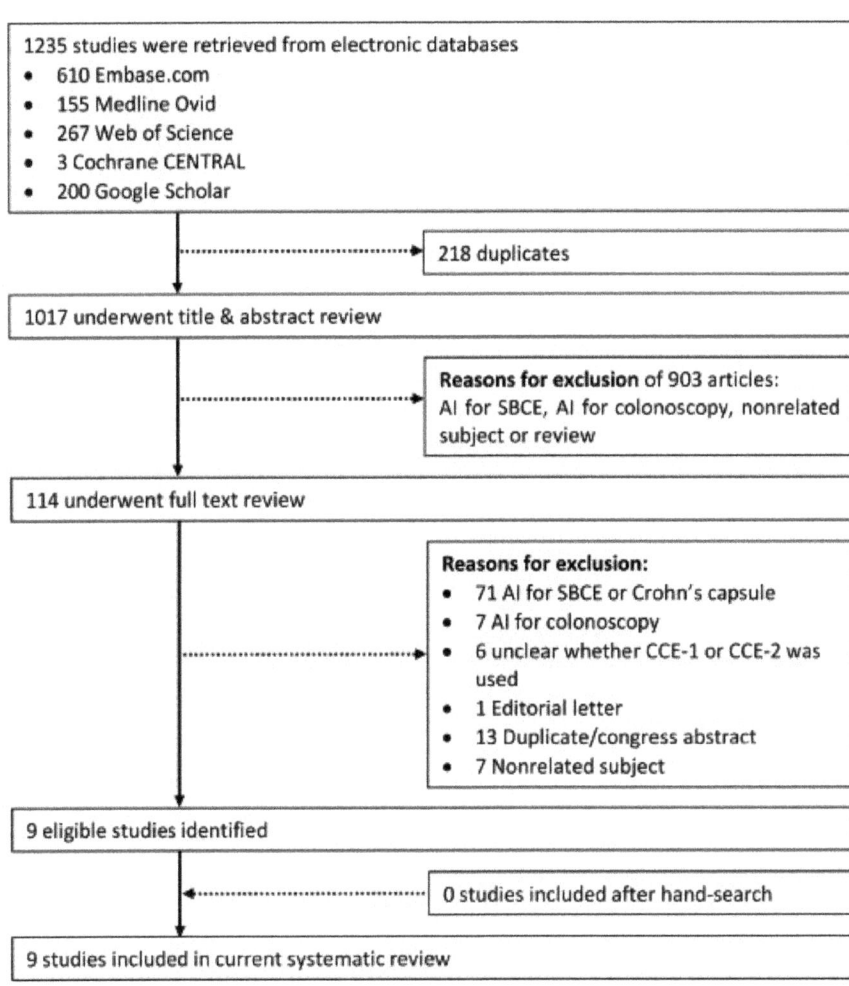

Figure 1. Flow chart of study selection.

3.2. Study Characteristics

Baseline characteristics of the included studies are shown in Table 2. All included studies were full-text papers presenting cohort studies reporting on AI for reviewing CCE-2 colonic images. Two studies reported on computed assessment of bowel cleansing, five studies reported on computed polyp or colorectal neoplasia detection, one study reported on computed blood detection and one study reported on computed capsule localization. For the studies reporting on bowel cleansing, one study evaluated bowel cleansing for each video frame while the other study evaluated bowel cleansing for the entire video. All other studies evaluated the presence of polyps, presence of blood or capsule localization for each frame. Regarding the AI method, five studies developed a SVM or CNN model, where a selection of frames is needed for the training of the model. To evaluate the performance of the proposed AI methods, all studies used a separate evaluation of the CCE images as a reference. Seven studies used the evaluation of CCE readers as a reference, one study used the known outcomes from a CCE database and one study used the findings from subsequent colonoscopy.

Table 2. Characteristics of the nine included studies.

First Author, Year of Publication, Country	Application	Type of AI Method	Evaluation for Each Frame or for Each Video	Included Videos, n	Frames Available from These Videos	Frames Available for Training the Model if Applicable	Selected Frames for Testing the Developed AI Method	Reference Group
Becq 2018 France [14]	Bowel cleansing assessment	1. Red over green (R/G ratio) 2. Red over brown (R/(R + G) ratio)	Frame	12	79,497	N/A	216 (R/G set) 192 (R/(R + G) set)	2 CCE readers
Buijs 2018 Denmark [16]	Bowel cleansing assessment	1. Non-linear index model 2. SVM model	Video	41	Unknown	Unknown	N/A	4 CCE readers
Figueiredo 2011 Portugal [17]	Polyp detection	Protrusion based algorithm	Frame	5	Unknown	N/A	1700	Subsequent colonoscopy
Mamonov 2014 USA [15]	Polyp detection	Binary classification after pre-selection	Frame	5	18,968	N/A	18,968	Known reviewed CCE dataset
Nadimi 2020 Denmark [19]	Polyp detection	CNN	Frame	255	11,300	7910	1695	Unknown amount of CCE readers
Yamada 2020 Japan [20]	Colorectal neoplasia detection	CNN	Frame	184	20,717	15,933	4784	3 CCE readers
Saraiva 2021 Portugal [21]	Protruding lesion detection	CNN	Frame	24	1,017,472	2912	728	2 CCE readers
Saraiva 2021 Portugal [22]	Blood detection	CNN	Frame	24	3,387,259	4660	1165	2 CCE readers
Herp 2021 Denmark [18]	Capsule localization	T-T model	Frame	84	Unknown	N/A	Unknown	Unknown amount of CCE readers

AI = Artificial Intelligence, SVM = Support Vector Machine; CNN = Convolutional Neural Network, CCE = Colon Capsule Endoscopy, N/A = Not Applicable, R/G = Red over Green, R/(R + G) = Red over Brown.

3.3. Quality of the Included Studies

The risk of bias and applicability concerns in the included studies, which were determined by using the QUADAS-2 tool, are presented in Table 3. All studies had a high risk of bias regarding patient selection, since they included CCE videos derived from previous trials or databases and information on the patient population behind the CCE videos was limited or lacking. One study regarding AI bowel cleansing assessment also raised applicability concerns regarding patient selection, since CCE videos were excluded when they were too poor in quality after the first lecture or when the CCE videos were incomplete [14]. Two studies had a high risk of bias regarding their index test, since they determined their models' optimal cut-off values yielding the highest diagnostic performance by using a ROC curve, which could have led to overoptimistic results, which could likely be poorer when using the same threshold in an independent sample [14,15]. Three studies raised applicability concerns regarding their index test, since they did not report on the performance of their AI models in terms of sensitivity and specificity [16–18].

Table 3. QUADAS-2 (Quality Assessment of Diagnostic Accuracy Studies) analysis for the assessment of the risk of bias in the included studies.

	Risk of Bias				Applicability Concerns		
	Patient Selection	Index Test	Reference Standard	Flow and Timing	Patient Selection	Index Test	Reference Standard
Becq [14]	+	+	−	−	+	−	−
Buijs [16]	+	−	−	−	−	+	−
Figueiredo [17]	+	−	−	−	−	+	−
Mamonov [15]	+	+	−	−	−	−	−
Nadimi [19]	+	−	−	−	−	−	−
Yamada [20]	+	−	−	−	−	−	−
Saraiva [21]	+	−	−	−	−	−	−
Saraiva [22]	+	−	−	−	−	−	−
Herp [18]	+	−	−	−	−	+	−

− = low risk of bias; + = high risk of bias.

3.4. Artificial Intelligence for the Assessment of Bowel Cleansing Quality in CCE-2

Two studies reported on computed assessment of bowel cleansing in CCE-2 (Table 4, Figure 2).

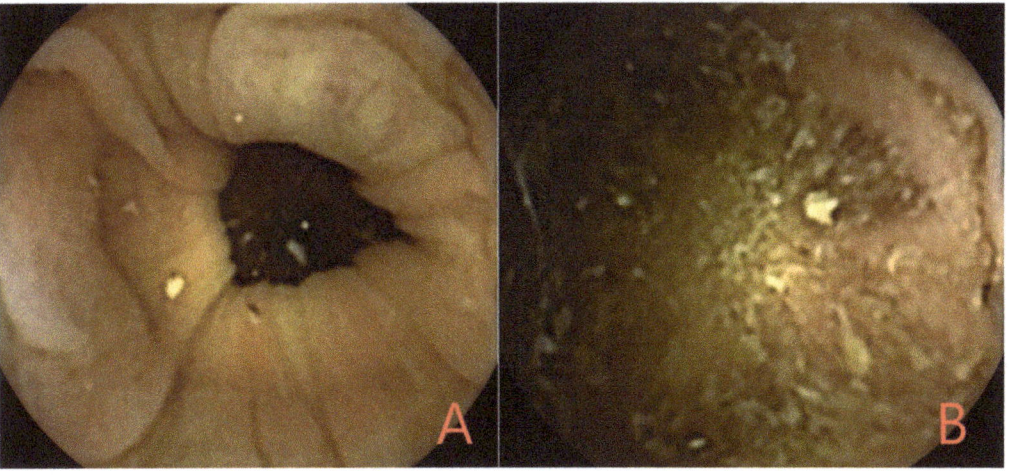

Figure 2. (**A**) Adequately cleansed CCE frame; (**B**) Inadequately cleansed CCE frame.

3.4.1. Development of the Proposed AI Models for Computed Assessment of Bowel Cleansing

The first study created two computed assessment of cleansing (CAC) scores using the ratio of color intensities red over green (R/G ratio) and red over brown (R/(R + G) ratio) [14]. After sorting and random selection, for each ratio a set of frames representative of the range of these ratios were obtained. These sets of frames were also evaluated by two experienced CCE readers who were blinded to the CAC scores. The experienced readers classified the frames as having either poor, fair, good or excellent bowel cleansing. Frames with poor or fair quality were defined as inadequately cleansed and frames with good or excellent quality were defined as adequately cleansed. Using the assessment of the experienced reviewers as a reference, the optimal cut-off values yielding the highest diagnostic performance for cleansing assessment were determined for both ratios using a receiver operating characteristic (ROC) curve.

The second study developed two CAC models, a non-linear index model and a support vector machine (SVM) model [16]. In both models, each pixel was defined as being clean or dirty, after which, the cleanliness of each frame was determined based on the number of clean and dirty pixels it contained. The cleansing level of the complete video was determined by the median cleansing of all frames and weighted based on the number of pixels in the frames. The non-linear index model classified pixels as either clean or dirty based on the distribution of the colors red, green and blue. The SVM model is based on machine learning concepts. A medical doctor classified pixels as being either clean or dirty. Using these evaluated pixels, a SVM algorithm was created through machine learning to assess the cleanliness of each pixel. For defining the cleanliness of each frame, and subsequently for each video, thresholds for unacceptable, poor, fair and good cleansing were predicted and corrected using learning techniques within the algorithm. To be able to evaluate both models, the bowel cleansing quality of each video was also classified by four CCE readers, including two international experts and two medical doctors with short formal training.

3.4.2. Performance of the Proposed AI Models for Computed Assessment of Bowel Cleansing

The CAC scores developed in the first study resulted in a bowel cleansing evaluation for each CCE frame defined as either adequately or inadequately cleansed [14]. The R/G ratio discriminated adequately cleansed frames from inadequately cleansed frames with a sensitivity of 86.5% and a specificity of 78.2%, whereas the R/(R + G) ratio did this with a higher sensitivity of 95.5% but a lower specificity of 63.0%.

The CAC models developed in the second study resulted in a bowel cleansing classification for each CCE video defined as either unacceptable, poor, fair or good [16]. Evaluation of the performance of their models was not expressed in terms of sensitivity and specificity, but in levels of agreement with the CCE readers. The non-linear index model classified 32% of the videos in agreement with the CCE readers, while the SVM model reached a higher agreement level of 47%. The non-linear index model misclassified 32% of the videos with more than one level of cleanliness compared to 12% in the SVM model.

3.5. Artificial Intelligence for Polyp Detection in CCE-2

Five studies reported on AI polyp detection in CCE-2 (Table 5, Figure 3).

Table 4. Results of the two included studies examining computed assessment of bowel cleansing in CCE.

Study	Type of AI	Frames/Videos Analyzed, n	Adequately Cleansed Frames/Videos, %	Sensitivity, %	Specificity, %	PPV, %	NPV, %	Level of Agreement AI with Readers, %	Videos Misclassified More than One Class
Becq * [14]	R/G ratio	216 frames	16.7%	86.5%	78.2%	45.1%	96.6%	-	-
	R/(R + G) ratio	192 frames	9.9%	95.5%	63.0%	25.0%	99.0%	-	-
Buijs ** [16]	Non-linear index model	41 videos	Unknown	-	-	-	-	32%	32%
	SVM model	41 videos	Unknown	-	-	-	-	47%	12%

AI = Artificial Intelligence, PPV = Positive Predictive Value, NPV = Negative Predictive Value, R/G = Red over Green, R/(R+G) = Red over Brown, SVM = Support Vector Machine, CCE = Colon Capsule Endoscopy. The computed assessment of cleansing (CAC) scores developed by Becq et al. resulted in a bowel cleansing evaluation for each frame defined as either adequately or inadequately cleansed. The CAC models developed by Buijs et al. resulted in a bowel cleansing classification for each video defined as unacceptable, poor, fair or good. * The percentage of adequately cleansed frames/videos was based on the evaluation by the reference group. ** 31 adequately cleansed (fair or good) and 10 inadequately cleansed (unacceptable or poor) videos were selected from a previous trial. The videos were re-evaluated by the reference group in this study, however, numbers on the adequate cleansing levels from these evaluations were not reported.

Table 5. Results of the five included studies examining computed polyp- or colorectal neoplasia detection in CCE.

Study	Type of AI	Application	Frames Analyzed, n	Amount of Polyps or Colorectal Neoplasia, n	Amount of Frames Containing Polyps, n	Cut-off Value	Accuracy	Sensitivity on a per Frame Basis, %	Specificity on a per Frame Basis, %	Sensitivity on a per Polyp Basis, %	Specificity on a per Polyp Basis, %
Figueiredo [17]	Protrusion based algorithm	Polyp detection	1700	10	Unknown	-	-	-	-	-	-
Mamonov [15]	Binary classification after pre-selection	Polyp detection	18,968	16	230	37	-	47.4%	90.2%	81.3%	90.2%
						40	-	-	-	81.3%	93.5%
Nadimi * [19]	CNN	Polyp detection	1695	Unknown	Unknown	-	98.0%	98.1%	96.3%	-	-
Yamada ** [20]	CNN	Colorectal neoplasia detection	4784	105	Unknown	-	83.9%	79.0%	87.0%	96.2%	Unknown
Saraiva [21]	CNN	Protruding lesion detection	728	Unknown	172	-	92.2%	90.7%	92.6%	-	-

AI = Artificial Intelligence, CNN = Convolutional Neural Network. Unknown means the numbers were not described. - means the numbers were not part of the outcomes of the study. * The entire dataset consisted of 11,300 CCE images of which 4800 contained colorectal polyps. Of the entire dataset, 15% was used to test the performance of the CNN. The amount of frames containing a polyp in this test dataset was not described. ** From the 105 observed colorectal neoplasia, 103 were polyps and 2 were colorectal cancers. 1850 images of patients with colorectal neoplasia were included. It was not described how many of the frames of the CCE-2 videos of these patients contained polyps or colorectal cancers.

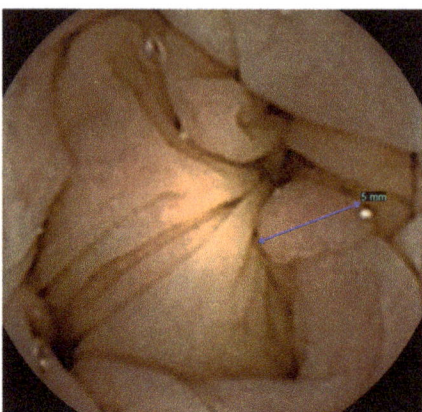

Figure 3. Polyp visualized in CCE.

3.5.1. Development of the Proposed AI Models for Polyp Detection

The first two studies developed algorithms for automated polyp detection based on the geometric characteristic of polyps that they have a roundish protrusion into the colonic lumen compared to the surrounding mucosal surface. In the first study, the amount of protrusion was gauged into a special function called P, where the value of P is closely related to the size of the protrusion in the images [17]. Findings from a subsequent colonoscopy were used as a reference to determine which frames contained polyps. In the second study, a binary classification algorithm was developed that resulted in the output "polyp" or "normal" [15]. Frames that potentially contained polyps were first pre-selected based on the texture content. The surface of polyps is often highly textured, however too much texture implies the presence of bubbles or trash liquid. Therefore, in the preselection procedure all frames with too little or too much texture were discarded. Subsequently, a measure of protrusion was created which was used as the decision parameter of the final binary classifier with pre-selection. From the used CCE dataset, it was known which frames contained polyps. Based on the entire dataset, the optimal threshold of the created binary classifier with pre-selection used to classify a frame as containing a polyp was determined by using a ROC curve. To limit the number of frames that need to be manually re-assessed by an expert, a desired level of 90% specificity was used.

The other three studies on CCE polyp detection developed a convolutional neural network (CNN) that classified frames as either "normal" or "containing a polyp/colorectal neoplasia/protruding lesion" [19–21]. CNN uses many images to develop and train a model by learning rich features from these images. Ideally, a large amount of data is needed to develop and train these models. However, available data in the form of CCE images is limited which makes it difficult to create a CNN for CCE polyp detection from scratch. To partially overcome this problem, all three studies used an existing CNN architecture and trained this model with CCE images to improve its performance. To test the performance of the proposed CNN models, all studies used separate images that were not used for the training of the models. The third study used manual analyses performed by trained nurses and gastro-enterologists as the reference group [19]. The fourth study used manual analyses performed by three expert gastroenterologists [20]. The fifth study used manual analyses performed by two expert gastroenterologists [21]. The proposed CNN model in the fourth study was not only developed to detect polyps but also colorectal cancer (colorectal neoplasia) and the CNN model in the fifth study was developed to detect protruding lesions such as polyps, epithelial tumors, submucosal tumors and nodes. These last two studies created a ROC curve to measure the performance of their CNN model.

3.5.2. Performance of the Proposed AI models for Polyp Detection

The first study did not evaluate the accuracy of their developed algorithm in terms of sensitivity and specificity [17]. They only provided a description of the amount of protrusion into the lumen of CCE images expressed in p-values for different colonic anomalies. 80% of all polyps had a p-value higher than 500. All polyps that expressed a p-value higher than 2000 were polyps that were larger than 1 cm. The p-value was always under 500 in frames with cecal ulcer, diverticula, bubbles or trash liquid. However, some examples were shown that some folds mimicked polyps and were associated with a high p-value.

The other studies did provide numbers on the accuracy of their AI models for automated polyp detection in CCE. The binary classifier with pre-selection developed in the second study resulted in a sensitivity of 47.4% and a specificity of 90.2% on a per frame basis using a threshold value of 37 [15]. Since in a clinical setting it is important that each polyp is detected in at least 1 frame, a ROC curve was also determined on a per polyp basis. At the same threshold value, this resulted in a sensitivity of 81.3% and a specificity of 90.2%. At a threshold of 40 a specificity of 93.5% was reached while maintaining the same per polyp sensitivity.

Even though the CNN model created in the third study was only evaluated on a per frame basis, their model resulted in an even better performance with a sensitivity of 98.1% and a specificity of 96.3% [19].

The fourth study also evaluated performance on both per frame and per lesion basis, but again this did not result in a better performance than the CNN model in the third study. The model from the fourth study resulted in a sensitivity of 79.0% and a specificity of 87.0% for colorectal neoplasia on a per frame basis. Per lesion analysis increased the sensitivity to 96.2% [20]. The CNN model in the fifth study was only evaluated on a per frame basis and resulted in a sensitivity of 90.7% and a specificity of 92.6% [21].

3.6. Other Artificial Intelligence for CCE-2

Besides the studies on artificial intelligence for the assessment of bowel cleansing and polyp detection in CCE-2, two other studies were included. One study reported on the detection of blood in the colonic lumen [22]. They developed a convolutional neural network (CNN) that classified frames as either "normal" or "containing blood." The same strategy for CNN development was used as in the previously mentioned study on polyp detection conducted by the same research group [21]. The CNN model only evaluated the presence of blood on a per frame basis and resulted in a sensitivity of 99.8% and a specificity of 93.2%.

Another study reported on artificial intelligence for the localization of CCE-2 [18]. A model describing the shape of the intestine was created and feature points such as edges, corners, blobs or ridges were identified. Subsequently, capsule movement and speed were estimated by determining movement towards, away or rotated from these feature points, also taken the capsule's frames per second (Hz) into account. The model was run many times and resulted in similar colonic shaped paths. Points usually associated with the ascending colon, hepatic flexure, transverse colon, splenic flexure and descending colon were identified. The model's predictions of colonic sections were compared to expert labeled sections. The average accuracy of the model for frame colonic section classification was 86%.

4. Discussion

To our knowledge, this is the first systematic review providing an overview on the use of AI methods for reviewing CCE-2 colonic images. CCE provides a non-invasive alternative to colonoscopy for exploration of the colonic mucosa, but its applicability is limited by the accompanying labor-intensive reviewing time and by the risk of inter-observer variability. Automated reviewing of CCE images is an important step in the evolution of CCE. AI methods show promising results, with high sensitivity but lower specificity for the assessment of bowel cleansing and high sensitivity and specificity for polyp or colorectal neoplasia detection and blood detection.

Only one study reported on the AI assessment of CCE-2 bowel cleansing in terms of sensitivity and specificity [14]. However, this study shows promising results for its two developed CAC scores yielding high sensitivities (86.5% and 95.5% respectively) but lower specificities (78.2% and 63.0% respectively) for discriminating adequately cleansed from inadequately cleansed images. Adequately cleansed frames were only observed in 16.7% and 9.9%, respectively. CCE videos were excluded when they were identified as being too poor in quality after the first lecture and when they were incomplete, so the actual overall adequate cleansing levels were even lower. In a previous meta-analysis on the accuracy of CCE compared to colonoscopy, the rate of adequate bowel preparation varied from 40–100%, where most studies reported adequate cleansing levels over 80% [4]. The low number of adequately cleansed frames in the study included in this current review makes the risk of falsely identifying frames as adequately cleansed higher, which could explain the lower specificities of the CAC scores compared to its sensitivities. Since this was the only study reporting on AI for CCE bowel cleansing assessment in terms of sensitivity and specificity, the observed accuracy of bowel cleansing assessment by the CAC scores in this study cannot be compared to previous literature. However, optimal cut-off values yielding the highest diagnostic performances were determined for scores using a ROC curve, which could have led to overoptimistic results, which could likely be poorer when using the same threshold in an independent sample [13].

The other study reporting on the AI assessment of CCE bowel cleansing did not report accuracy results of their proposed AI models in terms of sensitivity and specificity or the percentage of adequately cleansed videos [16]. However, the low agreement levels of the non-linear index model (32%) and the SVM model (47%) with the reference group CCE readers are alarming. More studies on the AI assessment of CCE bowel cleansing in terms of sensitivity of specificity, with realistic adequate cleansing levels, are needed to be able to evaluate newly developed AI models accurately.

The proposed AI models for polyp or colorectal neoplasia detection resulted in high sensitivities of 47.4–98.1% and high specificities of 87.0% to 96.3% in per-frame analysis [15,19–21]. Two studies performed per-lesion analysis, in addition to per-frame analysis, which improved sensitivity of polyp- or colorectal neoplasia detection to 81.3–98.1% [15,20]. It should be noted that the abovementioned results from four included AI studies were all compared to CCE-2 readers, so the concluded sensitivities and specificities represent the ability of the AI models to reach the same performance levels as CCE-2 readers. The previously mentioned meta-analysis on the accuracy of per-lesion detection by CCE-2 readers compared to colonoscopy reported a sensitivity of 85% and a specificity of 85% for polyps of any size [4].

One study determined the optimal threshold of their binary classifier with pre-selection by using a ROC curve, which may have led to overoptimistic estimates of its performance [15]. Still, the highest sensitivities were reached in the other three studies that developed a CNN model for polyp or colorectal neoplasia detection [19–21]. We believe future development of AI methods for reviewing CCE images should be focused on the creation of CNN models. While other AI methods fail to reach the same performance as humans, previous literature has shown that CNN is able to match human performance in different tasks [8,23]. However, optimal CNN requires training the algorithms with large amounts of data, which can be a challenge in the field of CCE for which the availability of data is limited.

Only one study reported on the computed detection of blood in the colonic lumen [22]. Even so, their CNN model shows a promising result with a high sensitivity of 99.8%. Computed localization of the capsule within the colon was also only reported in one study. The accuracy for classifying frames to a specific colonic section was high (86%), but further studies are needed to validate this application in terms of sensitivity and specificity.

While conducting our literature search, it was remarkable how many articles did not specify whether they used small bowel capsule endoscopy (SB-CE) or colon capsule endoscopy (CCE). Even when the use of CCE was reported, it was not always reported whether the first-generation (CCE-1) or second-generation (CCE-2) capsule was used. CCE-1 is an outdated version of the colon capsule with low sensitivity for detection of polyps compared to CCE-2. Therefore, articles not specifying the use of CCE-2 were excluded from this review. Future studies on the AI assessment of reviewing CCE images should report on the type of capsule that was used.

Overall, literature on AI for reviewing CCE-2 colonic images is scarce. Two studies reported on the AI assessment of bowel cleansing and five studies reported on AI polyp or colorectal neoplasia detection. Only one study reported on the detection of blood in the colonic lumen and only one study created a rough AI model for determining the location of the capsule within the colon. The AI methods and study designs used were heterogeneous. Therefore, we could not perform a formal meta-analysis. Most studies had a limited sample size to test the performance of their AI models. Especially for studies using machine or deep learning, a large proportion of CCE images is needed for training the model, limiting the amount of images left for testing the models. Three out of nine studies included in this review did not report on the performance of their AI models in terms of sensitivity and specificity, making it hard to determine their value [16–18].

Nevertheless, the studies presented in this systematic review show promising results for the use of AI for reviewing CCE-2 colonic images with high sensitivies for both bowel cleansing assessment as well as polyp or colorectal neoplasia detection and blood detection. Manual CCE review is time-consuming and faces problems regarding inter observer variability. Improvements in imaging recognition will improve the reading time and inter observer variability, and may accelerate the use of CCE. This systematic review gives hope that AI can provide a timesaving, objective and reproducible method for reviewing CCE images.

Necessary Action Points to Reach Implementation of AI Technology for CCE in Daily Practice

Actual implementation of AI for reviewing CCE-2 colonic images is a crucial step in the applicability of CCE in daily clinical practice. Future studies should preferably focus on CNN, because of its high potential for reaching human-like performance. In order to reach its implementation, several steps need to be taken. CNN algorithms need to be optimized and tested with more data, possibly requiring the set-up of a large international CCE database. To ensure adequate evaluation of the added value of the AI method, studies should always report the version of the capsule used and the accuracy of their models in terms of sensitivity and specificity. Additionally, studies should preferably only use the results from expert CCE readers to test the performance of their AI methods, since the concluded sensitivities and specificities represent the ability of the AI models to reach the same performance levels as these readers. Besides CNN, which requires an adequate number of coloscopy images, synthetic samples can also be used as artificial intelligence methods [24,25]. Finally, when these gaps and barriers have been overcome, prospective clinical trials have to confirm the accuracy of the optimized CNN models.

Author Contributions: Conceptualization, S.M.; M.C.W.S.; methodology, S.M. and F.E.R.V.; formal analysis, S.M. and F.E.R.V.; investigation, S.M.; data curation, S.M.; writing—original draft preparation, S.M.; writing—review and editing, S.M., F.E.R.V., M.C.W.S.; supervision, M.C.W.S. and E.J.K.; project administration, M.C.W.S.; All authors have read and agreed to the published version of the manuscript."

Funding: This research received no external funding.

Institutional Review Board Statement: Ethical review and approval were waived for this study due to retrospective aspect of this study.

Informed Consent Statement: Not applicable.

Data Availability Statement: No new data were created or analyzed in this study. Data sharing is not applicable to this article.

Acknowledgments: The authors wish to thank Wichor M. Bramer from the Erasmus MC Medical Library for developing and updating the search strategies.

Conflicts of Interest: The authors declare no conflict of interest.

Abbreviations

CCE = Colon Capsule Endoscopy; GI = Gastrointestinal; ESGE = European Society of Gastrointestinal Endoscopy; FDA = Food and Drug Administration; AI = Artificial Intelligence; SVM = Support Vector Machine; CNN = Convolutional Neural Network.

References

1. Spada, C.; Hassan, C.; Galmiche, J.P.; Neuhaus, H.; Dumonceau, J.M.; Adler, S.; Epstein, O.; Gay, G.; Pennazio, M.; Rex, D.K.; et al. Colon capsule endoscopy: European Society of Gastrointestinal Endoscopy (ESGE) Guideline. *Endoscopy* **2012**, *44*, 527–536. [CrossRef]
2. Spada, C.; Hassan, C.; Bellini, D.; Burling, D.; Cappello, G.; Carretero, C.; Dekker, E.; Eliakim, R.; de Haan, M.; Kaminski, M.F.; et al. Imaging alternatives to colonoscopy: CT colonography and colon capsule. European Society of Gastrointestinal Endoscopy (ESGE) and European Society of Gastrointestinal and Abdominal Radiology (ESGAR) Guideline—Update 2020. *Eur. Radiol.* **2021**, *31*, 2967–2982. [CrossRef] [PubMed]
3. Spada, C.; Pasha, S.F.; Gross, S.A.; Leighton, J.A.; Schnoll-Sussman, F.; Correale, L.; Gonzalez Suarez, B.; Costamagna, G.; Hassan, C. Accuracy of First- and Second-Generation Colon Capsules in Endoscopic Detection of Colorectal Polyps: A Systematic Review and Meta-analysis. *Clin. Gastroenterol. Hepatol.* **2016**, *14*, 1533–1543.e8. [CrossRef] [PubMed]
4. Kjolhede, T.; Olholm, A.M.; Kaalby, L.; Kidholm, K.; Qvist, N.; Baatrup, G. Diagnostic accuracy of capsule endoscopy compared with colonoscopy for polyp detection: Systematic review and meta-analyses. *Endoscopy* **2021**, *53*, 713–721. [CrossRef] [PubMed]
5. Vuik, F.E.; Moen, S.; Nieuwenburg, S.A.; Schreuders, E.H.; Kuipers, E.J.; Spaander, M.C. Applicability of Colon Capsule Endoscopy as Pan-endoscopy: From bowel preparation, transit- and rating times to completion rate and patient acceptance. *Endosc. Int. Open* **2021**, *9*, E1852–E1859. [CrossRef] [PubMed]
6. Buijs, M.M.; Kroijer, R.; Kobaek-Larsen, M.; Spada, C.; Fernandez-Urien, I.; Steele, R.J.; Baatrup, G. Intra and inter-observer agreement on polyp detection in colon capsule endoscopy evaluations. *United Eur. Gastroenterol. J.* **2018**, *6*, 1563–1568. [CrossRef] [PubMed]
7. Soffer, S.; Klang, E.; Shimon, O.; Nachmias, N.; Eliakim, R.; Ben-Horin, S.; Kopylov, U.; Barash, Y. Deep learning for wireless capsule endoscopy: A systematic review and meta-analysis. *Gastrointest. Endosc.* **2020**, *92*, 831–839.e8. [CrossRef] [PubMed]
8. Hosny, A.; Parmar, C.; Quackenbush, J.; Schwartz, L.H.; Aerts, H. Artificial intelligence in radiology. *Nat. Rev. Cancer* **2018**, *18*, 500–510. [CrossRef]
9. LeCun, Y.; Bengio, Y.; Hinton, G. Deep learning. *Nature* **2015**, *521*, 436–444. [CrossRef]
10. Hassan, C.; Spadaccini, M.; Iannone, A.; Maselli, R.; Jovani, M.; Chandrasekar, V.T.; Antonelli, G.; Yu, H.; Areia, M.; Dinis-Ribeiro, M.; et al. Performance of artificial intelligence in colonoscopy for adenoma and polyp detection: A systematic review and meta-analysis. *Gastrointest. Endosc.* **2021**, *93*, 77–85.e6. [CrossRef]
11. Antonelli, G.; Badalamenti, M.; Hassan, C.; Repici, A. Impact of artificial intelligence on colorectal polyp detection. *Best Pract. Res. Clin. Gastroenterol.* **2021**, *52–53*, 101713. [CrossRef]
12. Moher, D.; Liberati, A.; Tetzlaff, J.; Altman, D.G.; Group, P. Preferred reporting items for systematic reviews and meta-analyses: The PRISMA statement. *BMJ* **2009**, *339*, b2535. [CrossRef]
13. Whiting, P.F.; Rutjes, A.W.; Westwood, M.E.; Mallett, S.; Deeks, J.J.; Reitsma, J.B.; Leeflang, M.M.; Sterne, J.A.; Bossuyt, P.M.; QUADAS-2 Group. QUADAS-2: A revised tool for the quality assessment of diagnostic accuracy studies. *Ann. Intern. Med.* **2011**, *155*, 529–536. [CrossRef]
14. Becq, A.; Histace, A.; Camus, M.; Nion-Larmurier, I.; Abou Ali, E.; Pietri, O.; Romain, O.; Chaput, U.; Li, C.; Marteau, P.; et al. Development of a computed cleansing score to assess quality of bowel preparation in colon capsule endoscopy. *Endosc. Int. Open* **2018**, *6*, E844–E850. [CrossRef]
15. Mamonov, A.V.; Figueiredo, I.N.; Figueiredo, P.N.; Tsai, Y.H. Automated polyp detection in colon capsule endoscopy. *IEEE Trans. Med. Imaging* **2014**, *33*, 1488–1502. [CrossRef]
16. Buijs, M.M.; Ramezani, M.H.; Herp, J.; Kroijer, R.; Kobaek-Larsen, M.; Baatrup, G.; Nadimi, E.S. Assessment of bowel cleansing quality in colon capsule endoscopy using machine learning: A pilot study. *Endosc. Int. Open* **2018**, *6*, E1044–E1050. [CrossRef]
17. Figueiredo, P.N.; Figueiredo, I.N.; Prasath, S.; Tsai, R. Automatic polyp detection in pillcam colon 2 capsule images and videos: Preliminary feasibility report. *Diagn. Ther. Endosc.* **2011**, *2011*, 182435. [CrossRef]
18. Herp, J.; Deding, U.; Buijs, M.M.; Kroijer, R.; Baatrup, G.; Nadimi, E.S. Feature Point Tracking-Based Localization of Colon Capsule Endoscope. *Diagnostics* **2021**, *11*, 193. [CrossRef]

19. Nadimi, E.S.; Buijs, M.M.; Herp, J.; Kroijer, R.; Kobaek-Larsen, M.; Nielsen, E.; Pedersen, C.D.; Blanes-Vidal, V.; Baatrup, G. Application of deep learning for autonomous detection and localization of colorectal polyps in wireless colon capsule endoscopy. *Comput. Electr. Eng.* **2020**, *81*, 106531. [CrossRef]
20. Yamada, A.; Niikura, R.; Otani, K.; Aoki, T.; Koike, K. Automatic detection of colorectal neoplasia in wireless colon capsule endoscopic images using a deep convolutional neural network. *Endoscopy* **2021**, *53*, 832–836. [CrossRef]
21. Saraiva, M.M.; Ferreira, J.P.S.; Cardoso, H.; Afonso, J.; Ribeiro, T.; Andrade, P.; Parente, M.P.L.; Jorge, R.N.; Macedo, G. Artificial intelligence and colon capsule endoscopy: Development of an automated diagnostic system of protruding lesions in colon capsule endoscopy. *Technol. Coloproctol.* **2021**, *25*, 1243–1248. [CrossRef]
22. Mascarenhas Saraiva, M.; Ferreira, J.P.S.; Cardoso, H.; Afonso, J.; Ribeiro, T.; Andrade, P.; Parente, M.P.L.; Jorge, R.N.; Macedo, G. Artificial intelligence and colon capsule endoscopy: Automatic detection of blood in colon capsule endoscopy using a convolutional neural network. *Endosc. Int. Open* **2021**, *9*, E1264–E1268. [CrossRef]
23. Mnih, V.; Kavukcuoglu, K.; Silver, D.; Rusu, A.A.; Veness, J.; Bellemare, M.G.; Graves, A.; Riedmiller, M.; Fidjeland, A.K.; Ostrovski, G.; et al. Human-level control through deep reinforcement learning. *Nature* **2015**, *518*, 529–533. [CrossRef]
24. Adjei, P.E.; Lonseko, Z.M.; Du, W.; Zhang, H.; Rao, N. Examining the effect of synthetic data augmentation in polyp detection and segmentation. *Int. J. Comput. Assist. Radiol. Surg.* **2022**, *17*, 1289–1302. [CrossRef]
25. Ozyoruk, K.B.; Gokceler, G.I.; Bobrow, T.L.; Coskun, G.; Incetan, K.; Almalioglu, Y.; Mahmood, F.; Curto, E.; Perdigoto, L.; Oliveira, M.; et al. EndoSLAM dataset and an unsupervised monocular visual odometry and depth estimation approach for endoscopic videos. *Med. Image Anal.* **2021**, *71*, 102058. [CrossRef]

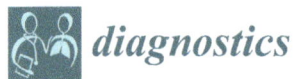

Article

Multi-Scale Hybrid Network for Polyp Detection in Wireless Capsule Endoscopy and Colonoscopy Images

Meryem Souaidi [1,*] and Mohamed El Ansari [1,2]

1 LABSIV, Computer Science, Faculty of Sciences, University Ibn Zohr, Agadir 80000, Morocco
2 Informatics and Applications Laboratory, Computer Science Department, Faculty of Sciences, University of Moulay Ismail, Meknès 50070, Morocco
* Correspondence: souaidi.meryem@gmail.com

Abstract: The trade-off between speed and precision is a key step in the detection of small polyps in wireless capsule endoscopy (WCE) images. In this paper, we propose a hybrid network of an inception v4 architecture-based single-shot multibox detector (Hyb-SSDNet) to detect small polyp regions in both WCE and colonoscopy frames. Medical privacy concerns are considered the main barriers to WCE image acquisition. To satisfy the object detection requirements, we enlarged the training datasets and investigated deep transfer learning techniques. The Hyb-SSDNet framework adopts inception blocks to alleviate the inherent limitations of the convolution operation to incorporate contextual features and semantic information into deep networks. It consists of four main components: (a) multi-scale encoding of small polyp regions, (b) using the inception v4 backbone to enhance more contextual features in shallow and middle layers, and (c) concatenating weighted features of mid-level feature maps, giving them more importance to highly extract semantic information. Then, the feature map fusion is delivered to the next layer, followed by some downsampling blocks to generate new pyramidal layers. Finally, the feature maps are fed to multibox detectors, consistent with the SSD process-based VGG16 network. The Hyb-SSDNet achieved a 93.29% mean average precision (mAP) and a testing speed of 44.5 FPS on the WCE dataset. This work proves that deep learning has the potential to develop future research in polyp detection and classification tasks.

Keywords: deep transfer learning; multi-scale encoding; weighted feature maps fusion; image augmentation; polyp; inception module; single-shot multibox detector (SSD); wireless capsule endoscopy images (WCE)

Citation: Souaidi, M.; El Ansari, M. Multi-Scale Hybrid Network for Polyp Detection in Wireless Capsule Endoscopy and Colonoscopy Images. *Diagnostics* **2022**, *12*, 2030. https://doi.org/10.3390/diagnostics12082030

Academic Editors: Eun-Sun Kim and Kwang-Sig Lee

Received: 26 July 2022
Accepted: 17 August 2022
Published: 22 August 2022

Publisher's Note: MDPI stays neutral with regard to jurisdictional claims in published maps and institutional affiliations.

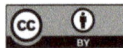

Copyright: © 2022 by the authors. Licensee MDPI, Basel, Switzerland. This article is an open access article distributed under the terms and conditions of the Creative Commons Attribution (CC BY) license (https://creativecommons.org/licenses/by/4.0/).

1. Introduction

Gastrointestinal cancer is the third major cause of death worldwide [1]. Colorectal cancer begins as a benign growth of glandular tissue in the colonic mucosa, known as adenomatous polyps, which may turn into malignant tumors over time. The number of patients affected by this disease has increased considerably in recent years [2–4]. The non-invasive technique of wireless capsule endoscopy (WCE) is widely utilized in clinics to examine the GI tract as an advanced medical imaging technology [5]. Contrary to traditional colonoscopy devices, it enables physicians to fully visualize the inner cavities of the small bowel from the inside without pain or sedation [6,7]. However, many circumstances hinder the diagnosis process; some polyps may be overlooked due to their small size, low illumination inside the GI tract, or the skills of the gastroenterologist. A WCE produces two or more color images per second, which lasts 8 hours, to capture an approximation of 55,000 frames per patient. A large amount of data makes the task of detection laborious and tedious for trained endoscopists to identify suspicious areas and manually locate polyp regions in each WCE frame. Therefore, a computer-aided system (CAD) is required, which may help clinicians automatically locate large and small polyps and reduce the miss rate. Even for highly-skilled clinical practitioners, the detection process is more difficult owing to the complicated characteristics of the polyp regions (shape, texture, size, and morphology). Recently, many polyp detection solutions have been proposed to assist endoscopists in providing an automated system acquiring some knowledge without requiring the physical presence of the specialists [8,9]. Deep learning (DL) architectures have rapidly grown in the medical image analysis field, owing to their superior performance in image classification compared to the handcrafted methods [10–14]. This study aimed to classify abnormalities and automatically detect and localize polyp regions on both colonoscopy and capsule endoscopic images [15–18]. The transfer of information between the CNN blocks can automatically learn features from raw data and avoid the obstacles of manual feature extraction. In WCE polyp detection, the lack of public and annotated datasets pushed most previous studies to utilize private data sets. Other studies on colonoscopy employed public data sets according to their initiatives (e.g., MICCAI 2015 sub-challenge on automatic polyp detection in the colonoscopy). Region-based object detection and scale variations are the primary focuses of computer vision. In this context, CNN-based object detectors can be divided into two categories: two-stage detectors, such as R-CNNs [19], and their many variants (Faster R-CNN [20], R-FCN [21], etc.), and one-stage detectors (YOLO [22], SSD [23], etc.). Two-stage detectors show low speed and high computation rates by selecting a one-scale feature map and using a fixed receptive field, which limits the practical application of deep learning in small polyp region detection. Thus, two-stage detectors are accurate but relatively slow compared to one-stage detectors that map image pixels directly to the coordinates of the bounding boxes. One-stage detectors are more accurate for speed and memory but sacrifice precision for small object detection. Recently, many researchers have effectuated corresponding research on improving the small object detection ability of SSD models. However, the trade-off between accuracy and speed is still the goal of object detection research in medical image analysis. The SSD model's detector succeeded in preserving the location information in either shallower or deep layer networks. However, semantic information may be lacking in feature maps generated by shallow layers, particularly for small polyp regions, resulting in performance degradation over time.

The motivation of this study is to achieve an encouraging mean average precision (mAP) for polyp detection purposes while reducing the running time by implementing tremendous deep learning frameworks. For that reason, we redesigned a new SSD model using the inception-v4 (as a backbone), which can solve the problem of over-fitting and increased computation during the optimization process. Thus, the inception frameworks can capture more target information compared to the VGG networks without increasing network complexity. The inception-v4 has a more uniform simplified architecture and more inception modules than inception-v3. However, it may not be necessary to add more inception layers to obtain significant increases in the performances as stated in [24]. Therefore, a weighted mid-fusion of two successive modified inception-A modules of inception v4 is introduced in order to replace the conv4_3 layer of the VGG16 network for further contextual and semantic information extraction. The modified version of inception v4 aims to reduce the number of layers used to speed up the run time with remarkable gain in precision.

Inspired by the feature fusion single-shot multibox detector (FSSD) [25] and the GoogLeNet inception v4 [26] Szegedy et al. 2017), this paper proposes a hybrid network-based single-shot multibox detector (Hyb-SSDNet) to tackle the problem of small polyp region detection in both WCE and colonoscopy frames. To achieve this goal, the proposed method benefits from the powerful architectural designs of inception modules to produce ultimate architecture used as the backbone of the SSD detector. Indeed, it replaces the classical strategy of alternating convolutional and pooling layers of the shallow part of the VGG16 network with stacked inception modules. Since inception networks tend to be very deep, it is natural to effectively redesign them in the higher part of inception v4 (backbone) consistent with the VGG16 architecture's small polyp target detection. This would allow the Hyb-SSDNet framework to reap all the benefits of inception blocks while retaining its computational efficiency; thus, enabling the network to detect polyp patterns of various sizes within the same layer and avoid heavy parameter redundancies. To give higher importance to the region of interest, we designed a weighted mid-fusion module (WFM) that enhances more contextual features in shallow layers by assigning weights to different channels and positions on the feature maps. The simplest strategy of concatenating mid-level inception modules is aimed at incorporating contextual and semantic information into deep networks and constructing a multi-scale feature map. Finally, a downsampling block was applied to generate a new feature pyramid that is fed to the multibox detectors to produce the final detection results consistent with the SSD process. Using proper fine-tuning parameters, we conducted extensive experiments on the WCE and the challenging CVC-ClinicDB and ETIS-Larib datasets. The results show that the Hyb-SSDNet obtains a higher mAP than the conventional SSD with gains of 16.09, 17.43, and 16.98 points on the WCE, CVC-ClinicDB, and ETIS-Larib datasets, respectively, especially for small polyp regions with small speed drops.

The main contributions of this paper are as follows:

1. The application of a lightweight version of inception v4 architecture as the backbone to improve the SSD detector ability in small polyp detection.
2. A weighted mid-fusion block of two adjacent modules of the modified version of inception-A is used to replace the Conv4_3 layer of the VGG16 network; thus, tackling the problem of missing target details.
3. The filter numbers of the first convolution layers in the stem part of the inception v4 backbone were modified from (32 to 64) to capture more patterns and relevant information similar to the original SSD.
4. The modification of the inception v4 model through the reduction of layers is used to achieve faster speed while maintaining the computational cost.
5. The Hyb-SSDNet uses a weighted mid-fusion block to add new convolution layers to construct the multi-scale feature pyramid differently from the conventional SSD.
6. The Hyb-SSDNet model robustness is verified through repeated experimentation on three well-known datasets in the field (WCE, CVC-ClinicDB, and ETIS-Larib) for a fair comparison with the competitor's state-of-the-art methods.
7. The discussion of the advantages and limitations of the proposed framework.

The remainder of this paper is organized as follows. Section 2 presents the related studies. Section 3 describes the proposed Hyb-SSDNet model in detail. Section 4 reports the experimental results and compares them with those of other models. Finally, the conclusions are presented in Section 5.

2. Literature Review
2.1. Hand-Crafted and CNN Methods

Automatically detecting polyps in WCE images is a challenging task because of their variations in terms of size, shape, and morphology. Recently, significant progress has been made in investigating handcrafted features for gastrointestinal classification purposes. In this regard, a framework-based pyramid histogram for polyp classification based on T-CWT and gamma parameters were presented in a previous study [6]. Understanding these biological mechanisms remains highly complex. Thus, handcrafted features encode only some parts and neglect the intrinsic information of the entire frame. Recently, with the rapid development of CNN, several attempts have been made to classify colonoscopy polyp abnormalities using existing deep learning frameworks, such as VGGNet [27], GoogLeNet [28], and ResNet [29]. Limited by the size of medical datasets owing to privacy concerns, a proper fine-tuning setting leads to good results in many fields compared to retraining architectures from scratch, especially in the context of colonoscopy/endoscopy polyp recognition [30]. This is the main motivation behind transferring knowledge to wireless capsule endoscopy polyp detection tasks.

2.2. SSD-Based and Other Object Detectors

Polyps localization in WCE/colonoscopy images by drawing a bounding box around the localized region is the purpose of this paper, whereas polyp classification is conducted directly as an internal stage of localization. The frameworks of domain-specific object detection methods are primarily categorized into two types. One is the two-stage algorithm that first generates region proposals and then classifies each proposal into different object categories (e.g., Faster R-CNN [31]). The second one is a one-stage algorithm based on regression (e.g., YOLO [32] and SSD [33]). The authors of [34] proposed an improved version of the mask R-CNN framework for polyp detection and segmentation tasks. Jia et al. [35] presented a two-stage framework based on deep learning for automatic polyp recognition in colonoscopy images. An improved version of the CNN algorithm was proposed by TASHK et al. [36], which used DRLSE to automatically locate polyps in an image. However, a meta-analysis showed that the detection speed of the two-stage algorithm is slow, making it difficult to meet the real-time requirements of polyp detection even if it performs high localization and object recognition performance. In contrast, the one-stage algorithm achieved a high inference speed by using the predicted boxes from the input images directly, without the region proposal step. Misawa et al. [37] proposed a polyp detection system based on YOLOv3, which achieved real-time detection with over 90% sensitivity and specificity. The advantages are that there is only one processing step, so a preliminary step to extract an ROI is not performed. However, the limitation of the YOLO algorithm is that it struggles with small objects within the image due to the spatial constraints of the algorithm, especially for small polyp detection purposes. Liu et al. [38] proposed a deep framework-based single-shot detector (SSD) that uses ResNet50 and VGG16 architectures as backbone networks to detect polyps in colonoscopy videos. However, the traditional SSD-based VGG16 network only uses a 1×1 and 3×3 convolution kernel for one convolution layer making its feature extraction ability inefficient. Therefore, a more powerful backbone (such as inception v4) is needed to strengthen the polyp detection process. Some attempts have been made to address the problems of small polyp detection using the SSD algorithm. Zhang et al. [39] presented an architecture (SSD-GPNet) based on the SSD model in which they combined low-level feature maps with the deconvolution of high-level feature maps. Jeong et al. [40] proposed an enhanced version of the SSD model, in which they fully utilized the direction information of the feature maps by performing a simple concatenation and deconvolution operation. These improvements made the Rainbow SSD suitable for small-target detection. Although some attempts have been made to improve the accuracy of small polyp region detection by simplifying the SSD architecture, the addition of deconvolution layers leads to excessive computational complexity at the expense of speed. Within the same scope, Sheping et al. [41] proposed an enhanced SSD network-based dense convolutional network (DenseNet), in which a residual block was established before object prediction to further improve the model performance. They performed a fusion mechanism of multi-scale feature layers to enhance the relationships between the levels in the feature pyramid. However, information from multiple scales was treated equally during fusion. For feature extraction enhancement, a weighted mid-fusion to capture more informative patterns and contextual information is needed, giving weight to more important features and reducing the model complexity while maintaining high execution speed; thus, reaching the requirements for a complete detection process. The ability to perform both real-time detection and high precision is an indispensable factor in clinical applications [42]. A lightweight concatenation of mid-level visual and semantic features is investigated to fully utilize the synthetic information that leads to the improvement in the performance of small polyp detection in WCE images.

2.3. Single-Shot Multibox Detector (SSD)

The single-shot multibox detector (SSD) uses VGG16 as the backbone network and is truncated with other convolutional layers [23]. SSD uses ConvNet to generate a series of fixed-size bounding boxes and scores. Subsequently, it employs a non-maximum suppression (NMS) method for final detection. Figure 1 shows the SSD300 design framework separated into two parts; backbone and pyramid networks. The input sizes of the original images are 300 × 300 × 3. The VGG-16 network is used in the SSD300 model as the backbone, the first part constitutes four layers, and the second part is the application of a convolution operation to the Conv4_3 layer of the VGG16 network to generate five additional layers [18]. Shallower layers are investigated to predict smaller regions, while deeper layers for bigger ones. However, the problem of small object detection persists as the semantic information is not well extracted in shallower layers.

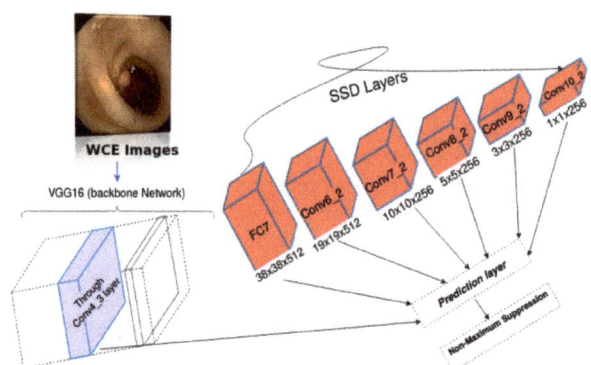

Figure 1. Framework of the traditional SSD.

2.4. Feature Pyramids Hierarchy

For object detection in medical imaging, various deep network architectures have been investigated to trade-off between precision and speed. Faster R-CNN [31] and R-FCN [21] perform one-scale feature maps to propose anchors for different scales. However, they cannot efficiently detect multi-scale objects as well as regions of small sizes. FPN [43] and DSSD [44] have used bottom-up and top-down architectures, respectively. For the rapid detection process, layer-by-layer feature map fusion is not recommended. The traditional SSD [23] uses the features of shallower layers, concatenates, and scales them from bottom to top to make predictions. Then, it generates a pyramidal feature map. Inspired by the feature fusion module, the proposal adopts the FSSD network structure [25]. However, the feature pyramid network has been altered to enhance the fusion effect in which an improved inception network is proposed to optimize SSD for improving the small object feature extraction ability in the shallow network and to tackle the problem of scale variations in detecting small polyp regions more effectively. The detailed information is presented in the following sections.

3. Materials and Methods

A systemic overview of the Hyb-SSDNet architecture for polyp detection is shown in Figure 2. The low-level feature layer with rich object information is not well reused in the conventional SSD using the VGG16 backbone, and the polyp region information is partially lost in the multi-layer transmission process. Therefore, the resulted feature information at each layer is unbalanced. To boost the detection effect of the model, an improved version of the SSD model-based inception v4 network (as the backbone) is proposed with further modification in regards to the deep network part. This study aimed to develop an optimization method for the detection results without sacrificing speed by fully utilizing the synthetic information of all the feature layers and increasing the effective receptive field. Thus, more object feature information can be extracted. We first describe the pre-processing step, in which the surrounding black regions in the WCE images are removed to extract the region of interest (ROI) patches that provide only useful information. The training phase of Hyb-SSDNet is divided into two parts: (i) data augmentation strategies to handle overfitting in deep learning models owing to the data insufficiency problem. Then, we pre-trained the Hyb-SSDNet model on the ILSVRC CLS-LOC dataset [45] and fine-tuned it on the WCE/colonoscopy polyp datasets. (ii) The backbone network inception v4 for feature extraction (including a weighted mid-fusion block of the inception modules) for small polyp detection and the classification sub-network on multi-scale feature maps.

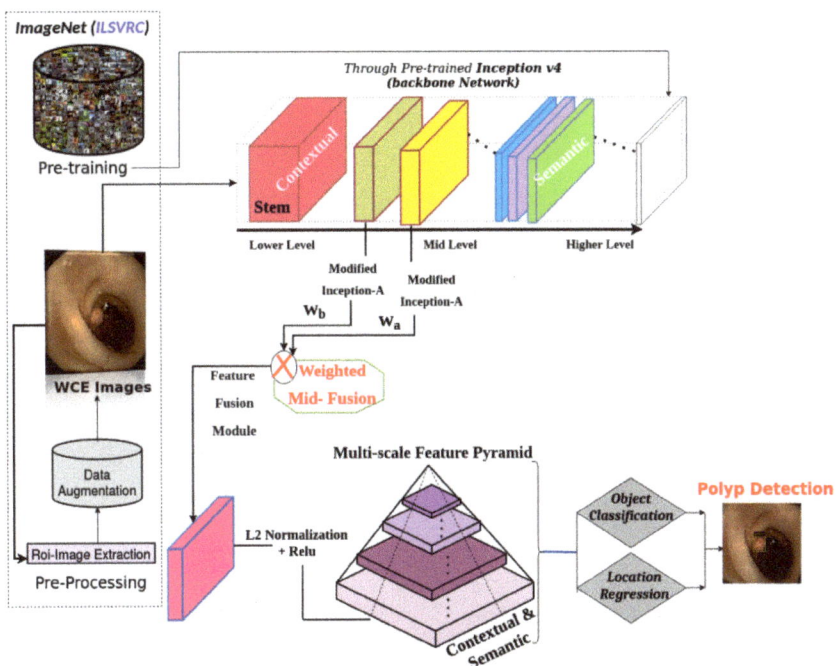

Figure 2. Flowchart of the proposed Hyb-SSDNet method for small polyp detection in WCE images.

3.1. Mid-Fusion Block

Different multi-modal fusions have been widely used in deep learning. Mid-fusion operates independently at each scale. It then merges and passes them to complete the network processes. However, information from multiple scales is treated equally during fusion. Capturing variance in visual patterns as well as more informative patterns in class prediction is one of the requirements of the complete classification approach. Besides, the traditional SSD-based VGG16 network only uses the 1×1 and 3×3 convolution kernel for one convolution layer, making its feature extraction ability inefficient. To address this shortcoming, two weighted inception-A modules based on inception v4 were adapted to the mid-fusion block, giving more weight to important features. The modified inception-A module is presented in Figure 3. To enhance the feature extraction, the network width is increased by exploiting sparsity in the network connectivity. A cascade convolution layer composed of two convolution kernels with different sizes and an average pooling layer are combined in parallel. First, the 1×1 convolution reduces the dimension before the convolution operation and after the pooling operation, which significantly reduces the calculation cost. The inception-A module of (inception v4 network) uses two 3×3 continuous convolutions instead of the 5×5 convolution kernel to extract more detailed object features and improve the calculation speed. Finally, the information of different receptive fields is concatenated in one single layer in order to improve the feature representation ability of the network. The L2 weight regularization is added to the convolutional layers, the most common type used for neural networks with a sensible default weighting of 0.00004 specifying the type of regularization as He_normal initializers. In addition, after the convolution layer, batch normalization (BN) and ReLU activation functions are used to accelerate the network training speed and enhance the detection robustness.

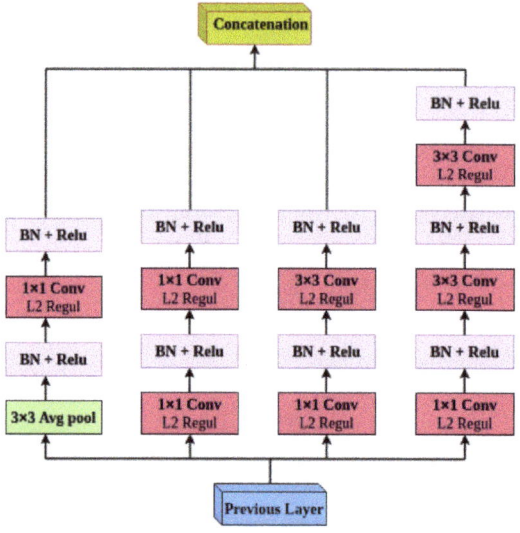

Figure 3. Modified inception structure.

The main fusion structure is shown in Figure 4. We considered S_{L_i} as the mid-level inception module feature and $S_{L_{i+1}}$ as its adjacent inception module feature maps. After extracting mid-level features at two scales, we apply the mSE-Network to each inception feature map in each channel (F) and spatial position, enabling the extraction of the most representative features in highlighting the region of interest computed as:

$$\tilde{S}_{L_i}^F = (mSE-Network(S_{L_i}); mSE-Network(S_{L_{i+1}})) \qquad (1)$$

The $\tilde{S}_{L_i}^F$ and $\tilde{S}_{L_{i+1}}^F$ have the same channel sizes and are fused using a simple concatenation strategy. In the literature, there are other fusion approaches, such as element-wise summation, element-wise multiplication, averaging process, etc. To verify the best concatenation strategy, several experiments were conducted. Inspired by the [46] connection module, a simple concatenation strategy was adopted in this study for the global feature fusion module, as it is more effective. The concatenation operation provides more feature representations for feature maps of the same size. The map merging operation can be described as:

$$S'_{HL} = D(\tilde{S}_{L_i}^F; \tilde{S}_{L_{i+1}}^F) \qquad (2)$$

where D is the feature concatenation operation, $\tilde{S}_{L_i}^F$ and $\tilde{S}_{L_{i+1}}^F$ are the channel-adjusted feature maps from two successive mid-level layers, and S'_{HL} is the fused feature map producing a new high-resolution image that contains both rich semantic features and location information. An L2 normalization operation and ReLU activation were then applied to all filters after the concatenation procedure because the feature values in the layers were significantly different in scale. The feature fusion module also localizes small polyp regions by assigning higher weights to pixels containing the object class. Furthermore, the fusion block tends to increase the discrimination capacity of the network by highlighting small polyp edges in some of the feature maps. Thus, the most informative features of the background were extracted and discriminated from the object in the weighted feature maps. In this study, the mid-fusion block is used to generate spatial and multi-scale score maps for the features extracted from two successive inception modules at the mid-level of the inception v4 network. Polyp regions show great variation in shape, size, and orientation at different scales. This is the main motivation behind using a heterogeneous weighted feature fusion of polyp regions. Thus, making the network sensitive to unique contextual image features improved the classification performance for polyp regions.

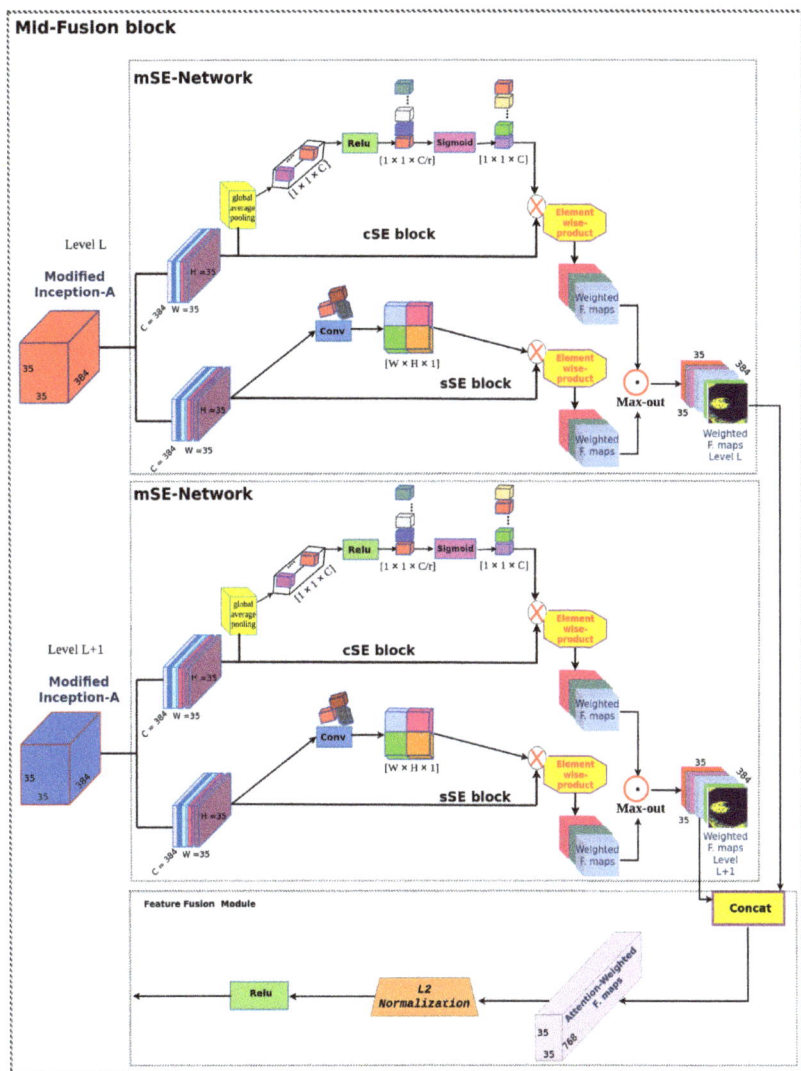

Figure 4. The mid-fusion framework. Input feature maps were created at two successive inception modules of the inception v4 network to encode contextual information. All scale sizes are $35 \times 35 \times 384$. Extracted features were passed to the mSE-Network to generate the score maps, reflecting the importance of features at different positions and scales. Weighted features were then concatenated and normalized to complete the network process.

mSE-Network

This is motivated by the squeeze-and-excitation network's success [47] in showing significant improvement in the performance related to medical image analysis. Hyb-SSDNet uses a learnable mechanism, highlighting the most salient feature maps, and avoiding no-useful information of background. The structure of the squeeze-and-excitation block (mSE-Network) used in this proposal is shown in Figure 4.

cSE Block The squeeze-and-excitation network uses a squeeze operation as a primary process by applying a global average pooling (Shen et al., 2015) to spatially compress the input feature maps, and reduce the dimensionality from $W \times H \times C$ to $1 \times 1 \times C$. The squeeze operation can be described in Equation (3) as follows: We consider the input feature map $Y = [y_1, y_2, y_3, \ldots, y_c], y_i \in \mathbb{R}^{H \times W}$

$$x_l = \frac{1}{W \times H} \sum_j^W \sum_k^H y_l(i,j). \quad (3)$$

where x is the vector output, $x \in \mathbb{R}^{1 \times 1 \times c}$ with its lth element. The spatial squeeze operation only embeds the global spatial information in the output vector (x). Therefore, the channel-wise dependencies will not be well encoded. Hence, the squeeze-and-excitation network uses the excitation operation to solve the channel's weight inefficiency. One of the more significant issues of the excitation operation is to properly learn the non-linear interaction between channels as they have to be activated simultaneously. Therefore, two fully-connected layers $F_1 \in \mathbb{R}^{C \times \frac{C}{r}}, F_2 \in \mathbb{R}^{\frac{C}{r} \times C}$, and the ReLU operation $\delta(.)$ were used. The excitation operation is calculated in Equation (4) as follows:

$$\tilde{x} = F_1(Relu(F_2 \times x)). \quad (4)$$

where C and r mean the number of channels and the scaling parameters, respectively. To reduce the computational complexity of the modified inception-A modules, the r parameter is set to 2. Finally, a channel-wise recalibration of the output vector was performed with the input feature maps to be scaled consistently to original sizes. We consider sig as the sigmoid activation. The final step reconstructs the spatial squeeze and channel excitation block (cSE). The merging operation expressed in Equation (5) is as follows:

$$\tilde{x} = [sig(\tilde{x}_1)y_1, sig(\tilde{x}_2)y_2, sig(\tilde{x}_3)y_3, \ldots, sig(\tilde{x}_C)y_C]. \quad (5)$$

sSE block: The channel squeeze and spatial excitation (sSE block) assume the importance of squeezing the input feature map along the channels and mutually exciting them spatially. Therefore, a convolutional layer is applied to compress the input feature map. The sigmoid function is activated to obtain spatially distributed information. Finally, the sSE block processed a concatenation operation for the feature map fusion with the input feature map, computed in Equation (6) as:

$$\ddot{x} = Sig(W_d, Y) \times Y. \quad (6)$$

where $Y = [y^{1,1}, y^{2,2}, y^{3,3}, \ldots, y^{H \times W}], y^{i,j} \in \mathbb{R}^{1 \times 1 \times C}$ is the input feature map and $W_d \in \mathbb{R}^{1 \times 1 \times C}$, generating a projection tensor $d \in \mathbb{R}^{W \times H}$, $\ddot{x}$ is the final vector for the sSE block. To mutually recalibrate feature information in both spatial and channel directions, the mSE-block performs a joint version of the spatial squeeze and channel excitation (cSE) block and channel squeeze and spatial excitation (sSE) block [48], which can be calculated in Equation (7) as follows:

$$Y_{scSE}(i,j,C) = max(\tilde{x}(i,j,C), \ddot{x}(i,j,C)). \quad (7)$$

This is based on the experiments conducted in the work of [48]. Concatenation obtains the best results compared to other strategies that target the spatial and channel squeeze excitation SE. However, it increases the channel number that implicitly increases the model complexity. Thus, we used the max-out strategy to merge the two blocks as it obtains approximately similar results to the concatenation procedure.

3.2. Multi-Scale Feature Pyramid

This is motivated by FSSD [18,25]. The feature maps from the weighted feature fusion module (Figure 4) using the inception v4 network (backbone) were considered as inputs for the multi-scale feature pyramid, as shown in Figure 5. The lightweight feature fusion module (S'_{HL}) is designed to utilize a spatially coarser but a semantically richer feature map from the middle pyramid level incorporating proprieties of both high level and its relatively lower-level features. Figure 5 presents a top-down Hyb-SSDNet architecture that incorporates semantic information of shallow and mid-level layers into textural features of high levels. The entire process is as follows: First, a mid-fusion block of two adjacent inception-A modules was performed. Then, L2 normalization and ReLU activation were applied. The input size of the WCE/colonoscopy images was 299 × 299, and the network structure of the Hyb-SSDNet could be divided into two parts: the backbone network inception v4 feature extraction and feature fusion module, and multi-scale feature pyramid for polyp region detection. The filter numbers of the first convolution layers in the stem part of the inception v4 backbone were modified from 32 to 64 to reinforce the model to capture more patterns and relevant information similar to the original SSD. Sequential experiments proved that these steps enrich the semantic information of shallow and mid-level features, and improve the model performance in small polyp regions. After concatenation, a batch normalization operation was performed. The detailed structure of the model is illustrated in Figure 6. Based on experiments conducted in the work of [25], a feature map of resolution smaller than 10 px × 10 px may not contain much information to reuse. This was inspired by the feature fusion SSD (FSSD) [25]. We constructed multi-scale feature layers based on the SSD network, which added new layers, Conv6_2, Conv7_2, Conv8_2, and Conv9_2, for object classification and location regression. To ensure precision and detection speed, the Hyb-SSDNet network investigated new feature fusion module layers based on the inception v4 network, Conv1_WF, Conv2_WF, Conv3_WF, Conv4_WF, Conv5_WF, and Conv6_WF, for the detection of small polyps. The target sizes of the resulting feature layers were 35 × 35, 18 × 18, 9 × 9, 5 × 5, 3 × 3, and 1 × 1, different from those of the FSSD model.

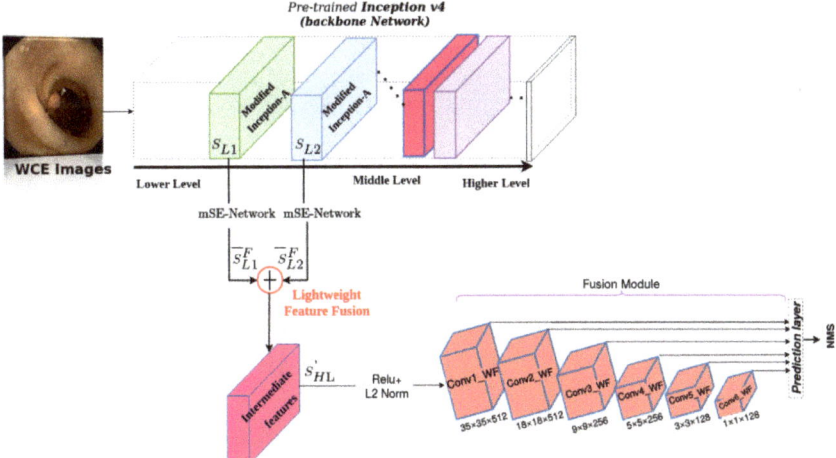

Figure 5. Overview of the Hyb-SSDNet architecture with a 299 × 299 × 3 input size and inception v4 as the backbone. Features from two successive modified inception-A layers (S_{L1}, S_{L2}) were fused by a mid-fusion block producing an intermediate feature representation (S'_{HL}).

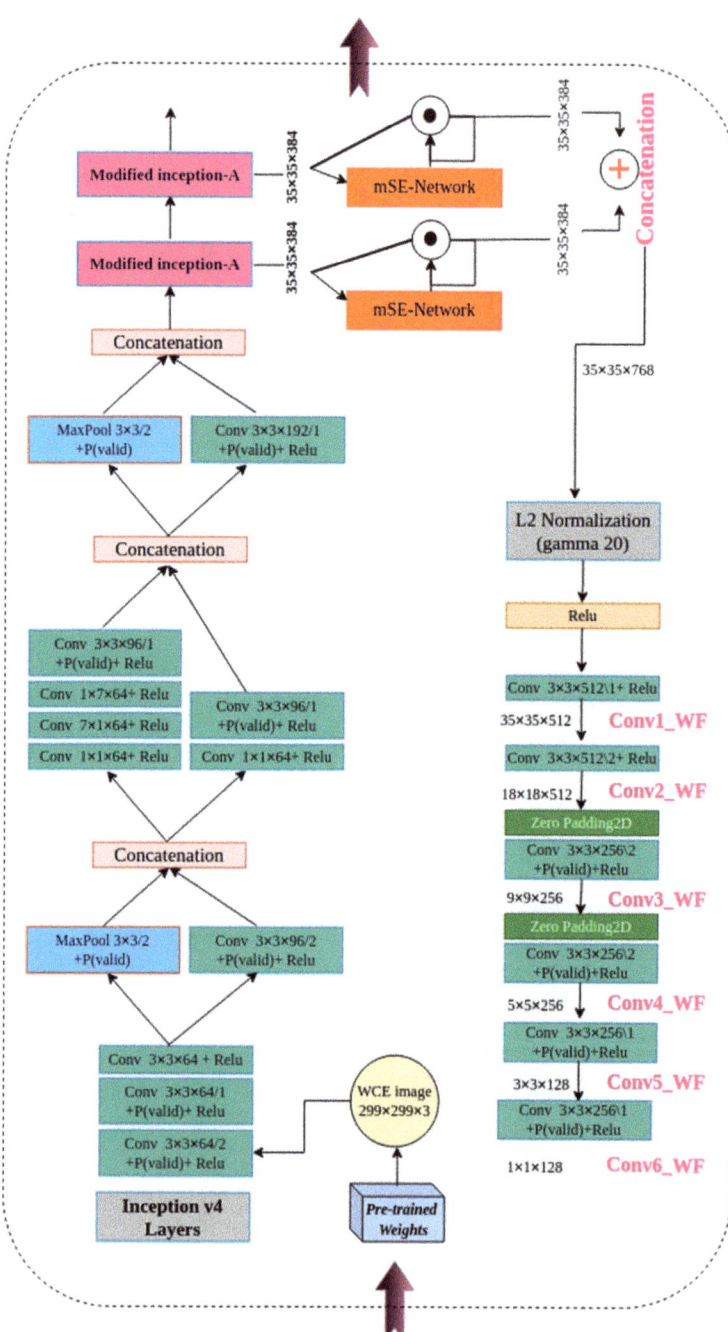

Figure 6. Detailed structure of the Hyb-SSDNet network.

4. Experiments

4.1. Datasets

The Fist WCE dataset was acquired from PillCam©COLON 2 polyps [49]. The original image's resolution was 256 pixels × 256 pixels. As depicted in Figure 7, the WCE dataset contains 120 polyps and 181 normal images obtained from one patient's VCE test. To avoid the overfitting problem owing to the small dataset size, we increased the training dataset size by the pre-processing step, as described in this section. Therefore, the revised dataset included 1250 polyp patches and 1864 normal patches. Subsequently, two trained experts reviewed and manually defined binary masks corresponding to the polyp regions covered to provide ground truths after being manually labeled and annotated as positive and negative samples. The ground truth bounding box was drawn based on the mask ground truth provided by specialists to meet the requirements of the polyp detection tools, using a graphical image annotation tool and label object bounding boxes in images (LabelImg) and corrected by experts. A popular colonoscopy dataset called CVC-ClinicDB [50] was also used in this work, which contained frames showing polyp regions of different shapes. A total of 25 colonoscopy videos were used by researchers to select at least 29 sequences containing one polyp region in every frame. Subsequently, a set of frames was selected for each sequence. As depicted in Figure 8, the CVC-ClinicDB dataset comprises 612 polyp images (size: 384 × 288; format: tiff). Experts created the ground truth by manually defining masks corresponding to the regions covered by the polyps in each frame. To meet the requirements of polyp detection tools, the ground truth bounding box was drawn based on the ground truth provided by specialists. The annotated ETIS-Larib [51] dataset was used to assess the detection results. A total of 34 colonoscopy videos were used to generate 196 polyp images of different shapes and sizes. The ground truths of the ETIS-Larib dataset were annotated by competent endoscopists members of clinical institutions as depicted in Figure 9. The colonoscopy CVC-ClinicDB [52] and ETIS-Larib [53] datasets were adopted in the 2015 MICCAI sub-challenge on automatic polyp detection. The normal and abnormal images were rescaled to 299 × 299 pixels to reach the pre-trained inception v4 network input size. We split the data into training 70%, validation 10%, and model testing 20%. The five-fold cross-validation [54] was used, in which the state and convergence of the model were checked after each epoch was completed. The hyperparameter number of iterations and learning rate were adjusted automatically during the validation data. In general, the validation set only adjusts the hyperparameters, such as the number of iterations and learning rate. Subsequently, they were adopted according to the five group performances in the models. The results were then averaged over the splits to estimate the mean average precision metric.

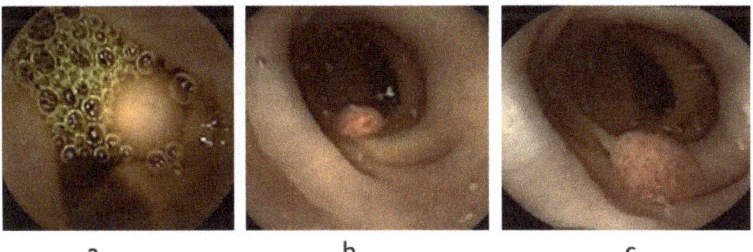

Figure 7. Example of WCE polyp images (**a**–**c**).

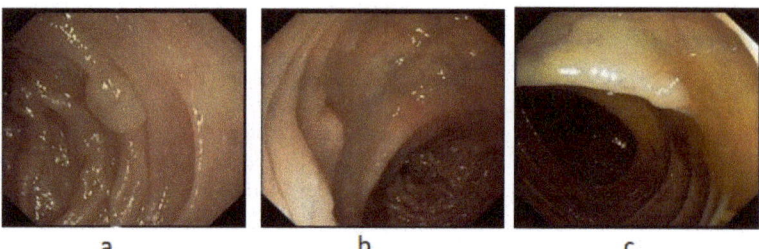

Figure 8. Example of CVC-ClinicDB polyp images (**a–c**).

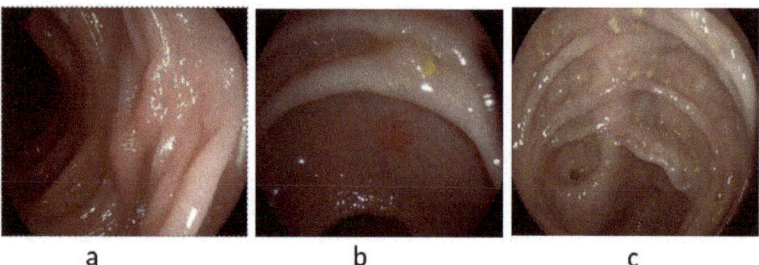

Figure 9. Example of ETIS-Larib polyp images (**a–c**).

4.2. Evaluation Indexes

In this study, the mean average precision (mAP) metric was adopted to evaluate polyp detection performance. Using an intersection over union (IoU) of 0.5, the mAP is defined as the average of the average precision (AP) of all object categories. It is formulated by Equation (8).

$$mAP = \frac{\sum_{q=1}^{Q} AveP(q)}{Q} \qquad (8)$$

where Q is the number of queries in the set and q is the query for average precision.

Given a set of ground truth bounding boxes annotated by the experts, and a set of predicted bounding boxes produced by the network with a confidence score above a specific threshold (for example, 0.5), *precision*, *recall*, and *F1-score* can be defined in Equations (9) and (10) as:

$$Precision = \frac{TP}{TP+FP} \quad Recall = \frac{TP}{TP+FN} \qquad (9)$$

$$F-measure/F1-score = \frac{(2 \times Recall \times Precision)}{Recall + Precision} \qquad (10)$$

where *TP* denotes true positives; that is, IoU > 0.5, *FP* indicates false positives and *FN* indicates false negatives. Frame per second (FPS) is used to measure the detection speed and indicates the number of frames transmitted per second. More details regarding the evaluation metrics can be found in [18].

4.3. Experimental Setup

4.3.1. Experimental Environment Configuration

The experiments were performed using Colab Pro Plus solution provided by Google, with a maximum RAM of 52 Gb and a disk of 166,83 Gb. All experiments were conducted using CUDA 8.0.61-1, CuDNN6.0, Keras 2.0.5, Python 3.5, h5py 2.10.0, NumPy 1.16.3, TensorFlow 1.15, TensorFlow-GPU 1.15, and OpenCV 3.1. According to the ground truth bounding boxes of the small polyp region, the same aspect ratio within a range of 1–2 was maintained for all employed datasets.

4.3.2. Model Training

To verify the capability of the Hyb-SSDNet model, various indicators and parameters in the field of medical imaging were investigated and adjusted. As a primary process, the surrounding black regions containing no useful information about the WCE polyp image were removed, as they may have degraded the performance of WCE polyp detection and increased the computation time. The input images were resized to $299 \times 299 \times 3$, and the batch size was 32. Concerning data augmentation strategies [55], we investigated flipping, rotation by 270°, and cropping schemes. Further details can be found in previous studies [56,57]. We pre-trained the model on the ImageNet Large Scale Visual Recognition Challenge (ILSVRC) dataset, as it showcased massive progress in large-scale object recognition over the past five years. We then fine-tuned the model on the WCE and colonoscopy datasets. This method dynamically decreases the learning rate based on the number of epochs, training times, and losses. Adaptive moment estimation (Adam) is an optimization method for the adaptive learning rate. Practically, the Adam optimizer is utilized in this work due to its efficiency with large problems. The initial learning rate is set to 0.0001, and the learning rate decay policy is approximately different from the original SSD with a drop of 0.5 and epochs_drop of 10. Other hyperparameters were adjusted, beta_1 = 0.9, epsilon of 1×10^{-8}, and beta_2 = 0.999. Using Keras, the learning rate schedule is defined as follows: 0.0001 if epoch < 50, 0.00001 if epoch < 80, and 0.000001 otherwise. Hyb-SSDNet is an improved model for the in-depth feature fusion of SSD300. For a fair comparison with the state-of-the-art approaches, target polyp detection was used [18]. The model uses 100 epochs and 500 steps per training epoch. The mean average precision (mAP), the number of picture frames that could be detected by the model per second (FPS), and other indicators were used to evaluate the detection performance. Similar to conventional SSD [23], the same loss function was used in the Hyb-SSDNet model. The hyper-parameter neg_pos_ratio was set to 3 and the α parameter was adjusted by cross-validation to 1. More SSD_Loss details are presented in [41].

4.4. Results and Discussion

4.4.1. Ablation Studies

In this section, we investigate the effectiveness of the different components that affected the experimental results of the main structure of the Hyb-SSDNet detector through an ablation study on the WCE, CVC-ClinicDB, and ETIS-Larib colonoscopy datasets. Different Hyb-SSDNet model settings are shown in Table 1 in which the inception v4 backbone was kept. A mid-fusion block was designed based on the middle part of the detection network to incorporate the semantic information of small polyps into the Hyb-SSDNet network. Training and testing were performed on the WCE images, or in the CVC-ClinicDB and ETIS-Larib joint training set and tested on the CVC-ClinicDB and ETIS-Larib test sets. First, we compare two mainstream normalization methods (Batch Normalization and L2 Normalization) and report their effects on the performance mAP (%) of the proposed system. As reported in Table 1 (row 5, row 7 and row10), L2 normalization yielded better results (90.11%, 93.29% and 92.53% mAP), whereas it is (88.42%, 89.96% and 89.75% mAP) using batch normalization on the WCE train and test. The CVC-ClinicDB and ETIS-Larib test sets support the results obtained on the WCE test set (col 5–row 17 and row 20) and (col 4–row 27 and row 30). Thus, it is reasonable to choose L2 normalization instead of batch normalization in mid-fusion design. Various feature fusion techniques have been investigated to determine the most appropriate one for the Hyb-SSDNet framework. Considering the WCE test set, it can be seen in Table 1 (rows 7) that the framework adopting simple concatenation to fuse and scale the feature maps of shallow and middle layers obtains the best result, 3.18 points higher than the average strategy and 4.6 points higher than element-wise summation while it costs low performances in term of mAP Table 1 (row 1 and row 8) without utilizing a weighted fusion structure. This means assigning a weighted score to each feature map in each layer and scale, giving them relative importance in contributing to small polyp detection. In addition, experiments on the CVC-ClinicDB and ETIS-Larib test set Table 1 (row 11–20) and (row 21–30) support the results obtained on the WCE images and demonstrate the high efficiency of the concatenation strategy for mid-level fusion with L2 normalization, highlighting more important features for small polyp detection.

Table 1. Effects of different design factors of the mid-fusion block on the Hyb-SSDNet performances. The mAP is measured on the WCE, CVC-ClinicDB, and ETIS-Larib test sets.

Training Data	Testing Data	Mid-Fusion Block	Weighted Feature Fusion	Normalization	Feature Fusion	mAP (%)
WCE	WCE	Inception-A (×2)	×	×	Concatenation	89.85
		Inception-A(× 2)	✓	×	Summation	88.69
		Stem & Inception-A(×1)	×	B.Norm	Concatenation	88.42
		Stem & Inception-A(×1)	✓	×	Summation	89.28
		Inception-A(×2)	✓	L2.Norm	Average	90.11
		Inception-A(×2)	✓	B.Norm	Average	89.96
		Inception-A(×2)	✓	L2.Norm	Concatenation	**93.29**
		Stem & Inception-A(×2)	×	B.Norm	Concatenation	89.75
		Stem & Inception-A(×2)	✓	×	Summation	91.42
		Stem & Inception-A(×2)	✓	L2.Norm	Average	92.53
CVC-ClinicDB & ETIS-Larib	CVC-ClinicDB	Inception-A (×2)	×	×	Concatenation	88.25
		Inception-A(×2)	✓	×	Summation	87.37
		Stem & Inception-A(×1)	×	B.Norm	Concatenation	88.21
		Stem & Inception-A(×1)	✓	×	Summation	88.98
		Inception-A(×2)	✓	L2.Norm	Average	89.74
		Inception-A(×2)	✓	B.Norm	Average	88.65
		Inception-A(×2)	✓	L2.Norm	Concatenation	**91.93**
		Stem & Inception-A(×2)	×	B.Norm	Concatenation	88.87
		Stem & Inception-A(×2)	✓	×	Summation	89.68
		Stem & Inception-A(×2)	✓	L2.Norm	Average	90.14
CVC-ClinicDB & ETIS-Larib	ETIS-Larib	Inception-A (×2)	×	×	Concatenation	88.49
		Inception-A(x2)	✓	×	Summation	88.03
		Stem & Inception-A(×1)	×	B.Norm	Concatenation	87.82
		Stem & Inception-A(x1)	✓	×	Summation	89.46
		Inception-A(×2)	✓	L2.Norm	Average	89
		Inception-A(×2)	✓	B.Norm	Average	88.94
		Inception-A(×2)	✓	L2.Norm	Concatenation	**91.10**
		Stem & Inception-A(×2)	×	B.Norm	Concatenation	87.73
		Stem & Inception-A(×2)	✓	×	Summation	89.41
		Stem & Inception-A(×2)	✓	L2.Norm	Average	90.05

Where B.Norm and L2. Norm mean batch normalization and L2 normalization, respectively. Concatenation is a simple concatenation strategy. Summation refers to an element-wise addition strategy, and average is an element-wise mean strategy.

Table 2 lists the results of the proposed method on the WCE, CVC-ClinicDB, and ETIS-Larib test sets, as well as some state-of-the-art detector-based SSDs. The (mAP) of SSD300 using VGG16 (backbone) were 77.2%, 74.5%, and 74.12% for the WCE, CVC-ClinicDB, and ETIS-Larib test sets, respectively. The feature fusion strategy provides richer details and semantic information, showing remarkable results compared to the conventional SSD. As depicted in Table 2 (rows 5–6 and rows 15–16), FSSD300 and FSSD500 frameworks were increased by (12.58% and 9.25%), (12.76% and 9.16%), and (12.18% and 11.47%) in terms of (mAP) in WCE, CVC-ClinicDB, and ETIS-Larib test sets. By replacing the backbone network VGGNet with DenseNet-S-32-1, the DF-SSD300 model exceeded the FSSD300 by 1.46%, 2.66%, and 0.54 mAP (91.24% vs. 89.78%), (89.92% vs. 87.26%), and (86.84% vs. 86.3%) for all test sets, respectively. The detection speed decreases by half. The VGG16 network was replaced with the ResNet-101 backbone in the L_SSD model (row 8 and row 18) to perform feature fusion, which contained rich details and semantic information. The mAP of ResNet-101 was slightly better than that of FSSD300 for both WCE and colonoscopy datasets. The proposed Hyb-SSDNet algorithm outperforms the FSSD300, DF-SSD300, and L_SSD models by 3.51 points (93.29% vs. 89.78%), 2.05 points (93.29% vs. 91.24%), and 3.31 points (93.29% vs. 89.98%) on WCE dataset, while it achieves almost similar performance with the MP-FSSD network on the WCE dataset; 0.22 points (93.29% vs. 93.4%). The Hyb-SSDNet framework achieved promising results, with a small drop in speed. However, it still achieved real-time detection with 44.5 FPS, compared with DF-SSD300 and L-SSD with 11.6 FPS and 40 FPS, respectively. Figure 10a–c supports the results obtained in Table 2 as it shows the recall vs. precision plots obtained for this experiment on WCE, CVC-ClinicDB, and ETIS-Larib test sets. The Hyb-SSDNet has strong feature reuse and extraction abilities. The mid-fusion block uses a weighted concatenation of spatial features at each location and scale. Therefore, the features of unrelated regions, such as the background, are suppressed. Thus, the fusion inception modules help the model focus on real targets and improve the precision of the detection of small polyps.

Table 2. Comparison with previously published methods based on SSD, WCE, CVC-ClinicDB, and ETIS-Larib test sets. Pre-train means that a pre-trained backbone was adopted to initialize the model or it was initialized from scratch. The speed (FPS) and the (mAP) performances were tested using google Colab pro+ GPU.

Training Data	Methods	Backbone	Input Size	Pre-Train	FPS	mAP@0.5(%)	
						WCE	
WCE	SSD300	VGG16	300 × 300 × 3	✓	46	77.2	
	SSD300	ResNet-101	300 × 300 × 3	✓	47.3	81.65	
	SSD500	VGG16	300 × 300 × 3	✓	19	79.45	
	SSD500	ResNet-101	300 × 300 × 3	✓	20	84.95	
	FSSD300	VGG16	300 × 300 × 3	✓	65.9	89.78	
	FSSD500	VGG16	500 × 500 × 3	✓	69.6	88.71	
	DF-SSD300 [41]	DenseNet-S-32-1	300 × 300 × 3	✓	11.6	91.24	
	L_SSD [58]	ResNet-101	224 × 224 × 3	✓	40	89.98	
	MP-FSSD [18]	VGG16	300 × 300 × 3	✓	62.57	93.4	
	Hyb-SSDNet (ours)	Inception v4	299 × 299 × 3	✓	44.5	93.29	
						CVC-ClinicDB	ETIS-Larib
CVC-ClinicDB & ETIS-Larib	SSD300	VGG16	300 × 300 × 3	✓	46	74.5	74.12
	SSD300	ResNet-101	300 × 300 × 3	✓	47.3	78.85	75.73
	SSD500	VGG16	500 × 500 × 3	✓	19	78.38	75.45
	SSD500	ResNet-101	500 × 500 × 3	✓	20	82.74	80.14
	FSSD300	VGG16	300 × 300 × 3	✓	65.9	87.26	86.3
	FSSD500	VGG16	500 × 500 × 3	✓	69.6	87.54	86.92
	DF-SSD300 [41]	DenseNet-S-32-1	300 × 300 × 3	✓	11.6	89.92	86.84
	L_SSD [58]	ResNet-101	224 × 224 × 3	✓	40	88.18	87.23
	MP-FSSD [18]	VGG16	300 × 300 × 3	✓	62.57	89.82	90
	Hyb-SSDNet (ours)	Inception v4	299 × 299 × 3	✓	44.5	91.93	91.10

4.4.2. Comparison with the State-of-the-Art Method

For fair comparison experiments with the proposed Hyb-SSDNet framework, we selected the most highlighted methods in the literature-based SSDs models, YOLOv3, and DSSD, as listed in Table 3. To quantitatively compare Hyb-SSDNet with other state-of-the-art models, the performances of the trained model on the ETIS-Larib and CVC-ClinicDB training sets were evaluated on the publicly available ETIS-Larib dataset. As depicted in Table 3, the Hyb-SSDNet model obtains encouraging results of the (mAP) metric on the WCE dataset compared with other models. This is attributable to the fact that polyp abnormalities exhibit great variation in terms of color and shape. In addition, WCE, CVC-ClinicDB, and ETIS-Larib images differ in nature, texture, and illumination acquisition conditions. However, they achieved similar metrics. Additionally, the colors of the polyps vary across different images within a patient's VCE and other patients' examinations. Compared to previous approaches targeting polyp detection, Hyb-SSDNet achieved the best mAP, which reached 93.29%, 91.93%, and 91.10%, respectively. The joint training of the ETIS-Larib and CVC-ClinicDB datasets exceeded some competitor models or achieved approximately similar metrics on the ETIS-Larib test set. Overall, the Hyb-SSDNet shows promising results in terms of the mAP with a slight speed drop.

Table 3. WCE or colonoscopy test detection results, or both (IOU > 0.5, batch-size 1).

Training Dataset	Methods	Testing Dataset	Backbone Network	Pre-Train	Input Size	Prec	Recall	F1 Score
WCE images	Hyb-SSDNet (ours)	WCE images	Inception v4	✓	299 × 299	93.29%(mAP)	89.4%(mAR)	91.5%(mAF)
ETIS-Larib+CVC-ClinicDB	Hyb-SSDNet (ours)	CVC-ClinicDB	Inception v4	✓	299 × 299	91.93%(mAP)	89.5%(mAR)	90.8%(mAF)
ETIS-Larib+CVC-ClinicDB	Hyb-SSDNet (ours)	ETIS-Larib	Inception v4	✓	299 × 299	91.10%(mAP)	87%(mAR)	89%(mAF)
WCE +CVC-ClinicDB	Souaidi et al., 2022 [18]	ETIS-Larib	VGG16	✓	300 × 300	90.02%(mAP)	×	×
CVC-ClinicDB + ETIS-Larib	Shin et al., 2018 [59]	ETIS-Larib	Inception ResNet	✓	768 × 576	92.2%	69.7%	79.4%
SUN+ PICCOLO+ CVC-ClinicDB	Ishak et al., 2021 [32]	ETIS-Larib	YOLOv3	✓	448 × 448	90.61%	91.04%	90.82%
CVC-ClinicDB	Liu et al., 2021 [60]	ETIS-Larib	ResNet-101	✓	384 × 288	77.80%	87.50%	82.40%
GIANA 2017	Wang et al., 2019 [61]	ETIS-Larib	AFP-Net(VGG16)	✓	1225 × 996	88.89%	80.7%	84.63%
CVC-ClinicDB	Qadir et al., 2021 [62]	ETIS-Larib	ResNet34	✓	512 × 512	86.54%	86.12%	86.33%
CVC-ClinicDB	Pacal and Karaboga, 2021 [63]	ETIS-Larib	CSPDarkNet53	✓	384 × 288	91.62%	82.55%	86.85%
CVC-ClinicDB	Wang et al., 2019 [61]	ETIS-Larib	Faster R-CNN (VGG16)	×	224 × 224	88.89%	80.77%	84.63%
CVC-VideoClinicDB	Krenzer et al., 2019 [64]	CVC-VideoClinicDB	YOLOv5	×	574 × 500	73.21%(mAP)	×	79.55%

4.4.3. Visualization of Detection Results

The main objective is to prove the efficiency of the proposed Hyb-SSDNet framework, not only for WCE polyp images detection but also for colonoscopy polyp localization cases (CVC-ClinicDB and ETIS-Larib). Polyp detection involves the identification of polyp regions and the rejection of parts containing normal, blurry tissues, and others showing feces or water jet sprays to clean the colon. Figures 11–13 show some detection cases of the FSSD and their analogs of the Hyb-SSDNet model on the WCE, CVC-ClinicDB, and ETIS-Larib polyp test sets, respectively. The false negative rate decreased because the Hyb-SSDNet model Figures 11h and 12b,d showed a relative improvement in small polyp localization from the normal intestinal mucosa in comparison with the FSSD model Figures 11g and 12a,c. Specifically, the FSSD model failed to observe the context information of the object because it uses a small receptive field that can only detect smaller objects from shallow layers. Other circumstances have hindered the identification of small polyp regions. Their similarity in appearance to the surrounding normal mucosa, their complicated characteristics (color, texture, contrast, and size), and the presence of air bubbles, food, and other debris, limits the visualization of the actual extent of the lumen by capsule endoscopy. Therefore, Hyb-SSDNet performs a weighted mid-fusion module of middle layers and embeds it into the final fusion block, which can capture scene contexts and differentiate polyp edge regions from normal mucosa. Figures 11e, 12g, and 13c,e show the false positive identifications of the FSSD model in the normal mucosa areas of the WCE, CVC-ClinicDB, and ETIS-Larib test sets. Compared to the Hyb-SSDNet framework, Figures 11f, 12h, and 13d,f show some true-positive identification cases of Hyb-SSDNet in different normal mucosa areas. Regarding the WCE images, the difference in appearance between the polyp regions and the normal mucosa was not obvious. Thus, the WCE frames captured in the case of insufficient light produced poor pixels, which hindered the detection process as depicted in Figure 11h. However, the proposed Hyb-SSDNet algorithm also shows a remarkable improvement in large polyp detection for the WCE, CVC-ClinicDB, and ETIS-Larib test sets, and accurately distinguishes them from the surrounding normal areas. Limited by different debris, Figures 12b and 13h show hard cases of small polyps behind the folds of the CVC-ClinicDB and ETIS-Larib test sets, respectively. Even specialists sometimes mistakenly recognize these parts when they are hidden from view behind a fold or wrapped around a fold in a clamshell fashion and find them difficult to 'resect'.

However, the proposed Hyb-SSDNet model successfully detected a hard polyp case in which the ground truth was not annotated by experts Figure 12b.

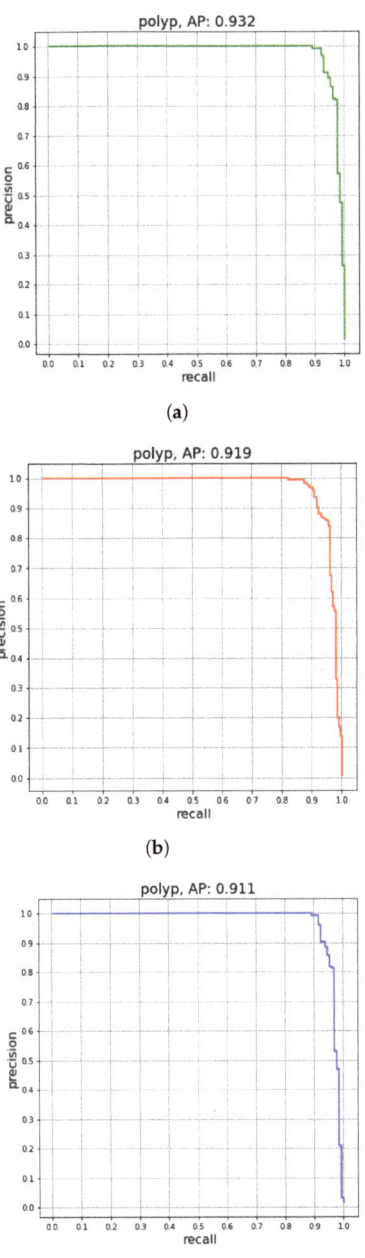

Figure 10. Precision vs. recall for (a) WCE test set, (b) CVC-ClinicDB test set, and (c) ETIS-Larib test set using the Hyb-SSDNet framework.

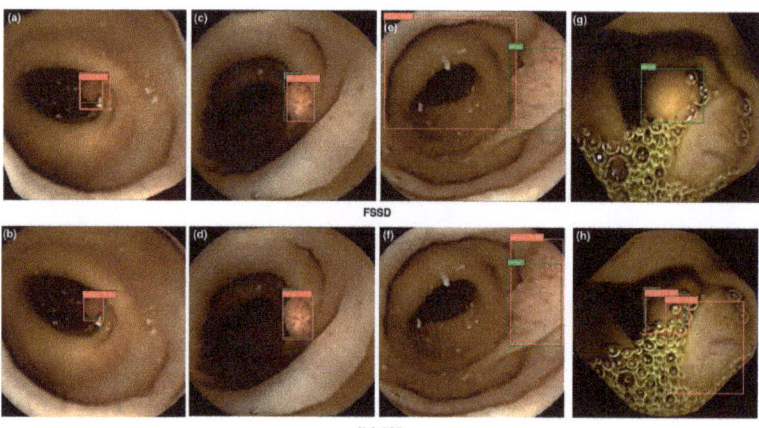

Figure 11. Qualitative results comparison between FSSD300 (**a,c,e,g**) and the proposed Hyb-SSDNet (**b,d,f,h**) on the WCE polyp test set. True bounding boxes with IoU of 0.5 or higher with the bounding predicted boxes are drawn in green and red colors, respectively.

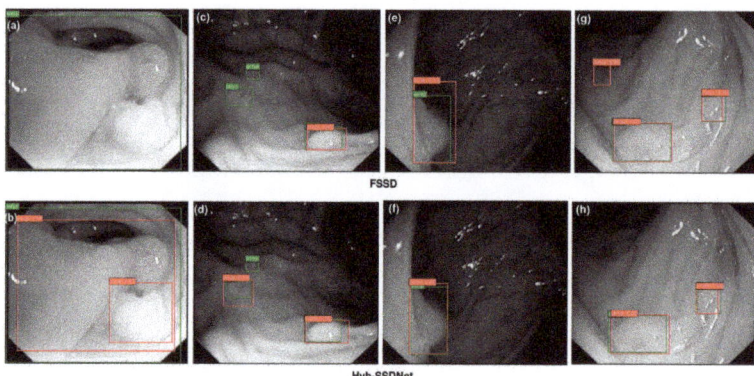

Figure 12. Qualitative results comparison between FSSD300 (**a,c,e,g**) and the proposed Hyb-SSDNet (**b,d,f,h**) on the CVC-ClinicDB polyp test set. True bounding boxes with IoU of 0.5 or higher with the bounding predicted boxes are drawn in green and red colors, respectively.

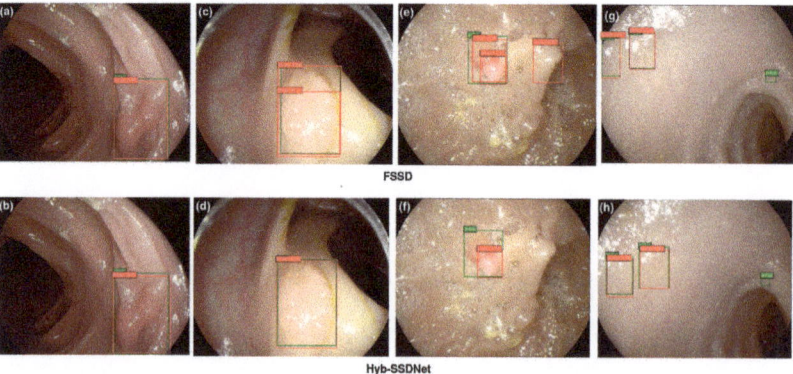

Figure 13. Qualitative results comparison between FSSD300 (**a,c,e,g**) and the proposed Hyb-SSDNet (**b,d,f,h**) on the ETIS-Larib polyp test set. True bounding boxes with IoU of 0.5 or higher with the bounding predicted boxes are drawn in green and red colors, respectively.

5. Conclusions

In this paper, an improved FSSD detection model (Hyb-SSDNet) was proposed for accurate polyp abnormality localization and detection in both WCE and colonoscopy datasets. In addition to the problem of medical ethics, researchers have been pushed to use their datasets for polyp detection owing to the lack of standard and public WCE datasets. Therefore, research in this field is limited and the performance metrics may be subjective. The lightweight version of the Hyb-SSDNet aims to model the visual appearance of small polyp regions via a weighted mid-fusion of inception modules for a polyp detection network using the inception v4 backbone. The mid-fusion block uses the modified inception-A modules to magnify the mid-level feature maps instead of using simple convolution layers. Therefore, the Hyb-SSDNet model shows promising results in the (mAP) metric with little speed drop. An efficient feature fusion module using a simple concatenation strategy and L2 normalization was applied to the SSD framework to combine the intermediate inception layers to further generate new pyramid feature maps. The effectiveness of the weighted feature fusion was confirmed on three annotated testing datasets: WCE, CVC-ClinicDB, and ETIS-Larib. The Hyb-SSDNet framework adequately integrates low- and mid-level details, and high-level semantic information using a novel top-down feature fusion module. It also adopts one horizontal connection to reduce the number of repetitive computations, which shortens the detection time. In the future, a filtration strategy will be investigated to regularize the intermediate layer and reduce the false negative rate. Although the proposed model achieves satisfactory detection precision, the presence of the circumstances (e.g., debris, feces, and other factors) certainly influence the results as they cannot be completely omitted. This shortcoming should be examined through subsequent work, such as how to improve the performance of the model while maintaining a higher detection speed.

Author Contributions: Conceptualization, M.S. and M.E.A.; methodology, M.S.; software, M.E.A.; validation, M.S. and M.E.A.; formal analysis, M.S.; investigation, M.S.; resources, M.S.; data curation, M.S. and M.E.A.; writing—original draft preparation, M.S.; writing—review and editing, M.S.; visualization, M.S and M.E.A.; supervision, M.E.A.; project administration, M.S. and M.E.A.; funding acquisition, M.S. and M.E.A. All authors have read and agreed to the published version of the manuscript.

Funding: This work was partially supported by the Ministry of National Education, Vocational Training, Higher Education and Scientific Research, the Ministry of Industry, Trade and Green and Digital Economy, the Digital Development Agency (ADD), and the National Center for Scientific and Technical Research (CNRST). Project number: ALKHAWARIZMI/2020/20.

Data Availability Statement: Publicly available datasets were analyzed in this study. The CVC-ClinicDB datasets are publicly available here: https://polyp.grand-challenge.org/CVCClinicDB/ (accessed on 15 August 2022). The ETIS-Larib dataset is publicly available here: https://polyp.grand-challenge.org/EtisLarib (accessed on 15 August 2022).

Conflicts of Interest: The authors declare no conflict of interest

References

1. Garrido, A.; Sont, R.; Dghoughi, W.; Marcoval, S.; Romeu, J.; Fernández-Esparrach, G.; Belda, I.; Guardiola, M. Automatic Polyp Detection Using Microwave Endoscopy for Colorectal Cancer Prevention and Early Detection: Phantom Validation. *IEEE Access* **2021**, *9*, 148048–148059. [CrossRef]
2. Dulf, E.H.; Bledea, M.; Mocan, T.; Mocan, L. Automatic Detection of Colorectal Polyps Using Transfer Learning. *Sensors* **2021**, *21*, 5704. [CrossRef] [PubMed]
3. Charfi, S.; El Ansari, M.; Balasingham, I. Computer-aided diagnosis system for ulcer detection in wireless capsule endoscopy images. *IET Image Process.* **2019**, *13*, 1023–1030. [CrossRef]
4. Lafraxo, S.; El Ansari, M. GastroNet: Abnormalities Recognition in Gastrointestinal Tract through Endoscopic Imagery using Deep Learning Techniques. In Proceedings of the 2020 8th International Conference on Wireless Networks and Mobile Communications (WINCOM), Reims, France, 27–29 October 2020; pp. 1–5.
5. Souaidi, M.; Abdelouahad, A.A.; El Ansari, M. A fully automated ulcer detection system for wireless capsule endoscopy images. In Proceedings of the 2017 International Conference on Advanced Technologies for Signal and Image Processing (ATSIP), Fez, Morocco, 22–24 May 2017; pp. 1–6.

6. Souaidi, M.; Charfi, S.; Abdelouahad, A.A.; El Ansari, M. New features for wireless capsule endoscopy polyp detection. In Proceedings of the 2018 International Conference on Intelligent Systems and Computer Vision (ISCV), Fez, Morocco, 2–4 April 2018; pp. 1–6.
7. Charfi, S.; El Ansari, M. Computer-aided diagnosis system for colon abnormalities detection in wireless capsule endoscopy images. *Multimed. Tools Appl.* **2018**, *77*, 4047–4064. [CrossRef]
8. Souaidi, M.; Abdelouahed, A.A.; El Ansari, M. Multi-scale completed local binary patterns for ulcer detection in wireless capsule endoscopy images. *Multimed. Tools Appl.* **2019**, *78*, 13091–13108. [CrossRef]
9. Charfi, S.; El Ansari, M. A locally based feature descriptor for abnormalities detection. *Soft Comput.* **2020**, *24*, 4469–4481. [CrossRef]
10. Souaidi, M.; El Ansari, M. Automated Detection of Wireless Capsule Endoscopy Polyp Abnormalities with Deep Transfer Learning and Support Vector Machines. In *Proceedings of the International Conference on Advanced Intelligent Systems for Sustainable Development*; Springer: Berlin/Heidelberg, Germany, 2020; pp. 870–880.
11. Lafraxo, S.; Ansari, M.E.; Charfi, S. MelaNet: an effective deep learning framework for melanoma detection using dermoscopic images. *Multimed. Tools Appl.* **2022**, *81*, 16021–16045. [CrossRef]
12. Lafraxo, S.; El Ansari, M. CoviNet: Automated COVID-19 Detection from X-rays using Deep Learning Techniques. In Proceedings of the 2020 6th IEEE Congress on Information Science and Technology (CiSt), Agadir, Morocco, 5–12 June 2021; pp. 489–494.
13. Lafraxo, S.; Ansari, M.E. Regularized Convolutional Neural Network for Pneumonia Detection Trough Chest X-Rays. In *Proceedings of the International Conference on Advanced Intelligent Systems for Sustainable Development*; Springer: Berlin/Heidelberg, Germany, 2020; pp. 887–896.
14. Xu, L.; Xie, J.; Cai, F.; Wu, J. Spectral Classification Based on Deep Learning Algorithms. *Electronics* **2021**, *10*, 1892. [CrossRef]
15. Nogueira-Rodríguez, A.; Domínguez-Carbajales, R.; Campos-Tato, F.; Herrero, J.; Puga, M.; Remedios, D.; Rivas, L.; Sánchez, E.; Iglesias, Á.; Cubiella, J.; et al. Real-time polyp detection model using convolutional neural networks. *Neural Comput. Appl.* **2021**, *34*, 10375–10396. [CrossRef]
16. Mohammed, A.; Yildirim, S.; Farup, I.; Pedersen, M.; Hovde, Ø. Y-net: A deep convolutional neural network for polyp detection. *arXiv* **2018**, arXiv:1806.01907.
17. Chen, X.; Zhang, K.; Lin, S.; Dai, K.F.; Yun, Y. Single Shot Multibox Detector Automatic Polyp Detection Network Based on Gastrointestinal Endoscopic Images. *Comput. Math. Methods Med.* **2021**, *2021*, 2144472. [CrossRef]
18. Souaidi, M.; El Ansari, M. A New Automated Polyp Detection Network MP-FSSD in WCE and Colonoscopy Images based Fusion Single Shot Multibox Detector and Transfer Learning. *IEEE Access* **2022**, *10*, 47124–47140. [CrossRef]
19. Girshick, R.; Donahue, J.; Darrell, T.; Malik, J. Rich feature hierarchies for accurate object detection and semantic segmentation. In Proceedings of the IEEE Conference on Computer Vision and Pattern Recognition, Columbus, OH, USA, 23–28 June 2014; pp. 580–587.
20. Ren, S.; He, K.; Girshick, R.; Sun, J. Faster R-CNN: towards real-time object detection with region proposal networks. *IEEE Trans. Pattern Anal. Mach. Intell.* **2016**, *39*, 1137–1149. [CrossRef]
21. Jifeng, D.; Yi, L.; Kaiming, H.; Jian, S. Object Detection via Region-Based Fully Convolutional Networks. *arXiv* **2016**, arXiv:1605.06409.
22. Redmon, J.; Divvala, S.; Girshick, R.; Farhadi, A. You only look once: Unified, real-time object detection. In Proceedings of the IEEE Conference on Computer Vision and Pattern Recognition, Las Vegas, NV, USA, 27–30 June 2016; pp. 779–788.
23. Liu, W.; Anguelov, D.; Erhan, D.; Szegedy, C.; Reed, S.; Fu, C.Y.; Berg, A.C. Ssd: Single shot multibox detector. In *Proceedings of the European Conference on Computer Vision*; Springer: Berlin/Heidelberg, Germany, 2016; pp. 21–37.
24. Hasanpour, S.H.; Rouhani, M.; Fayyaz, M.; Sabokrou, M.; Adeli, E. Towards principled design of deep convolutional networks: Introducing simpnet. *arXiv* **2018**, arXiv:1802.06205.
25. Li, Z.; Zhou, F. FSSD: Feature fusion single shot multibox detector. *arXiv* **2017**, arXiv:1712.00960.
26. Szegedy, C.; Ioffe, S.; Vanhoucke, V.; Alemi, A.A. Inception-v4, inception-resnet and the impact of residual connections on learning. In Proceedings of the Thirty-First AAAI Conference on Artificial Intelligence, San Francisco, CA, USA, 4–9 February 2017.
27. Simonyan, K.; Zisserman, A. Very deep convolutional networks for large-scale image recognition. *arXiv* **2014**, arXiv:1409.1556.
28. Szegedy, C.; Liu, W.; Jia, Y.; Sermanet, P.; Reed, S.; Anguelov, D.; Erhan, D.; Vanhoucke, V.; Rabinovich, A. Going deeper with convolutions. In Proceedings of the IEEE Conference on Computer Vision and Pattern Recognition, Boston, MA, USA, 7–12 June 2015; pp. 1–9.
29. He, K.; Zhang, X.; Ren, S.; Sun, J. Deep residual learning for image recognition. In Proceedings of the IEEE Conference on Computer Vision and Pattern Recognition, Las Vegas, NV, USA, 27–30 June 2016; pp. 770–778.
30. Shin, H.C.; Lu, L.; Kim, L.; Seff, A.; Yao, J.; Summers, R.M. Interleaved text/image deep mining on a very large-scale radiology database. In Proceedings of the IEEE Conference on Computer Vision and Pattern Recognition, Boston, MA, USA, 7–12 June 2015; pp. 1090–1099.
31. Chen, B.L.; Wan, J.J.; Chen, T.Y.; Yu, Y.T.; Ji, M. A self-attention based faster R-CNN for polyp detection from colonoscopy images. *Biomed. Signal Process. Control.* **2021**, *70*, 103019. [CrossRef]
32. Pacal, I.; Karaman, A.; Karaboga, D.; Akay, B.; Basturk, A.; Nalbantoglu, U.; Coskun, S. An efficient real-time colonic polyp detection with YOLO algorithms trained by using negative samples and large datasets. *Comput. Biol. Med.* **2021**, *141*, 105031. [CrossRef]

33. Hong-Tae, C.; Ho-Jun, L.; Kang, H.; Yu, S. SSD-EMB: An Improved SSD Using Enhanced Feature Map Block for Object Detection. *Sensors* **2021**, *21*, 2842.
34. Qadir, H.A.; Shin, Y.; Solhusvik, J.; Bergsland, J.; Aabakken, L.; Balasingham, I. Polyp detection and segmentation using mask R-CNN: Does a deeper feature extractor CNN always perform better? In Proceedings of the 2019 13th International Symposium on Medical Information and Communication Technology (ISMICT), Oslo, Norway, 8–10 May 2019; pp. 1–6.
35. Jia, X.; Mai, X.; Cui, Y.; Yuan, Y.; Xing, X.; Seo, H.; Xing, L.; Meng, M.Q.H. Automatic polyp recognition in colonoscopy images using deep learning and two-stage pyramidal feature prediction. *IEEE Trans. Autom. Sci. Eng.* **2020**, *17*, 1570–1584. [CrossRef]
36. Tashk, A.; Nadimi, E. An innovative polyp detection method from colon capsule endoscopy images based on a novel combination of RCNN and DRLSE. In Proceedings of the 2020 IEEE Congress on Evolutionary Computation (CEC), Glasgow, UK, 19–24 July 2020; pp. 1–6.
37. Misawa, M.; Kudo, S.e.; Mori, Y.; Hotta, K.; Ohtsuka, K.; Matsuda, T.; Saito, S.; Kudo, T.; Baba, T.; Ishida, F.; et al. Development of a computer-aided detection system for colonoscopy and a publicly accessible large colonoscopy video database (with video). *Gastrointest. Endosc.* **2021**, *93*, 960–967. [CrossRef]
38. Liu, M.; Jiang, J.; Wang, Z. Colonic polyp detection in endoscopic videos with single shot detection based deep convolutional neural network. *IEEE Access* **2019**, *7*, 75058–75066. [CrossRef]
39. Zhang, X.; Chen, F.; Yu, T.; An, J.; Huang, Z.; Liu, J.; Hu, W.; Wang, L.; Duan, H.; Si, J. Real-time gastric polyp detection using convolutional neural networks. *PLoS ONE* **2019**, *14*, e0214133. [CrossRef] [PubMed]
40. Jeong, J.; Park, H.; Kwak, N. Enhancement of SSD by concatenating feature maps for object detection. *arXiv* **2017**, arXiv:1705.09587.
41. Zhai, S.; Shang, D.; Wang, S.; Dong, S. DF-SSD: An improved SSD object detection algorithm based on DenseNet and feature fusion. *IEEE Access* **2020**, *8*, 24344–24357. [CrossRef]
42. Wang, T.; Shen, F.; Deng, H.; Cai, F.; Chen, S. Smartphone imaging spectrometer for egg/meat freshness monitoring. *Anal. Methods* **2022**, *14*, 508–517. [CrossRef] [PubMed]
43. Lin, T.Y.; Dollár, P.; Girshick, R.; He, K.; Hariharan, B.; Belongie, S. Feature pyramid networks for object detection. In Proceedings of the IEEE Conference on Computer Vision and Pattern Recognition, Honolulu, HI, USA, 21–26 July 2017; pp. 2117–2125.
44. Fu, C.Y.; Liu, W.; Ranga, A.; Tyagi, A.; Berg, A.C. Dssd: Deconvolutional single shot detector. *arXiv* **2017**, arXiv:1701.06659.
45. Russakovsky, O.; Deng, J.; Su, H.; Krause, J.; Satheesh, S.; Ma, S.; Huang, Z.; Karpathy, A.; Khosla, A.; Bernstein, M.; et al. Imagenet large scale visual recognition challenge. *Int. J. Comput. Vis.* **2015**, *115*, 211–252. [CrossRef]
46. Pan, H.; Jiang, J.; Chen, G. TDFSSD: Top-down feature fusion single shot MultiBox detector. *Signal Process. Image Commun.* **2020**, *89*, 115987. [CrossRef]
47. Hu, J.; Shen, L.; Sun, G. Squeeze-and-excitation networks. In Proceedings of the IEEE Conference on Computer Vision and Pattern Recognition, Salt Lake City, UT, USA, 18–23 June 2018; pp. 7132–7141.
48. Roy, A.G.; Navab, N.; Wachinger, C. Recalibrating fully convolutional networks with spatial and channel "squeeze and excitation" blocks. *IEEE Trans. Med Imaging* **2018**, *38*, 540–549. [CrossRef]
49. Prasath, V.S. Polyp detection and segmentation from video capsule endoscopy: A review. *J. Imaging* **2016**, *3*, 1. [CrossRef]
50. Bernal, J.; Sánchez, F.J.; Fernández-Esparrach, G.; Gil, D.; Rodríguez, C.; Vilariño, F. WM-DOVA maps for accurate polyp highlighting in colonoscopy: Validation vs. saliency maps from physicians. *Comput. Med Imaging Graph.* **2015**, *43*, 99–111. [CrossRef]
51. WE, O. ETIS-Larib Polyp DB. Available online: https://polyp.grand-challenge.org/EtisLarib/ (accessed on 27 march 2022).
52. Angermann, Q.; Bernal, J.; Sánchez-Montes, C.; Hammami, M.; Fernández-Esparrach, G.; Dray, X.; Romain, O.; Sánchez, F.J.; Histace, A. Towards real-time polyp detection in colonoscopy videos: Adapting still frame-based methodologies for video sequences analysis. In *Computer Assisted and Robotic Endoscopy and Clinical Image-Based Procedures*; Springer: Berlin/Heidelberg, Germany, 2017; pp. 29–41.
53. Silva, J.; Histace, A.; Romain, O.; Dray, X.; Granado, B. Toward embedded detection of polyps in wce images for early diagnosis of colorectal cancer. *Int. J. Comput. Assist. Radiol. Surg.* **2014**, *9*, 283–293. [CrossRef]
54. Picard, R.R.; Cook, R.D. Cross-validation of regression models. *J. Am. Stat. Assoc.* **1984**, *79*, 575–583. [CrossRef]
55. Jha, D.; Ali, S.; Tomar, N.K.; Johansen, H.D.; Johansen, D.; Rittscher, J.; Riegler, M.A.; Halvorsen, P. Real-time polyp detection, localization and segmentation in colonoscopy using deep learning. *IEEE Access* **2021**, *9*, 40496–40510. [CrossRef]
56. Chatfield, K.; Simonyan, K.; Vedaldi, A.; Zisserman, A. Return of the devil in the details: Delving deep into convolutional nets. *arXiv* **2014**, arXiv:1405.3531.
57. Mash, R.; Borghetti, B.; Pecarina, J. Improved aircraft recognition for aerial refueling through data augmentation in convolutional neural networks. In *Proceedings of the International Symposium on Visual Computing*; Springer: Berlin/Heidelberg, Germany, 2016; pp. 113–122.
58. Ma, W.; Wang, X.; Yu, J. A Lightweight Feature Fusion Single Shot Multibox Detector for Garbage Detection. *IEEE Access* **2020**, *8*, 188577–188586. [CrossRef]
59. Shin, Y.; Qadir, H.A.; Aabakken, L.; Bergsland, J.; Balasingham, I. Automatic colon polyp detection using region based deep cnn and post learning approaches. *IEEE Access* **2018**, *6*, 40950–40962. [CrossRef]
60. Liu, X.; Guo, X.; Liu, Y.; Yuan, Y. Consolidated domain adaptive detection and localization framework for cross-device colonoscopic images. *Med. Image Anal.* **2021**, *71*, 102052. [CrossRef]

61. Wang, D.; Zhang, N.; Sun, X.; Zhang, P.; Zhang, C.; Cao, Y.; Liu, B. Afp-net: Realtime anchor-free polyp detection in colonoscopy. In Proceedings of the 2019 IEEE 31st International Conference on Tools with Artificial Intelligence (ICTAI), Portland, OR, USA, 4–6 November 2019; pp. 636–643.
62. Qadir, H.A.; Shin, Y.; Solhusvik, J.; Bergsland, J.; Aabakken, L.; Balasingham, I. Toward real-time polyp detection using fully CNNs for 2D Gaussian shapes prediction. *Med. Image Anal.* **2021**, *68*, 101897. [CrossRef]
63. Pacal, I.; Karaboga, D. A robust real-time deep learning based automatic polyp detection system. *Comput. Biol. Med.* **2021**, *134*, 104519. [CrossRef]
64. Krenzer, A.; Banck, M.; Makowski, K.; Hekalo, A.; Fitting, D.; Troya, J.; Sudarevic, B.; Zoller, W.G.; Hann, A.; Puppe, F. A Real-Time Polyp Detection System with Clinical Application in Colonoscopy Using Deep Convolutional Neural Networks. 2022. Available online: https://www.researchsquare.com/article/rs-1310139/latest.pdf (accessed on 13 August 2022)

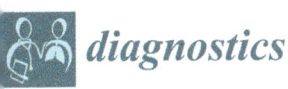

Article

Deep Learning for Automatic Differentiation of Mucinous versus Non-Mucinous Pancreatic Cystic Lesions: A Pilot Study

Filipe Vilas-Boas [1,2,3], Tiago Ribeiro [1,2], João Afonso [1,2], Hélder Cardoso [1,2,3], Susana Lopes [1,2,3], Pedro Moutinho-Ribeiro [1,2,3], João Ferreira [4,5], Miguel Mascarenhas-Saraiva [1,2,3,*] and Guilherme Macedo [1,2,3]

1. Department of Gastroenterology, São João University Hospital, Alameda Professor Hernâni Monteiro, 4200-427 Porto, Portugal
2. World Gastroenterology Organisation Gastroenterology and Hepatology Training Center, 4200-427 Porto, Portugal
3. Faculty of Medicine of the University of Porto, Alameda Professor Hernâni Monteiro, 4200-427 Porto, Portugal
4. Department of Mechanical Engineering, Faculty of Engineering of the University of Porto, Rua Dr. Roberto Frias, 4200-465 Porto, Portugal
5. INEGI—Institute of Science and Innovation in Mechanical and Industrial Engineering, Rua Dr. Roberto Frias, 4200-465 Porto, Portugal
* Correspondence: miguelmascarenhassaraiva@gmail.com

Abstract: Endoscopic ultrasound (EUS) morphology can aid in the discrimination between mucinous and non-mucinous pancreatic cystic lesions (PCLs) but has several limitations that can be overcome by artificial intelligence. We developed a convolutional neural network (CNN) algorithm for the automatic diagnosis of mucinous PCLs. Images retrieved from videos of EUS examinations for PCL characterization were used for the development, training, and validation of a CNN for mucinous cyst diagnosis. The performance of the CNN was measured calculating the area under the receiving operator characteristic curve (AUC), sensitivity, specificity, and positive and negative predictive values. A total of 5505 images from 28 pancreatic cysts were used (3725 from mucinous lesions and 1780 from non-mucinous cysts). The model had an overall accuracy of 98.5%, sensitivity of 98.3%, specificity of 98.9% and AUC of 1. The image processing speed of the CNN was 7.2 ms per frame. We developed a deep learning algorithm that differentiated mucinous and non-mucinous cysts with high accuracy. The present CNN may constitute an important tool to help risk stratify PCLs.

Keywords: pancreatic cystic lesions; mucinous cystic neoplasm; intraductal papillary mucinous neoplasm; endoscopic ultrasound; artificial intelligence

1. Introduction

Pancreatic cystic lesions (PCLs) are very common. A recent systematic review including 17 studies found a pooled prevalence of 8% [1]. PCLs include a wide range of entities, namely congenital, inflammatory, and neoplastic lesions. Patients with PCLs have an increased risk of pancreatic malignancy compared with the general population [2]. However, malignancy occurs virtually only in those with PCLs of mucinous phenotype. Intraductal papillary mucinous neoplasm (IPMN) is the most common pancreatic cystic neoplasia, accounting for nearly half of pancreatic resections due to cystic lesions at a reference academic hospital in the USA [3].

The diagnosis of PCLs based on endoscopic ultrasound (EUS) has important limitations [4]. In fact, the range of accuracy in differentiating mucinous from non-mucinous lesions is 48–94% with a sensitivity of 36–91% and a specificity of 45–81% [4]. However, one of the main limitations of EUS is its low interobserver agreement for the diagnosis of neoplastic versus non-neoplastic lesions and the determination of the specific type of PCL. These concerns remain valid for a wide spectrum of endoscopists, with different degrees of expertise in EUS (experts, semi-experts, or novices) [5,6].

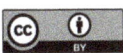

The application of artificial intelligence (AI) algorithms for the interpretation of medical imaging has been the focus of intense research across several areas [7,8]. The implementation of these automated systems for the automatic analysis of endoscopic images has provided promising results [9]. The ever-increasing computational power allows the analysis of large image datasets through deep learning algorithms. Convolutional neural networks (CNNs) are a type of multi-layer deep learning algorithm resembling the visual cortex, which is tailored for automatic image analysis [10].

To date, only a small number of studies reported the use of deep learning systems for the automatic interpretation of EUS images [11]. To optimize the diagnosis based on EUS morphology and mitigate the low interobserver agreement, we aimed to develop a CNN algorithm for the automatic diagnosis of mucinous PCLs using EUS images.

2. Materials and Methods

2.1. Patient Population and Study Design

We conducted a retrospective study using a prospectively maintained hospital database of patients submitted to EUS for PCL characterization. All patients whose EUS exam was recorded as a video file were included. All videos were recorded using the same EUS device. Images retrieved from these examinations were used for the development, training, and validation of a CNN-based model for the automatic identification of mucinous PCLs.

This study was approved by the ethics committee of São João University Hospital/Faculty of Medicine of the University of Porto (CE 41/2021) and was conducted respecting the Declaration of Helsinki. This study is of a non-interventional nature.

2.2. Data Collection

We retrieved the videos from 28 patients for high-quality EUS image analysis. These images comprised still frames acquired during the EUS procedure as well as images obtained through the decomposition of recorded videos into frames. The fragmentation of videos into still images was performed using the VLC media player (VideoLAN, Paris, France). The complete set of images was evaluated by an expert in EUS (FVB) with an experience of more than 1000 EUS exams. All non-relevant frames were excluded. A total of 5505 images were ultimately extracted. From this pool, 3725 depicted mucinous PCLs and 1780 showed non-mucinous PCLs.

Clinical and demographic data were obtained from the electronic clinical record of each patient. Any information deemed to potentially identify the subjects was omitted. Each patient was assigned a random number in order to guarantee effective data anonymization. A team with Data Protection Officer (DPO) certification confirmed the non-traceability of data and conformity with the general data protection regulation (GDPR).

2.3. Endoscopic Ultrasound Procedures and Definitions

All EUS procedures were performed under anesthesiologist-directed sedation using linear echoendoscopes (Olympus® GF-UCT180 and Olympus® GF-UC140) coupled with an Olympus® EU-ME2 ultrasound processor under anesthesiologist-directed sedation. Cyst type was determined based on surgical specimen, intracystic biopsy forceps samples (Moray® micro forceps, STERIS) or cyst fluid cytology combined with carcinoembryonic antigen (CEA) and glucose fluid levels. PCLs were considered mucinous if cytology revealed mucinous epithelial cells or, in their absence, CEA fluid levels >192 ng/mL and glucose levels <50 mg/dL. Patients with cystic neuroendocrine tumors and solid pseudopapillary neoplasms were excluded.

2.4. Development of the Convolutional Neural Network

A deep learning CNN was developed for the automatic identification and differentiation of mucinous and non-mucinous PCLs. In the former group, we included IPMNs and mucinous cystic neoplasms (MCN), while the latter included neoplastic (serous cystadenoma) and non-neoplastic (pseudocyst) lesions. From the collected pool of images

(n = 5505), 3725 depicted mucinous and 1780 showed non-mucinous lesions. This pool of images was divided for the constitution of training and validation datasets. The training dataset was composed of 80% of the extracted images (n = 4404). The remaining 20% was used as the validation dataset (n = 1101). The performance of the CNN was assessed using the validation dataset. A flowchart summarizing the study design is presented in Figure 1.

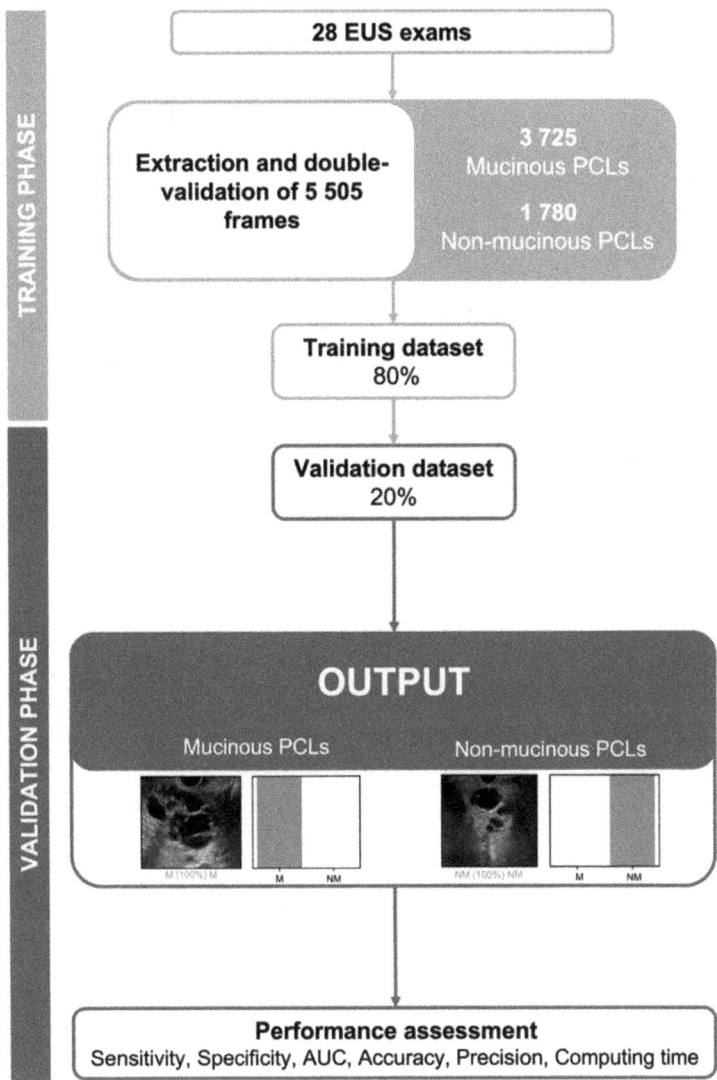

Figure 1. Study design for the construction of the convolutional neural network and subsequent evaluation of its performance. EUS—endoscopic ultrasound; PCLs—pancreatic cystic lesions; M—mucinous pancreatic cystic lesion; NM—non-mucinous pancreatic cystic lesion; AUC—area under the receiving operator curve.

The CNN was created using the *Xception* model with its weights trained on *ImageNet* (a large-scale image dataset aimed for use in development of object recognition software). To transfer this learning to our data, we kept the convolutional layers of the model. We removed the last fully connected layers and attached fully connected layers based on the number of classes we used to classify our endoscopic images. We used two blocks, each having a fully connected layer followed by a dropout layer of 0.25 drop rate. Following these two blocks, we add a dense layer with a size defined as the number of categories to classify (three: normal pancreatic parenchyma, mucinous PCLs and non-mucinous PCLs). The learning rate of 0.00015, batch size of 32, and the number of epochs of 30 was set by trial and error. We used *Tensorflow* 2.3 and *Keras* libraries to prepare the data and run the model. The analyses were performed with a computer equipped with a 2.1 GHz Intel® Xeon® Gold 6130 processor (Intel, Santa Clara, CA, USA) and a double NVIDIA Quadro® RTX™ 4000 graphic processing unit (NVIDIA Corporate, Santa Clara, CA, USA).

2.5. Model Performance and Statistical Analysis

The primary outcome measures included sensitivity, specificity, positive and negative predictive values (PPV and NPV, respectively), and the accuracy in differentiating mucinous and non-mucinous lesions. Moreover, we used receiver operating characteristic (ROC) curves analysis and area under the ROC curves (AUC) to measure the performance of our model in the distinction between categories. The classification provided by the CNN was compared to the definitive diagnosis (mucinous or non-mucinous cyst), the latter being considered the gold standard. For each image, the trained CNN calculated the probability for each category. A higher probability translated in a greater confidence in the CNN prediction. The category with the highest probability score was outputted as the CNN's predicted classification (Figure 2). Additionally, the image processing performance of the network was determined by calculating the time required for the CNN to provide output for all images in the validation image dataset. Clinical and demographic data are presented as median (interquartile range) or frequency (percent). Continuous data were compared using the Mann–Whitney U test. Differences in the distribution of categorical variables were assessed using the chi-square test. Statistical analysis was performed using Sci-Kit learn v0.22.2 [12].

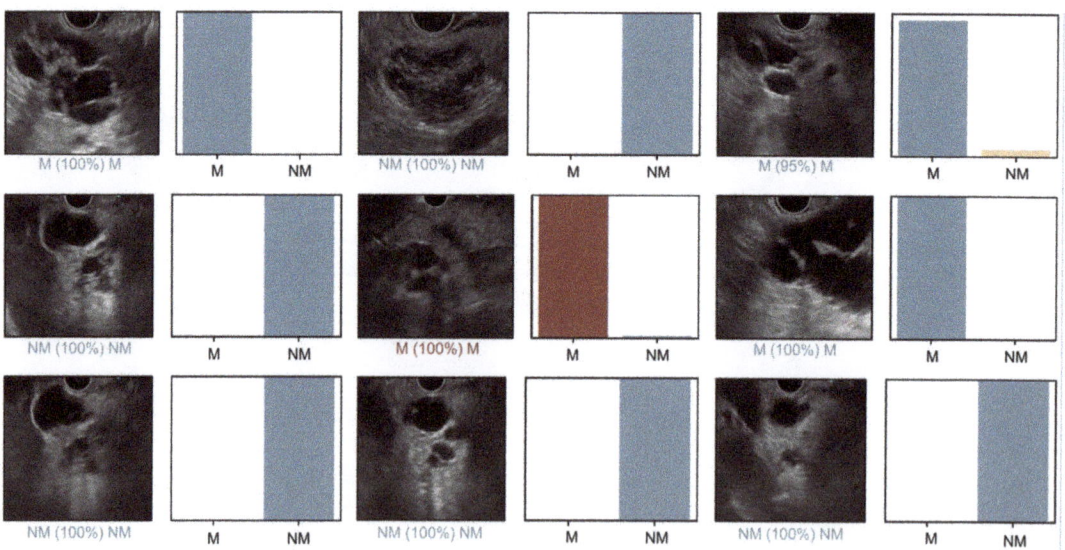

Figure 2. Output provided during the validation phase of the convolutional neural network. The bars represent the probability estimated by the algorithm. The finding with the highest probability was outputted as the predicted classification. A blue bar represents a correct prediction. Red bars represent an incorrect prediction. M—mucinous pancreatic cystic lesion; NM—non-mucinous pancreatic cystic lesion.

3. Results

3.1. Clinical and Demographic Data

A total of 28 videos from patients submitted to EUS for pancreatic cystic lesion characterization between November 2017 and August 2021 were used for image retrieval. From these patients, 16 were female (57%) and had a median age of 65 years (IQR 53–70). A total of 17 (61%) individuals had a final diagnosis of mucinous cysts, while 11 (39%) were ultimately diagnosed with a non-mucinous lesion. Surgical specimens were reported for eight lesions. Histology using intracystic biopsy forceps samples (Moray® micro forceps, STERIS) was available for five patients. The remaining cysts ($n = 15$) were considered mucinous based on fluid cyst analysis (cytology plus CEA and glucose levels). Concerning cyst histotype, we included 16 IPMNs, 1 mucinous cystic neoplasm (MCN), 8 SCA (five of which were of the macrocystic variant), and 3 pseudocysts (PC). The median follow-up time was 18 months (3–29). The characteristics of the patients and lesions including demographic data and lesion size and location are summarized in Table 1. Most lesions (86%) were incidentally found, 30% were located in the head and neck of the pancreas and the median size was 34.5 mm (19.3–44.8 mm). In this cohort, 14 patients underwent EUS for presumed mucinous lesions with worrisome features as per international consensus guidelines and 14 because of indeterminate cyst type after clinical and imaging integration (unilocular/oligocystic lesion without clear communication with the main pancreatic duct). Mucinous cysts were smaller in size compared to non-mucinous lesions, respectively, 26.0 mm (IQR 17.5–44.5) vs. 37.0 mm (IQR 26.0–46.0), although this difference was not statistically significant ($p = 0.29$). The location of the lesions had a similar distribution for mucinous and non-mucinous lesions ($p = 0.90$) and were more frequently found in the head and neck of the pancreas (47% and 55%, respectively). No adverse events were reported for the EUS procedures, nor for EUS-FNA (including through-the-needle biopsies).

Table 1. Baseline clinical and demographic data.

	Mucinous PCLs ($n = 17$)	Non-Mucinous PCLs ($n = 11$)	*p* Value
Sex			0.57
Female, *n* (%)	10 (58.8)	6 (54.5)	
Age			0.64
Years, median (IQR)	64.0 (53.0–69.5)	65.0 (53.0–72.0)	
Presentation			0.22
Incidental, *n* (%)	13 (76.5)	11 (100.0)	
Abdominal pain, *n* (%)	2 (11.8)	-	
Pancreatitis, *n* (%)	2 (11.8)	-	
Indication for EUS			<0.01
Worrisome features, *n* (%)	13 (76.5)	1 (9.1)	
Indeterminate cyst type, *n* (%)	4 (23.5)	10 (90.9)	
Cyst location on EUS			0.90
Pancreatic head, *n* (%)	8 (47.1)	6 (54.5)	
Pancreatic body, *n* (%)	6 (35.3)	3 (27.3)	
Pancreatic tail, *n* (%)	3 (17.6)	2 (18.2)	
Cyst morphology			0.63
Unilocular, *n* (%)	6 (35.3)	4 (36.4)	
Multilocular, *n* (%)	11 (64.7)	7 (63.6)	
Cyst diameter			
mm, median (IQR)	26.0 (17.5–44.5)	37.0 (26.0–46.0)	0.29

Abbreviations: EUS—endoscopic ultrasound; PCLs—pancreatic cystic lesions; IQR—interquartile range.

Overall, a total of 5505 frames were extracted for the construction of the CNN: 3725 of mucinous cysts (IPMNs and MCN) and 1780 of non-mucinous lesions (SCA and PC). The accuracy of the algorithm increased as data were repeatedly input into the multi-layer architecture of the CNN (Figure 3).

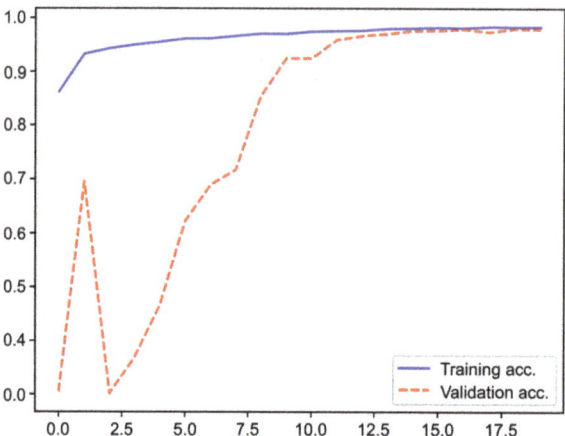

Figure 3. Evolution of the accuracy of the convolutional neural network during training and validation phases, as the training and validation datasets were repeatedly input in the neural network.

3.2. Performance of the Convolutional Neural Network

The full-size dataset was split for the constitution of training and validation datasets as follows: 80% of the retrieved images were used as a training dataset, and the remaining 20% were used as a validation dataset for evaluation of the CNN's performance. The confusion matrix between the trained CNN and final diagnosis is shown in Table 2. Overall, the algorithm had an accuracy of 98.5%. The sensitivity, specificity, PPV and NPV for the detection and differentiation of mucinous cysts versus normal or non-mucinous structures were, respectively, 98.3%, 98.9%, 99.5% and 96.4%. The AUC of the CNN for the discrimination of mucinous and non-mucinous cystic lesions was 1.00 (Figure 4).

Table 2. Confusion matrix of the automatic detection versus final diagnosis.

		Final Diagnosis	
		Mucinous	Non-Mucinous
CNN	Mucinous	743	9
	Non-mucinous	12	337

Abbreviations: CNN—convolutional neural network; Mucinous—mucinous pancreatic cystic lesions; Non-mucinous—non-mucinous pancreatic cystic lesions.

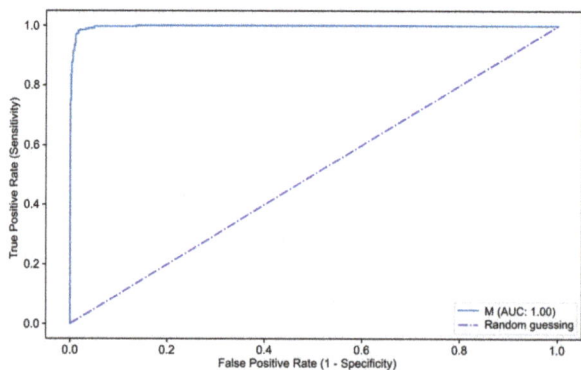

Figure 4. ROC analysis of the network's performance in the detection of mucinous pancreatic cystic lesions. AUC—area under the receiver operating characteristic curve. M—mucinous pancreatic cystic lesion.

3.3. Computational Performance of the CNN

The CNN completed the reading of the validation dataset in 6 seconds at a speed of 5.2 ms/frame. This translates into an approximated reading rate of 191 frames per second.

4. Discussion

The development of AI algorithms is a hot topic in medical literature. Several reports show promising results regarding gains in diagnostic accuracy, particularly for medical specialties highly dependent on imaging [9]. The application of machine learning (ML) in endoscopy has shown encouraging results [10].

In this proof-of-concept study, we have developed a CNN for the automatic identification of mucinous pancreatic cysts during EUS. The algorithm demonstrated an excellent discriminatory ability with 98.5% accuracy for the differentiation of mucinous cysts from non-mucinous lesions. This proof-of-concept study represents a pilot effort to minimize the limited interobserver agreement regarding the EUS characterization of pancreatic cysts. Evidence on the application of AI to EUS for the study of pancreatic lesions is limited. Particularly, studies focusing on the detection and differentiation between mucinous and non-mucinous pancreatic cystic lesions based on EUS images are scarce. To the authors' knowledge, only one study focusing on this subject has been previously published [13]. Nevertheless, the development of AI algorithms for the evaluation of pancreatic diseases is a subject of increasing interest [14–19].

The development of a deep learning model accurately predicting the phenotype of PCLs during EUS procedures may have a substantial impact on patient management. The main goals when approaching these lesions is defining their type (mucinous vs. non-mucinous) and, subsequently, attaining a definite histotype. The first step of this sequence is of particular relevance, as the malignant potential is virtually restricted to mucinous lesions. Therefore, we developed a deep learning algorithm for the automatic classification of PCLs as mucinous vs. non-mucinous. Nguon and coworkers implemented a CNN model to differentiate MCN and SCA using EUS images [13]. Their algorithm achieved an overall accuracy around 80%, which is in line with the classification performance of experienced endosonographers. The authors explained this suboptimal accuracy as the result of the inclusion of EUS images obtained using both radial and linear echoendoscopes as well as variations in the demarcation of single or multiple regions of interest (ROI), which included the cyst as well as surrounding tissue. This study differs from ours as we only included linear EUS images and our CNN model included complete images, without pre-selected ROI. Nevertheless, the main difference between the studies resides in the spectrum of included lesions, as our study focuses on group classification rather than differentiating between two different cyst types. Our model was built including EUS images from IPMNs in the mucinous group, in addition to MCN. IPMNs are the most frequent pancreatic cystic neoplasia and constitute a big challenge when it comes to correctly risk stratifying the malignant potential of each lesion. The work by Kuwahara et al. expands the reach of our study [15]. This group developed a deep learning algorithm to predict the malignancy potential of IPMNs using images from patients with malignant and non-malignant IPMNs. The authors used the output value of deep learning calculated after training as the predictive value of malignancy (AI value). The mean AI value of malignant lesions was higher than that of benign IPMNs. In this study, the CNN had a higher diagnostic performance than that of the endoscopists diagnosis and the predictive factors provided by scientific societies guidelines. Further studies on deep learning tools for application to EUS should expand the knowledge in this issue and address the challenge of automatic detection of cysts with advanced neoplasia, therefore minimizing the need for cyst puncture, ultimately preventing unnecessary surgeries.

The development of AI solutions for PCLs differentiation has expanded to other endoscopic tools complementary to conventional EUS. Confocal laser endomicroscopy (CLE) has been proven useful for differentiating various types of PCLs and more recently was shown to outperform international guidelines in the prediction of malignancy in IPMNs.

However, image interpretation is observer dependent, and CLE is not widely available [20]. Recently, Machicado et al. described the development of a CNN algorithm based on CLE images to risk stratify IPMNs [16]. They used CLE videos from 35 histopathologically confirmed IPMNs and developed two CNN algorithms whose accuracy was compared to International Consensus Guidelines and American Gastroenterology Association criteria for advanced lesion/surgical indication. The results showed the higher accuracy of the CNN algorithm compared with the guidelines.

We conducted a proof-of-concept study assessing the potential of deep learning tools for the differentiation of mucinous and non-mucinous PCLs. This study has several highlights. First, to our knowledge, it is the first study to provide a clinically useful tool for the differentiation of PCLs as mucinous or non-mucinous. The accurate differentiation between both entities allows a prompt estimate of malignant potential, which has significant impact in patient management and follow-up. Second, our model was demonstrated to be highly sensitive, specific, and accurate. Finally, our algorithm had a high image processing performance with an approximate reading rate of 139 frames per second. An adequate image processing performance is a key element for subsequent real-time implementation of this proof-of-concept CNN model.

This study has several limitations. First, a small number of patients were enrolled and, therefore, some cyst types were underrepresented. The inclusion of a large pool of frames extracted from full-length videos, in addition to the routine still frames included in the standard EUS report, with distinct resolution and viewing angles contributed to provide an adequate variability to our dataset. Second, we performed a single-center retrospective study. Subsequent robust multicenter prospective studies are required to assess the clinical significance of our results. Further development of this technology will require the inclusion of large numbers of patients. Additionally, the refinement of the algorithm will require the inclusion of other types of pancreatic cysts as this should be required before it reaches clinical practice, providing automatic differentiation between several classes. Third, our proof-of-concept algorithm was developed and assessed using a single EUS suite. Therefore, our results may not be generalizable to other EUS platforms. Finally, the absence of surgical specimens or histological samples as the gold standard for all the included cysts is a significant limitation for establishing a reliable and reproducible gold standard for the development of the automated algorithm. An automated predictive model can only be as good as the gold standard for defining the true classification. Furthermore, the future application of AI tools into real-life EUS practice will require going through a strict regulatory pathway. The Food and Drug Administration (FDA) has approved several AI/ML-based Software as medical device (SaMD) with locked algorithms and changes beyond original market authorization requiring FDA premarket review [21]. Additionally, the FDA accepts the evolving and changing nature of AI/ML-based SaMD, namely convolutional neural networks. This particular matter constitutes a change from the previous paradigm for medical device regulation, as it was not initially designed for adaptive deep learning models. Indeed, a new framework is being gradually developed to provide appropriate regulatory oversight.

Artificial intelligence is gradually changing the landscape in digestive health care. Indeed, accurate, faster, and tireless AI tools will disrupt clinical practice and play a key role in endoscopic ultrasound. The potential of deep learning algorithms to impact the care of patients with pancreatic disease is vast and may contribute to improving the prognosis of these patients. We believe this AI model constitutes a significant milestone in the phenotypic differentiation of PCLs. Indeed, this work highlights the technological feasibility of accurately achieving morphologic pattern identification of pleomorphic pancreatic lesions.

Author Contributions: F.V.-B. and T.R.: equal contribution in study design, revision of EUS videos, image extraction and labelling, data interpretation and drafting of the manuscript; M.M.-S. and J.F.: development and invention of the endoscopic ultrasound CNN model; J.A. and H.C.: study design, statistical analysis; S.L., P.M.-R. and G.M.: study design, revision of the scientific content of the manuscript. All authors have read and agreed to the published version of the manuscript.

Funding: The authors acknowledge Fundação para a Ciência e Tecnologia (FCT) for supporting the computational costs related to this study through the grant CPCA/A0/7363/2020. This entity had no role in study design, data collection, data analysis, preparation of the manuscript and publishing decision.

Institutional Review Board Statement: The study was conducted in accordance with the Declaration of Helsinki and approved by the Ethics Committee of São João University Hospital (No. CE 41/2021, 19 March 2021).

Informed Consent Statement: Patient consent was waived as no potentially identifiable patient data was used.

Data Availability Statement: Data will be made available upon reasonable request.

Acknowledgments: The authors acknowledge the Portuguese Group of Ultrasound in Gastroenterology (GRUPUGE) for the scholarship awarded to this study protocol.

Conflicts of Interest: The authors declare no conflict of interest.

References

1. Zerboni, G.; Signoretti, M.; Crippa, S.; Falconi, M.; Arcidiacono, P.G.; Capurso, G. Systematic review and meta-analysis: Prevalence of incidentally detected pancreatic cystic lesions in asymptomatic individuals. *Pancreatology* **2019**, *19*, 2–9. [CrossRef] [PubMed]
2. Munigala, S.; Gelrud, A.; Agarwal, B. Risk of pancreatic cancer in patients with pancreatic cyst. *Gastrointest. Endosc.* **2016**, *84*, 81–86. [CrossRef] [PubMed]
3. Valsangkar, N.P.; Morales-Oyarvide, V.; Thayer, S.P.; Ferrone, C.R.; Wargo, J.A.; Warshaw, A.L.; Fernandez-del Castillo, C. 851 resected cystic tumors of the pancreas: A 33-year experience at the Massachusetts General Hospital. *Surgery* **2012**, *152*, S4–S12. [CrossRef] [PubMed]
4. European Study Group on Cystic Tumours of the Pancreas. European evidence-based guidelines on pancreatic cystic neoplasms. *Gut* **2018**, *67*, 789–804.
5. Ahmad, N.A.; Kochman, M.L.; Brensinger, C.; Brugge, W.R.; Faigel, D.O.; Gress, F.G.; Kimmey, M.B.; Nickl, N.J.; Savides, T.J.; Wallace, M.B.; et al. Interobserver agreement among endosonographers for the diagnosis of neoplastic versus non-neoplastic pancreatic cystic lesions. *Gastrointest. Endosc.* **2003**, *58*, 59–64. [CrossRef]
6. de Jong, K.; Verlaan, T.; Dijkgraaf, M.; Poley, J.; van Dullemen, H.; Bruno, M.; Fockens, P. Interobserver agreement for endosonography in the diagnosis of pancreatic cysts. *Endoscopy* **2011**, *43*, 579–584. [CrossRef]
7. Gargeya, R.; Leng, T. Automated Identification of Diabetic Retinopathy Using Deep Learning. *Ophthalmology* **2017**, *124*, 962–969. [CrossRef]
8. Dey, D.; Slomka, P.J.; Leeson, P.; Comaniciu, D.; Shrestha, S.; Sengupta, P.P.; Marwick, T.H. Artificial Intelligence in Cardiovascular Imaging: JACC State-of-the-Art Review. *J. Am. Coll. Cardiol.* **2019**, *73*, 1317–1335. [CrossRef]
9. Le Berre, C.; Trang-Poisson, C.; Bourreille, A. Small bowel capsule endoscopy and treat-to-target in Crohn's disease: A sys-tematic review. *World J. Gastroenterol.* **2019**, *25*, 4534–4554. [CrossRef]
10. Van den Sommen, F.; de Groof, J.; Struyvenberg, M.; van der Putten, J.; Boers, T.; Fockens, K.; Schoon, E.J.; Curvers, W.; de With, P.; Mori, Y.; et al. Machine learning in GI endoscopy: Practical guidance in how to interpret a novel field. *Gut* **2020**, *69*, 2035–2045. [CrossRef]
11. Kuwahara, T.; Hara, K.; Mizuno, N.; Haba, S.; Okuno, N.; Koda, H.; Miyano, A.; Fumihara, D. Current status of artificial intelligence analysis for endoscopic ultrasonography. *Dig. Endosc.* **2021**, *33*, 298–305. [CrossRef] [PubMed]
12. Pedregosa, F.; Varoquaux, G.; Gramfort, A.; Michel, V.; Thirion, B.; Grisel, O.; Blondel, M.; Prettenhofer, P.; Weiss, R.; Dubourg, V.; et al. Scikit-learn: Machine Learning in Python. *J. Mach. Learn. Res.* **2011**, *12*, 2825–2830.
13. Nguon, L.S.; Seo, K.; Lim, J.-H.; Song, T.-J.; Cho, S.-H.; Park, J.-S.; Park, S. Deep Learning-Based Differentiation between Mucinous Cystic Neoplasm and Serous Cystic Neoplasm in the Pancreas Using Endoscopic Ultrasonography. *Diagnostics* **2021**, *11*, 1052. [CrossRef] [PubMed]
14. Tonozuka, R.; Mukai, S.; Itoi, T. The Role of Artificial Intelligence in Endoscopic Ultrasound for Pancreatic Disorders. *Diagnostics* **2020**, *11*, 18. [CrossRef]
15. Kuwahara, T.; Hara, K.; Mizuno, N.; Okuno, N.; Matsumoto, S.; Obata, M.; Kurita, Y.; Koda, H.; Toriyama, K.; Onishi, S.; et al. Usefulness of Deep Learning Analysis for the Diagnosis of Malignancy in Intraductal Papillary Mucinous Neoplasms of the Pancreas. *Clin. Transl. Gastroenterol.* **2019**, *10*, e00045-8. [CrossRef]
16. Machicado, J.D.; Chao, W.-L.; Carlyn, D.E.; Pan, T.-Y.; Poland, S.; Alexander, V.L.; Maloof, T.G.; Dubay, K.; Ueltschi, O.; Middendorf, D.M.; et al. High performance in risk stratification of intraductal papillary mucinous neoplasms by confocal laser endomicroscopy image analysis with convolutional neural networks (with video). *Gastrointest. Endosc.* **2021**, *94*, 78–87.e2. [CrossRef]

17. Tonozuka, R.; Itoi, T.; Nagata, N.; Kojima, H.; Sofuni, A.; Tsuchiya, T.; Ishii, K.; Tanaka, R.; Nagakawa, Y.; Mukai, S. Deep learning analysis for the detection of pancreatic cancer on endosonographic images: A pilot study. *J. Hepato-Biliary-Pancreatic Sci.* **2021**, *28*, 95–104. [CrossRef]
18. Zhang, J.; Zhu, L.; Yao, L.; Ding, X.; Chen, D.; Wu, H.; Lu, Z.; Zhou, W.; Zhang, L.; An, P.; et al. Deep learning–based pancreas segmentation and station recognition system in EUS: Development and validation of a useful training tool (with video). *Gastrointest. Endosc.* **2020**, *92*, 874–885.e3. [CrossRef]
19. Marya, N.B.; Powers, P.D.; Chari, S.T.; Gleeson, F.C.; Leggett, C.L.; Abu Dayyeh, B.K.; Chandrasekhara, V.; Iyer, P.G.; Majumder, S.; Pearson, R.K.; et al. Utilisation of artificial intelligence for the development of an EUS-convolutional neural network model trained to enhance the diagnosis of autoimmune pancreatitis. *Gut* **2021**, *70*, 1335–1344. [CrossRef]
20. Krishna, S.G.; Hart, P.A.; DeWitt, J.M.; DiMaio, C.J.; Kongkam, P.; Napoleon, B.; Othman, M.O.; Tan, D.M.Y.; Strobel, S.G.; Stanich, P.; et al. EUS-guided confocal laser endomicroscopy: Prediction of dysplasia in intraductal papillary mucinous neoplasms (with video). *Gastrointest. Endosc.* **2020**, *91*, 551–563.e5. [CrossRef]
21. Chawla, S.; Schairer, J.; Kushnir, V.; Hernandez-Barco, Y.G.; ACG FDA-Related Matters Committee. Regulation of Artificial Intelligence-Based Applications in Gastroenterology. *Am. J. Gastroenterol.* **2021**, *116*, 2159–2162. [PubMed]

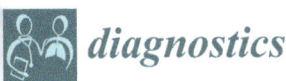

Article

Diagnosis of Inflammatory Bowel Disease and Colorectal Cancer through Multi-View Stacked Generalization Applied on Gut Microbiome Data

Sultan Imangaliyev [1,2], Jörg Schlötterer [1,2], Folker Meyer [1] and Christin Seifert [1,2,*]

1 Institute for Artificial Intelligence in Medicine, University of Duisburg-Essen, 45131 Essen, Germany
2 Cancer Research Center Cologne Essen (CCCE), 45147 Essen, Germany
* Correspondence: christin.seifert@uni-due.de

Abstract: Most of the microbiome studies suggest that using ensemble models such as Random Forest results in best predictive power. In this study, we empirically evaluate a more powerful ensemble learning algorithm, multi-view stacked generalization, on pediatric inflammatory bowel disease and adult colorectal cancer patients' cohorts. We aim to check whether stacking would lead to better results compared to using a single best machine learning algorithm. Stacking achieves the best test set Average Precision (AP) on inflammatory bowel disease dataset reaching AP = 0.69, outperforming both the best base classifier (AP = 0.61) and the baseline meta learner built on top of base classifiers (AP = 0.63). On colorectal cancer dataset, the stacked classifier also outperforms (AP = 0.81) both the best base classifier (AP = 0.79) and the baseline meta learner (AP = 0.75). Stacking achieves best predictive performance on test set outperforming the best classifiers on both patient cohorts. Application of the stacking solves the issue of choosing the most appropriate machine learning algorithm by automating the model selection procedure. Clinical application of such a model is not limited to diagnosis task only, but it also can be extended to biomarker selection thanks to feature selection procedure.

Keywords: gut microbiome; machine learning; classification; inflammatory bowel disease; colorectal cancer; stacked generalization; ensemble learning

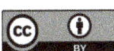

1. Introduction

The human microbiota are connected to health and disease in many clinical applications [1,2], e.g., cancer [3] or immune-mediated inflammatory diseases [4] including e.g., inflammatory bowel disease [5]. Traditionally, the medical microbiology community used univariate statistical hypothesis tests to identify significantly different species across patient cohorts [6]. Such methods have their limitations since they neither include complex non-linear interactions among species, nor do they provide a prognostic value for a new unseen dataset [7]. Hence, most of the modern human microbiome studies rely on machine learning models to identify biomarkers of health and disease [7,8]. Machine learning also provides tools to integrate microbial data with other -omics datasets and to identify the most important species involved in health and disease [9,10]. For example, inflammatory bowel diseases such as Crohn's disease or ulcerative colitis have similar symptoms, but their etiology and hence the treatment regimens are different [6]. Cancer treatment is another example where finding a prognostic microbial marker can be important. For instance, due to the tumor growth, the microbiota composition changes and one can detect such changes early enough to diagnose and hence intervene when treatment has the best effect on patients [11].

The choice of the machine learning algorithm for microbial and clinical data-driven problems is methodologically and computationally challenging. Since both microbial and clinical features are represented as tabular data, specialized neural network models e.g., Convolutional Neural Networks [12–14] are not directly suitable on such datasets. In terms of predictive performance, due to the so-called "no free lunch" theorem there is no universally best algorithm which would perform equally well across all datasets [15]. Therefore, most of the microbiome studies related to looking for solution to this challenge are empirical and often apply a large suite of models on microbial data one-by-one with the aim of finding a model which performs the best [16–19]. Such studies often suggest that using ensemble models such as Random Forest or Gradient Boosted Decision Trees results in best predictive power. However, this is still a heuristic choice and even application of such complex models individually might still lead to suboptimal results.

Moreover, the application of machine learning on practical microbiology problems must be done with great care, because the consequences of wrong decisions based on model predictions can harm patients during treatment. For example, it has been shown that black-box models like Neural Networks can make accurate predictions even when they exploit clinically undesired data patterns [20,21]. Therefore, model interpretability becomes an important issue next to the model accuracy. It is known that there is a trade-off between model interpretability and model accuracy [7]. For example, complex black-box models such as Extreme Gradient Boosting [22] or Random Forest [23] are accurate but not interpretable, whilst simple models like Logistic Regression are interpretable, but often slightly less accurate [17]. To understand how the model makes its predictions and consequently increase trust in the model, *Explainable* (also sometimes interchangeably called *Intelligible* or *Interpretable*) machine learning models [24] should be used in biomedical applications involving microbiome data.

In summary, a clinically applicable machine learning diagnostic model must be (a) accurate, (b) explainable, (c) capable of integrating multiple data sources and d) reasonably efficient in terms of computation time. Generalized stacking [25] (often called stacking for the sake of simplicity) satisfies these requirements and solves the problem of selecting the most suitable machine learning model. Like Random Forest, stacking is also an ensemble learning algorithm, but instead of aggregating weak learners, i.e., decision trees, stacking combines the output of strong learners. Those strong learners make prediction errors on different subsets of samples, i.e., stacking directly benefits from a diversity of classifiers in terms of their predictions. Each of the base learners is akin a judge in a jury committee, which sees something unseen by other of his/her colleagues, but collectively using a higher level judge's help, entire committee achieves best judgement. The output of the base learners is not combined by simple averaging, but learnt using a so-called meta learner. Meta learning has been shown to improve predictive power, because the meta learner combines strengths of each base learner and compensates their weaknesses [26,27]. Additionally, the flexible approach of stacking allows to train base learners on different subsets of features stemming from various data views, resulting in a multi-view learning setting [28]. Moreover, stacking delivers a computational trade-off between running a single powerful machine learning algorithm (hence achieving possibly suboptimal result) and running virtually all possible algorithms one-by one (hence not achievable on practice).

In this study, we evaluate stacking on two different patient cohorts, a pediatric inflammatory bowel disease cohort [29,30] and adult patients of colorectal cancer [31]. We demonstrate that stacking leads to better result (Test Average Precision = 0.69 on inflammatory bowel disease dataset and Test Average Precision = 0.81 on colorectal cancer dataset) than using a single best machine learning algorithm, despite that each dataset poses its unique challenges from both medical and machine learning aspects. On the one hand, classifying two diseases such as Crohn's disease and ulcerative colitis is expected to be a more difficult task rather than comparing healthy patients and patients diagnosed with cancer. On the other hand, microbiota classification of newly-onset inflammatory bowel disease in treatment-naive children should be easier than classification of adult cancer patients who have undergone various treatments during their disease progression. Comparing results on both datasets, we assess reasons why stacking can be an alternative to applying a single model. We also evaluate empirically how base learners are mutually similar to each other with respect to predictions as well as how multi-view settings can potentially lead to an improved predictive performance. For model interpretability, we also provide feature importance values retrieved from both the meta learner and the entire stacking pipeline.

2. Materials and Methods

2.1. Datasets and Preprocessing

Table 1 provides an overview of basic characteristics of both datasets, including number of features included in both clinical and microbial views as well as number of unique values on genus taxonomic level in microbial view.

Table 1. Dataset characteristics for inflammatory bowel disease and colorectal cancer.

	Clinical View Features		Microbial View Features	
	# Numerical	# Categorical	# Total	# Unique Genera
Inflammatory bowel disease	1	6	6737	533
Colorectal cancer	2	7	5982	239

The 16s rRNA microbial data features and clinical patient data features for inflammatory bowel disease patient's cohort dataset were retrieved using the *MicrobeDS* R-library [32]. Only samples from a pediatric RISK cohort were included, excluding any patients who had any prior treatment using steroids and/or antibiotics. Among this subset, only samples of patients with ulcerative colitis and Crohn's disease were included. To prevent overoptimistic model performance and prevent training label's leakage, we removed disease-related features which implicitly disclose patient status e.g., disease subtype, disease extent in bowel, disease duration etc. Full list of removed features is provided in Appendix Table A1. Full list of included features is provided in Appendix Table A2. With this feature choice, we prevent the model learning shortcuts, e.g., that all patients diagnosed with certain subtype of ulcerative colitis are indeed patients diagnosed with ulcerative colitis. Moreover, from a clinical viewpoint, diagnosing a patient for whom the disease subtype is known becomes a trivial task. Our final data set consists of 535 examples with 7 features for the clinical data view and 6737 features for the microbiology view. Clinical data contains 223 missing values and no data imputation was applied. 443 samples are labeled with Crohn's disease (negative class) and 92 labeled with ulcerative colitis (positive class).

The 16s rRNA microbial data features and clinical patient data features for colorectal cancer were retrieved from the GitHub repository [33] referred to by the authors of the original paper [31]. Only samples of patients with colorectal cancer and healthy controls were included, excluding all patients with adenoma. To prevent training labels' leakage, disease-related features e.g., history of cancer, history of polyps etc., were removed. Full list of removed features is provided in Appendix Table A3. Full list of included features is provided in Appendix Table A4. As a result, the dataset prepared for colorectal cancer classification consists of 291 examples with 9 features for the clinical data view and 5982 features for the microbiology view. Clinical data contains 5 missing values and no data imputation was applied. 172 samples are labeled as healthy controls (negative class) and 119 samples are labeled as with cancer patients (positive class).

Both datasets were randomly split into 80% training and 20% test sets. To be able to assess overfitting, we held out the test set completely during model training, including the cross-validation experiments.

2.2. Machine Learning Model and Training Procedure

The multi-view stacked model consists of base learners which are trained independently from each other on original features per each view of the training set and a meta learner which is trained on predictions of base learners. To reduce computational time, the microbial features were filtered during training procedure. Namely, the microbial data was prepared as input for base learners by removing features which had zero variance, i.e., features with constant values. Furthermore, data was pre-filtered using ANOVA corrected by multiple test correction procedure after being power-transformed to achieve normal distribution [34]. To get a better error estimation, the training set was split into k folds and in k sequential iterations $k − 1$ folds were used for training. During each round of stratified cross-validation, the remaining fold was used as validation set and only those validation set predictions were combined, subsequently stacked and provided as a training data to the meta learner. This procedure reduces overfitting, since meta learner is trained on predictions made on validation set, not on training set. As training features for the meta learner, the predicted probabilities of the base learners were used instead of predicted classification labels. The illustrative example of a multi-view stacked generalization framework is depicted in Figure 1.

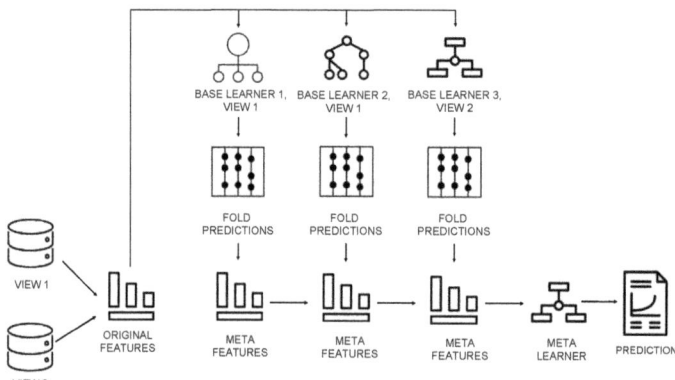

Figure 1. Multi-view stacked generalization framework's illustrative example. Methodologically this computational framework's example consists of three base machine learning models and a meta learner. The predictions of the base learners on validation folds are stacked together as meta features and presented for training to the meta learner model which outputs the final prediction. The illustrative example pipeline was trained on two subsets of features that allowed multi-view setting by training base learners 1 and 2 on features of view 1 and the base learner 3 on features of view 2. For the sake of simplicity, the example using only two views and three base learners is explained. In principle, number of views and base learners is not limited.

We selected a diverse set of classifiers from different model classes as candidates for the base learners. The linear classifiers are Stochastic Gradient Descent classifier with Logistic Loss (SGD_LL), Stochastic Gradient Descent classifier with modified Huber Loss (SGD_HL) and the K-nearest Neighbors Classifier (KNN). The non-linear classifiers are Multi-layer Perceptron (MLP), Quadratic Discriminant Analysis (QDA), Random Forest (RF) and Histogram-based Gradient Boosting Classification (HGBC). Since HGBC is the only classifier in this suite which can directly be applied on data with missing values and categorical features, HGBC was applied on both microbial data (HGBC_otu) and clinical data (HGBC_clin). All other models were applied to microbial data only, because their applications to clinical data would require imputing missing values with a risk of introducing mistakes and one-hot encoding of categorical features, which would hugely increase the feature space and hence it might increase possible overfitting. Stacking provides a simple, yet powerful pipeline with reasonable development effort by combining and learning outputs of suboptimal base learners, hence we did not perform hyperparameter tuning of base learners.

As a meta learner, we chose Logistic Regression with Elastic Net regularization with exhaustive grid search hyperparameter optimization and k-fold cross-validation. Logistic Regression is advantageous to black-box models, because it is more interpretable and empirically it results in comparable performance to black-box models [28]. We additionally applied a soft voting procedure (SoftVote) on output of base classifiers, which returns the class label as argmax of the sum of predicted probabilities for comparison. All models were trained using Python v3.7 programming language, scikit-learn v1.0.2 package [35].

2.3. Performance Metrics and Handling Class Imbalance

Both of the datasets exhibit class imbalance, because the number of negative classes is larger than number of positive ones. The dataset for inflammatory bowel disease has a high class imbalance with only 17% examples labeled with a positive class, while for the dataset of colorectal cancer this number is 41%. Such imbalanced data requires specialized performance metrics, because using metrics like Area Under Receiver Operating Characteristic (AUROC) curve may lead to misleading results with over-optimistic performance evaluation [36]. To obtain a more relevant performance estimate, we used Precision-Recall (PR) curves, because they should be preferred to the Receiver Operating Characteristic (ROC) curves in classification of rare diseases [37] and their summarization as Average Precision (AP) values [38]. We report values on training, validation and test sets. For training and validation, we report the median values over the cross-validation folds. Test set values are calculated on the hold-out test set. The training set values are calculated on the entire training set using hyperparameters found during cross-validation. To estimate diversity and prediction errors of classifiers, Matthews's Correlation Coefficient (MCC) was calculated, which was recommended as a more informative score in evaluating imbalanced binary classifications than accuracy and F1 score [39]. Unlike AP, MCC values are bound by $[-1; +1]$, where +1 represents a perfect prediction, 0 an average random prediction and -1 an inverse prediction.

In addition to choosing performance metric appropriate to imbalanced class data, we also applied data space weighting approach, which allows obtaining a modified distribution biased towards the costly rare classes during training base learners [40]. We did not apply any under-sampling methods, because this may eliminate useful examples which might contain rare microbial species as potential disease biomarkers. Neither we applied any over-sampling methods, because they may increase the likelihood of overfitting and increase computational effort [36].

2.4. Model Interpretability

Conceptually, we are interested in model interpretation on two levels, i.e., on the level of meta learner features and on the level of original features. The former shows which of the base learners contributed to which extend to the final prediction. The latter shows how the model including the base learners uses the original input features for the prediction.

Firstly, the regression weights of the meta learner were retrieved and normalized by dividing by the absolute maximum value, so that the top feature importance absolute value would be equal to one, which simplifies comparison between values. These normalized values were then ranked in decreasing order and presented as a model explanation for meta learner, providing insight on relative contribution of each base classifier on final prediction. Secondly, to evaluate feature importance of the entire model, permutation feature importance values were calculated. To calculate a permutation feature importance a baseline metric is evaluated on a training dataset, i.e., features of both clinical and microbiology views. Then, a feature column is permuted and the metric is evaluated again without retraining the full model. The permutation importance is defined as the difference between the baseline metric and metric from permuting the feature column [23]. For a feature that does not contribute to the model's decision, the model should be robust to changes in its value. For a highly important feature, we expect—on average—large changes in prediction for a data point if this feature values are changed.

3. Results

3.1. Classification of Gut Microbiota from Inflammatory Bowel Disease Patients

Figure 2 provides an overview of the performance of the stacked classifier and its independent base models. Figure 2a,b depict PR curves and the corresponding AP values of base classifiers, the SoftVote aggregation and the stacked classifier. On test set, the stacked classifier demonstrates the best performance (AP = 0.69), outperforming the best base classifier (MLP; AP = 0.61) and the simple ensemble meta learner (SoftVote; AP = 0.63). All models show signs of overfitting, their performance is worse on test set than on the training set.

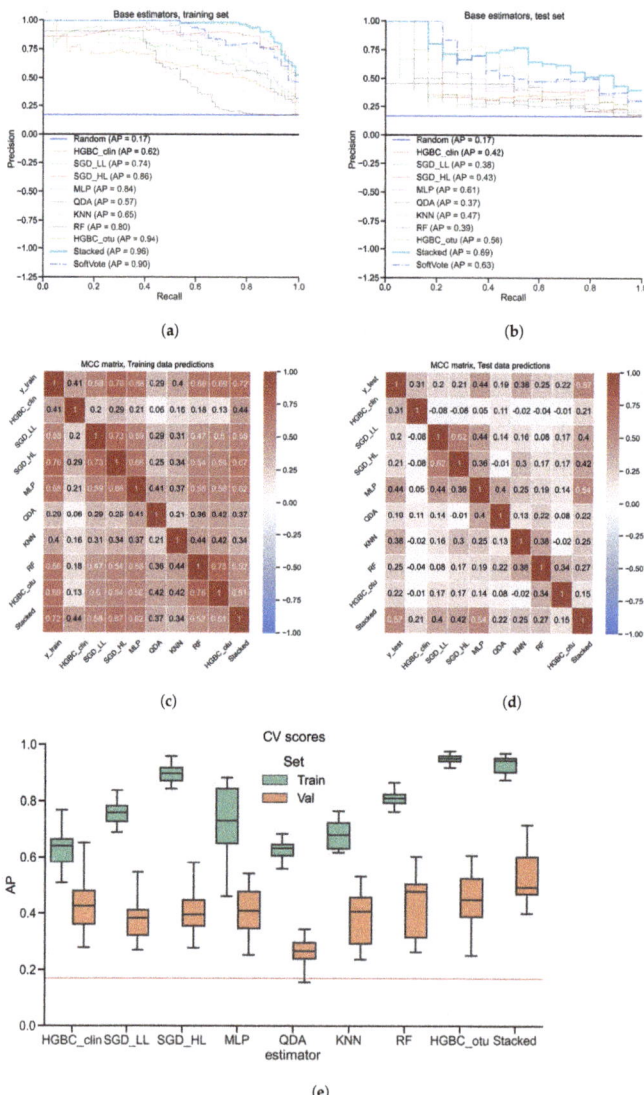

Figure 2. Model performance comparison between base learners and stacked model, inflammatory bowel disease dataset. (**a**) Precision-Recall (PR) curves and corresponding Average Precision (AP)

values of base classifiers, SoftVote classifier and the stacked classifier applied on training set; (**b**) PR curves and corresponding AP values of base classifiers, SoftVote classifier and the stacked classifier applied on test set; (**c**) Matthews's Correlation Coefficient (MCC) values matrix heatmap of base classifier predictions, classification labels and the stacked classifier predictions applied on training set; (**d**) MCC values matrix heatmap of base classifier predictions, classification labels and the stacked classifier predictions applied on test set; (**e**) AP values of each model during cross-validation on training and validation sets. Red horizontal line refers to AP value obtained from a random classifier.

Figure 2c,d depict the MCC values as heatmap. On the training set, the highest agreement among base classifiers is observed between RF and HGBC_otu (MCC = 0.75), while the lowest agreement is observed between QDA and HGBC_clin (MCC = 0.06). We observe a general low agreement between base classifiers, indicating that they learn different patterns which can be exploited by a meta learner. On test set, we observe the highest agreement between SGD_LL and SGD_HL (MCC = 0.62), and the lowest between SGD_LL and HGBC_clin (MCC = −0.08). The stacked classifier does not demonstrate the highest correlation with the training set labels reaching MCC = 0.72, but the highest correlation of its predictions with the test set labels (MCC = 0.57) outperforming best base classifier (MLP; MCC = 0.44). This indicates that the stacked classifier learns patterns that are better generalizable to unseen test data.

Figure 2e depicts the AP values of cross-validation on training and validation sets. The stacked classifier demonstrates the highest median AP on validation sets ($\approx$0.49), outperforming all base models with QDA being the closest to random guessing (AP of 0.17). None of the models is free from overfitting with HGBC_clin having the least difference between median AP on training and validation sets. To estimate overfitting, we calculated AP difference between median AP on training and validation sets for both stacked model and all base learners split by the data view. Those median values are depicted on Appendix Figure A1.

Figure 3 shows most important features of the predictive model, with Figure 3a showing the sorted normalized regression weights of the meta learner. HGBC_clin demonstrates the highest importance value followed by SGD_HL and KNN which have roughly equal weight values of around 0.4 each. QDA classifier's importance value though being non-zero is negligible, indicating that meta learner ignored predictions made by QDA base classifier. Figure 3b depicts the permutation feature importance values. The top 3 highest scores were assigned to the clinical features such as inflammation status, age and race with median importance values of about 0.10, 0.05 and 0.02 respectively. All other features in the top 10 list have lower feature importance scores (less than 0.02) and most of them are microbial features. Among them are microorganisms which are identified belonging to the taxonomic families *Ruminococcaceae*, *Comamonadaceae* and *Alcaligenaceae*, while two features are identified belonging to taxonomic order of *Clostridiales*.

3.2. Classification of Gut Microbiota from Colorectal Cancer Patients

Figure 4 shows an overview of the performance of the stacked classifier and its base models. Figure 4a,b depict PR curves and corresponding AP values of base classifiers, SoftVote aggregation and the stacked classifier. On test set, the stacked classifier demonstrates the best performance (AP = 0.81) outperforming both the best base classifier (SGD_LL; AP = 0.79) and simple ensemble meta learner (SoftVote; AP = 0.75). The best base learner performs better than a simple ensemble meta learner on test set (SoftVote; AP = 0.75 vs. SGD_LL; AP = 0.79). Overall, all models perform worse on test set compared to training set, which indicates overfitting.

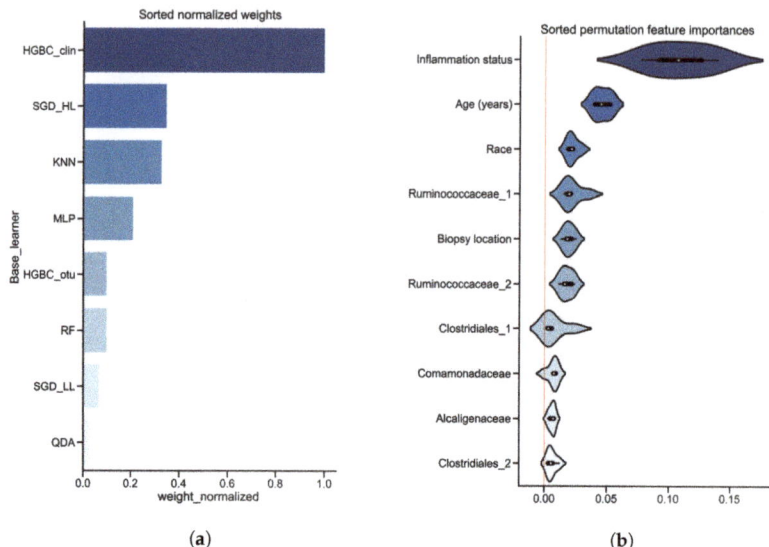

Figure 3. Sorted feature importance values, inflammatory bowel disease dataset, training set. (**a**) Normalized regression weights obtained from a meta learner used in stacked classifier; (**b**) Violin plots of permutation feature importance values obtained from a stacked classifier. Red vertical line represents zero importance value.

Figure 4c,d depict MCC values as heatmap. The stacked classifier demonstrates the best correlation of its predictions with the test set labels reaching MCC=0.55, outperforming best base classifier (HGBC_otu; MCC = 0.43). The highest agreement can be observed between linear methods (SGD_LL vs. SGD_HL, MCC = 0.59), while KNN shows an overall low agreement with other base learners. HGBC_clin MCC values indicate lowest correlation with any other base classifier trained on microbial data often reaching negative MCC values. The mutual agreement between base classifiers is generally low, because the predictions made by base models are diverse enough to correctly predict different subsets of data.

Figure 4e depicts the AP values of cross-validation on training and validation sets. The stacked classifier demonstrates the highest median AP on validation set (≈ 0.83). All base models achieve lower median validation set AP, with QDA and MLP classifiers being the closest to the random AP of 0.41. None of the models is free from overfitting with HGBC_clin having the least difference between median AP on training and validation sets. To estimate overfitting, we calculated AP difference between median AP on training and validation sets for both stacked model and all base learners split by the data view. Those median values are depicted on Appendix Figure A2.

Figure 5 shows most important features of the predictive model, with Figure 5a showing sorted normalized regression weights of the meta learner. HGBC_clin demonstrates the highest importance value followed by SGD_LL and HGBC_otu which have weight values of around 0.6 and 0.5 respectively. The importance score of KNN is negative, indicating that meta learner used predictions made by KNN base classifier, but considered them as negatively correlated to the positive class probability prediction. This aligns with the finding in Figure 4c where KNN MCC values show the lowest correlation with any other base classifiers, and it indicates that the stacked classifier can learn to utilize incorrect predictions by negating their influence. Figure 5b shows the importance of input features calculated by permutation feature importance. The highest score is assigned to the patients' age with median importance value of about 0.05. All other features in the top 10 list have lower feature importance score (less than 0.01) and most of them are microbial features. Among them are microorganisms which are identified belonging to the taxonomic families *Porphyromonadaceae*, *Bacteroidaceae*, *Prevotellaceae*, *Peptostreptococcaceae* and *Lachnospiraceae*.

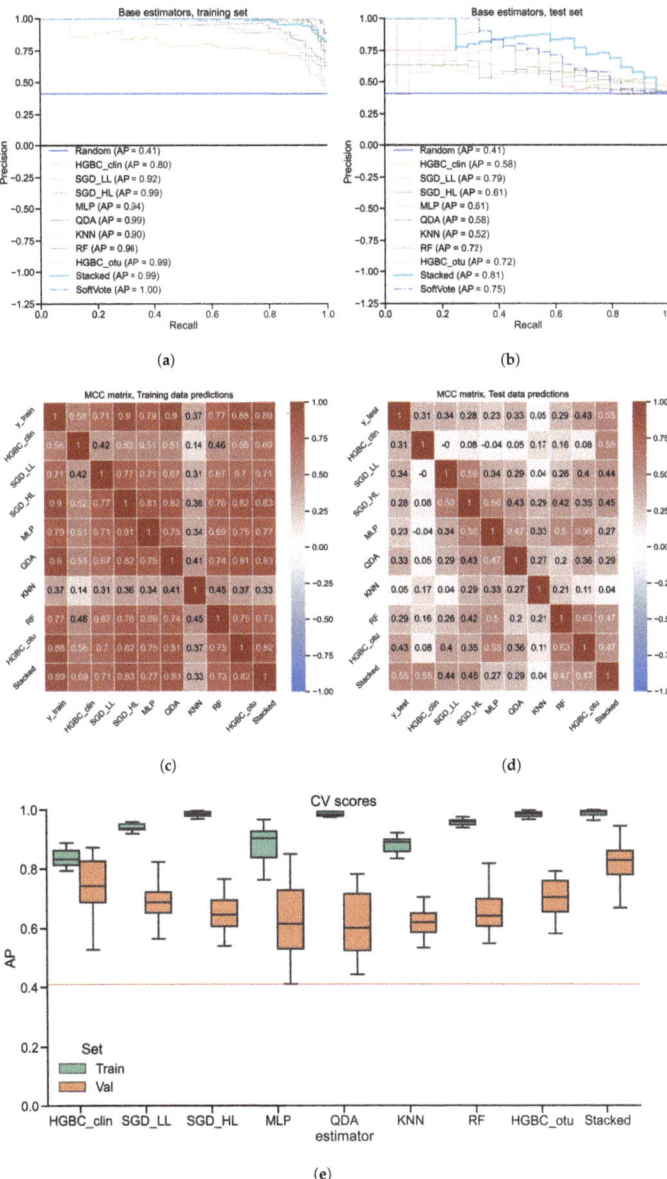

Figure 4. Model performance comparison between base learners and stacked model, colorectal cancer dataset. (**a**) PR curves and corresponding AP values of base classifiers, SoftVote classifier and the stacked classifier applied on training set; (**b**) PR curves and corresponding AP values of base classifiers, SoftVote classifier and stacked classifier applied on test set; (**c**) MCC values matrix heatmap of base classifier predictions, classification labels and the stacked classifier predictions applied on training set; (**d**) MCC values matrix heatmap of base classifier predictions, classification labels and stacked classifier predictions applied on test set; (**e**) AP values of each model during cross-validation on training and validation sets. Red horizontal line refers to AP value obtained from a random classifier.

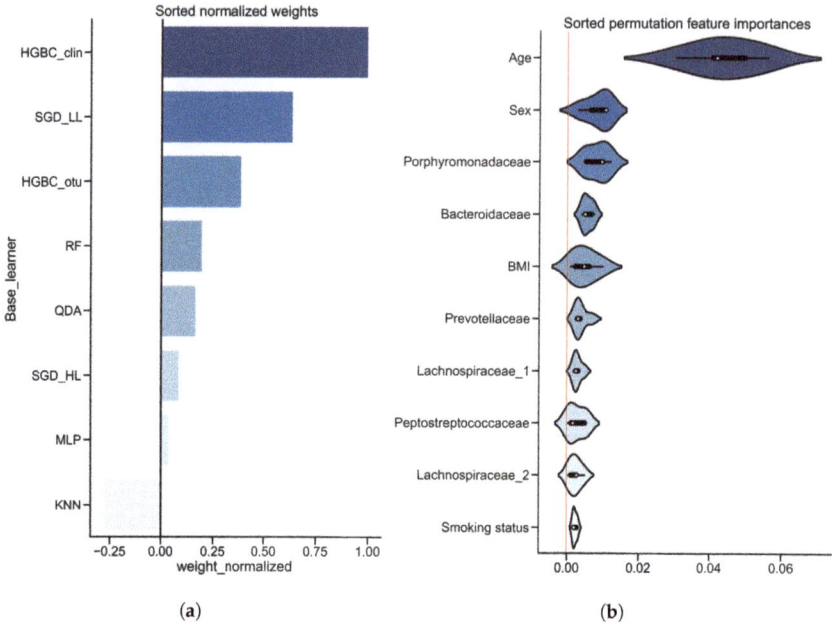

Figure 5. Sorted feature importance values, colorectal cancer dataset, training set. (**a**) Normalized regression weights obtained from a meta learner used in stacked classifier; (**b**) Violin plots of permutation feature importance values obtained from a stacked classifier. Red vertical line represents zero importance value.

4. Discussion

4.1. Stacking as a More Powerful Ensemble Method than Random Forest

The aim of this study was to investigate whether stacking would lead to better performance than a single model when applied to multi-view microbiome data. Previous similar studies [16–19] compared multiple machine learning models one-by-one and concluded that RF is often the best model in terms of predictive performance. We showed on two different real-world datasets that stacking outperforms RF in terms of generalization error, i.e., performance on unseen test data. Consistency of results among both inflammatory bowel disease and colorectal cancer datasets is particularly encouraging taking into account differences in patient cohorts and disease types. Higher performance of stacking seems logical because much like RF which combines output of multiple weak learners, stacking also combines output of multiple base learners. However, unlike RF, stacking combines the predictions of strong and diverse learners using training labels. If stacking is better than applying a single model, there must be a reason why it is not yet widely applied in microbiome community. In subsequent subsections we hypothesize reasons why stacking worked well on these two datasets and which recommendations we can conclude from our results.

4.2. Meta Learner's Role in Stacking

Application of stacking on real-world datasets requires making certain choices and tricks which were referred to as 'black art' [27]. Even when stacking is applied correctly, it might still perform only as well as best base classifier [26] or with marginal improvement of about 3% compared to the best individual base classifier [41]. In our study, we achieved results higher than a single base classifier, with improvement of over 8% on test set for inflammatory bowel disease, possibly due to combining prediction probabilities rather than predicted classification labels themselves, which is in line with general recommendations [42]. Moreover, we showed that even a simple meta learner like soft voting can still result in a good performance, if base classifier probabilities are well calibrated. The study addressing issues in stacking [42] also recommends using a linear model as a meta learner, which is in line with another empirical study on microbiome [28] where Logistic Regression was recommended to aggregate predictions of base learners. For comparison, we additionally trained stacking using RF as a meta learner. PR curves for both data sets are depicted in Appendix Figure A3. RF as meta learner did not result in improvement of test AP on any of the datasets: compared to the stacked model with Logistic Regression as meta learner, test AP degraded from 0.69 to 0.56 on inflammatory bowel disease dataset (Appendix Figure A3a) and from 0.81 to 0.77 on colorectal cancer dataset (Appendix Figure A3b). Besides achieving better AP values, applying linear model like Logistic Regression is also advantageous due to better interpretability of stacking. This is helpful for understanding which base learner models contributed highest for the final model prediction. For example, we observed in Figure 3a that the meta learner ignored predictions made by QDA base classifier. Looking back at Figure 2c,d we observed that QDA had a poor predictive performance, and the agreement with other classifiers was also low. Hence, the QDA base classifier mostly made wrong predictions which the meta learner learned to ignore. This demonstrates why stacking is more preferable than average voting.

4.3. Diversity of Base Learner's Role in Stacking

Another issue is the choice of base learners. Generally, it is recommended that base classifiers should be both accurate and diverse [27], though notion of diversity is rather vague and has no formal definition. In this study, we used domain knowledge by combining classifiers which are diverse based on their underlying mathematical roots, e.g., we trained linear models, ensemble models and a neural network model. The diversity of the classifiers outputs was confirmed empirically by large difference in MCC values between each model's prediction, while their high accuracy was confirmed by similarly high MCC values w.r.t. classification labels. Based on performance of base learners, we would discourage blindly using RF as a single classifier, because it did not always result in better performance compared to other models.

The diversity of classifiers can be increased by applying base classifiers on different sets of variables or, in biomedical applications, on different -omics views. In fact, multiple microbiome studies often encourage integration of multi-omics data [8–10,43] in a single model. One of the previous studies [43] combined multiple -omics views using stacking, but unlike in our study, authors used exactly the same linear model across all views instead of applying different models. Both of the previous studies [30,31] from which we extracted datasets for this study, lack access to other -omics views, but they provide us access to clinical patient metadata which we successfully used as a complementary view for stacking. Previous study on Crohn's Disease [30] did not use clinical traits data. On the contrary, the colorectal cancer study [31] used some of the clinical variables in a separately trained model. Authors of that study concluded that extra dataset can be complementary to microbial data as a source of diagnostic information. We demonstrated that stacking benefits from adding extra view for both colorectal cancer and inflammatory bowel disease datasets. MCC values, hence the mutual agreement, of base models trained on clinical data tend to be lower compared to the ones obtained from training base models on microbial data, meaning that those classifiers make errors on different subsets of samples. This improves the diversity of classifiers, hence improving overall stacking performance. The importance of adding clinical data is also indirectly confirmed by higher feature importance of the base learner trained on a clinical data. Such a diversity can potentially stem from the fact that clinical data reflects traits with long term effects on disease e.g., adaptive immune responses [6], race-related [44] or sex-related [31] differences, while microbial features reflect more dynamic traits, e.g., microbial dysbiosis [4,29] or response to treatment [11]. The performance of stacking model trained on inflammatory bowel disease can be further improved by including more clinical features. For instance, adding extra features which implicitly indicate the extent of the disease in a gut can help the model to learn differences between Crohn's disease and ulcerative colitis. Ulcerative colitis starts at the rectum and progresses continuously through the colon and it affects only colon. Crohn's disease is different, as it has a discontinuous pattern of spread and can affect entire gastrointestinal tract [45]. Such localization-related clinical features were explicitly excluded from the datasets in our experiments and are marked in Appendix Table A1 as "Implicit training label leakage". The PR curves on training and test sets of the stacking model trained on such an extended dataset are provided on Appendix Figure A6. Training AP increased to 0.93, Test AP also improved to 0.73, largely because HGBC_clin performance improved (Training AP = 0.65, Test AP = 0.48). We would generally discourage using such localization-related clinical features during training, since such model does not use complex interactions between microbial and clinical features. Diagnosis of two diseases is a challenging task and microbial traits are more interesting to discover from a research point of view [6,46]. We consider that Test AP value of 0.69 is high for such a complex classification task, because the random AP value for such an imbalanced dataset is 0.17. Hence stacking model's performance improved more than three times compared to the one of the random predictor.

Analysis of median AP values on validation and training sets of each base learner for both datasets indicates moderate or high level of overfitting. This can also be observed while comparing PR curves between training and test sets. Higher overfitting of the base learners trained on microbial data compared to base learners trained on clinical data is expected due to higher feature numbers in microbial view. Nevertheless, on test set stacking performs the best, indicating that training meta learner on overfitted base learner predictions operates like a regularizer by assigning lower weights on models with higher generalization error, i.e., on the ones trained using microbial data. This information is usually not known beforehand and it can be discovered empirically by training models and comparing their performance values on a validation set. In a case of using a single model, data practitioner has to manually choose the best model among all base learners. However, this task is taken care of by a meta learner in stacked model. During training the stacked model, only the meta learner hyperparameters were extensively optimized, while base learners were trained using default hyperparameters. Taking into account smaller dimensionality of the dataset presented to the meta learner and simplicity of the meta-learner itself, training time of entire stacking pipeline was low and it still yielded a reasonable generalization error. Hence, stacking might be a good alternative to an extensive hyperparameter tuning of a single model when quick insights are preferable to the highest possible model performance.

Based on these conclusions, we would recommend to apply stacking as a tool to achieve increased performance by using diverse classifiers trained on diverse data views. This recommendation is empirical and we cannot guarantee that stacking is going to work better or worse on other diseases or patient cohorts, because there is no consensus on the most optimal stacking configuration [27]. However, conclusions and examples provided in this subsection suggest that stacking would perform better than a single model on complex biomedical phenomena with multiple processes involved on molecular level, e.g., aging [28], head and neck cancer [41], pregnancy [43] or protein sequence compression [47]. Such biological processes can have patterns which can be reflected on multiple levelse.g., proteomics, metabolomics, metagenomics, patient history data etc. Those patterns can be modeled using diverse set of machine learning models which are complementary to each other, i.e., they show similar performance but make different decisions for the same data points reflected by low mutual agreement scores depicted on Figures 2c,d and 4c,d.

4.4. Overfitting Analysis

AP values depicted on Figures 2a,b and 4a,b indicate moderate overfitting of the stacked model, because the Test AP values are lower than Training AP values. However, such an observation is possible only when the proper model testing is implemented, i.e., when the model is applied on unseen test set. Both of the previous studies which used those two datasets [30,31] lack any indication of using independent test sets. Inflammatory bowel disease study [30] reports average cross-validation scores on training set, while colorectal cancer study [31] reports out-of-bag scores. The latter is shown to be as an unreliable measure of the classification performance [48]. We performed extensive analysis of overfitting using cross-validation and independent test set. We found out that stacking achieves better AP on training and validation sets compared to any of the base classifiers. Main source of overfitting comes from base learners trained on microbial data rather than from ones trained on clinical data (Appendix Figures A1 and A2). This might be due to the "curse of dimensionality" because the number of features in microbial view is magnitudes higher than the number of features in clinical view (Table 1). Hence, reducing input dimensionality of the microbial view data is one of the simplest and computationally inexpensive ways to reduce overfitting. This step is essentially a feature selection method often called variable ranking or filtering [49]. We used statistical filtering, but due to large number of features a multiple test correction procedure is essential to reduce false discovery rate [50,51]. By using multiple test corrected pre-filtering procedure on microbial features, overfitting can be further decreased for both inflammatory bowel disease dataset to Training AP = 0.78; Test AP = 0.66 (Appendix Figure A4) and for colorectal cancer dataset to Training AP = 0.96; Test AP = 0.79 (Appendix Figure A5). However, such a strict univariate filtering can miss potentially important microbial features which otherwise would have been detected by multivariate base learners. Moreover, although overfitting decreased, so did the Test AP on both datasets. Therefore, such a decreased overfitting comes with the price of reduced test performance and it should be considered balancing all of the associated compromises attached to it. As mentioned in Section 4.3, the meta learner in stacking framework takes care of regularization task and it can be considered as an efficient replacement for extensive hyperparameter tuning of base learners to achieve improved performance on test set.

4.5. Model Interpretation and Further Examples of Stacking

As for the model interpretation, it can be done in several ways thanks to flexibility of stacking framework. We calculated feature importance values in a meta learning scale by retrieving weights of Logistic Regression used as a meta learner. This gave us insight into which of the base models were the most contributing ones. Those results confirmed "no free lunch" theorem empirically, because different base models were identified as important ones between two different datasets. We also retrieved feature importance values of the entire pipeline using permutation feature importance. Those results indicated that clinical variables are the most important ones across both datasets, despite being underrepresented in terms of feature cardinality in feature space. Previous study on Crohn's disease [30] identified a few microbial features among which microorganisms belonging to taxonomic order of *Clostridiales*. Microbes of the same order were also identified as important ones using permutation importance on stacking classifier used in our study. Direct comparison of results between previous study and our study is not possible, because the clinical research question of our study is different, i.e., comparing Crohn's disease patients with ulcerative colitis patients instead of comparing Crohn's disease patients with healthy patients. In previous study of colorectal cancer [31], authors found associations of microorganisms belonging to order of *Porphyromonadaceae* and *Lachnospiraceae*. In our study, we also identified a few features belonging to the same taxonomic order along with a few others such as *Bacteroidaceae*, *Prevotellaceae* and *Peptostreptococcaceae*.

In a broader sense, stacking is not a single algorithm, but rather a family of ensemble algorithms with many variants [27]. Moreover, stacking can be performed in multiple stages of modeling and it is not limited to combining predictions only. For example, stacked ensemble of learners can be used as a tool to improve feature selection [52,53], achieve better protein sequence compression [47], integrate outputs of multiple neural networks [54] or integrate input of neural network from several normalization methods [55] when applied on microbiome data.

4.6. Study Limitations

This study has two major limitations. First of all, it might have not achieved the best possible predictive performance on either of the datasets. Hyperparameters of base learners were not extensively optimized, because it would be computationally expensive, but most importantly because achieving highest AP on test set for each base learner was not our goal. We aimed to demonstrate that stacking performs better than application of a single machine learning algorithm and there is no need to choose one "best" model which is not possible due to "no free lunch" theorem. Instead, we showed that application of a machine learning can help to identify which other machine learning algorithms can perform best and let the practitioner focus on model interpretation. Thus, based on our findings we would recommend to apply stacking as a tool for model selection, for multi-view data integration and as an alternative to extensive hyperparameter optimization of a single model.

Another limitation is that we used only two datasets. Those datasets are very different from each other, but stacking demonstrated similar patterns on both of them. Since we aimed to get an understanding of stacking, we limited ourselves on a detailed analysis of the internal mechanics applied to two most representative datasets, providing data practitioners with tips why stacking worked well and what can we learn from it.

5. Conclusions

This study presents an application of the multi-view stacked machine learning model on two microbial datasets from different diseases, i.e., inflammatory bowel disease and colorectal cancer. The model combines multiple heterogeneous machine learning models and it achieves best predictive performance on the test set outperforming the best single classifier. Detailed analysis of the model provided insight on why stacking achieves such a high performance, mainly due to diversity of classifiers as well as using a meta learner which regularizes overfitted prediction labels from base learners. Thanks to the flexibility of the stacked model, combined usage of multiple views is possible and clinical data usage is encouraged as a complementary view to the microbial data.

From a practical point of view, the results of the study suggest that the stacked model partially solves the issue of choosing the most appropriate machine learning model by automating the selection using the meta learner algorithm. Results empirically confirmed the "no free lunch" theorem on two different microbial datasets with rather different patient cohorts and disease types. Clinical application is not limited to diagnosis task only, but it also can be extended to biomarker selection thanks to model interpretation using permutation feature selection procedure.

Author Contributions: Conceptualization, S.I. and C.S.; methodology, S.I., J.S., F.M. and C.S.; software, S.I.; formal analysis, S.I. and C.S.; writing—original draft preparation, S.I.; writing—review and editing, S.I., J.S., F.M. and C.S.; visualization, S.I.; supervision, C.S.; funding acquisition, C.S. All authors have read and agreed to the published version of the manuscript.

Funding: This research received no external funding.

Institutional Review Board Statement: Not applicable.

Informed Consent Statement: Not applicable.

Data Availability Statement: Data and code to reproduce results of the paper are available at https://github.com/imansultan (accessed on 13 October 2022). Publicly available datasets were analyzed in this study. These data can be found here: https://github.com/twbattaglia/MicrobeDS (accessed on 13 October 2022) and https://github.com/SchlossLab/Baxter_glne007Modeling_GenomeMed_2015 (accessed on 13 October 2022).

Acknowledgments: We thank Andrea Tonk and Meike Nauta as their efforts in managing administrative tasks proved to be very helpful. We also thank Osman Koras for providing his opinion on the methodology during our internal discussions. We acknowledge support by the Open Access Publication Fund of the University of Duisburg-Essen.

Conflicts of Interest: The authors declare no conflict of interest.

Abbreviations

The following abbreviations are used in this manuscript:

AP	Average Precision
AUROC	Area Under Receiver Operating Characteristic
MCC	Matthews's Correlation Coefficient
SGD_LL	Stochastic Gradient Descent classifier with Logistic Loss
SGD_HL	Stochastic Gradient Descent classifier with modified Huber Loss
KNN	K-nearest Neighbors Classifier
MLP	Multi-layer Perceptron
QDA	Quadratic Discriminant Analysis
RF	Random Forest
HGBC	Histogram-based Gradient Boosting Classification

Appendix A

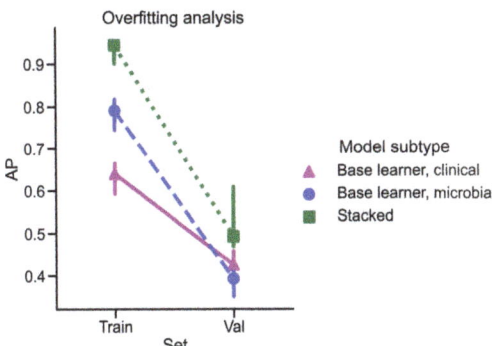

Figure A1. **Overfitting analysis for inflammatory bowel disease dataset comparing stacked model's and base learners' performance separated by view during cross-validation.** Point values refer to median AP values and bars refer to estimated confidence intervals. Values for base learners trained on microbial view are aggregated together without distinction with regard to an individual base learner.

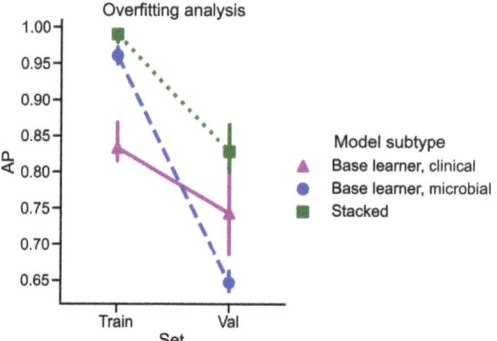

Figure A2. Overfitting analysis for colorectal cancer dataset comparing stacked model's and base learners' performance separated by view during cross-validation. Point values refer to median AP values and bars refer to estimated confidence intervals. Values for base learners trained on microbial view are aggregated together without distinction with regard to an individual base learner.

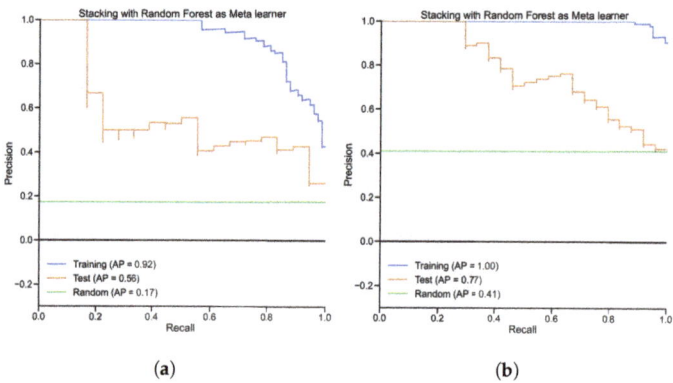

Figure A3. Training and Test set PR curves for stacked model with Random Forest as a meta learner. (**a**) Inflammatory bowel disease dataset; (**b**) Colorectal cancer dataset.

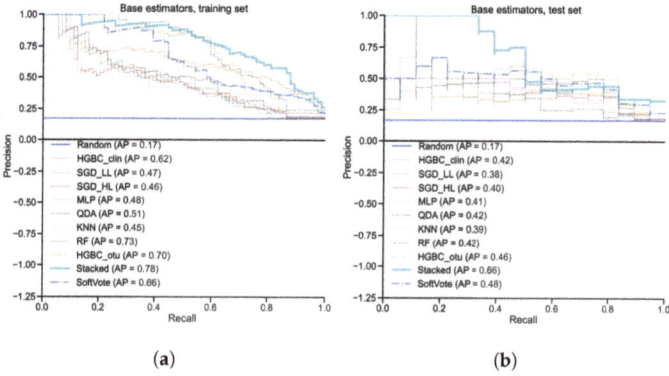

Figure A4. PR curves for stacked model applied on inflammatory bowel disease dataset with strict pre-filtering of microbial features. (**a**) Training set; (**b**) Test set.

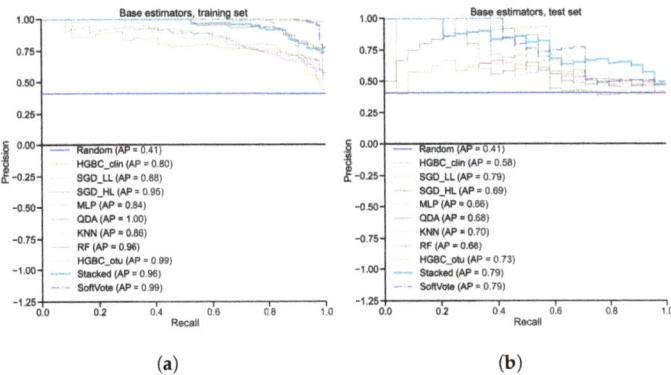

Figure A5. PR curves for stacked model applied on colorectal cancer dataset with strict pre-filtering of microbial features. (**a**) Training set; (**b**) Test set.

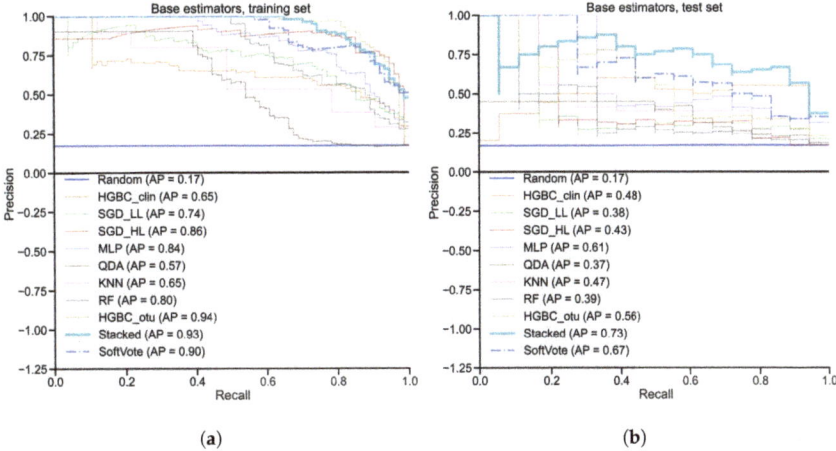

Figure A6. PR curves for stacked model applied on inflammatory bowel disease dataset with additional clinical features. (**a**) Training set; (**b**) Test set.

Table A1. List of features removed from the inflammatory bowel disease clinical view dataset.

Feature name	Type	Reason
diagnosis	Categorical	Training label
external_id	Categorical	Irrelevant
run_prefix	Categorical	Irrelevant
body_site	Categorical	Training label leakage
diseasesubtype	Categorical	Explicit training label leakage
gastrointest_disord	Categorical	Explicit training label leakage
host_subject_id	Categorical	Irrelevant
disease_stat	Categorical	Implicit training label leakage
disease_extent	Categorical	Implicit training label leakage
ileal_invovlement	Categorical	Implicit training label leakage
gastric_involvement	Categorical	Implicit training label leakage
antibiotics	Categorical	Irrelevant
steroids	Categorical	Irrelevant
collection	Categorical	Irrelevant
biologics	Categorical	Irrelevant
birthdate	Categorical	Irrelevant
body_habitat	Categorical	Implicit training label leakage
body_product	Categorical	Irrelevant
disease_duration	Numerical	Irrelevant
immunosup	Categorical	Irrelevant
mesalamine	Categorical	Irrelevant
sample_type	Categorical	Irrelevant
smoking	Categorical	Irrelevant

Table A2. List of features included in the inflammatory bowel disease clinical view dataset.

Feature Name	Type	Description
Age	Numerical	Age in years
b_cat	Categorical	Montreal classification of inflammatory bowel disease
biopsy_location	Categorical	Location of biopsy
inflammationstatus	Categorical	Inflammation status
perianal	Categorical	Extension to anal area
race	Categorical	Race
sex	Categorical	Biological gender

Table A3. List of features removed from the colorectal cancer clinical view dataset.

Feature Name	Type	Reason
Dx_Bin	Categorical	Training label
Site	Categorical	Irrelevant
Location	Categorical	Irrelevant
Ethnic	Categorical	Irrelevant
fit_result	Numerical	Training label leakage
Hx_Prev	Categorical	Training label leakage
Hx_Fam_CRC	Categorical	Training label leakage
Hx_of_Polyps	Categorical	Training label leakage
stage	Categorical	Training label leakage
Gender	Categorical	Encoded as "Sex"
White	Categorical	Encoded as "Ethnicity"
Native	Categorical	Encoded as "Ethnicity"
Black	Categorical	Encoded as "Ethnicity"
Pacific	Categorical	Encoded as "Ethnicity"
Asian	Categorical	Encoded as "Ethnicity"
Other	Categorical	Encoded as "Ethnicity"
Weight	Numerical	Encoded as "BMI"
Height	Numerical	Encoded as "BMI"

Table A4. List of features included in the colorectal cancer clinical view dataset.

Feature name	Type	Description
BMI	Numerical	Body Mass Index
Age	Numerical	Age in years
Smoke	Categorical	Smoking
Diabetic	Categorical	Diabetes Melitus
NSAID	Categorical	Anti-inflammatory medication
Diabetes_Med	Categorical	Anti-diabetes medication
Abx	Categorical	Antibiotic medication
Ethnicity	Categorical	Race
Sex	Categorical	Biological gender

References

1. Cho, I.; Blaser, M.J. The human microbiome: At the interface of health and disease. *Nat. Rev. Genet.* **2012**, *13*, 260–270. [CrossRef]
2. Lynch, S.V.; Pedersen, O. The human intestinal microbiome in health and disease. *N. Engl. J. Med.* **2016**, *375*, 2369–2379. [CrossRef]
3. Lv, G.; Cheng, N.; Wang, H. The gut microbiota, tumorigenesis, and liver diseases. *Engineering* **2017**, *3*, 110–114. [CrossRef]
4. Forbes, J.D.; Chen, C.Y.; Knox, N.C.; Marrie, R.A.; El-Gabalawy, H.; de Kievit, T.; Alfa, M.; Bernstein, C.N.; Van Domselaar, G. A comparative study of the gut microbiota in immune-mediated inflammatory diseases—Does a common dysbiosis exist? *Microbiome* **2018**, *6*, 1–15. [CrossRef]
5. Aldars-García, L.; Chaparro, M.; Gisbert, J.P. Systematic review: The gut microbiome and its potential clinical application in inflammatory bowel disease. *Microorganisms* **2021**, *9*, 977. [CrossRef]
6. Alexander, K.L.; Zhao, Q.; Reif, M.; Rosenberg, A.F.; Mannon, P.J.; Duck, L.W.; Elson, C.O. Human microbiota flagellins drive adaptive immune responses in Crohn's disease. *Gastroenterology* **2021**, *161*, 522–535. [CrossRef]
7. Ghannam, R.B.; Techtmann, S.M. Machine learning applications in microbial ecology, human microbiome studies, and environmental monitoring. *Comput. Struct. Biotechnol. J.* **2021**, *19*, 1092–1107. [CrossRef]
8. Sudhakar, P.; Machiels, K.; Verstockt, B.; Korcsmaros, T.; Vermeire, S. Computational biology and machine learning approaches to understand mechanistic microbiome-host interactions. *Front. Microbiol.* **2021**, *12*, 618856. [CrossRef]
9. Douglas, G.M.; Hansen, R.; Jones, C.; Dunn, K.A.; Comeau, A.M.; Bielawski, J.P.; Tayler, R.; El-Omar, E.M.; Russell, R.K.; Hold, G.L.; et al. Multi-omics differentially classify disease state and treatment outcome in pediatric Crohn's disease. *Microbiome* **2018**, *6*, 1–12. [CrossRef] [PubMed]
10. Knight, R.; Vrbanac, A.; Taylor, B.C.; Aksenov, A.; Callewaert, C.; Debelius, J.; Gonzalez, A.; Kosciolek, T.; McCall, L.I.; McDonald, D.; et al. Best practices for analysing microbiomes. *Nat. Rev. Microbiol.* **2018**, *16*, 410–422. [CrossRef] [PubMed]
11. Heshiki, Y.; Vazquez-Uribe, R.; Li, J.; Ni, Y.; Quainoo, S.; Imamovic, L.; Li, J.; Sørensen, M.; Chow, B.K.; Weiss, G.J.; et al. Predictable modulation of cancer treatment outcomes by the gut microbiota. *Microbiome* **2020**, *8*, 1–14. [CrossRef]
12. Vilas-Boas, F.; Ribeiro, T.; Afonso, J.; Cardoso, H.; Lopes, S.; Moutinho-Ribeiro, P.; Ferreira, J.; Mascarenhas-Saraiva, M.; Macedo, G. Deep Learning for Automatic Differentiation of Mucinous versus Non-Mucinous Pancreatic Cystic Lesions: A Pilot Study. *Diagnostics* **2022**, *12*, 2041. [CrossRef]
13. Mascarenhas, M.; Afonso, J.; Ribeiro, T.; Cardoso, H.; Andrade, P.; Ferreira, J.P.; Saraiva, M.M.; Macedo, G. Performance of a deep learning system for automatic diagnosis of protruding lesions in colon capsule endoscopy. *Diagnostics* **2022**, *12*, 1445. [CrossRef]
14. Nogueira-Rodríguez, A.; Reboiro-Jato, M.; Glez-Peña, D.; López-Fernández, H. Performance of Convolutional Neural Networks for Polyp Localization on Public Colonoscopy Image Datasets. *Diagnostics* **2022**, *12*, 898. [CrossRef]
15. Wolpert, D.H.; Macready, W.G. No free lunch theorems for optimization. *IEEE Trans. Evol. Comput.* **1997**, *1*, 67–82. [CrossRef]
16. Pasolli, E.; Truong, D.T.; Malik, F.; Waldron, L.; Segata, N. Machine learning meta-analysis of large metagenomic datasets: Tools and biological insights. *PLoS Comput. Biol.* **2016**, *12*, e1004977. [CrossRef]
17. Topçuoğlu, B.D.; Lesniak, N.A.; Ruffin IV, M.T.; Wiens, J.; Schloss, P.D. A framework for effective application of machine learning to microbiome-based classification problems. *MBio* **2020**, *11*, e00434-20. [CrossRef]
18. Bourel, M.; Segura, A. Multiclass classification methods in ecology. *Ecol. Indic.* **2018**, *85*, 1012–1021. [CrossRef]
19. Statnikov, A.; Henaff, M.; Narendra, V.; Konganti, K.; Li, Z.; Yang, L.; Pei, Z.; Blaser, M.J.; Aliferis, C.F.; Alekseyenko, A.V. A comprehensive evaluation of multicategory classification methods for microbiomic data. *Microbiome* **2013**, *1*, 1–12. [CrossRef]
20. Caruana, R.; Lou, Y.; Gehrke, J.; Koch, P.; Sturm, M.; Elhadad, N. Intelligible models for healthcare: Predicting pneumonia risk and hospital 30-day readmission. In Proceedings of the 21th ACM SIGKDD International Conference on Knowledge Discovery and Data Mining, Sydney, Australia, 10–13 August 2015; pp. 1721–1730.
21. Nauta, M.; Walsh, R.; Dubowski, A.; Seifert, C. Uncovering and correcting shortcut learning in machine learning models for skin cancer diagnosis. *Diagnostics* **2021**, *12*, 40. [CrossRef]
22. Chen, T.; Guestrin, C. Xgboost: A scalable tree boosting system. In Proceedings of the 22nd ACM SIGKDD International Conference on Knowledge Discovery and Data Mining, San Francisco, CA, USA, 13–17 August 2016; pp. 785–794.

23. Breiman, L. Random forests. *Mach. Learn.* **2001**, *45*, 5–32. [CrossRef]
24. Lou, Y.; Caruana, R.; Gehrke, J.; Hooker, G. Accurate intelligible models with pairwise interactions. In Proceedings of the 19th ACM SIGKDD international conference on Knowledge Discovery and Data Mining, Chicago, IL, USA, 11–14 August 2013; pp. 623–631.
25. Wolpert, D.H. Stacked generalization. *Neural Netw.* **1992**, *5*, 241–259. [CrossRef]
26. Džeroski, S.; Ženko, B. Is combining classifiers with stacking better than selecting the best one? *Mach. Learn.* **2004**, *54*, 255–273. [CrossRef]
27. Sesmero, M.P.; Ledezma, A.I.; Sanchis, A. Generating ensembles of heterogeneous classifiers using stacked generalization. *WIley Interdiscip. Rev. Data Min. Knowl. Discov.* **2015**, *5*, 21–34. [CrossRef]
28. Chen, Y.; Wang, H.; Lu, W.; Wu, T.; Yuan, W.; Zhu, J.; Lee, Y.K.; Zhao, J.; Zhang, H.; Chen, W. Human gut microbiome aging clocks based on taxonomic and functional signatures through multi-view learning. *Gut Microbes* **2022**, *14*, 2025016. [CrossRef]
29. Gevers, D.; Kugathasan, S.; Knights, D.; Kostic, A.D.; Knight, R.; Xavier, R J. A microbiome foundation for the study of Crohn's disease. *Cell Host Microbe* **2017**, *21*, 301–304. [CrossRef]
30. Gevers, D.; Kugathasan, S.; Denson, L.A.; Vázquez-Baeza, Y.; Van Treuren, W.; Ren, B.; Schwager, E.; Knights, D.; Song, S.J.; Yassour, M.; et al. The treatment-naive microbiome in new-onset Crohn's disease. *Cell Host Microbe* **2014**, *15*, 382–392. [CrossRef]
31. Baxter, N.T.; Ruffin, M.T.; Rogers, M.A.; Schloss, P.D. Microbiota-based model improves the sensitivity of fecal immunochemical test for detecting colonic lesions. *Genome Med.* **2016**, *8*, 1–10. [CrossRef]
32. Battaglia, T. A Repository for Large-Scale Microbiome Datasets. 2022. Available online: https://github.com/twbattaglia/MicrobeDS (accessed on 13 October 2022)
33. The Laboratory of Pat Schloss at the University of Michigan. 2022. Available online: https://github.com/SchlossLab/Baxter_glne007Modeling_GenomeMed_2015 (accessed on 13 October 2022)
34. Yeo, I.K.; Johnson, R.A. A new family of power transformations to improve normality or symmetry. *Biometrika* **2000**, *87*, 954–959. [CrossRef]
35. Pedregosa, F.; Varoquaux, G.; Gramfort, A.; Michel, V.; Thirion, B.; Grisel, O.; Blondel, M.; Prettenhofer, P.; Weiss, R.; Dubourg, V.; et al. Scikit-learn: Machine Learning in Python. *J. Mach. Learn. Res.* **2011**, *12*, 2825–2830.
36. Branco, P.; Torgo, L.; Ribeiro, R.P. A survey of predictive modeling on imbalanced domains. *ACM Comput. Surv. Csur* **2016**, *49*, 1–50. [CrossRef]
37. Ozenne, B.; Subtil, F.; Maucort-Boulch, D. The precision–recall curve overcame the optimism of the receiver operating characteristic curve in rare diseases. *J. Clin. Epidemiol.* **2015**, *68*, 855–859. [CrossRef] [PubMed]
38. Su, W.; Yuan, Y.; Zhu, M. A relationship between the average precision and the area under the ROC curve. In Proceedings of the 2015 International Conference on The Theory of Information Retrieval, Northampton, MA, USA, 27–30 September 2015; pp. 349–352.
39. Chicco, D.; Jurman, G. The advantages of the Matthews correlation coefficient (MCC) over F1 score and accuracy in binary classification evaluation. *BMC Genom.* **2020**, *21*, 1–13. [CrossRef] [PubMed]
40. Zadrozny, B.; Langford, J.; Abe, N. Cost-sensitive learning by cost-proportionate example weighting. In Proceedings of the Third IEEE International Conference on Data Mining, Melbourne, FL, USA, 22 November 2003; pp. 435–442.
41. Chang, C.C.; Huang, T.H.; Shueng, P.W.; Chen, S.H.; Chen, C.C.; Lu, C.J.; Tseng, Y.J. Developing a Stacked Ensemble-Based Classification Scheme to Predict Second Primary Cancers in Head and Neck Cancer Survivors. *Int. J. Environ. Res. Public Health* **2021**, *18*, 12499. [CrossRef]
42. Ting, K.M.; Witten, I.H. Issues in stacked generalization. *J. Artif. Intell. Res.* **1999**, *10*, 271–289. [CrossRef]
43. Ghaemi, M.S.; DiGiulio, D.B.; Contrepois, K.; Callahan, B.; Ngo, T.T.; Lee-McMullen, B.; Lehallier, B.; Robaczewska, A.; Mcilwain, D.; Rosenberg-Hasson, Y.; et al. Multiomics modeling of the immunome, transcriptome, microbiome, proteome and metabolome adaptations during human pregnancy. *Bioinformatics* **2019**, *35*, 95–103. [CrossRef]
44. Klang, E.; Freeman, R.; Levin, M.A.; Soffer, S.; Barash, Y.; Lahat, A. Machine Learning Model for Outcome Prediction of Patients Suffering from Acute Diverticulitis Arriving at the Emergency Department—A Proof of Concept Study. *Diagnostics* **2021**, *11*, 2102. [CrossRef]
45. Baumgart, D.C. The diagnosis and treatment of Crohn's disease and ulcerative colitis. *Dtsch. ÄRzteblatt Int.* **2009**, *106*, 123. [CrossRef]
46. Sartor, R.B. Mechanisms of disease: Pathogenesis of Crohn's disease and ulcerative colitis. *Nat. Clin. Pract. Gastroenterol. Hepatol.* **2006**, *3*, 390–407. [CrossRef]
47. Silva, M.; Pratas, D.; Pinho, A.J. AC2: An Efficient Protein Sequence Compression Tool Using Artificial Neural Networks and Cache-Hash Models. *Entropy* **2021**, *23*, 530. [CrossRef]
48. Janitza, S.; Hornung, R. On the overestimation of random forest's out-of-bag error. *PloS ONE* **2018**, *13*, e0201904. [CrossRef]
49. Guyon, I.; Elisseeff, A. An introduction to variable and feature selection. *J. Mach. Learn. Res.* **2003**, *3*, 1157–1182.
50. Benjamini, Y.; Hochberg, Y. Controlling the false discovery rate: A practical and powerful approach to multiple testing. *J. R. Stat. Soc. Ser. Methodol.* **1995**, *57*, 289–300. [CrossRef]
51. Benjamini, Y.; Yekutieli, D. The control of the false discovery rate in multiple testing under dependency. *Ann. Stat.* **2001**, *29*, 1165–1188. [CrossRef]

52. Zhu, Q.; Li, B.; He, T.; Li, G.; Jiang, X. Robust biomarker discovery for microbiome-wide association studies. *Methods* **2020**, *173*, 44–51. [CrossRef] [PubMed]
53. Bakir-Gungor, B.; Hacılar, H.; Jabeer, A.; Nalbantoglu, O.U.; Aran, O.; Yousef, M. Inflammatory bowel disease biomarkers of human gut microbiota selected via different feature selection methods. *PeerJ* **2022**, *10*, e13205. [CrossRef] [PubMed]
54. Sharma, D.; Paterson, A.D.; Xu, W. TaxoNN: Ensemble of neural networks on stratified microbiome data for disease prediction. *Bioinformatics* **2020**, *36*, 4544–4550. [CrossRef]
55. Mulenga, M.; Kareem, S.A.; Sabri, A.Q.M.; Seera, M. Stacking and chaining of normalization methods in deep learning-based classification of colorectal cancer using gut microbiome data. *IEEE Access* **2021**, *9*, 97296–97319. [CrossRef]

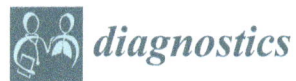 *diagnostics*

Review

Explainable Artificial Intelligence in the Early Diagnosis of Gastrointestinal Disease

Kwang-Sig Lee [1,*] and Eun Sun Kim [2,*]

1. AI Center, Korea University Anam Hospital, Seoul 02841, Korea
2. Department of Gastroenterology, Korea University Anam Hospital, Seoul 02841, Korea
* Correspondence: ecophy@hanmail.net (K.-S.L.); silverkes@naver.com (E.S.K.)

Abstract: This study reviews the recent progress of explainable artificial intelligence for the early diagnosis of gastrointestinal disease (GID). The source of data was eight original studies in PubMed. The search terms were "gastrointestinal" (title) together with "random forest" or "explainable artificial intelligence" (abstract). The eligibility criteria were the dependent variable of GID or a strongly associated disease, the intervention(s) of artificial intelligence, the outcome(s) of accuracy and/or the area under the receiver operating characteristic curve (AUC), the outcome(s) of variable importance and/or the Shapley additive explanations (SHAP), a publication year of 2020 or later, and the publication language of English. The ranges of performance measures were reported to be 0.70–0.98 for accuracy, 0.04–0.25 for sensitivity, and 0.54–0.94 for the AUC. The following factors were discovered to be top-10 predictors of gastrointestinal bleeding in the intensive care unit: mean arterial pressure (max), bicarbonate (min), creatinine (max), PMN, heart rate (mean), Glasgow Coma Scale, age, respiratory rate (mean), prothrombin time (max) and aminotransferase aspartate (max). In a similar vein, the following variables were found to be top-10 predictors for the intake of almond, avocado, broccoli, walnut, whole-grain barley, and/or whole-grain oat: *Roseburia* undefined, *Lachnospira* spp., *Oscillibacter* undefined, *Subdoligranulum* spp., *Streptococcus salivarius* subsp. *thermophiles*, *Parabacteroides distasonis*, *Roseburia* spp., *Anaerostipes* spp., Lachnospiraceae *ND3007* group undefined, and *Ruminiclostridium* spp. Explainable artificial intelligence provides an effective, non-invasive decision support system for the early diagnosis of GID.

Keywords: gastrointestinal disease; early diagnosis; artificial intelligence

Citation: Lee, K.-S.; Kim, E.S. Explainable Artificial Intelligence in the Early Diagnosis of Gastrointestinal Disease. *Diagnostics* 2022, 12, 2740. https://doi.org/10.3390/diagnostics12112740

Academic Editor: Dechang Chen

Received: 3 October 2022
Accepted: 6 November 2022
Published: 9 November 2022

Publisher's Note: MDPI stays neutral with regard to jurisdictional claims in published maps and institutional affiliations.

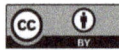

Copyright: © 2022 by the authors. Licensee MDPI, Basel, Switzerland. This article is an open access article distributed under the terms and conditions of the Creative Commons Attribution (CC BY) license (https://creativecommons.org/licenses/by/4.0/).

1. Introduction

1.1. Gastrointestinal Disease

Gastrointestinal disease (GID) is a major cause of disease burden in the world [1–6]. GID is defined as the disease of the gastrointestinal tract, e.g., the esophagus, liver, stomach, small and large intestines, gallbladder, and pancreas. Common GIDs are gastroesophageal reflux disease (GERD), cancer, irritable bowel syndrome, lactose intolerance, and hiatal hernia. Their common symptoms are bleeding, bloating, constipation, diarrhea, heartburn, nausea, pain, and vomiting [1]. GID is reported to contribute to 8 million deaths across the globe every year [2] and USD 120 billion of total expenditure in the United States as of 2018 [3]. Likewise, its disability-adjusted life years (1730 per 100,000, 5.9%) ranked 8th among 21 disease groups in Korea for the year 2015 [4], whereas its medical cost amounted to USD 4 billion or 13% of all medical costs in the country for the year 2007 [5]. GID has a variety of causes including: (1) bad health behavior, e.g., low-fiber diet, insufficient exercise, disrupted routine, high-dairy diet, excessive stress; (2) unhealthy bowel habits; (3) excessive anti-diarrheal/antacid medication; and (4) pregnancy [6].

There are two types of GID, functional and structural. In the case of functional GID, the gastrointestinal tract looks normal but reveals motility problems in medical examination. Its common examples include bloating, constipation, diarrhea, gas, GERD, irritable bowel syndrome, nausea, and poisoning. In the case of structural GID, the gastrointestinal tract has the issues of an abnormal outlook and motility at the same time. Colorectal polyps, colorectal cancers, diverticular disease, hemorrhoids, inflammatory bowel disease, stenosis, and strictures belong to the category of structural GID. GID can be prevented based on sound health behaviors, healthy bowel habits, and regular health screening such as regular colonoscopies from the age of 45. For instance, a majority of colorectal cancers develop when colorectal polyps, non-cancerous growths of colorectal tissues, begin to invade their surrounding tissues. Most of these colorectal polyps can be removed with no pain based on colonoscopy, whereas more advanced colorectal cancers require more complex surgical operations [1,6].

1.2. Explainable Artificial Intelligence

Recently, the notions of artificial intelligence and machine learning have garnered global attention. The definition of artificial intelligence is "the capability of a machine to imitate intelligent human behavior" (the Merriam–Webster dictionary). As a division of artificial intelligence, machine learning is denoted as "extracting knowledge from large amounts of data" [7]. The artificial/deep neural network, the decision tree, the naïve Bayesian predictor, the random forest, and the support vector machine are popular machine learning approaches (See [7] for a detailed explanation of these approaches). Specifically, a random forest is a group of decision trees which make majority votes on the dependent variable ("bootstrap aggregation"). Let us take a random forest with 1000 decision trees as an example. Let us assume that the original data include 10,000 participants. Then, the training and test of this random forest takes two steps. First, new data with 10,000 participants are created based on random sampling with the replacement, and a decision tree is created based on these new data. Here, some participants in the original data would be excluded from the new data, and these leftovers are called out-of-bag data. This process is repeated 1000 times, i.e., 1000 new data are created, 1000 decision trees are created, and 1000 out-of-bag data are created. Second, the 1000 decision trees make predictions on the dependent variable of every participant in the out-of-bag data, their majority vote is taken as their final prediction on this participant, and the out-of-bag error is calculated as the proportion of wrong votes on all participants in the out-of-bag data [7]. An artificial neural network is a group of neurons (information units) that are networked based on weights. It normally has one input layer, one, two, or three intermediate layers, and one output layer. A deep neural network is an artificial neural network with a large number of intermediate layers, e.g., 5, 10, or even 1000 [8].

Conventional research covers a limited range of predictors for the early diagnosis of disease, using logistic regression with an unrealistic assumption of *ceteris paribus*, i.e., "all the other variables staying constant". For this reason, emerging literature employs artificial intelligence for the early diagnosis of disease, e.g., arrhythmia [8], birth outcome [9,10], cancer [11,12], comorbidity [13], depression [14], liver transplantation [15], menopause [16,17], and temporomandibular disease [18,19]. It is free from unrealistic assumptions of "all the other variables staying constant". It delivers the importance values and rankings of predictors for the early diagnosis of the dependent variable. Moreover, the notion of explainable artificial intelligence is enjoying immense popularity now. Explainable artificial intelligence can be defined as "artificial intelligence to identify major predictors of the dependent variable", and there are four approaches of explainable artificial intelligence at this point, i.e., random forest impurity importance, random forest permutation importance [20,21], machine learning accuracy importance, and Shapley additive explanations (SHAP) [15,22–32]. Random forest impurity importance calculates the node impurity decrease from the creation of a branch on a certain predictor. It is a sum over all trees in a random forest with the range of 0 and the number of all trees. Random forest permutation importance measures the overall accuracy decrease from the permutation of data on the predictor. It is an average over all trees in the random forest with a value of 0 to 1 [20,21]. Machine learning accuracy importance (an extension of random forest permutation importance) calculates the accuracy decrease from the exclusion of data on the predictor. The SHAP value of a predictor for a participant measures the difference between what machine learning predicts for the probability of GID with and without the predictor [15,22–32]. For example, let us assume in a hypothetical figure (Figure 1) that the SHAP values of diabetes (x033) for GERD have the range of (−0.05, 0.30). Here, some participants have SHAP values as low as −0.05, and other participants have SHAP values as high as 0.30. The inclusion of a predictor (diabetes) into machine learning will decrease or increase the probability of the dependent variable (GERD) by the range of −0.05 and 0.30. In other words, there exists a positive association between diabetes and GERD in general. Random forest impurity importance and random forest permutation importance had been the only explainable artificial intelligence methods before machine learning accuracy importance, and the SHAP was introduced as their extension or alternative very recently.

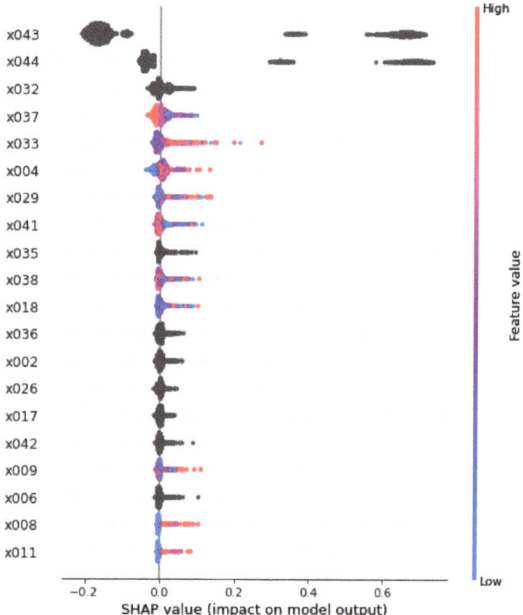

Figure 1. SHAP summary plot. The SHAP value of a predictor for a participant measures the difference between what machine learning predicts for the probability of GERD with and without the predictor. For example, in this hypothetical figure, the SHAP values of diabetes (x033) for GERD have the range of (−0.05, 0.30). Here, some participants have SHAP values as low as −0.05, and other participants have SHAP values as high as 0.30. The inclusion of a predictor (diabetes) into machine learning will decrease or increase the probability of the dependent variable (GERD) by the range of −0.05 and 0.30. In other words, there exists a positive association between diabetes and GERD in general.

In practice, experts in artificial intelligence use random forest impurity importance, random forest permutation importance, or machine learning accuracy importance to derive the rankings and values of all predictors for the prediction of the dependent variable. Then, they employ the SHAP plots to evaluate the directions of associations between the predictors and the dependent variable. Linear or logistic regression used to play this role before the SHAP approach took it over. This is because the SHAP approach has a notable strength compared to linear or logistic regression: the former considers all realistic scenarios, unlike the latter. Let us assume that there are three predictors of GERD, i.e., age, diabetes, and (calcium channel blocker) medication. As defined above, the SHAP value of diabetes for GERD for a particular participant is the difference between what machine learning predicts for the probability of GERD with and without diabetes for the participant. Here, the SHAP value for the participant is the average of the following four scenarios for the participant: (1) age excluded, medication excluded; (2) age included, medication excluded; (3) age excluded, medication included; and (4) age included, medication included. In other words, the SHAP value combines the results of all possible sub-group analyses, which are ignored in linear or logistic regression with an unrealistic assumption of *ceteris paribus*, i.e., "all the other variables staying constant". In this context, the purpose of this study is to review the recent progress of explainable artificial intelligence for the early diagnosis of GID.

2. Methods

Figure 2 shows the flow diagram of this study. Eight original studies were selected for review out of twenty-four original studies in PubMed with the search terms "gastrointestinal" (title) together with "random forest" or "explainable artificial intelligence" (abstract). The inclusion criteria of this review were: (1) the intervention(s) of the artificial/deep neural network, the decision tree, the naïve Bayesian predictor, the random forest, and/or the support vector machine; (2) the outcome(s) of accuracy and/or the area under the receiver operating characteristic curve for the early diagnosis of GID or a strongly associated disease; (3) the outcome(s) of variable importance and/or the SHAP for the early diagnosis of GID or a strongly associated disease; (4) a publication year of 2020 or later; and (5) the publication language of English. The following summary measures were adopted: artificial intelligence methods, sample size, data type, performance measures, and important predictors. Accuracy denotes the proportion of correct predictions over all observations. The area under the receiver operating characteristic curve (AUC) represents the area under the plot of the true positive rate (sensitivity) against the false positive rate (1-specificity) at various threshold settings.

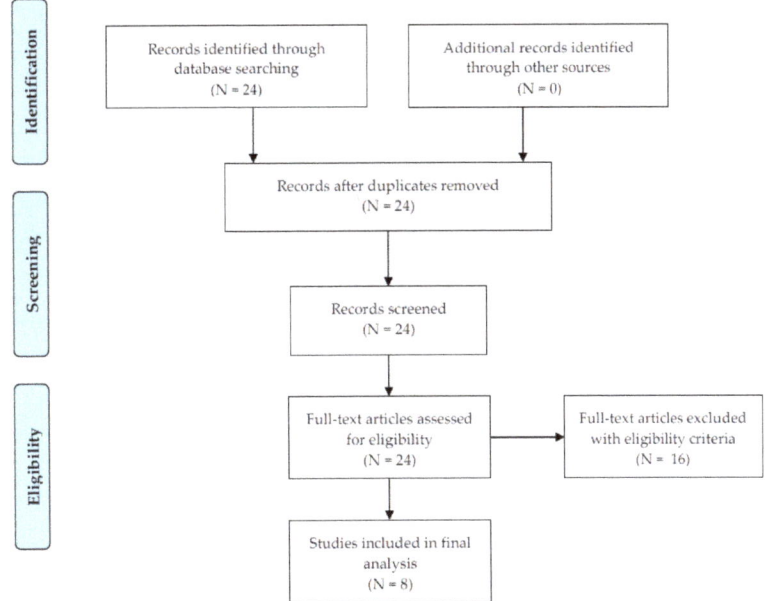

Figure 2. Flow diagram.

3. Results

3.1. Summary

The summary of the review for the eight original studies [33–40] is presented in Table 1. The table includes five summary measures such as artificial intelligence methods, sample size, data type, performance measures, and important predictors (independent variables). The ranges of performance measures were reported to be 0.70–0.98 for accuracy, 0.04–0.25 for sensitivity, and 0.54–0.94 for the AUC. The following determinants were discovered to be top-10 predictors of gastrointestinal bleeding in the intensive care unit: mean arterial pressure (max), bicarbonate (min), creatinine (max), PMN, heart rate (mean), Glasgow Coma Scale, age, respiratory rate (mean), prothrombin time (max), and aminotransferase aspartate (max). In a similar vein, the following factors were found to be top-10 predictors for the intake of almond, avocado, broccoli, walnut, whole-grain barley, and/or whole-grain oat: *Roseburia* undefined, *Lachnospira* spp., *Oscillibacter* undefined, *Subdoligranulum* spp., *Streptococcus salivarius* subsp. *thermophiles*, *Parabacteroides distasonis*, *Roseburia* spp., *Anaerostipes* spp., *Lachnospiraceae ND3007* group undefined, and *Ruminiclostridium* spp. The most important predictors for the prediction of early intestinal resection with Crohn's disease were clinical variables of age and disease behavior as well as the single nucleotide polymorphisms of rs28785174, rs60532570, rs13056955, and rs7660164. However, artificial intelligence is a data-driven approach, and more research is needed for more general conclusions.

Table 1. Summary of review.

ID	Method	Sample Size	Data Type	Performance	Important Predictor
[33]	ANN DT LR * NB RF * SVM	731	Numeric	Accuracy 0.79–0.87 AUC 0.54–0.76	RFVI for the prediction of preterm birth, which has a strong association with GERD: Age, education, upper gastrointestinal tract symptom, Helicobacter pylori, region
[34]	APACHE XGB *	5691	Numeric	Sensitivity 1.00 Specificity 0.04–0.27 AUC 0.80–0.85	SHAP for the prediction of mortality from gastrointestinal bleeding in the intensive care unit: mean arterial pressure (max), bicarbonate (min), creatinine (max), PMN, heart rate (mean), Glasgow Coma Scale, age, respiratory rate (mean), prothrombin time (max), aminotransferase aspartate (max), albumin (min), oxygen saturation (mean), white blood cell, AlkPhos (max), platelet (min), lactate (max), intubation, bilirubin (max), international normalized ratio (max), vasopressor, glucose (max), blood urea nitrogen (max), PTT (max), hemoglobin (min), potassium
[35]	RF *	340	Genomic	Accuracy 0.70 AUC 0.92	RFVI for the prediction of food intake (almond, avocado, broccoli, walnut, whole-grain barley, whole-grain oat): *Roseburia* undefined, *Lachnospira* spp., *Oscillibacter* undefined, *Subdoligranulum* spp., *Streptococcus salivarius* subsp. *thermophiles*, *Parabacteroides distasonis*, *Roseburia* spp., *Anaerostipes* spp., *Lachnospiraceae ND3007* group undefined, *Ruminiclostridium* spp.
[36]	CB *	337	Genomic	AUC 0.81–0.84	SHAP for the prediction of early intestinal resection with Crohn's disease: age, disease behavior (clinical predictors), rs28785174, rs60532570, rs13056955, rs7660164 (single nucleotide polymorphisms)
[37]	RF *	71	Radiomic	Accuracy 0.78–0.94	RFVI for the prediction of pneumatosis: dissecting gas in the bowel wall, intramural gas beyond a gas-fluid/fecal level, a circumferential gas pattern

Table 1. Cont.

ID	Method	Sample Size	Data Type	Performance	Important Predictor
[38]	ANN * LR * RF *	405,586	Numeric	Accuracy 0.93–0.98	RFVI for the prediction of preterm birth, which has a strong association with GERD: socioeconomic status, age, region (city)
[39]	RF *	710	Numeric	AUC 0.76–0.80	RFVI for the prediction of COVID-19 hospitalization based on gastrointestinal factors: aspartate transaminase, diabetes mellitus, chronic liver disease, alanine transaminase, diarrhea, age, bloating
[40]	RF *	590	Numeric	AUC 0.68	RFVI for the prediction of gastrointestinal sequelae months after COVID-19 infection: acute diarrhea, antibiotics administration

ANN—Artificial Neural Network, AUC—Area under the Receiver Operating Characteristic Curve, CB—CatBoost, DT—Decision Tree, LR—Logistic Regression, NB—Naïve Bayes, RF—Random Forest, RFVI—Random Forest Variable Importance, SHAP—Shapley Additive Explanations, SVM—Support Vector Machine, XGB—XGBoost, * Method with the best performance.

3.2. Numeric Data

This section summarizes original studies with numeric data regarding explainable artificial intelligence for the early diagnosis of GID or a strongly associated disease. A recent study [33] used single-center data and random forest permutation importance for the prediction of preterm birth, which has a strong association with GERD. Data on 36 demographic, socioeconomic, and clinical determinants came from Anam Hospital in Seoul, Korea, with 731 obstetric patients during January 1995—August 2018. In terms of accuracy, the random forest (0.8681) was similar with the logistic regression (0.8736). Based on random forest permutation importance, the major predictors of preterm birth were age (0.1211), education (0.0332), upper gastrointestinal tract symptom (0.0274), GERD (0.0242), Helicobacter pylori (0.0151), and region (0.0139). Likewise, a follow-up study [38] employed population data and random forest impurity importance to confirm these findings. Retrospective cohort data on 29 demographic, socioeconomic, and clinical determinants came from Korea National Health Insurance Service claims data for all women who were aged 25–40 years and gave birth for the first time as a singleton pregnancy during 2015–2017 (405,586 women). According to random forest impurity importance, the main predictors of preterm birth during 2015–2017 were socioeconomic status in 2014 (240.28), age in 2014 (221.13), GERD for the years 2012 (42.24), 2014 (38.86), 2010 (37.76), 2013 (36.64), 2007 (35.01), and 2009 (34.39), region in 2014 (34.36), and GERD for the year 2006 (31.98). These studies conclude that preterm birth has a stronger association with GERD than it does with periodontitis, and it would be vital to promote active counseling for general GERD symptoms (neglected by pregnant women).

A recent study [34] used multi-center data and the SHAP for the prediction of mortality from gastrointestinal bleeding in the intensive care unit. The source of the data on 34 demographic and clinical factors was 5691 patients of gastrointestinal bleeding registered in the Electronic Intensive Care Unit Collaborative Research Database. The XGBoost outperformed the APACHE IVa for prediction: specificity 0.27 vs. 0.04 at 1.00 sensitivity; AUC 0.85 vs. 0.80. Based on the SHAP, the major predictors of mortality from gastrointestinal bleeding in the intensive care unit were mean arterial pressure (max), bicarbonate (min), creatinine (max), PMN, heart rate (mean), Glasgow Coma Scale, age, respiratory rate (mean), prothrombin time (max), aminotransferase aspartate (max), albumin (min), oxygen saturation (mean), white blood cell, AlkPhos (max), platelet (min), lactate (max), intubation, bilirubin (max), international normalized ratio (max), vasopressor, glucose (max), blood urea nitrogen (max), PTT (max), hemoglobin (min), and potassium. In conclusion, explainable artificial intelligence provides an effective, non-invasive decision support system for the prediction of high-risk gastrointestinal bleeding in the intensive care unit.

Two recent studies [39,40] highlight the effectiveness of explainable artificial intelligence in investigating strong associations of gastrointestinal factors with COVID-19 hospitalization or infection. The first study [39] employed single-center data and random forest permutation importance for the prediction of COVID-19 hospitalization based on gastrointestinal factors. Data on 19 demographic and clinical variables came from the University Hospital in Martin, Slovakia, with 710 participants in the COVID-19 test during February 2021–May 2021. The AUC range of the random forest was (0.76, 0.80). Based on random forest permutation importance, the major predictors of COVID-19 hospitalization were aspartate transaminase (0.1451), diabetes mellitus (0.0248), chronic liver disease (0.0169), alanine transaminase (0.0110), diarrhea (0.0068), age (0.0139), and bloating (0.0011). In a similar vein, the second study [40] utilized single-center data and random forest permutation importance for the prediction of gastrointestinal sequelae months after COVID-19 infection. The source of data on 23 demographic and clinical variables was the University Hospital in Martin, Slovakia, with 590 participants in the COVID-19 test during February 2021–October 2021. The AUC of the random forest was 0.68. According to random forest permutation importance, the main predictors of gastrointestinal sequelae months were acute diarrhea (0.066) and antibiotics administration (0.058).

3.3. Genomic and Radiomic Data

This section summarizes original studies with genomic and radiomic data regarding explainable artificial intelligence for the early diagnosis of GID or a strongly associated disease. A recent study [35] used existing literature and random forest permutation importance for the prediction of intake for almond, avocado, broccoli, walnut, whole-grain barley, and whole-grain oat. The data on 4375 amplicon sequence variants came from five randomized control trials with 340 observations on microbiota composition. The accuracy and AUC of the random forest were 0.70 and 0.92, respectively. Based on random forest permutation importance, the top 10 predictors for the intake of almond, avocado, broccoli, walnut, whole-grain barley, and/or whole-grain oat were *Roseburia* undefined (0.097), *Lachnospira* spp. (0.043), *Oscillibacter* undefined (0.039), *Subdoligranulum* spp. (0.039), *Streptococcus salivarius* subsp. *thermophiles* (0.039), *Parabacteroides distasonis* (0.032), *Roseburia* spp. (0.026), *Anaerostipes* spp. (0.023), Lachnospiraceae ND3007 group undefined (0.022), and *Ruminiclostridium* spp. (0.022).

A recent study [36] employed multi-center data and the SHAP for the prediction of early intestinal resection with Crohn's disease. The source of the data on seven demographic/clinical factors and 102 single nucleotide polymorphisms was the IMPACT Study with 337 Crohn's disease patients during May 2017–May 2020. The AUC range of the CatBoost was (0.81, 0.84). Based on the SHAP, the major predictors of early intestinal resection with Crohn's disease were the clinical variables of age and disease behavior as well as the single nucleotide polymorphisms of rs28785174, rs60532570, rs13056955, and rs7660164. Another study [37] utilized single-center data and random forest permutation importance for the prediction of pneumatosis. The source of data on four radiomic factors was the radiological reports of 71 pneumatosis patients between 2012 and 2019. The accuracy range of the random forest was (0.78, 0.94). According to random forest permutation importance, the main predictors of pneumatosis were dissecting gas in the bowel wall (0.19), intramural gas beyond a gas–fluid/faecal level (0.15), and a circumferential gas pattern (0.12). These studies conclude that explainable artificial intelligence, together with genomic or radiomic data, also provides an effective, non-invasive decision support system for the prediction of GID or a strongly associated disease.

4. Discussion

Previous studies on the early diagnosis of GID based on explainable artificial intelligence had some limitations. Firstly, existing literature was characterized by single-center data with small sample sizes. Using multi-center or population data (e.g., national health insurance claims data) will further the horizon of research in this direction. Secondly, the AUC of some studies (0.68) might not be optimal as a diagnostic test yet. Thirdly, the four approaches of explainable artificial intelligence at this point (i.e., random forest impurity importance, random forest permutation importance, machine learning accuracy importance, and SHAP) can lead to different results in certain circumstances. Random forest impurity importance can vary depending on how variables are categorized, whereas random forest permutation importance is relatively free from this possible variation [21]. This would explain why only one of the eight original studies reviewed here used random forest impurity importance. It can be noted, however, that the random forest has a unique strength of incorporating sequential information and that this strength is much more apparent with impurity importance than with permutation importance. In this context, a comprehensive comparison for the four approaches of explainable artificial intelligence would be a great contribution for this line of research. Fourthly, the eight original studies reviewed above were selected with the search terms "gastrointestinal" (title) together with "random forest" or "explainable artificial intelligence" (abstract). These terms would be quite specific or broad. Employing a greater variety of search terms and comparing their results would make a great contribution to this line of research. Fifthly, this review did not consider other types of explainable artificial intelligence including local interpretable model-agnostic explanations (LIME) [41].

Indeed, some suggestions for this line of research are presented here. Firstly, combining different types of explainable artificial intelligence for different types of GID data would break new ground and bring more profound clinical insights. An increasing number of research endeavors combine image, genetic, and numeric artificial intelligence for disease diagnosis, prognosis, prevention, and management (wide and deep learning). This strand of research involves the extensive employment of multi-input multi-out models with Tensorflow or Keras. For example, one recent study [42] developed a glaucoma prediction system based on convolutional neural networks extracting key image features from multiple video inputs and recurrent neural networks predicting glaucoma outcomes from the trajectory of the key image features over time. In the convolutional neural network, feature detectors slide across input data, and their detections of certain features (their operations of "convolution") predict the status of a cell as normal vs. GID. In the recurrent neural network, the current output is determined, in a "recurrent" pattern, by the current input and the previous hidden state (here, the previous hidden state is the memory of all the past inputs) [7,8]. Little literature is available, and more examination is needed regarding the combination of different types of explainable artificial intelligence for different types of GID data.

Secondly, little research has been conducted and more examination is needed on explainable artificial intelligence for reinforcement learning. Reinforcement learning is a branch of machine learning in which (1) the environment presents a series of rewards, (2) an agent takes a series of actions to maximize the cumulative reward in response, and (3) the environment moves to the next period with given transition probabilities [43]. In fact, it has been reinforcement learning that has brought the notion of artificial intelligence to worldwide popularity since the publication of a seminal article on Alpha-Go in 2016. Two revolutionary ideas behind reinforcement learning were that artificial intelligence (e.g., Alpha-Go) starts like a human player, i.e., takes a series of actions and maximizes the cumulative reward (chance of victory) from the limited information available in limited periods only, and that it moves far beyond the best human player ever based on the sheer power of big data covering all human players to date. In other words, it is reinforcement learning (or temporal difference learning in a professional language) that epitomizes the salient characteristics of artificial intelligence as "being similar with but superior to human intelligence" [43]. Reinforcement learning has gained immense popularity in finance given that it does not require unrealistic assumptions but does register superb performance compared to conventional statistical models [44]. This success has been replicated in healthcare, covering treatment recommendation, diagnosis automation, resource allocation, and other domains of service in chronic disease and critical care alike from both structured data and unstructured information [45]. However, little literature has been available, and more investigation is needed on explainable reinforcement learning. A recent review reports that there have been a few studies on this issue, and these studies have relied on simplified models with easy interpretation but insufficient performance and little consideration of the psychological and social factors behind optimization processes [46].

In summary, this study reviewed the recent progress of explainable artificial intelligence for the early diagnosis of GID. The ranges of performance measures were 0.70–0.98 for accuracy, 0.04–0.25 for sensitivity, and 0.54–0.94 for the AUC. The following determinants were top-10 predictors of gastrointestinal bleeding in the intensive care unit: mean arterial pressure (max), bicarbonate (min), creatinine (max), PMN, heart rate (mean), Glasgow Coma Scale, age, respiratory rate (mean), prothrombin time (max), and aminotransferase aspartate (max). The following factors were top-10 predictors for the intake of almond, avocado, broccoli, walnut, whole-grain barley, and/or whole-grain oat: *Roseburia* undefined, *Lachnospira* spp., *Oscillibacter* undefined, *Subdoligranulum* spp., *Streptococcus salivarius* subsp. *thermophiles*, *Parabacteroides distasonis*, *Roseburia* spp., *Anaerostipes* spp., Lachnospiraceae *ND3007* group undefined, and *Ruminiclostridium* spp. Likewise, most important predictors for the prediction of early intestinal resection with Crohn's disease were the clinical variables of age and disease behavior as well as the single nucleotide polymorphisms of rs28785174, rs60532570, rs13056955, and rs7660164. In conclusion, explainable artificial intelligence provides an effective, non-invasive decision support system for the early diagnosis of GID.

Author Contributions: K.-S.L. and E.S.K. designed the study, collected, analyzed, and interpreted the data, and wrote and reviewed the manuscript. K.-S.L. and E.S.K. approved the final version of the manuscript. All authors have read and agreed to the published version of the manuscript.

Funding: This work was supported by the Korea University College of Medicine grant (K2209721), Korea Health Industry Development Institute grants (No. HI21C156001; HI22C1302 (Korea Health Technology R&D Project)) funded by the Ministry of Health and Welfare of South Korea, and the Technology Innovation Program (20001533) funded by the Ministry of Trade, Industry & Energy of South Korea.

Conflicts of Interest: The authors declare no conflict of interest.

References

1. Johns Hopkins Medicine. Health: Digestive Disorders. Available online: https://www.hopkinsmedicine.org/health/wellness-and-prevention/digestive-disorders (accessed on 28 September 2022).
2. Milivojevic, V.; Milosavljevic, T. Burden of Gastroduodenal Diseases from the Global Perspective. *Curr. Treat. Options Gastroenterol.* **2020**, *18*, 148–157. [CrossRef] [PubMed]
3. Peery, A.F.; Crockett, S.D.; Murphy, C.C.; Jensen, E.T.; Kim, H.P.; Egberg, M.D.; Lund, J.L.; Moon, A.M.; Pate, V.; Barnes, E.L.; et al. Burden and Cost of Gastrointestinal, Liver, and Pancreatic Diseases in the United States: Update 2021. *Gastroenterology* **2022**, *162*, 621–644. [CrossRef] [PubMed]
4. Kim, Y.-E.; Park, H.; Jo, M.-W.; Oh, I.-H.; Go, D.-S.; Jung, J.; Yoon, S.-J. Trends and Patterns of Burden of Disease and Injuries in Korea Using Disability-Adjusted Life Years. *J. Korean Med Sci.* **2019**, *34* (Suppl. S1), e75. [CrossRef] [PubMed]
5. Jung, H.-K.; Jang, B.; Kim, Y.H.; Park, J.; Park, S.Y.; Nam, M.-H.; Choi, M.-G. Health Care Costs of Digestive Diseases in Korea. *Korean J. Gastroenterol.* **2011**, *58*, 323–331. [CrossRef]
6. Cleveland Clinic. Health: Gastrointestinal Diseases. Available online: https://my.clevelandclinic.org/health/articles/7040-gastrointestinal-diseases (accessed on 28 September 2022).
7. Lee, K.-S.; Ahn, K.H. Application of Artificial Intelligence in Early Diagnosis of Spontaneous Preterm Labor and Birth. *Diagnostics* **2020**, *10*, 733. [CrossRef]
8. Lee, K.-S.; Jung, S.; Gil, Y.; Son, H.S. Atrial fibrillation classification based on convolutional neural networks. *BMC Med. Informatics Decis. Mak.* **2019**, *19*, 1–6. [CrossRef]
9. Lee, K.-S.; Korean Society of Ultrasound in Obstetrics and Gynecology Research Group; Kim, H.Y.; Lee, S.J.; Kwon, S.O.; Na, S.; Hwang, H.S.; Park, M.H.; Ahn, K.H. Prediction of newborn's body mass index using nationwide multicenter ultrasound data: A machine-learning study. *BMC Pregnancy Childbirth* **2021**, *21*, 1–10. [CrossRef]
10. Lee, K.-S.; Song, I.-S.; Kim, E.S.; Kim, H.-I.; Ahn, K.H. Association of preterm birth with medications: Machine learning analysis using national health insurance data. *Arch. Gynecol. Obstet.* **2022**, *305*, 1369–1376. [CrossRef]

11. Lee, J.Y.; Lee, K.S.; Seo, B.K.; Cho, K.R.; Woo, O.H.; Song, S.E.; Kim, E.K.; Lee, H.Y.; Kim, J.S.; Cha, J. Radiomic machine learning for pre-dicting prognostic biomarkers and molecular subtypes of breast cancer using tumor heterogeneity and angiogenesis prop-erties on MRI. *Eur. Radiol.* **2022**, *32*, 650–660. [CrossRef]
12. Lee, K.-S.; Jang, J.-Y.; Yu, Y.-D.; Heo, J.S.; Han, H.-S.; Yoon, Y.-S.; Kang, C.M.; Hwang, H.K.; Kang, S. Usefulness of artificial intelligence for predicting recurrence following surgery for pancreatic cancer: Retrospective cohort study. *Int. J. Surg.* **2021**, *93*, 106050. [CrossRef]
13. Lee, K.S.; Park, K.W. Social determinants of association among cerebrovascular disease, hearing loss and cognitive impair-ment in a middle-aged or old population: Recurrent-neural-network analysis of the Korean Longitudinal Study of Aging (2014–2016). *Geriatr. Gerontol. Int.* **2019**, *19*, 711–716. [CrossRef] [PubMed]
14. Lee, K.-S.; Kim, G.; Ham, B.-J. Original Article: Associations of antidepressant medication with its various predictors including particulate matter: Machine learning analysis using national health insurance data. *J. Psychiatr. Res.* **2022**, *147*, 67–78. [CrossRef] [PubMed]
15. Yu, Y.D.; Lee, K.S.; Kim, J.; Ryu, J.H.; Lee, J.G.; Lee, K.W.; Kim, B.W.; Kim, D.S.; Korean Organ Transplantation Registry Study Group. Artificial intelligence for predicting survival following deceased donor liver transplantation: Retrospective multi-center study. *Int. J. Surg.* **2022**, *105*, 106838. [CrossRef] [PubMed]
16. Ryu, K.-J.; Yi, K.W.; Kim, Y.J.; Shin, J.H.; Hur, J.Y.; Kim, T.; Seo, J.B.; Lee, K.-S.; Park, H. Machine Learning Approaches to Identify Factors Associated with Women's Vasomotor Symptoms Using General Hospital Data. *J. Korean Med. Sci.* **2021**, *36*, e122. [CrossRef]
17. Ryu, K.J.; Yi, K.W.; Kim, Y.J.; Shin, J.H.; Hur, J.Y.; Kim, T.; Seo, J.B.; Lee, K.S.; Park, H. Artificial intelligence approaches to the determi-nants of women's vaginal dryness using general hospital data. *J. Obstet. Gynaecol.* **2022**, *42*, 1518–1523. [CrossRef]
18. Lee, K.S.; Kwak, H.J.; Oh, J.M.; Jha, N.; Kim, Y.J.; Kim, W.; Baik, U.B.; Ryu, J.J. Automated detection of TMJ osteoarthritis based on artificial intelligence. *J. Dent. Res.* **2020**, *99*, 1363–1367. [CrossRef]
19. Lee, K.-S.; Jha, N.; Kim, Y.-J. Risk factor assessments of temporomandibular disorders via machine learning. *Sci. Rep.* **2021**, *11*, 1–11. [CrossRef]
20. R Package Randomforest. Available online: https://cran.r-project.org/web/packages/randomForest/randomForest.pdf (accessed on 28 September 2022).
21. Python Package sklearn.ensemble. Random Forest Classifier. Available online: https://scikit-learn.org/stable/modules/generated/sklearn.ensemble.RandomForestClassifier.html (accessed on 28 September 2022).
22. Lundberg, S.; Lee, S.I. A unified approach to interpreting model predictions. *arXiv* **2017**, arXiv:1705.07874.
23. Python Package Shap. Available online: https://github.com/slundberg/shap (accessed on 10 August 2021).
24. Mokhtari, K.E.; Higdon, B.P.; Basar, A. Interpreting financial time series with SHAP values. In Proceedings of the 29th Annual International Conference on Computer Science and Software Engineering, Markham, ON, Canada, 4–6 November 2019; pp. 166–172.
25. Mangalathu, S.; Hwang, S.-H.; Jeon, J.-S. Failure mode and effects analysis of RC members based on machine-learning-based SHapley Additive exPlanations (SHAP) approach. *Eng. Struct.* **2020**, *219*, 110927. [CrossRef]
26. Parsa, A.B.; Movahedi, A.; Taghipour, H.; Derrible, S.; Mohammadian, A. (Kouros) toward safer highways, application of XGBoost and SHAP for real-time accident detection and feature analysis. *Accid. Anal. Prev.* **2020**, *136*, 105405. [CrossRef]
27. Kha, Q.-H.; Le, V.-H.; Hung, T.N.K.; Le, N.Q.K. Development and Validation of an Efficient MRI Radiomics Signature for Improving the Predictive Performance of 1p/19q Co-Deletion in Lower-Grade Gliomas. *Cancers* **2021**, *13*, 5398. [CrossRef] [PubMed]
28. Manikis, G.; Ioannidis, G.; Siakallis, L.; Nikiforaki, K.; Iv, M.; Vozlic, D.; Surlan-Popovic, K.; Wintermark, M.; Bisdas, S.; Marias, K. Multicenter DSC–MRI-Based Radiomics Predict IDH Mutation in Gliomas. *Cancers* **2021**, *13*, 3965. [CrossRef] [PubMed]
29. Laios, A.; Kalampokis, E.; Johnson, R.; Munot, S.; Thangavelu, A.; Hutson, R.; Broadhead, T.; Theophilou, G.; Leach, C.; Nugent, D.; et al. Factors predicting surgical effort using explainable artificial intelligence in advanced stage epithelial ovarian cancer. *Cancers* **2022**, *14*, 3447. [CrossRef]
30. Buergel, T.; Steinfeldt, J.; Ruyoga, G.; Pietzner, M.; Bizzarri, D.; Vojinovic, D.; Zu Belzen, J.U.; Loock, L.; Kittner, P.; Christmann, L.; et al. Metabolomic profiles predict individual multidisease outcomes. *Nat. Med.* **2022**, 1–12. [CrossRef] [PubMed]
31. Song, S.I.; Hong, H.T.; Lee, C.; Lee, S.B. A machine learning approach for predicting suicidal ideation in post stroke patients. *Sci. Rep.* **2022**, *12*, 15906. [CrossRef] [PubMed]
32. Kruk, M.; Goździejewska, A.M.; Artiemjew, P. Predicting the effects of winter water warming in artificial lakes on zooplankton and its environment using combined machine learning models. *Sci. Rep.* **2022**, *12*, 16145. [CrossRef]
33. Lee, K.-S.; Song, I.-S.; Kim, E.-S.; Ahn, K.H. Determinants of Spontaneous Preterm Labor and Birth Including Gastroesophageal Reflux Disease and Periodontitis. *J. Korean Med. Sci.* **2020**, *35*, e105. [CrossRef]
34. Deshmukh, F.; Merchant, S.S. Explainable Machine Learning Model for Predicting GI Bleed Mortality in the Intensive Care Unit. *Am. J. Gastroenterol.* **2020**, *115*, 1657–1668. [CrossRef]
35. Shinn, L.M.; Li, Y.; Mansharamani, A.; Auvil, L.S.; Welge, M.E.; Bushell, C.; Khan, N.A.; Charron, C.S.; Novotny, J.A.; Baer, D.J.; et al. Fecal Bacteria as Biomarkers for Predicting Food Intake in Healthy Adults. *J. Nutr.* **2020**, *151*, 423–433. [CrossRef]

36. Kang, E.A.; Jang, J.; Choi, C.H.; Kang, S.B.; Bang, K.B.; Kim, T.O.; Seo, G.S.; Cha, J.M.; Chun, J.; Jung, Y.; et al. Development of a clinical and genetic prediction model for early intestinal resection in pa-tients with Crohn's disease: Results from the IMPACT Study. *J. Clin. Med.* **2021**, *10*, 633. [CrossRef]
37. Esposito, A.A.; Zannoni, S.; Castoldi, L.; Giannitto, C.; Avola, E.; Casiraghi, E.; Catalano, O.; Carrafiello, G. Pseudo-pneumatosis of the gastrointestinal tract: Its incidence and the accuracy of a checklist supported by artificial intelligence (AI) techniques to reduce the misinterpretation of pneumatosis. *Emerg. Radiol.* **2021**, *28*, 911–919. [CrossRef] [PubMed]
38. Lee, K.-S.; Kim, E.S.; Kim, D.-Y.; Song, I.-S.; Ahn, K.H. Association of Gastroesophageal Reflux Disease with Preterm Birth: Machine Learning Analysis. *J. Korean Med. Sci.* **2021**, *36*. [CrossRef] [PubMed]
39. Lipták, P.; Banovcin, P.; Rosoľanka, R.; Prokopič, M.; Kocan, I.; Žiačiková, I.; Uhrik, P.; Grendar, M.; Hyrdel, R. A machine learning approach for identification of gastrointestinal predictors for the risk of COVID-19 related hospitalization. *PeerJ* **2022**, *10*, e13124. [CrossRef] [PubMed]
40. Liptak, P.; Duricek, M.; Rosolanka, R.; Ziacikova, I.; Kocan, I.; Uhrik, P.; Grendar, M.; Hrnciarova, M.; Bucova, P.; Galo, D.; et al. Gastrointestinal sequalae months after severe acute respiratory syndrome corona virus 2 infection: A prospective, observational study. *Eur. J. Gastroenterol. Hepatol.* **2022**, *34*, 925–932. [CrossRef] [PubMed]
41. Ribeiro, M.T.; Singh, S.; Guestrin, C. Why should I trust you? Explaining the predictions of any classifier. *arXiv* **2016**, arXiv:1602.04938.
42. Gheisari, S.; Shariflou, S.; Phu, J.; Kennedy, P.J.; Agar, A.; Kalloniatis, M.; Golzan, S.M. A combined convolutional and recurrent neural network for enhanced glaucoma detection. *Sci. Rep.* **2021**, *11*, 1945. [CrossRef] [PubMed]
43. Silver, D.; Huang, A.; Maddison, C.J.; Guez, A.; Sifre, L.; van den Driessche, G.; Schrittwieser, J.; Antonoglou, I.; Panneershelvam, V.; Lanctot, M.; et al. Mastering the game of Go with deep neural networks and tree search. *Nature* **2016**, *529*, 484–489. [CrossRef]
44. Hambly, B.; Xu, R.; Yang, H. Recent advances in reinforcement learning in finance. *arXiv* **2022**, arXiv:2112.04553. [CrossRef]
45. Yu, C.; Liu, J.; Nemati, S. Reinforcement learning in healthcare: A survey. *arXiv* **2020**, arXiv:1908.08796. [CrossRef]
46. Puiutta, E. Veith EMSP. Explainable reinforcement learning: A survey. *arXiv* **2020**, arXiv:2005.06247.

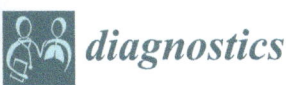

Article

GAR-Net: Guided Attention Residual Network for Polyp Segmentation from Colonoscopy Video Frames

Joel Raymann [1] and Ratnavel Rajalakshmi [2,*]

[1] Faculty of Mathematics, University of Waterloo, Waterloo, ON N2L 3G1, Canada
[2] School of Computer Science and Engineering, Vellore Institute of Technology, Chennai 600127, India
* Correspondence: rajalakshmi.r@vit.ac.in

Abstract: Colorectal Cancer is one of the most common cancers found in human beings, and polyps are the predecessor of this cancer. Accurate Computer-Aided polyp detection and segmentation system can help endoscopists to detect abnormal tissues and polyps during colonoscopy examination, thereby reducing the chance of polyps growing into cancer. Many of the existing techniques fail to delineate the polyps accurately and produce a noisy/broken output map if the shape and size of the polyp are irregular or small. We propose an end-to-end pixel-wise polyp segmentation model named Guided Attention Residual Network (GAR-Net) by combining the power of both residual blocks and attention mechanisms to obtain a refined continuous segmentation map. An enhanced Residual Block is proposed that suppresses the noise and captures low-level feature maps, thereby facilitating information flow for a more accurate semantic segmentation. We propose a special learning technique with a novel attention mechanism called Guided Attention Learning that can capture the refined attention maps both in earlier and deeper layers regardless of the size and shape of the polyp. To study the effectiveness of the proposed GAR-Net, various experiments were carried out on two benchmark collections viz., CVC-ClinicDB (CVC-612) and Kvasir-SEG dataset. From the experimental evaluations, it is shown that GAR-Net outperforms other previously proposed models such as FCN8, SegNet, U-Net, U-Net with Gated Attention, ResUNet, and DeepLabv3. Our proposed model achieves 91% Dice co-efficient and 83.12% mean Intersection over Union (mIoU) on the benchmark CVC-ClinicDB (CVC-612) dataset and 89.15% dice co-efficient and 81.58% mean Intersection over Union (mIoU) on the Kvasir-SEG dataset. The proposed GAR-Net model provides a robust solution for polyp segmentation from colonoscopy video frames.

Keywords: medical image analysis; polyp segmentation; colonoscopy; deep learning; attention mechanism; semantic segmentation; healthcare informatics

1. Introduction

Colorectal Cancer is one of the most common variants of cancer found in human beings. The predecessor of this cancer is the formation of polyps which are found in the colon region. The malignancy degree assessment of colorectal adenocarcinoma consists of two stages. The first stage involves the detection and delineation of polyps from the colon region via colonoscopy examinations. In this stage, the polyps are identified and delineated by an expert clinician. The second stage involves biopsy sample analysis from the segmented polyps using Hematoxylin and Eosin (H&E) staining technique. To reduce the risk of colorectal cancer, the polyps are often analyzed under H&E Staining to assess the malignancy degree and eventually resected [1]. The morphological segmentation of the gland for histopathology is commonly performed by pathologists to determine the stage of cancer/tumor. Accurate segmentation of the glands is a crucial stage in obtaining reliable morphological statistics for quantitative diagnosis. Hence, this is generally performed by the expert pathologist who segments and studies the structure of the glands in the biopsy sample. However, to proceed with the H&E staining on the biopsy sample, there is a need to

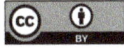

detect, segment, and delineate polyps from colonoscopy video frames. Unfortunately, even with the careful perusal of each frame in a colonoscopy video, an expert clinician might miss some polyps [2]. Hence, there is a need for a real-time Computer-Aided Detection (CAD) system that can detect and segment polyps in the first stage itself, which is the focus of this research work. The development of such a system can assist clinicians with the delineation of polyps from the colon and can reduce the miss-rate of polyps.

Automated polyp segmentation is a challenging task mainly due to the varied appearance, shape, and size of polyps. Even though there is a progressive change in the texture, size, and shape of the colorectal polyps in the later stages, it is small and may have no obvious differentiating texture appearance in the earlier stages. This makes it difficult to differentiate with intestinal tissue. Some polyps might even take the entire field of view in the colonoscopy camera. Also, each frame is susceptible to image artifacts, the pattern of shadows, highlights, and even occlusions due to the illuminations in colon screening. In some types of polyps, there is no obvious boundary between a polyp and the surrounding tissue, and the same polyp may look significantly different depending on the camera angle. So, the reliability of polyp segmentation by manual delineation is greatly affected by the lab's guidelines and the experience of the clinician. Hence, it is hard to determine the gold standard for an automatic segmentation method to deal with all possible types of polyps efficiently, thereby increasing the difficulty of developing a reliable polyp segmenting CAD system. The earlier techniques, such as template matching, contour detections, and texture-based analysis, required manual intervention. Many machine learning and computer vision techniques were applied to solve the polyp segmentation problem. Ref. [3] studied the application of active contours for the segmentation of polyps. As the above approach relies heavily on pre-defined template and shape models, it failed to detect small polyps. Ref. [4] introduced the "depth of valley" concept to detect more general polyp shapes-segmenting the polyps through evaluation of their relationship between the detected edge and the pixels. Their region segmentation algorithm could not handle all types of polyps and lacked robustness. It not only fails to identify some of the small polyps but also segments the endoluminal scene incorrectly as a polyp. To address the challenges in the measurement of segmented colon, different image processing techniques along with statistical analysis were performed [5], but it is a time-consuming and tedious process and could not detect a new type of polyps. Also, the above approaches do not consider contextual information and are not robust.

Recently, deep learning techniques have proven to solve many real-world problems with high robustness. Many variants of deep neural network architectures have been reported in the literature for the task of semantic segmentation for various applications, viz., remotely sensed data segmentation [6], road-scene segmentation, indoor scene segmentation [7], and biomedical image segmentation [8]. The study by [9] shows the superior performance of a Fully Convolutional Network (FCN) for semantic segmentation in colonoscopy images but is not able to yield an accurate prediction in the case of noisy images. In another work by [10], FCNs are employed for the segmentation of polyps along with a probabilistic-based post-processing algorithm. In this approach, a heuristic-based threshold was used to differentiate the polyp from the normal tissues, which is error-prone and could not characterize well all types of polyps that are irregular in shape and size.

The incorporation of the attention mechanism in deep neural networks can help the model generate a less noisy and more refined output map. For the diagnosis of coronary artery diseases [11], the attention-based vessel segmentation approach has been applied by adding low-level and high-level features. The sparse contour attention mechanism has been applied to obtain accurate region boundaries for liver segmentation in abdominal CT images [12]. They combined the sparse contour attention along with an auto-context algorithm and applied the self-supervised algorithm to improve the performance of segmentation.

In this research work, we propose a novel deep end-to-end architecture for segmenting polyps from colon screening frames by employing a modified residual network with a special attention mechanism. In the proposed approach, the lower semantic information captured in initial layers is also considered to handle different sizes, and shapes of polyps and to suppress the noise in the input. A novel Guided Attention mechanism is proposed that allows the model to generate and apply attention maps for each feature map in the input to obtain a refined and accurate segmentation output. We evaluated our model on two datasets, viz., the CVC-ClinicDB polyp dataset and the recent Kvasir-Seg [13] dataset and achieved state-of-the-art performance over other proposed deep learning models. Our significant contributions to this research work are summarized below:

- A novel end-to-end deep learning framework for segmenting polyps from colonoscopy video frames.
- A modified and enhanced Residual Block is proposed that suppresses the noise and preserves the low-level feature maps for a more accurate semantic segmentation.
- A special learning technique is introduced with a novel attention mechanism for obtaining an accurate segmentation map.
- A novel attention mechanism to capture the refined attention maps regardless of the size and shape of the polyp, also under improper illumination conditions.
- Design of a competitive and robust model with consistent performance over the benchmark CVC-ClinicDB dataset and the Kvasir-SEG Dataset.

This paper is organized as follows: The related works are discussed in Section 2. The proposed methodology is elaborated on in Section 3. The results and discussions of all experiments are presented in Section 4 followed by a conclusion in Section 5.

2. Related Works

Many machine learning and deep learning methods were proposed by various researchers in the field of medical image analysis that includes, including lesion identification in pulmonary nodules, lung nodules, colonial cancer, brain lesion segmentation, polyp segmentation, etc. Ref. [14] presented a detailed survey on image-based cancer detection using various deep learning architectures. In their study, they have outlined the methods suitable for different types of cancers, including breast cancer, lung cancer, skin cancer, prostate cancer, brain cancer, colonial cancer, cervical cancer, bladder cancer, etc. They discussed the issues of the lack of large data sets required for training the better models and the various available solutions like image augmentation and transfer learning to address the same. Computer Aided Detection (CAD) plays a major role in detecting lesions by providing assistance in the workflow of the radiologist. Ref. [15] studied the problems in identifying lesions in pulmonary nodules. To address the issues of highly imbalanced data and to reduce the false negatives in classification, they have proposed a multi-kernel approach. In their work, feature fusion and oversampling have been employed to select the important subset of relevant features. Ref. [16] proposed a deep learning-based technique for lung nodule detection on low-dose thoracic helical CT (LDCT) dataset and exploited the Convolutional Neural Network (CNN) and the traditional Artificial Neural Network (ANN). In their study, they observed that CNN architecture is good at capturing low-level and high-level features compared to ANN.

In this research work, we mainly focus on the polyp segmentation problem. Many solutions were proposed to automate the segmentation process of polyps in colon screening. In many cases, polyps have well-defined shapes and structures. Hence, earlier methods tried to leverage this to perform polyp segmentation. Ref. [17] proposed the usage of the canny edge detector technique to process the images and identify relevant edges with the assistance of template matching techniques. Following this, Ref. [3] studied the application of active contours for the segmentation of polyps, but these template-based models are not suitable for detecting small polyps.

Many texture-based methods were also introduced as a solution to the polyp segmentation problem. Karkanis et al. [18] used Grey-Level Co-occurrence Matrix (GLCM) and wavelet methods to detect polyps. Ref. [19] proposed an SVM-based method to detect and classify the abnormalities in endoscopic images. They mainly focused on feature extraction and developed an algorithm that can assign the weights for the relevant features and to remove the useless ones from the hand-crafted features that were extracted from the endoscopic image. With their deep sparse SVM-based approach, they were able to reduce the feature dimension and build a better model for classifying the endoscopic images on their own dataset. In another work, an SVM-based approach with hand-crafted features was applied [19] to detect the abnormalities in endoscopic images. As their SVM model could not handle the noisy and poor-quality images, they introduced a rejection stage. The image quality was pre-assessed based on its pixels, and only if it was at an acceptable level was it fed to the next segmentation stage by SVM. Otherwise, the image was rejected in the pre-processing stage itself, thereby limiting its usage. Ref. [20] attempted to characterize the polyps by traditional methods such as edge detection, feature extraction, and feature reduction and then applying an ensemble-based approach for classification. But these handcrafted features were not accurate for delineating the polyp boundary.

For colonic polyp measurement, Ref. [21] followed a topographical height map approach. They computed the topographic features from the generated height maps of the polyp. The concentric patterns from the height maps were then used for the texture analysis. By applying the SVM classifier, the normal surface of the colon was differentiated from the colonic polyps. They analyzed the experimental measurements with that of the height map approach, and it was found to be more efficient than the other methods. Recently, a rapid change has been observed in these tasks as Convolutional Neural Networks (CNN) are being employed to provide more robustness compared to hand-crafted features.

All the above approaches are not sufficient for the polyp segmentation task, as they fail to capture the contextual information from the images. To address the above problems, Fully Convolutional Networks (FCN) proposed by [22] were adapted for semantic segmentation. Later, U-Net [8] architecture was widely used for developing an end-to-end model for semantic segmentation. Following these works, Ref. [9] proposed a standard FCN for the segmentation of polyps and used the Random Forest algorithm to decrease the false positive results.

From neural machine translation to sentence classification, applying the attention mechanism has allowed models to focus on important features, resulting in less noisy, more refined feature maps [23]. Recently, Ref. [24] tried to incorporate an attention mechanism, and their study suggests that attention mechanisms can substantially reduce the noise in the output and help the model generate a more refined output map. Hence, it can be concluded that a better attention mechanism can further improve the performance of the models. Ref. [25] tried various methods, from Machine Learning to Deep CNN models, and suggested various methods for classifying Gastrointestinal (GI) tract diseases.

As deep learning methods have proven to learn robust features for segmentation problems, we have applied them to get a robust model for the segmentation of polyps of varied textures, shapes, and sizes. However, recent deep learning approaches in polyp segmentation output noisy outputs and broken segmentation maps. Hence, the incorporation of a better attention mechanism can help the model generate a less noisy and more refined output map. In this work, we have proposed a Guided Attention Residual Network (GAR-Net) by employing both residual blocks and attention mechanisms to obtain a refined segmentation map for polyp segmentation.

Materials and Methods should be described with sufficient details to allow others to replicate and build on the published results. Please note that the publication of your manuscript implies that you must make all materials, data, computer code, and protocols associated with the publication available to readers. Please disclose at the submission stage any restrictions on the availability of materials or information. New methods and protocols should be described in detail, while well-established methods can be briefly described and appropriately cited.

Research manuscripts reporting large datasets that are deposited in a publicly available database should specify where the data have been deposited and provide the relevant accession numbers. If the accession numbers have not yet been obtained at the time of submission, please state that they will be provided during review. They must be provided prior to publication.

Interventional studies involving animals or humans, and other studies that require ethical approval, must list the authority that provided approval and the corresponding ethical approval code.

3. Proposed Methodology

The proposed Guided Attention Residual Network (GAR-Net) architecture for polyp segmentation is presented here with its building blocks. We present our novel Guided Attention Learning (GAL) along with the proposed loss function of the proposed GAR-Net model.

3.1. Building Blocks of GAR-Net

The basic residual block, which is incorporated in the proposed model, is presented below. It is followed by our modified residual block and the Guided Attention Module (GAM)-the attention mechanism that we have proposed in this research.

3.1.1. Residual Block

The residual block, ResNet [26], provides an exceptional performance boost and faster convergence because of the skip connections present in the block. The authors have shown that, even if the network depth increases by stacking many layers, it is not guaranteed to get an increase in accuracy. Because the network depth is limited by the issue of vanishing gradients. The gradient becomes very small, or even zero, in the earlier layers, and in such cases, even the shallow networks perform better than the deeper networks. To address this issue, the concept of skip connections was introduced, which provides better gradient flow and helps in avoiding exploding and vanishing gradients. By using skip connections, the information captured in the initial layers can be allowed to the later layers, thereby enabling the later layers to learn the lower semantic information captured in earlier layers. It is incorporated in many deep learning models to improve the performance of classification and semantic segmentation problems [6]. Figure 1 shows the overview of the used residual block.

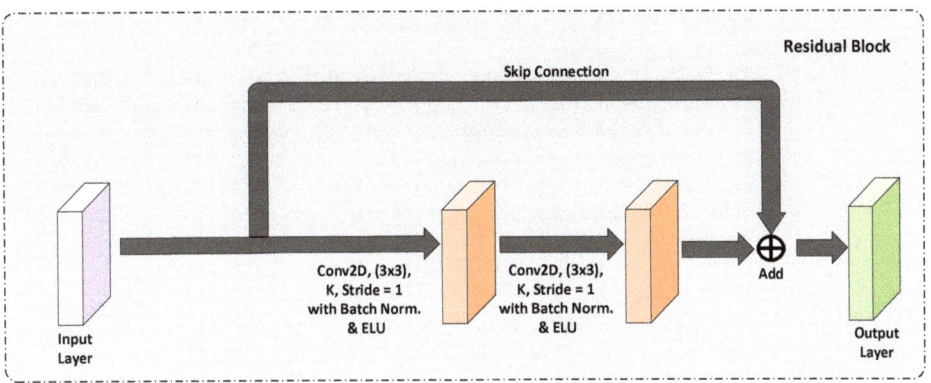

Figure 1. The overview of the Residual Block used.

The K in Figure 1 is the number of filters applied in the convolution operation used in the residual block. Although residual networks have shown great performance, they have a drawback of noise added to the low-level features captured in the earlier stages of the network due to the plain addition of the skip connection. The ResNet adds the skip connection bypassing the non-linear transformations with an identify function, which helps the gradient to flow directly to the earlier layers from later layers. Even though it preserves the information from earlier layers by additive identity transformation, noise is also added.

To suppress that noise, we have modified this architecture to learn the refined low-level feature maps by adding a convolutional block in the skip connection, as explained below.

3.1.2. Modified Residual Block

We proposed a modified residual block and applied it in our GAR-Net model to alleviate the problem found in normal residual networks. We have introduced a convolution layer in the skip connection before the addition, and this helps the model in two ways, (i) suppresses the amount of noise added in the feature maps and (ii) helps the model to learn in the skip connection and to capture refined low-level feature maps. The overview of the modified residual block is shown in Figure 2.

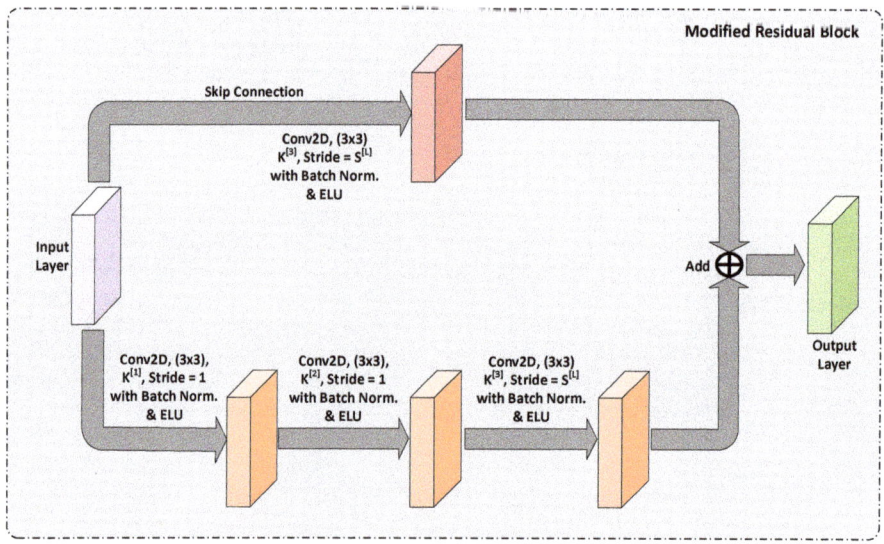

Figure 2. The overview of the Modified Residual Block.

In the proposed modified residual block, the two important parameters are $K^{[i]}$ and $S^{[L]}$. $K^{[i]}$ is the number of filters applied at the ith convolution operation in the main flow. $S^{[L]}$ indicates the striding for the last convolution layer. The input layer is taken through two paths-main paths and a skip path. In the main path, a series of convolutions are applied, and the last convolution alone with a stride of $S^{[L]}$. In the skip connection, a single convolution is introduced with a stride of $S^{[L]}$. Finally, the output of both paths is added to get the final output feature maps.

3.1.3. Guided Attention Module

Attention mechanisms can drastically improve the performance of deep learning models. A general attention mechanism consists of a $query(Q)$ and a $value(V)$ and it boosts the set of features present in the values to which the query is related. In other words, the attention lets the model focus on the information it needs from the values using the query. Ref. [24] proposed an attention-gated mechanism for semantic segmentation tasks on medical images. The major drawback of this work is that a single attention map is broadcasted and multiplied across the entire set of feature maps. This can lead to a noisy feature map at the beginning of the training making the entire training process slower with a higher convergence time. Furthermore, this can disrupt the feature map set, as each feature map consists of information that facilitates the model to output more refined output. To address the above drawbacks, we propose a new attention mechanism called Guided Attention Module (GAM), which allows the model to generate and apply attention maps for each feature map in the input feature sets. Furthermore, GAM is fine-tuned to generate a more refined attention map with a special technique called Guided Attention Learning (GAL). The overview of the proposed Guided Attention Module is presented in Figure 3.

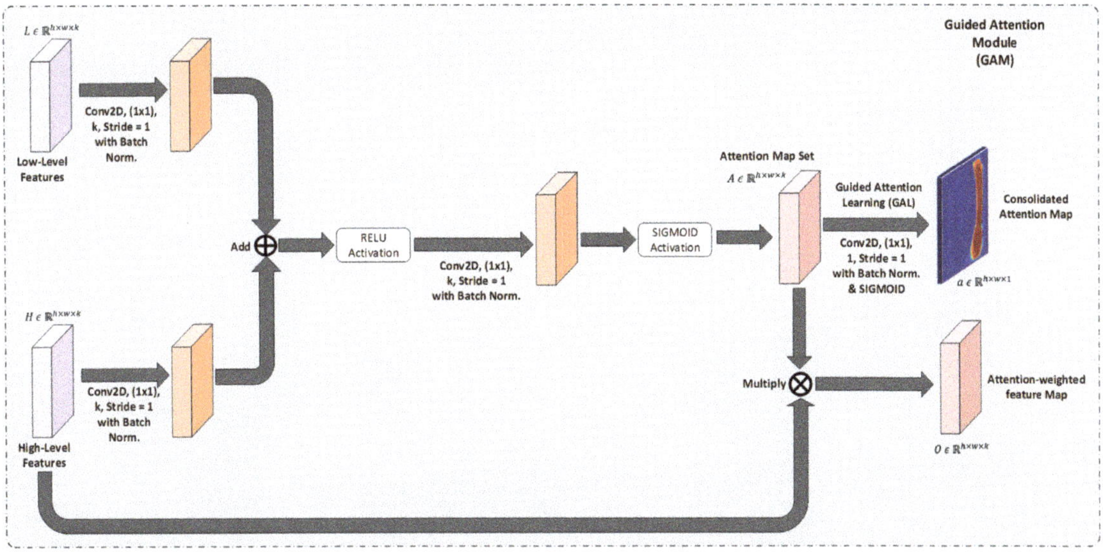

Figure 3. The overview of the Guided Attention Module with Guided Attention Learning.

Consider a low-level feature map $L \in \mathbb{R}^{h \times w \times k}$ and a high-level feature map $H \in \mathbb{R}^{h \times w \times k}$, where h, w, k denote the height, width and number of channels in the feature map set. To apply GAM, a 1×1 convolution with k filters is applied on the low-level feature map L and another 1×1 convolution with k filters is applied on high-level feature map H, simultaneously. The outputs of these two operations are added together and activated with a non-linear $relu()$ function. This output is passed through a 1×1 convolution with k filters and is activated with a non-linear $sigmoid()$ function to obtain the attention map set $A \in \mathbb{R}^{h \times w \times k}$. A is then multiplied elementwise with the up-sampled low-level features to get the final attention-weighted feature maps $O \in \mathbb{R}^{h \times w \times k}$. Batch-Normalization [27] is applied before every non-linear activation function to improve the training process. With the attention map set A, we obtain individual pixel-wise attention maps for each feature map, thereby allowing the noise due to multiplying a single attention map. To further refine the attention maps, we train this set of attention maps A using our proposed Guided Attention Learning (GAL) technique.

3.2. GAR-Net for Polyp Segmentation

The working principle of the proposed Guided Attention Learning (GAL), along with the loss function used in our GAR-Net architecture, is presented below.

3.2.1. GAR-Net Architecture

The overview of GAR-Net architecture is shown in Figure 4. The input of the proposed GAR-Net architecture is $256 \times 256 \times 3$ normalized between [0.0, 1.0]. The encoder learns the features from the given input, which is then fed to a set of bottleneck layers to get the consolidated encoded feature maps. The decoder reconstructs the output from the encoded feature maps. The skip connection plays a crucial step in the reconstruction process as it helps the decoder access the low-level information from the encoder layers. These low-level feature maps consist of the spatial/location information and help the decoder reconstruct the output map, viz., the skip connection. We incorporated a Guided Attention Module (GAM) with GAL to effectively reconstruct a refined output map at each stage in the decoder. The GAM takes the up-sampled High-Level feature maps and the low-level feature maps from the skip connection and merges the map efficiently to reconstruct a refined output map in the decoder.

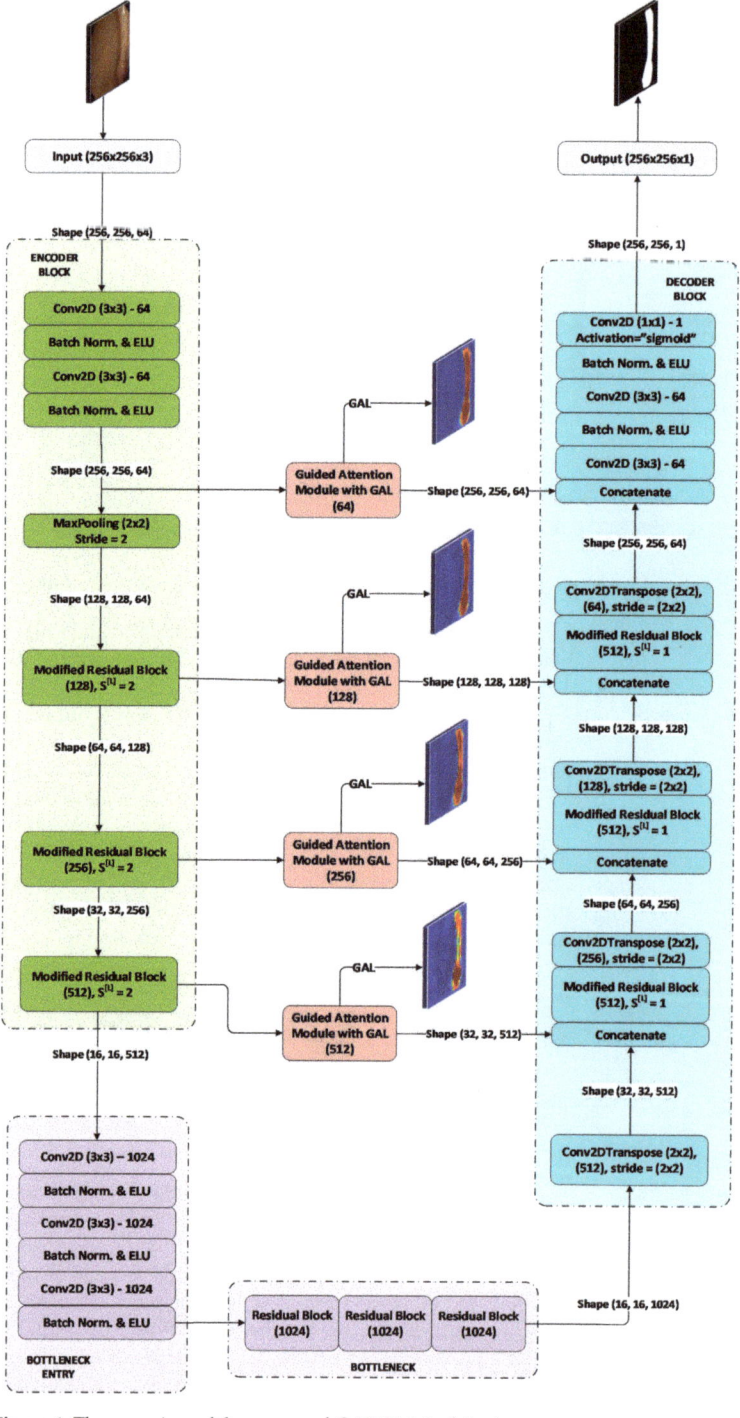

Figure 4. The overview of the proposed GAR-Net Architecture.

3.2.2. Guided Attention Learning

The high-level features consist of more information pertinent to the segmentation task, while the low-level features consist of information that helps the model reconstruct the output segmentation map. The purpose of attention is to use the information from the high-level coarse feature map, and spatial/location information from the low-level feature maps to reconstruct a more refined set of feature maps, hence, combining both high-level and low-level feature maps effectively. However, an attention mechanism can be detrimental to the performance of the model if it fails to capture meaningful information from the training set. To address this issue, we propose Guided Attention Learning (GAL) mechanism. Guided Attention Learning is a training mechanism that allows one to train the attention map according to their needs and to have control over its focus on specific features. To implement GAL, a simple 1×1 convolution is applied with a single filter over the attention map set A. It is then followed by batch normalization and a non-linear $sigmoid()$ activation. GAL results in a consolidated single attention map $a \in \mathbb{R}^{height \times width \times 1}$ representing all the information present in the attention map set A. Next, we train the output a using binary cross-entropy to suit our desired attention map. The incorporation of GAL in the loss function for our proposed GAR-Net is elaborated below.

3.2.3. Loss Function for GAR-Net

The model proposed in Figure 4 gives five outputs, namely: The main segmentation map output (y_{pred}), and the attention maps (a_1, a_2, a_3, a_4) from the GAM module. For training the model, the dice loss L_{main} for our main output (y_{pred}) is initially calculated using the following equation:

$$L_{main} = 1.0 - \frac{2 \left| y_{pred} \cap y_{gnd} \right|}{\left| y_{pred} \right| + \left| y_{gnd} \right|} \qquad (1)$$

where, y_{pred} is the set of pixels in the predicted output map, y_{gnd} is the set of pixels in the ground truth segmentation map.

In general, the attention layer is allowed to train on its own. But in this proposed work, Guided Attention Learning is introduced to control what must be focused on by the attention mechanism. The crux of GAL is to train the attention mechanism on where to focus. To focus on the region of interest using the proposed attention mechanism (GAM), each attention layer is trained alongside the main objective in a multi-tasked learning approach. For each attention map $a_i \in [a_1, a_2, a_3, a_4]$, the binary cross-entropy loss is calculated. At this stage, the following question arises in our mind: With respect to what will we find the loss? What is the ground truth attention map? This can be answered by understanding what a perfect attention map is. The main reason for applying attention at each up-sampling stage is that we wish to reconstruct higher resolution feature maps effectively using the up-sampled high-level features maps and the low-level skip connection feature maps. A perfect attention map, in such cases, must resemble the segmentation map. Hence, the ground truth for the attention maps will simply be the segmentation map itself but resized to the size of that attention map a_i. For example, let's take $a_3 \in \mathbb{R}^{64 \times 64}$ and $y_{gnd} \in \mathbb{R}^{256 \times 256}$ be the ground-truth segmentation map, then the ground truth attention map for a_3 will be y_{gnd} itself but resized to 64×64 to match the dimension of a_3. By using this method, we can train all four attention mechanisms using binary cross-entropy. The guided attention loss L_{a_i} for each attention map $a_i \in [a_1, a_2, a_3, a_4]$ can be calculated by the following equation:

$$L_a = - \sum_{x \in \Omega} \log\left(P\left(a_{i_{pred}}(x), a_{i_{gnd}}(x)\right)\right) \qquad (2)$$

where Ω implies the image space from which each pixel x is considered. $P\left(a_{i_{pred}}(x), a_{i_{gnd}}(x)\right)$ is the calculated sigmoid probability of the attention map a_i on the corresponding pixel x.

The total loss L_{total} is the aggregation of all these loss functions and can be calculated by the following equation:

$$L_{total} = L_{main} + \sum_{i=1}^{4} L_{a_i} \qquad (3)$$

4. Results and Discussion:

To evaluate the performance of the proposed method, various experiments were carried out. A detailed discussion of the experimental setup and results are presented in this section, along with the attention visualization.

4.1. Dataset

For the polyp segmentation task from images, each pixel in the training images must be labeled as either the polyp class or the non-polyp class. For evaluating our proposed GAR-Net model, we have used two benchmark datasets-the CVC-ClinicDB [28] and the Kvasir-SEG [13]. The CVC-ClinicDB is an open-access dataset of 612 images, each with a resolution of 384 × 288, acquired from 31 colonoscopy sequences. The Kvasir-SEG dataset is a considerably huge dataset of 1000 polyp images given along with their annotated ground truth masks. The annotations of these masks were performed by expert endoscopists from the Oslo University Hospital (Norway). The resolution of the individual images in the Kvasir-SEG dataset varies from 300 × 300 to 1920 × 1080 and beyond in certain cases.

4.2. Experimental Setup

All the architectures used for comparison and evaluation in this research were implemented in TensorFlow version 2.0. The models were built using the high-level Keras API, while the training process was performed with TensorFlow 2.0's gradient tape training mechanism. The loss and metrics were evaluated using TensorLayer [29]. The models were trained with an Intel i7-7700HQ CPU with 16GB DDR4-2400MHz RAM and an Nvidia GTX 1060 GPU with 6GB VRAM. The system environment is Windows 10 OS and had the latest Nvidia CUDA v10.2 installed with CuDNN v7.6.5. The implementation code is developed in python version 3.6.8.

4.3. Training Setup

The size of the image within the same dataset varies significantly. Hence, for effective GPU utilization and to reduce the training time, we resized the training images to 270 × 270 and applied a series of augmentation techniques to increase the training dataset. The final input training images of size 256 × 256 are acquired from random cropping of the augmented training images. We extensively used data augmentation techniques such as random HSV saturation, random brightness, random contrast, random horizontal and vertical flip, random scaling, and random rotation (rotation range ϵ [0°, 90°]). We also used noise and blurring augmentation techniques such as median blur, gaussian blur, motion blur, and gaussian noise. It is to be noted that augmentation techniques were applied only during the training process and not for testing and validation. For validation and testing, we resized the input image to 256 × 256 using a bicubic resizing algorithm [30] before feeding the images to the model.

For all the experiments, 80% of the dataset was used for training, 10% for validation, and the remaining 10% for testing. All the models were trained for 120 epochs with a batch size of 4. We used Adam optimizer and Dice loss to train the model. The initial learning rate was set to 1.0×10^{-4} and was eventually reduced upon reaching a plateau in the validation loss. This type of learning rate reduction is called learning rate plateau-a technique that monitors the validation loss and reduces the learning rate upon no improvement in the validation loss for the corresponding epoch. For testing and evaluating the model after training, we used the models which gave the least validation loss. All hyper-parameters were tuned manually and found that the above setting helped all the models perform well on both datasets.

4.4. Results

We implemented and compared the proposed model with the existing techniques to study the effectiveness of this approach. We compared our proposed GAR-Net model with FCN [22], U-Net [8], U-Net with gated attention [24], SegNet [7], ResUNet [6], and DeepLabv3 [31]. We implemented all the aforementioned models on our own except the DeepLabv3 model. The implementation code for the DeepLabv3 model was taken from their GitHub repository [*GitHubRepo*]. We trained all the models on both the CVC-ClinicDB dataset and the Kvasir-SEG dataset. We used the dice coefficient and meant Intersection over Union (mIoU) as our main metric of evaluation, as these metrics are much more suitable for evaluating semantic segmentation tasks.

4.4.1. Results on CVC-ClinicDB Dataset

The models were evaluated with the CVC-ClinicDB dataset, and the results are shown in Table 1.

Table 1. The Results on the CVC-ClinicDB Dataset.

S No	Model	Dice Score	mIoU	Pixel Accuracy
1	FCN8	0.8724981	0.74308	0.9757281
2	SegNet	0.73168665	0.811956	0.97676927
3	UNet	0.8803434	0.767874	0.97531813
4	UNet-Attn	0.89131886	0.783651	0.97713906
5	ResUNet	0.89080334	0.781462	0.97680587
6	DeepLabv3	0.90001955	0.819477	0.9817561
7	**GAR-Net**	0.9100929	0.831234	0.9831491

From Table 1, our proposed model outperforms other models with the highest dice coefficient (0.910) and mIoU score (0.831). Even in the pixel-wise accuracy (0.983), the proposed model outperforms all the other models.

The performance of the proposed GAR-Net was analyzed by plotting a graph with the obtained Dice Coefficient and mIoU for the training set (left side of the graph) and validation set (right side of the graph), respectively. From Figure 5, it is observed that DeepLabv3 performs well only on the training set (depicted in the top-left and bottom-left of the graph) but lacks generalization, which has led to poor performance on the validation set (top-right and bottom-right). But our proposed model GAR-Net shows its superiority in the validation set also with a competitive performance in the training set, hence, providing a robust solution on the CVC-ClinicDB dataset. Similarly, other existing models also fail to provide a robust solution, and the performance on the validation set is not as good as the proposed GAR-Net. So, we can conclude that our proposed model provides consistent performance in terms of Dice Co-efficient and mIoU over both the training and validation set.

4.4.2. Results on Kvasir-SEG Dataset

All the models were also evaluated on the Kvasir-SEG dataset, and the results are summarized in Table 2.

Table 2. The Results for the Kvasir-SEG Dataset.

S No	Model	Dice Score	mIoU	Pixel Accuracy
1	FCN8	0.73635364	0.548514	0.9176181
2	SegNet	0.78634053	0.784731	0.9607266
3	UNet	0.85862905	0.750284	0.959373
4	UNet-Attn	0.8637741	0.754757	0.9587085
5	ResUNet	0.86858636	0.761282	0.9630264
6	DeepLabv3	0.87866044	0.805872	0.9693878
7	**GAR-Net**	0.8915458	0.815802	0.9717203

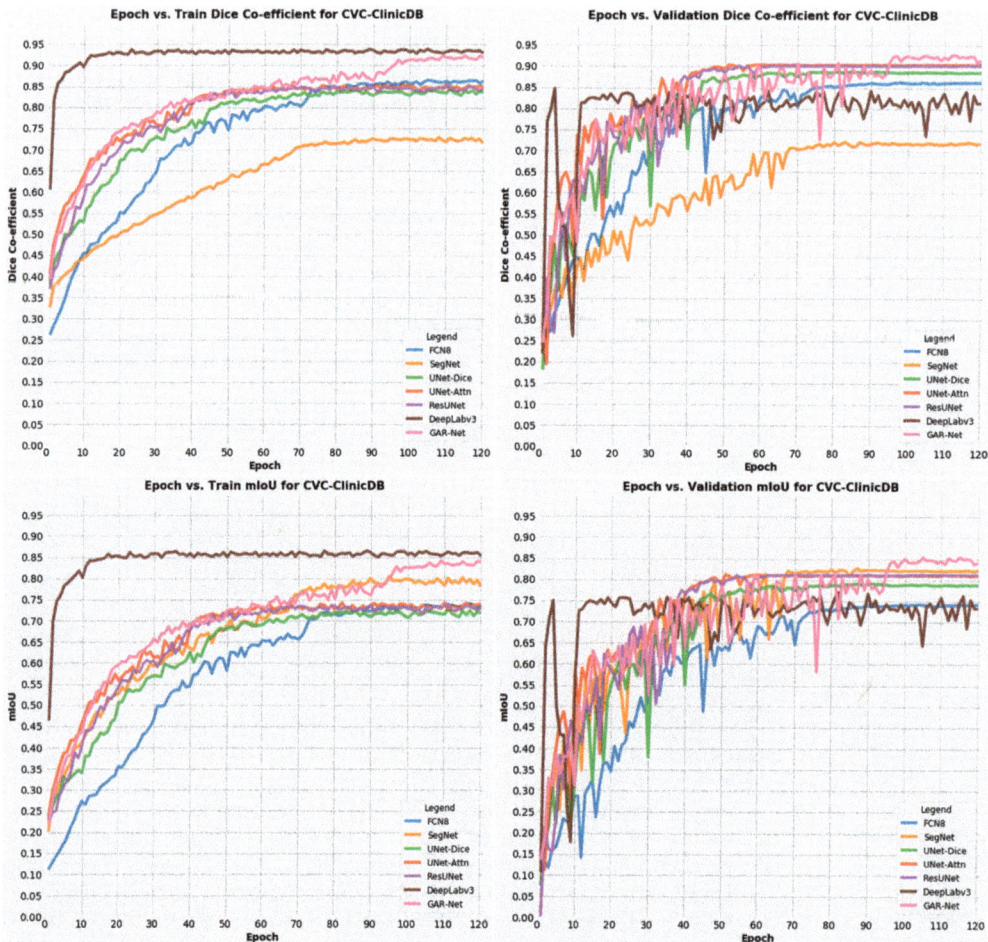

Figure 5. Training and Validation results on the CVC-ClinicDB dataset.

From the results, it is evident that our proposed model outperforms all the other models with the highest dice coefficient (0.891), mIoU score (0.815), and pixel-wise accuracy (0.971).

From the plotted graphs, as shown in Figure 6, we can observe that our model performance is consistent in both the training and validation set on the Kvasir-SEG dataset also. Our proposed model shows competitive performance in terms of dice coefficient and outperforms all other models in mIoU in the validation set, thus providing a robust solution.

4.5. Further Discussions

To evaluate the significance of the proposed Guided Attention mechanism, we present the visualization of the outputs of all the models for some test samples randomly taken from both datasets and compare its performance with existing methods

4.5.1. Output Visualization for CVC-ClinicDB Dataset

A set of random test samples were taken from the CVC-ClinicDB dataset and is visualized. The comparison with all the other trained models is depicted in Figure 7.

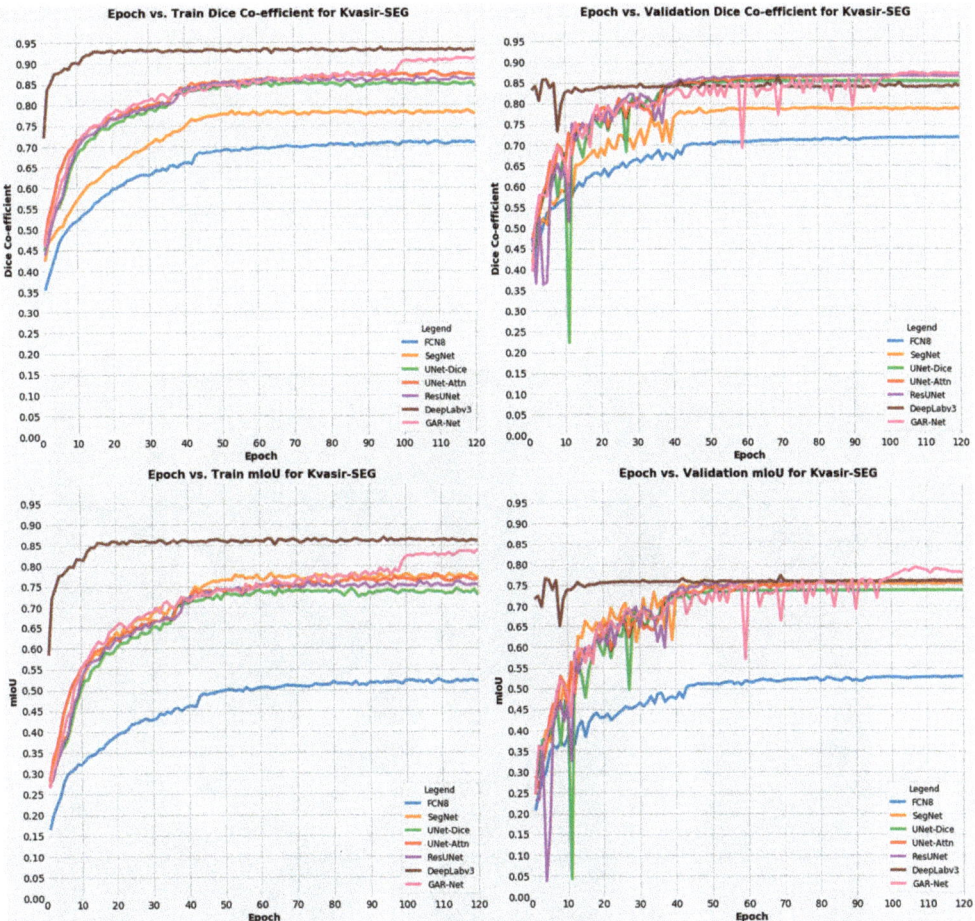

Figure 6. The Training and Validation Graphs for the Kvasir-SEG Dataset training.

From Figure 7, it can be observed that our proposed model produces a more refined map than all other models. It is also evident that almost all models predict well for samples 1 and 2. In sample 3, DeepLabv3 predicts with noise, while in sample 4 and sample 5, the DeepLabv3 model fails to provide proper continuous maps. All models, except our proposed GAR-Net model, fail to capture a refined output map for the Sample 6 model. This is due to improper illumination. However, our proposed model adapts to it to an extent and provides an overall refined output map. Hence, we can conclude that our model outperforms all the other models showing the superiority of the proposed GAR-Net architecture on the CVC-ClinicDB dataset.

4.5.2. Output Visualization for Kvasir-SEG dataset

A set of random test samples were taken from the Kvasir-SEG dataset and visualized (Figure 8) and compared with all the trained models.

From Figure 8, one can quickly notice the visual noises present in the Kvasir-SEG input images. These noises include writings, random color patches, etc., which make the Kvasir-SEG dataset, a challenging dataset. FCN8 fails to provide any refined output for all the samples. Most models perform well on sample 1, but UNet and UNet-Attention fail to handle the visual noises present in the input image of samples 2, 3, and 7, hence, resulting in a broken and irregular output map. SegNet provides a decent output compared to UNet and UNet-Attention on all the samples except sample 6, where it fails to find two separate polyp objects. DeepLabv3 outputs decent maps but fails to capture any output from sample 3 and sample 7. Also, DeepLabv3 completely misses the smaller polyp in sample 6. Our proposed GAR-Net model outputs a refined segmentation map for all the samples. There is a small noise in the output map of sample 6 from our GAR-Net model. However, considering all the samples, our model outperforms other models with high efficacy, thus showing the superior performance of the proposed GAR-Net architecture on the Kvasir-SEG dataset also.

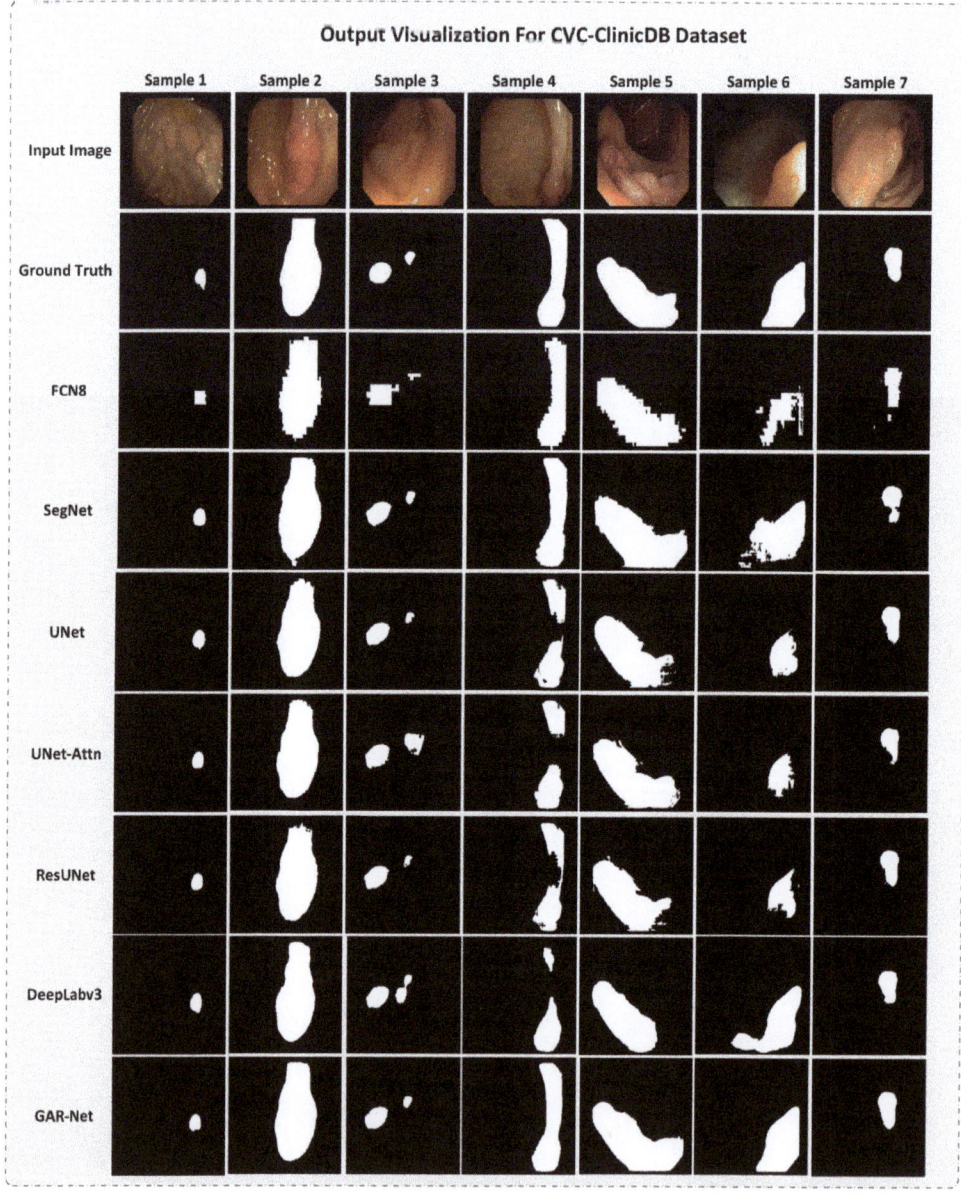

Figure 7. The output comparison for all the models on the CVC-ClinicDB Dataset.

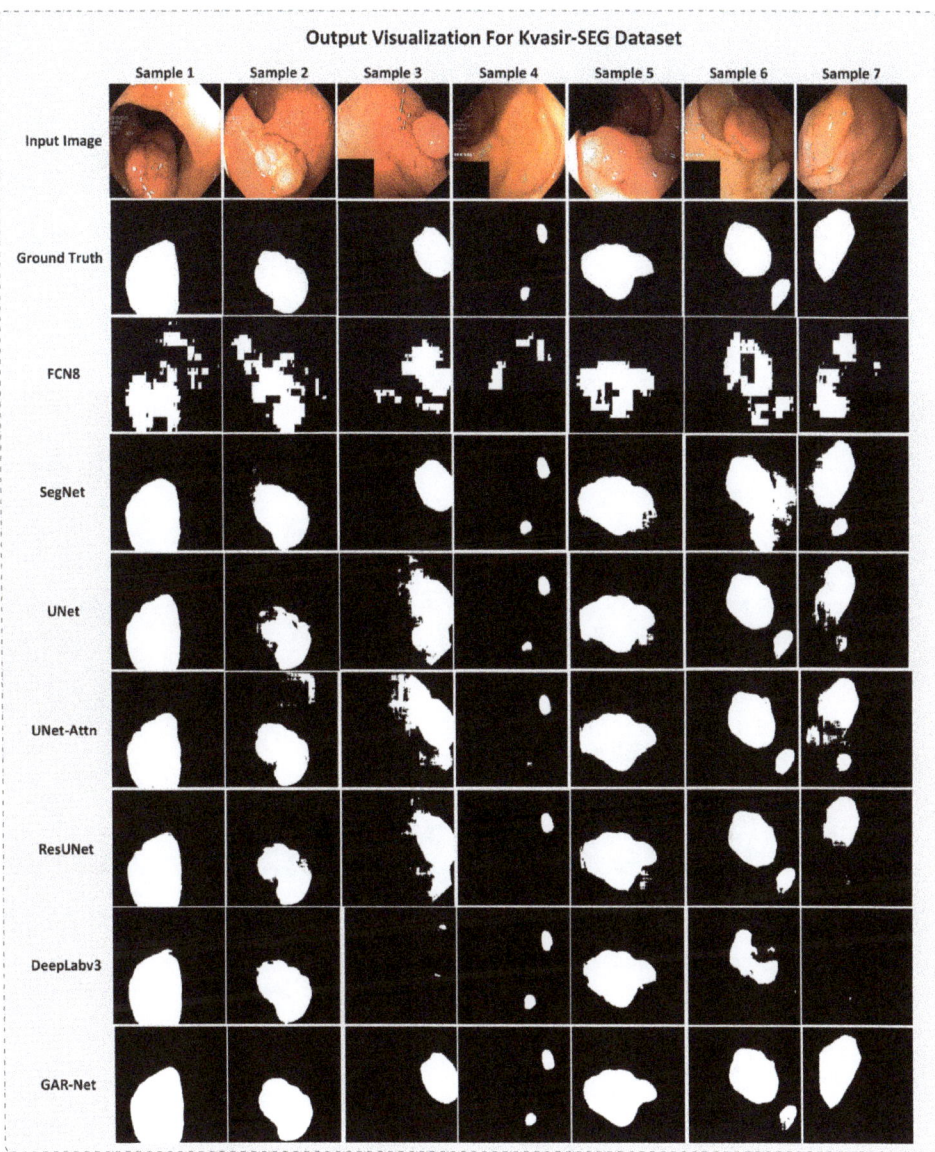

Figure 8. The output comparison for all the models on the Kvasir-SEG Dataset.

From Figures 7 and 8, we can conclude that the proposed GAR-Net provides a more refined output map regardless of the noise or improper illuminations, providing a robust model for segmenting polyps from colonoscopy video frames.

4.5.3. Strength of the Proposed Guided Attention Learning

To understand the significance of Guided Attention Learning in our GAR-Net architecture, we compared and visualized the attention map from the existing Attention Gated Mechanism [24] and the proposed GAM with GAL by taking a random test sample from both datasets. The attention visualization is presented in Figures 9 and 10 for a random test sample in the CVC-ClinicDB dataset and Kvasir-SEG dataset, respectively.

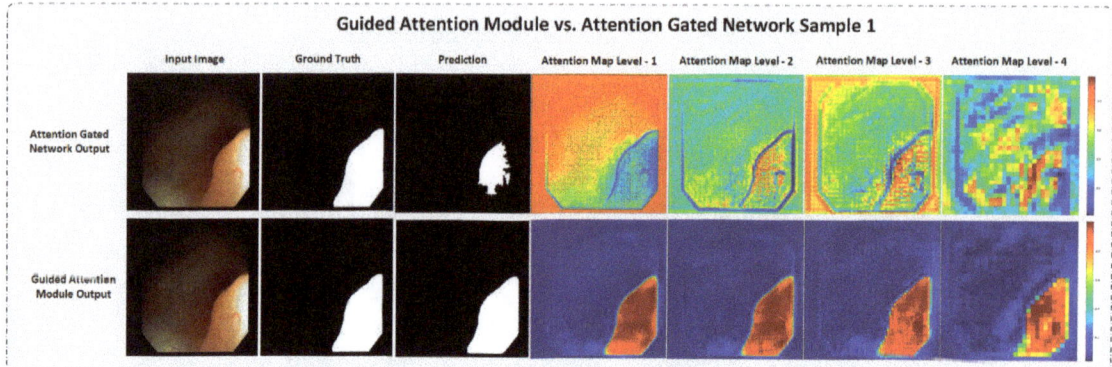

Figure 9. The attention visualization comparison: Attention Gated Network vs. Guided Attention Module with a test sample from CVC-ClinicDB dataset. Even in deeper layers, GAM is still able to capture refined attention maps, while Attention Gated Network only outputs coarse and broken attention maps.

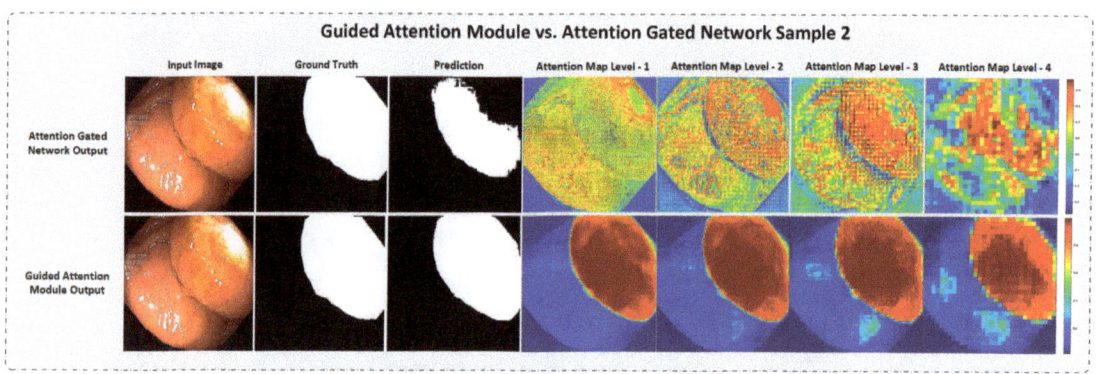

Figure 10. The attention visualization comparison compares Attention Gated Network vs. Guided Attention Module with a test sample from the Kvasir-SEG dataset. Notice even in deeper layers, GAM is still able to capture refined attention maps, while Attention Gated Network-only outputs coarse and broken attention maps.

From Figure 9, it is evident that the attention map of the Attention-Gated Network fails to capture the entire region of interest, hence, resulting in a broken, uneven output map. Moreover, as we go deeper into the network, the attention-gated network fails to provide a refined map and results in a very coarse attention map. However, the attention maps from our proposed GAM with GAL are highly refined even in the deeper layers of the network. Hence, we can get a more refined continuous output map.

From Figure 10, it is again evident that the attention-gated network completely fails to capture the region of interest at low-level layers (early stages of the network). However, in the deeper layers of the network, we can see that the attention-gated network results in a coarse feature map with a lot of noise, as it captures only some part of the output and lacks to obtain a refined attention map. But our proposed Guided Attention Learning successfully captures a refined attention map both in earlier and in deeper layers of the model. Hence, we can conclude that our Guided Attention Module with Guided Attention Learning outperforms the previously proposed Attention-gated network and boosts the model's performance by capturing refined output maps.

5. Conclusions

In this paper, we presented GAR-Net: Guided Attention-based Residual Network, which is an architecture designed to address the need for a more accurate and refined segmentation map for the colorectal polyps found in colonoscopy examinations. The proposed architecture takes advantage of residual blocks, and attention mechanisms to output refined segmentation maps. We have modified the residual block by including a convolution layer in the skip connection to suppress the noise and capture the refined low-level feature map. We have proposed a new attention mechanism that successfully captures a refined attention map both in earlier and in deeper layers of the model. The Guided Attention mechanism proposed for this GAR-Net architecture generates a more refined output map regardless of improper illuminations, providing a robust model for segmenting polyps from colonoscopy video frames.

Comprehensive examinations and experiments were conducted using the benchmark CVC-ClinicDB dataset and Kvasir-SEG dataset to evaluate and assess the proposed model with the existing state-of-art architectures. Through experimental results, it is shown that our proposed GAR-Net model can provide a reliable and robust model with the highest Dice co-efficient and mIoU score, outperforming other proposed semantic segmentation models such as FCN8, U-Net, U-Net with Gated Attention, ResUNet, SegNet, and DeepLabv3. The computation overload is slightly high in our proposed GAR-Net architecture, as we used normal convolution over depth-wise separable convolution. We did an experiment with depth-wise separable convolution and found it quite detrimental, especially to the attention mechanisms. There is further research scope to improve this model by making it lightweight and incorporating spatial information in Guided Attention Learning. We can conclude that the proposed GAR-Net architecture can be considered a strong baseline for further investigation in the direction of developing a robust and clinically useful method for polyp segmentation from colonoscopy video frames.

Author Contributions: Development, Validation, and Manuscript Preparation—J.R.; Methodology, Validation, and Manuscript Preparation/Reviewing—R.R. All authors have read and agreed to the published version of the manuscript.

Funding: This research has been carried out in collaboration with Mithraa Hospital, Madurai, and with financial support.

Institutional Review Board Statement: Not applicable.

Informed Consent Statement: Not applicable.

Data Availability Statement: The dataset used in this research is a benchmark dataset and is publicly available for researchers.

Acknowledgments: The authors would like to thank the Mithraa Hospital, Madurai, for carrying out the collaborative research and for their financial support.

Conflicts of Interest: The authors declare no conflict of interest.

References

1. Lawton, C. Colonoscopic Polypectomy and Long-Term Prevention of Colorectal-Cancer Deaths. *Yearb. Oncol.* **2013**, *2013*, 128–129. [CrossRef]
2. van Rijn, J.C.; Reitsma, J.B.; Stoker, J.; Bossuyt, P.M.; van Deventer, S.J.; Dekker, E. Polyp Miss Rate Determined by Tandem Colonoscopy: A Systematic Review. *Am. J. Gastroenterol.* **2006**, *101*, 343–350. [CrossRef]
3. Breier, M.; Gross, S.; Behrens, A.; Stehle, T.; Aach, T. Active contours for localizing polyps in colonoscopic NBI image data. *Med. Imaging 2011 Comput.-Aided Diagn.* **2011**, *7963*, 79632M. [CrossRef]
4. Bernal, J.; Sánchez, J.; Vilariño, F. Towards automatic polyp detection with a polyp appearance model. *Pattern Recognit.* **2012**, *45*, 3166–3182. [CrossRef]
5. Manjunath, K.N.; Prabhu, G.K.; Siddalingaswamy, P.C. A quantitative validation of segmented colon in virtual colonoscopy using image moments. *Biomed. J.* **2020**, *43*, 74–82. [CrossRef]
6. Diakogiannis, F.I.; Waldner, F.; Caccetta, P.; Wu, C. ResUNet-a: A deep learning framework for semantic segmentation of remotely sensed data. *ISPRS J. Photogramm. Remote Sens.* **2020**, *162*, 94–114. [CrossRef]

7. Badrinarayanan, V.; Kendall, A.; Cipolla, R. SegNet: A Deep Convolutional Encoder-Decoder Architecture for Image Segmentation. *IEEE Trans. Pattern Anal. Mach. Intell.* **2017**, *39*, 2481–2495. [CrossRef]
8. Ronneberger, O.; Fischer, P.; Brox, T. U-net: Convolutional networks for biomedical image segmentation. In *Medical Image Computing and Computer-Assisted Intervention*; Lecture Notes in Computer Science (Including subseries Lecture Notes in Artificial Intelligence and Lecture Notes in Bioinformatics); Springer: Cham, Switzerland, 2015; Volume 9351, pp. 234–241. [CrossRef]
9. Vázquez, D.; Bernal, J.; Sánchez, F.J.; Fernández-Esparrach, G.; López, A.M.; Romero, A.; Drozdzal, M.; Courville, A. A Benchmark for Endoluminal Scene Segmentation of Colonoscopy Images. *J. Healthc. Eng.* **2017**, *2017*, 4037190. [CrossRef]
10. Haj-Manouchehri, A.; Mohammadi, H.M. Polyp detection using CNNs in colonoscopy video. *IET Comput. Vis.* **2020**, *14*, 241–247. [CrossRef]
11. Hao, D.; Ding, S.; Qiu, L.; Lv, Y.; Fei, B.; Zhu, Y.; Qin, B. Sequential vessel segmentation via deep channel attention network. *Neural Netw.* **2020**, *128*, 172–187. [CrossRef]
12. Chung, M.; Lee, J.; Park, S.; Lee, C.E.; Lee, J.; Shin, Y.-G. Liver segmentation in abdominal CT images via auto-context neural network and self-supervised contour. *Artif. Intellingence Med.* **2021**, *113*, 102023. [CrossRef]
13. Jha, D.; Smedsrud, P.H.; Riegler, M.A.; Halvorsen, P.; de Lange, T.; Johansen, D.; Johansen, H.D. Kvasir-SEG: A Segmented Polyp Dataset. In *MultiMedia Modeling*; Springer: Cham, Switzerland, 2020; pp. 451–462. [CrossRef]
14. Aina, O.E.; Adeshina, S.A.; Aibinu, A.M. Deep learning for image-based cervical cancer detection and diagnosis—A survey. In Proceedings of the 2019 15th International Conference on Electronics, Computer and Computation, ICECCO 2019, Abuja, Nigeria, 10–12 December 2019. [CrossRef]
15. Zaiane, O.; Liu, X.; Zhao, D.; Li, W. A multi-kernel based framework for heterogeneous feature selection and over-sampling for computer-aided detection of pulmonary nodules. *Pattern Recognit.* **2017**, *64*, 327–346. [CrossRef]
16. Tajbakhsh, N.; Suzuki, K. Comparing two classes of end-to-end machine-learning models in lung nodule detection and classification: MTANNs vs. CNNs. *Pattern Recognit.* **2017**, *63*, 476–486. [CrossRef]
17. Gross, S.; Kennel, M.; Stehle, T.; Wulff, J.; Tischendorf, J.; Trautwein, C.; Aach, T. Polyp segmentation in NBI colonoscopy. In *Informatik Aktuell*; Springer: Berlin/Heidelberg, Germany, 2009; pp. 252–256. [CrossRef]
18. Karkanis, S.A.; Iakovidis, D.K.; Maroulis, D.E.; Karras, D.A.; Tzivras, M. Computer-Aided Tumor Detection in Endoscopic Video Using Color Wavelet Features. *IEEE Trans. Inf. Technol. Biomed.* **2003**, *7*, 141–152. [CrossRef]
19. Cong, Y.; Wang, S.; Liu, J.; Cao, J.; Yang, Y.; Luo, J. Deep sparse feature selection for computer aided endoscopy diagnosis. *Pattern Recognit.* **2015**, *48*, 907–917. [CrossRef]
20. Sánchez-González, A.; García-Zapirain, B.; Sierra-Sosa, D.; Elmaghraby, A. Automated colon polyp segmentation via contour region analysis. *Comput. Biol. Med.* **2018**, *100*, 152–164. [CrossRef]
21. Yao, J.; Li, J.; Summers, R.M. Employing topographical height map in colonic polyp measurement and false positive reduction. *Pattern Recognit.* **2009**, *42*, 1029–1040. [CrossRef]
22. Long, J.; Shelhamer, E.; Darrell, T. Fully convolutional networks for semantic segmentation. In Proceedings of the IEEE Computer Society Conference on Computer Vision and Pattern Recognition, Boston, MA, USA, 7–12 June 2015; pp. 3431–3440. [CrossRef]
23. Vaswani, A.; Shazeer, N.; Parmar, N.; Uszkoreit, J.; Jones, L.; Gomez, A.N.; Kaiser, Ł.; Polosukhin, I. Attention is all you need. *Adv. Neural Inf. Process. Syst.* **2017**, *2017*, 5999–6009.
24. Schlemper, J.; Oktay, O.; Schaap, M.; Heinrich, M.; Kainz, B.; Glocker, B.; Rueckert, D. Attention gated networks: Learning to leverage salient regions in medical images. *Med. Image Anal.* **2019**, *53*, 197–207. [CrossRef]
25. Thambawita, V.; Jha, D.; Riegler, M.; Halvorsen, P.; Hammer, H.L.; Johansen, H.D.; Johansen, D. The Medico-Task 2018: Disease detection in the gastrointestinal tract using global features and deep learning. *CEUR Workshop Proc.* **2018**, *2283*.
26. He, K.; Zhang, X.; Ren, S.; Sun, J. Deep residual learning for image recognition. In Proceedings of the IEEE Computer Society Conference on Computer Vision and Pattern Recognition, Las Vegas, NV, USA, 27–30 June 2016; pp. 770–778. [CrossRef]
27. Ioffe, S.; Szegedy, C. Batch normalization: Accelerating deep network training by reducing internal covariate shift. In Proceedings of the 32nd International Conference on Machine Learning, ICML 2015, Lille, France, 6–11 July 2015; Volume 1, pp. 448–456.
28. Bernal, J.; Sánchez, F.J.; Fernández-Esparrach, G.; Gil, D.; Rodríguez, C.; Vilariño, F. WM-DOVA maps for accurate polyp highlighting in colonoscopy: Validation vs. saliency maps from physicians. *Comput. Med. Imaging Graph.* **2015**, *43*, 99–111. [CrossRef]
29. Dong, H.; Supratak, A.; Mai, L.; Liu, F.; Oehmichen, A.; Yu, S.; Guo, Y. TensorLayer: A versatile library for efficient deep learning development. In Proceedings of the 2017 ACM Multimedia Conference, Mountain View, CA, USA, 23–27 October 2017; pp. 1201–1204. [CrossRef]
30. Keys, R. Cubic convolution interpolation for digital image processing. *IEEE Trans. Acoust.* **1981**, *29*, 1153–1160. [CrossRef]
31. Chen, L.C.; Papandreou, G.; Kokkinos, I.; Murphy, K.; Yuille, A.L. DeepLab: Semantic Image Segmentation with Deep Convolutional Nets, Atrous Convolution, and Fully Connected CRFs. *IEEE Trans. Pattern Anal. Mach. Intell.* **2018**, *40*, 834–848. [CrossRef]

Disclaimer/Publisher's Note: The statements, opinions and data contained in all publications are solely those of the individual author(s) and contributor(s) and not of MDPI and/or the editor(s). MDPI and/or the editor(s) disclaim responsibility for any injury to people or property resulting from any ideas, methods, instructions or products referred to in the content.

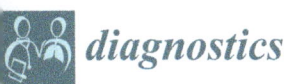

Article

A Multiscale Polyp Detection Approach for GI Tract Images Based on Improved DenseNet and Single-Shot Multibox Detector

Meryem Souaidi [1,*], Samira Lafraxo [1], Zakaria Kerkaou [1], Mohamed El Ansari [1,2] and Lahcen Koutti [1]

1. LABSIV, Computer Science, Faculty of Sciences, University Ibn Zohr, Agadir 80000, Morocco
2. Informatics and Applications Laboratory, Computer Science Department, Faculty of Sciences, University of Moulay Ismail, Meknès 50070, Morocco
* Correspondence: souaidi.meryem@gmail.com

Abstract: Small bowel polyps exhibit variations related to color, shape, morphology, texture, and size, as well as to the presence of artifacts, irregular polyp borders, and the low illumination condition inside the gastrointestinal GI tract. Recently, researchers developed many highly accurate polyp detection models based on one-stage or two-stage object detector algorithms for wireless capsule endoscopy (WCE) and colonoscopy images. However, their implementation requires a high computational power and memory resources, thus sacrificing speed for an improvement in precision. Although the single-shot multibox detector (SSD) proves its effectiveness in many medical imaging applications, its weak detection ability for small polyp regions persists due to the lack of information complementary between features of low- and high-level layers. The aim is to consecutively reuse feature maps between layers of the original SSD network. In this paper, we propose an innovative SSD model based on a redesigned version of a dense convolutional network (DenseNet) which emphasizes multiscale pyramidal feature maps interdependence called DC-SSDNet (densely connected single-shot multibox detector). The original backbone network VGG-16 of the SSD is replaced with a modified version of DenseNet. The DenseNet-46 front stem is improved to extract highly typical characteristics and contextual information, which improves the model's feature extraction ability. The DC-SSDNet architecture compresses unnecessary convolution layers of each dense block to reduce the CNN model complexity. Experimental results showed a remarkable improvement in the proposed DC-SSDNet to detect small polyp regions achieving an mAP of 93.96%, F1-score of 90.7%, and requiring less computational time.

Keywords: polyp; wireless capsule endoscopy images (WCE); single-shot multibox detector (SSD); image augmentation; multiscale DenseNet

Citation: Souaidi, M.; Lafraxo, S.; Kerkaou, Z.; El Ansari, M.; Koutti, L. A Multiscale Polyp Detection Approach for GI Tract Images Based on Improved DenseNet and Single-Shot Multibox Detector. *Diagnostics* **2023**, *13*, 733. https://doi.org/10.3390/diagnostics13040733

Academic Editors: Eun-Sun Kim and Kwang-Sig Lee

Received: 16 January 2023
Revised: 7 February 2023
Accepted: 9 February 2023
Published: 15 February 2023

Copyright: © 2023 by the authors. Licensee MDPI, Basel, Switzerland. This article is an open access article distributed under the terms and conditions of the Creative Commons Attribution (CC BY) license (https://creativecommons.org/licenses/by/4.0/).

1. Introduction

Recently, small bowel tumors have been the third leading cause of death in the word. Adenomatous polyps formed by glandular tissue are considered as one of the most common cases of colorectal cancer. Contrary to hyperplastic polyps, which have no malignant potential, adenomas are considered precancerous and can transform into malignant structures despite being benign tumors. The prevalence of this disease is expected to rise in the coming years [1]. For that reason, the endoscopic removal of benign and early malignant polyp regions in the GI tract in their early stage is required. Thus, doctors need a full direct visualization of the GI tract [2]. Wireless capsule endoscopy (WCE) is an advanced tool that revolutionizes the diagnosis technology [3]. It provides a feasible noninvasive method for detecting the entire gastrointestinal (GI) tract without pain and sedation compared with traditional colonoscopies. However, its short working time, low image resolution, and low frame rates restrict its wide application. In fact, the large quantity of data produced per examination per patient (approximation 55,000 images) is a laborious task for physicians to accurately locate the polyp regions in each WCE frame. An automated tumor detection technique is required to relieve specialists of the time-consuming task of reviewing the whole video before making a diagnosis. The presence of artifacts and complex characteristics (e.g., texture, shape, size, and morphology) inside the GI tract may hinder the detection process of polyp regions, as shown in Figure 1. As a result, small polyp regions are invisible to the naked eye, preventing doctors from identifying suspicious areas and manually locating polyp regions in each WCE frame. With the rise of artificial intelligence, deep learning (DL) frameworks, as opposed to handcrafted methods, have widely been investigated in medical image analysis due to their superior performance in image classification [4–6]. Many CAD systems have been proposed for polyp detection purposes to assist endoscopists by providing an automated tool that acquires some knowledge without requiring their physical attendance [7]. Therefore, they help clinicians to correctly determine the polyp frame's ground truth and make the correct decision by reducing human error. Some manuscripts aimed to automatically detect and localize polyp regions on both colonoscopy and capsule endoscopic images [8–10]. The lack of public and annotated datasets for polyp detection purpose is a common issue in the field. However, researchers use their own dataset, and the results may lack of subjectivity. According to their initiative, other studies on colonoscopy have used public data sets (e.g., the MICCAI 2015 subchallenge on automatic polyp detection in colonoscopy). Based on their architecture, preexisting cross-domain image object detectors are split into two categories: one-stage detectors, such as YOLO [11], SSD [12], etc., and two-stage detectors (R-CNNs [13] and their numerous variations (Faster R-CNN [14], R-FCN [15], etc.)). One-stage detectors are generally faster but less accurate. Even though speed-focused object detection research in medical image analysis runs in real time on high-end GPUs, a trade-off between precision and speed prevents SSD models from detecting small objects quickly. Even though it succeeds in keeping location information in shallow/deeper layers of the network, the SSD model's detector fails to preserve semantic information for small polyp regions. Two-stage detectors are typically more accurate but slower, and using a fixed receptive field limits deep learning's practical application in detecting small polyp regions. The main motivation of this work is to improve the performance of the polyp detection task in term of mean average precision (mAP) with less computational cost, using more powerful deep learning frameworks. Thence, a new SSD model is redesigned based on a modified version of DenseNet. The original backbone network, VGG16, is replaced by DenseNet-46, which can address the issue of high computational runs and overfitting during the optimization process. The redesigned DenseNet framework significantly reduces the number of model parameters while improving the backbone network's feature extraction capability. It can also capture more target information than VGG networks. The unnecessary convolution layers of each dense block are compressed to get significant increases in performance without increasing network complexity. The DenseNet-46 design reduces the number of layers used to speed up the run time while gaining significant precision, and the front stem is improved to enable the extraction of more powerful contextual information. Inspired by the DenseNet-S-32-1 [16], this manuscript presents a densely connected single-shot multibox detector (DC-SSDNet) for detecting small polyp regions in WCE and colonoscopy frames. To reach the main target, the proposed network takes advantage of the power architectural design of dense blocks to create an ultimate architecture that serves as the backbone of the SSD detector. It changes the traditional procedure of the shallow part of the VGG16 network's alternating convolutional and pooling layers with a couple of dense blocks and transition blocks. The DenseNet architecture tends to be very deep, and an effective DenseNet compression is essential for reaping all the benefits of dense blocks, consistent with the VGG16 architecture, to target the small polyp detection while retaining computational efficiency. As a result, an entire extraction of polyp patterns of various sizes within the same layer is possible while avoiding heavy parameter redundancy. The strategy of altering dense blocks and transition blocks is aimed at incorporating contextual and semantic information into deep networks and construct a multiscale feature map. Inspired by stacking-based models, the proposal adopts the SSD network structure [12]. The backbone pyramidal network is modified to reuse missed information. Moreover, we propose a new DenseNet network to optimize the SSD network's ability to improve small object feature extraction in the shallower network and to overcome scale variation limitations in detecting small polyp regions. Properly tuning the hyperparameters of the proposed DC-SSDNet, our experiments yield a higher mAP than the conventional SSD, with gains of 16.76, 17.74, and 16.74 points on the WCE, CVC-ClinicDB, and Etis-Larib datasets, respectively, with an enhancement of the speed–precision trade-off for the detection of small polyp regions.

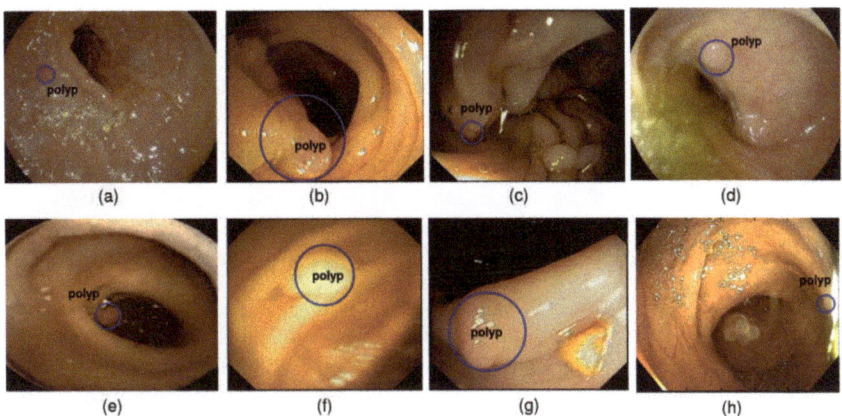

Figure 1. Examples of polyp image artifacts used in the current study. (**a**) Bubbles; (**b**) images with medical instruments; (**c**) white liquid and specular reflections; (**d**) cloudy liquid and specular reflections; (**e**) debris; (**f**) blurry images caused by different factors; (**g**) bile and specularity; (**h**) low contrast between polyp region and normal tissues.

The following are the primary contributions of this study:

1. The application of a modified version of DenseNet called DenseNet-46 as a backbone and smoothly adapted to the SSD detector to improve its ability for small polyp detection.
2. Based on the inception v4 stem part, the backbone DenseNet-46 front stem is improved, allowing the extraction of highly relevant features and contextual information.
3. To capture enough patterns and representative information, we increased the filter numbers of the first convolution layers in the stem part of the DenseNet-46 backbone from 32 to 64.
4. We omitted the unnecessary convolution layers of each dense block of the DenseNet-46 backbone to reduce the DC-SSDNet model's complexity and to achieve a faster speed while preserving a lesser computation time.
5. DC-SSDNet adds a couple of new dense and transition blocks to match the structure of SSD that detects targets in images using a single deep neural network.
6. DC-SSDNet introduces additional convolution layers to the multiscale feature pyramid, which is consistent with the traditional SSD.
7. The proposed model is trained from scratch.
8. We conducted several experiments on three well-known datasets in the field (WCE, CVC-ClinicDB, and Etis-Larib) to verify the DC-SSDNet model's effectiveness for a fair comparison with previously published methods of the literature.
9. This manuscript provides a thorough examination of the benefits and drawbacks of the proposed framework.

The rest of this paper is structured as follows: Section 2 contains references to related works. The proposed DC-SSDNet model is presented in detail in Section 3. The experimental results are reported and compared to those of other models in Section 4. Finally, Section 5 discusses the conclusions.

2. Literature Review

WCE images exhibit great variations in terms of size, shape, and morphology making the automated polyp detection process more difficult. Handcrafted features have been widely investigated, showing a significant progress for gastrointestinal classification tasks. A previous study [17] presented a model-based pyramid histogram for polyp classification using T-CWT and gamma. The major problem is the misunderstanding of biological mechanisms. They rely heavily on prior knowledge and have limited generalizability. Thus, handcrafted methods encode only a portion of the image and ignore the intrinsic data of the whole frame. They use low-level features created manually to describe the structures of regions that are not sufficiently robust to be applied for automatic polyp detection. Recently, the development of deep learning and powerful computing devices made the realization of deep CNNs (DCNNs) feasible. Several attempts have been made to use existing deep-learning frameworks to classify colonoscopy polyp abnormalities: VGGNet repeatedly stacked 3×3 convolution layers and 2×2 pooling layers to reach a maximum depth of 19 layers; GoogleNet [18] increased both the network depth and the width to enhance the feature representation by parallelly performing multiple convolution and pooling operations at each layer; and ResNet [19]. However, the vanishing-gradient problem always persists when training DCNNs. Inspired by the end-to-end frameworks for the polyp recognition task, Yuan et al. [16] used the most recent DenseNet model in 2019 as the basic model to directly calculate representative features from image information rather than using low-level handcrafted features to characterize the WCE image. Thus, they improved feature propagation through dense connections and significantly reduced the number of tuning while maintaining a high performance. The main proposal was to localize polyps in WCE/colonoscopy images by drawing a bounding box around the emphasis region, whereas polyp classification was a localization interstage conducted directly. In general, CNN-based methods are divided into two categories: the two-stage algorithms that generate region proposals as a first step and then classify them into different object categories (e.g., Faster R-CNN [20]), and the one-stage algorithms based on regression (e.g., YOLO [21] and SSD [22]). The Faster R-CNN [20] and R-FCN [23]) proposed anchors for different scales using a one-scale feature map. However, they failed to detect multiscale objects of small sizes. The FPN [24] and DSSD [25] methods used bottom-up and top-down frameworks, respectively; however, using the layer-by-layer feature map fusion results slowed the detection process. As a solution, the conventional SSD [12] made predictions by utilizing the feature of shallower layers and scaling them from the bottom to the top to generate a new pyramidal feature map. In this context, a two-stage framework based on deep learning was presented by Jia et al. [26] for automatic polyp recognition in colonoscopy images. The authors of [27] presented a modified version of the mask R-CNN model for performing polyp detection and for segmentation purposes. TASHK et al. [28] proposed an improved version of the CNN algorithm based on DRLSE to automatically locate polyps within a frame. However, two-stage algorithms sacrifice speed for a high-performing localization and object recognition performance. Thus, they hardly meet the real-time requirements of polyp detection. Oppositely, the one-stage algorithms achieve a high inference speed by ignoring the region proposal step and using the predicted boxes directly from the input images. To detect polyps in colonoscopy videos, Liu et al. [29] investigated the potential of the ResNet50 and VGG16 frameworks used as a backbone to propose a new architecture-based single-shot detector (SSD). However, the traditional SSD using the VGG16 network as a backbone repeatedly stacks convolution and pooling layers, and its feature extraction ability is inefficient due to its use of only 1×1 and 3×3 convolution kernels. Improving the polyp detection process necessitates a robust backbone (such as DenseNets [30]). Regarding the advantages of you only look once (YOLO) algorithms in real-time detection speed at the expense of precision, they eliminate a preprocessing step to obtain an ROI and abandon the process of proposal generation. Misawa et al. [31] presented a YOLOv3-based polyp detection system that achieved real-time detection with greater than 90% sensitivity and specificity. However, the spatial constraints of the algorithm limited it to perform with small regions within the image. Researchers made many efforts based on SSD algorithms to tackle the limitations of small polyp detection and localization. In this context, the authors of [32] proposed a rainbow SSD-based method. It applied a simple concatenation and deconvolution operation of feature maps produced from SSD layers. Zhang et al. [33] presented an SSD-GPNet-model-based SSD network by combining feature maps of the low level with the deconvolution of high-level feature maps. However, adding deconvolution layers increased the computational complexity of the SSD architectures at the expense of speed, even if it improved the performance of small polyp region detection. Regarding the success of DenseNet frameworks in many fields, Zhai et al. [16] presented an improved SSD network that used the residual prediction block and switched the network backbone to DenseNet. They then used a multiscale feature layer fusion mechanism to reinforce the relationships between the levels in the feature pyramid. However, it exhibited a decrease in detection speed by using a complex network and adding complicated feature fusion modules. To extract more semantic information while keeping the detection speed constant, we propose a densely connected single-shot detector called DC-SSDNet. The characteristic ramification of the feature maps within the same block would become quite beneficial if the purpose was to reuse them to perform stacked dense and transition blocks with the capacity of the SSD network to be more compact while going deeper. A typical compression method of a network's feature maps is to remove unnecessary layers by reducing parameter dimensions. Concretely, there is no need for feature extraction enhancement using a lightweight feature fusion of shallower and deeper layers due to the power of dense networks for capturing more representative patterns and reassembling contextual and semantic information. Indeed, meeting the requirements of a detection process involves the reduction of the model complexity while preserving a high detection speed. Thus, clinical applications require a real-time detection and promising precision [34].

3. Proposed Method

Figure 2 depicts the network structure of DC-SSDNet for the polyp detection task. A redesigned SSD-detector-based compact DenseNet-46 network used as a backbone is proposed to strengthen the network detection ability. The conventional SSD with the VGG16 as a backbone fails to preserve contextual information in the multilayer transmission process. Therefore, unbalanced feature maps appear at each layer. To reuse the rich object information of low-level layers and incorporate it with high-level layers, DC-SSDNet splits the network structure into two sections: a compact version of DenseNet (a DenseNet-46 network as a backbone) for feature reuse and extraction and the front-end network to perform multiscale object detection. Firstly, a preprocessing step is performed to remove the black regions in the WCE images and keep only useful information. Then, a data augmentation strategy is investigated to handle overfitting in deep learning models due to the data insufficiency problem. The model input size is 299×299. For object classification and location regression, the conventional SSD model selects VGG-16 layers Conv4_3 and Conv_7 and adds new ones Conv8_2, Conv9_2, Conv10_2, and Conv11_2. Consistent with the SSD network, we construct a multiscale feature pyramid under the premise of maximizing the use of synthetic information from all feature layers and improving precision without sacrificing speed. To improve the model's detection ability, we use our own multiscale feature pyramid Dense_C1, Dense_C2, Dense_C3, Dense_C4, Dense_C5, and Dense_C6. The main parts of the DC-SSDNet detector are described in detail below.

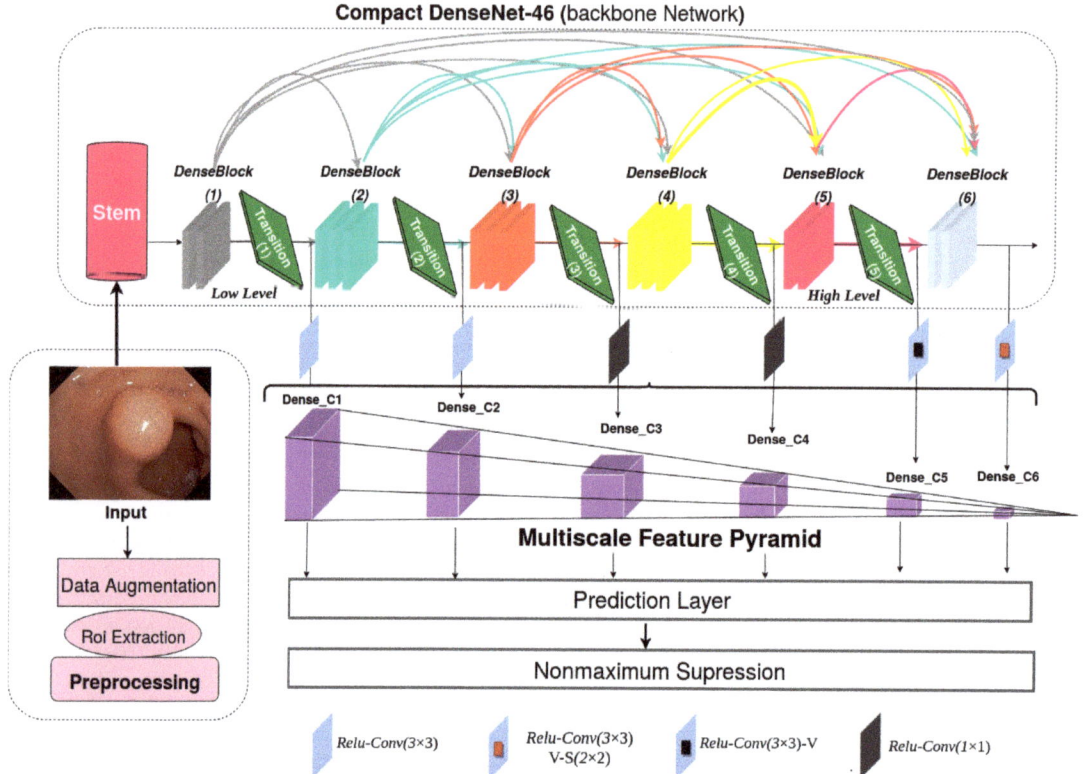

Figure 2. Architecture of the proposed densely connected single shot multibox detector (DC-SSDNet).

3.1. Compact DenseNet-46

A deep CNN uses many repeated convolution layers resulting in the bottom-level features being destroyed. Many medical imaging applications utilize DenseNet to improve precision caused by the vanishing gradient in high-level neural networks. DenseNet reuses some not-useful redundant information to concatenate the high-level features with the residual sparse low-level ones, even if it does not propagate them effectively. In this paper, we propose a compact DenseNet-46 as a backbone network of DC-SSDNet by applying certain modifications to DenseNet. Table 1 depicts the main structure based on the number of layers. DenseNet-46 use the feature maps from all previous layers as input in the next layer to alleviate the lack of region location information of high-level features, as depicted in Table 1. Despite the success of deep DenseNets applications in many fields, we believe that using this network directly as an ultimate SSD backbone is probably not going to be an effective solution for small polyp detection. Compared to other deep DenseNet versions, the compact DenseNet-46 compresses some repeated dense connections in each dense block to allow fewer feature propagations and reduce the destruction of low-level features. Compressing each block's unnecessary convolution layers, the compact DenseNet-46 avoids generating more redundant information, preventing the small polyp's features from being submerged, and reducing the system's complexity. Unlike the commonly used structure in the DenseNet model design, the backbone network consists of a stem block and six phases of dense and transition blocks. Only the sixth phase does not use a transition block.

Table 1. Compact DenseNet-46 architecture (growth rate k = 32) in each dense block.

Phase	Layer	Setting	Output Size (Input 299 × 299 × 3)
	Stem block		75 × 75 × 96
Phase 1	Dense block (1)	$\begin{pmatrix} 1 \times 1 & Conv \\ 3 \times 3 & Conv\lfloor Pad - Valid \rfloor \end{pmatrix} \times 2$	75 × 75 × 160
	Transition block (1)	$1 \times 1 \quad Conv\lfloor Pad - valid \rfloor$	75 × 75 × 160
		$2 \times 2 \quad AveragePool\lfloor stride2 \rfloor$	38 × 38 × 160
Phase 2	Dense block (2)	$\begin{pmatrix} 1 \times 1 & Conv \\ 3 \times 3 & Conv\lfloor Pad - Valid \rfloor \end{pmatrix} \times 3$	38 × 38 × 256
	Transition block (2)	$1 \times 1 \quad Conv\lfloor Pad - valid \rfloor$	38 × 38 × 256
		$2 \times 2 \quad AveragePool\lfloor stride2 \rfloor$	19 × 19 × 256
Phase 3	Dense block (3)	$\begin{pmatrix} 1 \times 1 & Conv \\ 3 \times 3 & Conv\lfloor Pad - Valid \rfloor \end{pmatrix} \times 3$	19 × 19 × 352
	Transition block (3)	$1 \times 1 \quad Conv\lfloor Pad - valid \rfloor$	19 × 19 × 352
		$2 \times 2 \quad AveragePool\lfloor stride2 \rfloor$	10 × 10 × 352
Phase 4	Dense block (4)	$\begin{pmatrix} 1 \times 1 & Conv \\ 3 \times 3 & Conv\lfloor Pad - Valid \rfloor \end{pmatrix} \times 3$	10 × 10 × 448
	Transition block (4)	$1 \times 1 \quad Conv\lfloor Pad - valid \rfloor$	10 × 10 × 448
		$2 \times 2 \quad AveragePool\lfloor stride2 \rfloor$	5 × 5 × 448
Phase 5	Dense block (5)	$\begin{pmatrix} 1 \times 1 & Conv \\ 3 \times 3 & Conv\lfloor Pad - Valid \rfloor \end{pmatrix} \times 2$	5 × 5 × 512
	Transition block (5)	$1 \times 1 \quad Conv\lfloor Pad - valid \rfloor$	5 × 5 × 512
		$2 \times 2 \quad AveragePool\lfloor stride2 \rfloor$	3 × 3 × 512
Phase-6	Dense block (6)	$\begin{pmatrix} 1 \times 1 & Conv \\ 3 \times 3 & Conv\lfloor Pad - Valid \rfloor \end{pmatrix} \times 2$	3 × 3 × 576

3.1.1. Stem Block

The motivation behind the DenseNet-46 stem block design originates from the considerable success of the Inception-v4 structure [35] in small polyp detection. It is designed in the same manner before the first dense block, as depicted in Figure 3. Experimentally, the DenseNet-46 stem block can slightly reduce the information loss from input frames compared with the conventional structure of DenseNet, which includes a 7 × 7 convolutional layer and a 3 × 3 max pooling before the first dense block. The redesigned stem block can also reinforce the DC-SSDNet network's ability for feature extraction with less computational cost. However, the DenseNet-46 stem block structure excerpted from the asymmetric convolution kernel structure used in Inception-v4 reduces the model complexity while maintaining a small loss of feature information.

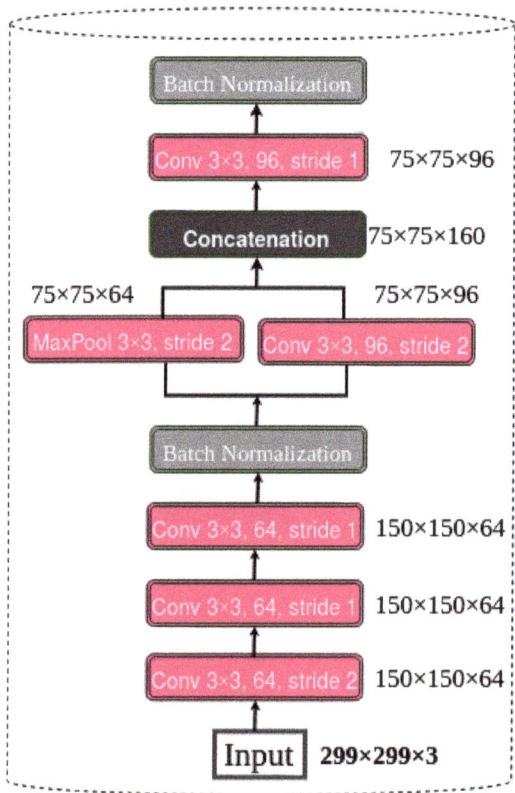

Figure 3. Structure of stem block.

3.1.2. Dense Block

The dense block is the basic unit of the compact DenseNet-46 structure, as shown in Figure 4. We denote the feature maps of the K − 1 layer as $m \times n \times p_0$, where m and n represent the width and height of feature maps, and p_0 means the number of channels. R(·) represents a nonlinear transformation consisting of a rectified linear unit (Relu) as an activation function, a 1 × 1 convolution layer, and a 3 × 3 convolution layer. It changes the number of channels to k (k = 32) without altering the size of the feature maps. To reduce the number of channels, we used the 1 × 1 convolution operation, and we adopted the 3 × 3 convolution operation for feature restructuring and to improve the network performance. Each dense block reduces the redundancy of dense connectivity represented by the long dashed arrow, in which feature maps of the K − 1 layer are connected directly to those of the K layer and then make a concatenation with the output of R(·), thus resulting in $m \times n \times (p_0 + p)$. The output of the K + 1 layer is $m \times n \times (p_0 + 2p)$. Previous studies based on DenseNet used a fixed number of dense blocks (4 dense blocks in all DenseNet architectures) to keep the same scale of outputs. They also added new layers to each DenseNet network's dense blocks to increase framework depth. A connectivity increase may decrease network performance due to contextual and semantic information redundancy. For this reason, the proposed DenseNet-46 backbone structure adds two additional dense blocks to increase the network depth rather than increasing the connections of each dense block. The DenseNet-46 backbone structure used in this work has two base blocks in dense blocks (1), three in dense blocks (2), three in dense blocks (3), three in dense blocks (4), two in dense blocks (5), and two in dense blocks (6).

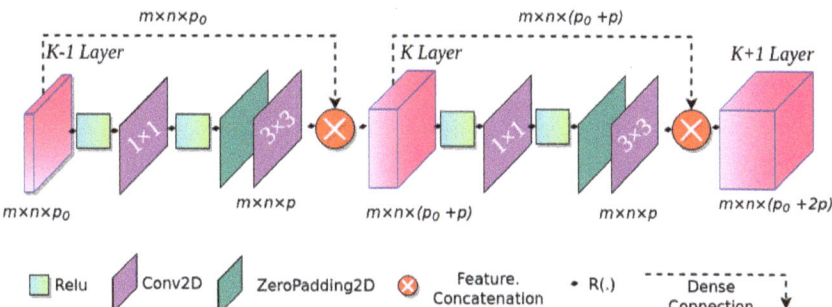

Figure 4. Structure of dense block.

3.1.3. Transition Block

After several dense connections, the number of feature maps of the DenseNet-46 grows dramatically. Consistent with the original DenseNet, we designed transition layer blocks to reduce the dimension of previous dense blocks' features, as depicted in Figure 5. The transition block includes a 1×1 convolution layer with valid padding to reduce the number of channels of the previous layers. Then, it performs a 2×2 average pooling layer to decrease half of the feature map sizes. In the last phase, the transition block is not used to not reduce the final feature map resolution for further modification related to the SSD output requirements.

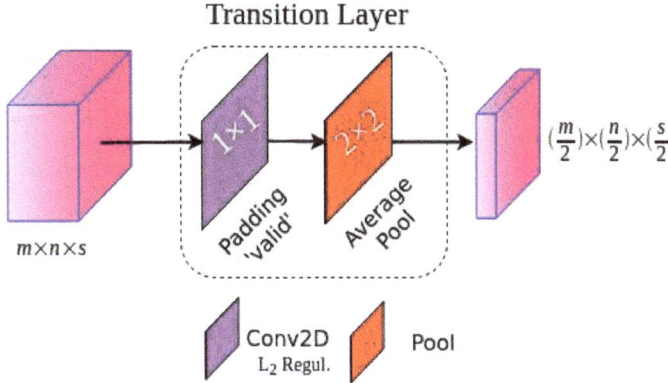

Figure 5. Structure of transition block.

3.1.4. Growth Rate

Table 1 shows the details of the compact DenseNet-46 backbone. The growth rate of the DenseNet denoted as 'k' is referred to as the number of 3×3 convolution kernels in each dense block. It changes the number of channels of the input feature maps in each dense block. Since each dense block is concatenating to its previous ones, the succeeding layer channels grow by k after each dense block. The number of base blocks in the dense block, which consists of 4k 1×1 convolutions and 1k 3×3 convolutions, varies depending on the dense block location. It is well known an increase in growth rate gives good performance due to the large amount of information circulating in the network. This assumption is not always verified as it depends on the context environment, and the system complexity will also increase. In the DenseNet-64 base model used in this proposal, we utilized three settings: k = 16, k = 32, and k = 48. The growth rate choice was validated experimentally.

3.2. Multiscale Feature Pyramid Network

Several feature layers (Conv6_2, Conv7_2, Conv8_2, and Conv9_2) are added to the original SSD via the base network's end (VGG16) for object classification and location regression from multiple feature maps at different depths. Inspired by the pyramidal feature hierarchy, the proposed approach adopts the SSD network structure [12]. However, the original backbone network VGG-16 of SSD is replaced with DenseNet-46 to enhance the feature extraction ability of the SSD model and address the problem of scale variations in detecting small polyp regions. The DC SSDNet network uses the output of each transition block as the input of the multiscale feature pyramidal except for the sixth phase, to keep the final feature map resolution not reduced. Convolutional layers are used to perform pyramidal feature maps for small polyp detection but with different configurations. Consistent with the SSD model, the final feature layers have target sizes of 38×38, 19×19, 10×10, 5×5, 3×3, and 1×1.

4. Experiments

4.1. Datasets and Experimental Environments

The WCE dataset is from PillCam©COLON 2 polyps [36]. It consists of 120 polyps and 181 normals images collected from one patient's VCE test with a resolution of 256 pixels × 256 pixels, as shown in Figure 6. A preprocessing stage was performed to avoid overfitting and increase the training dataset size. Hence, the regenerated dataset comprised 1250 polyp patches and 1864 normal ones. Two highly qualified experts manually labeled and annotated frames as positive and negative samples. To provide ground truths, they defined binary masks corresponding to the polyp regions covered. To meet the needs of polyp detection tools, the bounding boxes of polyp regions were delimited using the specialists' ground-truth mask using a graphical image annotation tool to label objects' bounding boxes in images (LabelImg). Then, experts corrected them. The second dataset was the popular CVC-ClinicDB [37]. In this regard, researchers reviewed 25 colonoscopy videos to choose at least 29 sequences with at least one polyp region and selected a set of frames for each of them. The CVC-ClinicDB dataset contains 612 polyp images with a resolution of 384 × 288. The specialists manually defined masks for the polyp-covered regions in each image to provide the ground truths. Then, they were drawn based on the ground truth provided by the specialists using advanced medical annotation tools. To confirm the proposed model's credibility, we used the annotated ETIS-Larib dataset [38] in which 34 colonoscopy videos produced 196 polyp images of various shapes and sizes, as shown in Figure 6. Skilled experts annotate the ETIS-Larib dataset ground truths. The colonoscopy images were from the MICCAI 2015 subchallenge on the automatic polyp detection task. Polyps' images were rescaled to 299 × 299 pixels. We divided the data into 70% for training, 10% for validation, and 20% for model testing. We employed a fivefold cross-validation to validate the model's state and convergence after each epoch. The validation data step automatically adjusted the iterations and the learning rate. The model adopted a validation set according to the five group performances in the models. Finally, the performances were averaged across the splits to calculate the mean average precision measure.

In this study, we performed the training and testing phases using the Colab Pro Plus solution provided by Google, with a maximum RAM of 52 Gb and a disk of 166.83 Gb. The CUDA 8.0.61-1, CuDNN6.0, Keras 2.1.0, Python 3.7, protobuf 3.20.*, h5py 2.10.0, NumPy 1.16.3, TensorFlow 1.14, TensorFlow-GPU 1.14, OpenCV-python, scikit-learn, scikit-image, tqdm, beautifulsoup4, lxml, html5lib, bs4, ipykernel, and OpenCV 3.1 packages were used to implement the algorithm. For all used datasets, an aspect ratio between one and two was adopted depending on the small polyp regions' true bounding boxes.

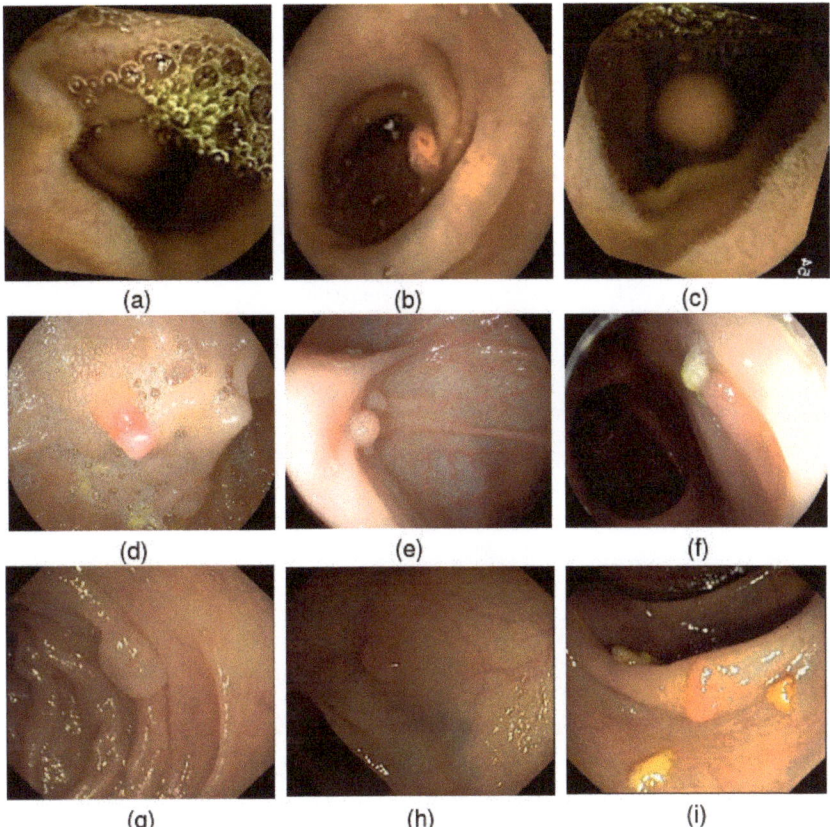

Figure 6. Example of samples: (**a–c**) WCE polyp images; (**d–f**) Etis-Larib polyp images; (**g–i**) CVC-ClinicDB polyp images.

4.2. Training

Many training hyperparameters were adjusted to strengthen the DC-SSDNet capability for detecting polyp abnormalities in WCE and colonoscopy frames as shown in Table 2. The presence of black regions in WCE images may impair detection performance and lengthen computation time. Hence, the original capsule endoscopy image was reduced to a center square-shaped image in the peripheral area as a first preprocessing step in order to remove unwanted black regions. We used a batch size of 32 and rescaled the input images to (299 × 299 × 3). The model employed 100 training epochs and 500 steps per epoch. The motivation behind the data augmentation was a lack of data for the WCE classification and detection tasks. Moreover, data access was tightly restricted owing to privacy concerns. In this regard, we applied popular augmentation methods used in recent studies [10,35]. We applied geometric methods which altered the geometry of the resulted region-of-interest (ROI) image as a second preprocessing step, by mapping the individual pixel values to new destinations. To perform data augmentation techniques, the flipping approach was examined in order to mirror the ROI WCE frames across their vertical and horizontal axes at first, then across both in the second pass. Finally, we rotated the ROI WCE images by 270° about their center, as shown in Figure 7.

Table 2. Hyperparameter settings of the densely connected single-shot multibox detector (DC-SSDNet).

Hyperparameters	Values
Optimizer	Adam
beta_1	0.9
beta_2	0.999
epsilon	1×10^{-8}
Initial learning rate	0.0001
Learning rate decay drop factor	0.5
Epoch drop factor	10
Learning rate	epoch < 80: 0.0001 epoch < 100: 0.00001 0.000001 otherwise
α parameter	1
neg_pos_ratio	3
Batch size	32
Training epochs	100
Steps per epoch	500
Aspect ratio	1–2

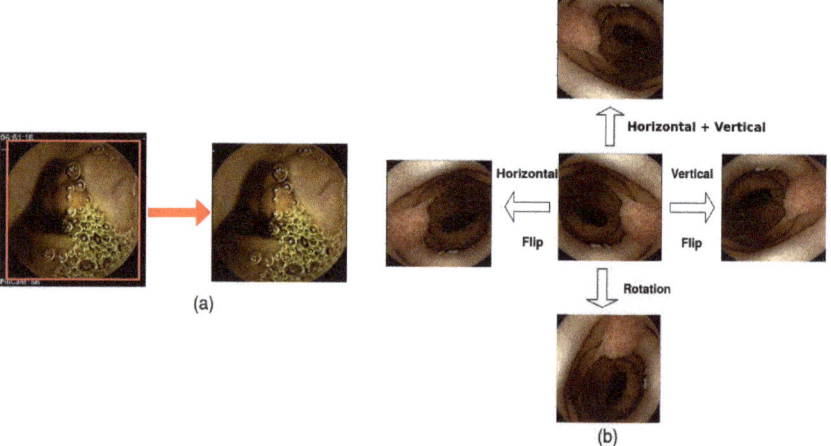

Figure 7. A flow-chart of the preprocessing steps: (**a**) acquiring the region of interest (ROI) of the WCE polyp image (**b**); sample of image from the WCE dataset with geometric transformation.

We trained the proposed model from scratch to not rely on any model pretrained on classification tasks to initialize the network, as commonly known visual purposes of classification and detection are distinct. For training DC-SSDNet, we used adaptive moment estimation (Adam) as the optimizer (beta_1 of 0.9, beta_2 of 0.999, and an epsilon of 1×10^{-8}). The learning rate was initially set to 0.0001, and the learning rate decay policy differed slightly from the original SSD with a drop of 0.5 and an epoch drop of 10, which allowed the network to converge by controlling its learning rate. If the epoch number was less than 80, the learning rate was 0.0001, 0.00001 if the epoch number was less than 100, and 0.000001 otherwise. Recent state-of-the-art approaches targeting polyp detection were investigated in this study to compare them with the proposed model [10]. We used a loss function consistent with that used in the traditional SSD [12]. The cross-validation method adjusted the α parameter to one and the neg_pos_ratio to three. More information about SSD_Loss can be found in [16]. The proposal evaluated the detection performance with the most used metrics in the field, the mean average precision (mAP), the number of frames per second (FPS), and other indicators.

4.3. Evaluation Indexes

This study evaluated polyp detection performance using the mean average precision (mAP) and frames per second (FPS), which are well-known in target object detection. The mAP represents the average of all object categories' average precision (AP), expressed as:

$$mAP = \frac{\sum_{s=1}^{S} AveP(s)}{S} \quad (1)$$

where S denotes the number of queries in the set and s denotes the average precision query.

The precision indicator represents a measure of exactness and the recall a measure of completeness. The expected overlap between the ground-truth bounding box annotated by the experts and the predicted one produced by the network expresses the intersection over union (IoU). The following equations formulate the precision, recall, and F1-score indicators as follows:

$$Precision = \frac{TP}{TP+FP} \quad Recall = \frac{TP}{TP+FN} \quad (2)$$

$$F-measure/F1-score = \frac{(2 \times Recall \times Precision)}{Recall + Precision} \quad (3)$$

where TP represents the true positives with an IoU greater than 0.5, FP represents the false positives, and FN represents the false negatives. The frames per second (FPS) metric measures the detection speed and denotes the number of frames sent per second. A detailed evaluation metric of the model's performance is provided in the work of [10].

4.4. Results and Discussion

4.4.1. Ablation Studies

On the WCE, CVC-ClinicDB, and ETIS-Larib colonoscopy datasets, we performed an ablation study to investigate the impact of each component of the DC-SSDNet detector on performance. Table 3 shows different model settings using the compact DenseNet-46 as a backbone, where the training was conducted on the WCE images, the CVC-ClinicDB+ETIS-Larib joint training sets, and tested on the WCE, CVC-ClinicDB, and ETIS-Larib test sets. Using three values of the growth rate K, the performance was 81.96% when K = 16 and improved to 85.41% mAP at K = 32. The use of a small growth rate produced better results for K = 32, and a larger K = 48 could also provide a better model performance according to the DF-SSD as it showed a smaller mean AP of 84.54% than K = 32. It is highly recommended not to set a higher growth rate to reduce network complexity and computing costs. The growth rate of DC-SSDNet was set to 32. Table 3 demonstrates that the stem block improved the model's mAP performance by 7.78% (89.74% vs. 81.96%) at K = 16, 8.55% (93.96% vs. 85.41%) at K = 32, and 7.08% (91.62% vs. 84.54%) at K = 48 on the WCE dataset. The results proved the relative importance of stem blocks in preserving information in the original input image and contributing to small polyp detection. Then, we evaluated transition pooling techniques (average pooling and max pooling) and report their influence on the proposed system's performance mAP (%). We can see from Table 3 that an average pooling on the WCE test set obtained a higher mAP of 93.96% compared with max pooling (90.56% mAP) using the stem block at K = 32. Consistent with the traditional DenseNet, we used the average pooling layer to decrease the resolution of the feature maps. As reported in Table 3 (row 5, row 6, and row 8), without batch normalization for each conv layer, the proposed approach obtained better results (mAP of 85.41%, 90.56%, and 93.96%) at K = 32, whereas the mAP was 83.54% and 84.97% when utilizing batch normalization on the WCE training and test sets at K = 32 and K = 48, respectively. The ETIS-Larib and CVC-ClinicDB test sets in Table 3 (rows 11–20 and 21–30) complement the WCE image results and illustrate the efficacy of the stem block and growth rate parameters in emphasizing more salient aspects for small polyp identification.

Table 3. Results of an ablation study on the WCE and colonoscopy datasets. BN denotes the addition of a batch normalization layer to each convolution layer. K refers to the growth rate. The stem block represents the front layers of the DenseNet-46 backbone. The transition pool is either an average pooling layer or a max pooling layer. The mAP represents the mean average precision on the WCE, Etis-Larib, and CVC-ClinicDB test sets.

Training Data	Test Data	Stem Block	K	BN	Transition Pool	mAP (%)
WCE	WCE	×	16	×	Average	81.96
		×	32	✓	Max	83.54
		✓	48	✓	Average	91.62
		×	48	✓	Max	84.97
		×	32	×	Average	85.41
		✓	32	×	Max	90.56
		✓	16	×	Max	88.16
		✓	32	×	Average	**93.96**
		✓	16	×	Average	89.74
		×	48	×	Average	84.54
CVC-ClinicDB joint Etis-Larib	CVC-CLinicDB	×	16	×	Average	80.68
		×	32		Max	81.32
		✓	48	✓	Average	89.22
		×	48	✓	Max	83.14
		×	32	×	Average	83.75
		✓	32	×	Max	88.09
		✓	16	×	Max	87.09
		✓	32	×	Average	**92.24**
		✓	16	×	Average	89.36
		×	48	×	Average	84.77
CVC-ClinicDB joint Etis-Larib	Etis-Larib	×	16	×	Average	79.98
		×	32	✓	Max	81
		✓	48	✓	Average	89.46
		×	48	✓	Max	83.98
		×	32	×	Average	84.52
		✓	32	×	Max	87.55
		✓	16	×	Max	87.14
		✓	32	×	Average	**90.86**
		✓	16	×	Average	89.34
		×	48	×	Average	82.72

4.4.2. SSD Results on WCE and Colonoscopy Datasets

We trained the detector-based SSDs on the WCE, CVC-ClinicDB, and ETIS-Larib combined training set and tested on each dataset separately as depicted from Tables 4 and 5. SSD300 with VGG16 (as a backbone) showed that the WCE, CVC-ClinicDB, and ETIS-Larib test sets had mAPs of 77.2%, 74.5%, and 74.22%, respectively. Tables 4 and 5 (rows 5–6) prove that the FSSD300 and FSSD500 models showed gains of 12.58% and 9.25%, 12.76% and 9.16%, and 12.18% and 11.47% in terms of mAP compared to the original SSD. DenseNet-S-32-1 replaces VGGNet as the backbone network on the DF-SSD300. Thus, for the WCE, CVC-CLinicDB, and Etis-Larib data sets, it outperformed the FSSD300 model by 1.46%, 2.66%, and 0.54% for the mAP with 91.24% vs. 89.78%, 89.92% vs. 87.26%, and 86.84% vs. 86.3%, respectively. To incorporate contextual and semantic information, the L_SSD model in Tables 4 and 5 (row 8) replaced the VGG16 network with the ResNet-101 backbone showing an improvement in terms of mAP compared to the FSSD model for all employed datasets. The DF-SSD300 algorithm outperformed the L_SSD algorithm in terms of mAP with a gain of 1.26 points (91.24 % vs. 89.98%), 1.74 points (89.92 % vs. 88.18%) on the WCE and CVC-ClinicDB test sets, respectively, due to the power of DenseNet in feature reuse and extraction abilities. However, it showed a slight drop in mAP on the Etis-Larib test set. The proposed DC-SSDNet model surpassed the DF-SSD300, MP-FSSD, and Hyb-SSDNet networks by 2.72 points (93.96% vs. 91.24%), 0.56 points (93.96% vs. 93.4%), and

0.67 points (93.96% vs. 93.29%) on the WCE dataset. The DC-SSDNet framework achieved a 32.5 FPS real-time detection, compared to 11.6 FPS, 17.4 FPS, and 40 FPS for the DF-SSD300, DSOD300, and L-SSD, respectively.

Table 4. SSD comparison with previously reported approaches based on the WCE test set. Pretrain denotes a pretrained backbone to initialize the model, as opposed to starting from scratch. The Google Colab pro+ GPU was used to assess the speed (FPS) and performance (mAP).

Training Data	Methods	Backbone	Input Size	Pretrain	FPS	mAP@0.5 (%)
WCE	SSD300	VGG16	$300 \times 300 \times 3$	✓	46	77.2
	SSD300	ResNet-101	$300 \times 300 \times 3$	✓	47.3	81.65
	SSD500	VGG16	$300 \times 300 \times 3$	✓	19	79.45
	SSD500	ResNet-101	$300 \times 300 \times 3$	✓	20	84.95
	FSSD300	VGG16	$300 \times 300 \times 3$	✓	65.9	89.78
	FSSD500	VGG16	$500 \times 500 \times 3$	✓	69.6	88.71
	DF-SSD300 [16]	DenseNet-S-32-1	$300 \times 300 \times 3$	✗	11.6	91.24
	L_SSD [39]	ResNet-101	$224 \times 224 \times 3$	✓	40	89.98
	MP-FSSD [10]	VGG16	$300 \times 300 \times 3$	✓	62.57	93.4
	Hyb-SSDNet [35]	Inception v4	$299 \times 299 \times 3$	✓	44.5	93.29
	DSOD300 [40]	DS/64-192-48-1	$300 \times 300 \times 3$	✗	17.4	91.70
	DC-SSDNet (ours)	DenseNet-46	$299 \times 299 \times 3$	✗	32.5	**93.96**

Table 5. SSD comparison with previously reported approaches based on CVC-ClinicDB and Etis-Larib test sets. Pretrain denotes a pretrained backbone to initialize the model, as opposed to starting from scratch. The Google Colab pro+ GPU was used to assess the speed (FPS) and performance (mAP).

Training Data	Methods	Backbone	Input Size	Pretrain	FPS	mAP@0.5 (%)	
						CVC-ClinicDB	ETIS-Larib
CVC-ClinicDB joint ETIS-Larib	SSD300	VGG16	$300 \times 300 \times 3$	✓	46	74.5	74.12
	SSD300	ResNet-101	$300 \times 300 \times 3$	✓	47.3	78.85	75.73
	SSD500	VGG16	$500 \times 500 \times 3$	✓	19	78.38	75.45
	SSD500	ResNet-101	$500 \times 500 \times 3$	✓	20	82.74	80.14
	FSSD300	VGG16	$300 \times 300 \times 3$	✓	65.9	87.26	86.3
	FSSD500	VGG16	$500 \times 500 \times 3$	✓	69.6	87.54	86.92
	DF-SSD300 [16]	DenseNet-S-32-1	$300 \times 300 \times 3$	✗	11.6	89.92	86.84
	L_SSD [39]	ResNet-101	$224 \times 224 \times 3$	✓	40	88.18	87.23
	MP-FSSD [10]	VGG16	$300 \times 300 \times 3$	✓	62.57	89.82	90
	Hyb-SSDNet [35]	Inception v4	$299 \times 299 \times 3$	✓	44.5	91.93	91.10
	DSOD300 [40]	DS/64-192-48-1	$300 \times 300 \times 3$	✗	17.4	90	89.3
	DC-SSDNet (ours)	DenseNet-46	$299 \times 299 \times 3$	✗	32.5	**92.24**	**90.86**

4.4.3. Comparison with Existing Detection Methods

We compared the performance of the proposed DC-SSDNet approach to the most prominent networks in the literature-based SSDs models, YOLOv3 and Faster R-CNN, as shown in Table 6. For further comparing DC-SSDNet with previous studies' target polyp detection, we trained the model on the joint ETIS-Larib and CVC-ClinicDB training sets and evaluated it on the publicly accessible ETIS-Larib dataset. The DC-SSDNet model achieved promising results or similar metrics in the worst cases on the three employed test sets compared to other state-of-art approaches. One of the main reasons for the difference in results was that the nature, texture, and lighting conditions of the WCE and colonoscopy images change inside the GI tract. Following a series of improvements to the initial SSD model, DC-SSDNet achieved an mAP of 93.96% utilizing only the WCE for both training and test sets, and outperforming other methods on the CVC-ClinicDB and Etis-Larib test sets by 92.24% and 90.86%, respectively. Due to the fact the WCE images were gathered from a single patient's VCE test, and CVC-ClinicDB images were acquired from 25 colonoscopy recordings to choose at least 29 sequences with at least one polyp area and a series of frames for each of them, even if the WCE was accurately divided into training, validation, and testing sets, there would be some overlap. As a result, the network might have been familiar with certain hard cases. Moreover, it showed superior performance compared to the YOLOv3 model [21] and close to that of Hyb-SSDNet [35]. DC-SSDNet yielded good results in terms of mAP while maintaining the computational cost and a small speed drop.

Table 6. Results of the WCE or the colonoscopy test with an IoU greater than 0.5 and a batch size of 1.

Training Dataset	Methods	Testing Dataset	Backbone Network	Pretrain	Input Size	Prec (%)	Recall (%)	F1 Score (%)
WCE	DC-SSDNet (ours)	WCE	DenseNet-46	×	299 × 299	93.96%	90.82%	90.7%
CVC-ClinicDB + ETIS-Larib	DC-SSDNet (ours)	CVC-ClinicDB	DenseNet-46	×	299 × 299	92.24%	91%	88.40%
CVC-ClinicDB + ETIS-Larib	DC-SSDNet (ours)	ETIS-Larib	DenseNet-46	×	299 × 299	90.86%	90.4%	89.12%
CVC-ClinicDB + ETIS-Larib	Shin et al., 2018 [2]	ETIS-Larib	Inception ResNet	✓	768 × 576	92.2%	69.7%	79.4%
ETIS-Larib+CVC-ClinicDB	Souaidi et al., 2022 [35]	ETIS-Larib	Inception v4	✓	299 × 299	91.10%	87%	89%
SUN+ PICCOLO+ CVC-ClinicDB	Ishak et al., 2021 [21]	ETIS-Larib	YOLOv3	✓	448 × 448	90.61%	91.04%	90.82%
WCE +CVC-ClinicDB	Souaidi et al., 2022 [10]	ETIS-Larib	VGG16	✓	300 × 300	90.02%	×	×
CVC-ClinicDB	Liu et al., 2021 [41]	ETIS-Larib	ResNet-101	✓	384 × 288	77.80%	87.50%	82.40%
GIANA 2017	Wang et al., 2019 [42]	ETIS-Larib	AFP-Net(VGG16)	✓	1225 × 996	88.89%	80.7%	84.63%
CVC-ClinicDB	Qadir et al., 2021 [43]	ETIS-Larib	ResNet34	✓	512 × 512	86.54%	86.12%	86.33%
CVC-ClinicDB	Pacal and Karaboga, 2021 [44]	ETIS-Larib	CSPDarkNet53	✓	384 × 288	91.62%	82.55%	86.85%
CVC-ClinicDB	Wang et al., 2019 [42]	ETIS-Larib	Faster R-CNN (VGG16)	×	224 × 224	88.89%	80.77%	84.63%
CVC-VideoClinicDB	Krenzer et al., 2019 [45]	CVC-VideoClinicDB	YOLOv5	×	574 × 500	73.21%	×	79.55%

4.4.4. Visualization

The main objective of this study was to show the impact of the condensed model in highlighting small polyp regions for the detection and localization tasks on the WCE, Etis-Larib, and CVC-ClinicDB test sets. Polyp detection aims at selecting polyp areas and ignoring normal parts, feces, artifacts, and water jet sprays to clean the colon. Some examples of polyp detection of the SSD model and DC-SSDNet network on the employed datasets are depicted in Figures 8–10. Compared to DC-SSDNet (Figures 8b,f, 9b,d, and 10b,d,h), Figures 8a,e, 9a,c, and 10a,c,g show false negative results in which the conventional SSD failed to detect small and flat polyp regions. The polyp region appeared similar to the surrounding normal mucosa as well the existence of food, air bubbles, and other debris may have hindered its localization process. Polyp areas showed variations related to color, texture, size, and shape and required more compact models to limit the number of false negatives and avoid missed detection. DC-SSDNet performed feature reuse by directly connecting shallower and deeper layers to distinguish polyp edge areas from normal ones. Figure 9g shows a false positive case of the SSD model on the ETIS-Larib test set with an error in detecting the polyp region while it was not there, whereas Figures 8b,f, 9b,d,g, and 10b,d,h show the correct identifications of the DC-SSDNet network. Besides small polyp detection, the proposed DC-SSDNet network achieved promising performance even for detecting large polyps on the WCE, CVC-ClinicDB, and ETIS-Larib test sets; see Figure 8b. With the presence of multiple polyps in one frame and a low contrast between the polyps and the background regions, both SSD and DC-SSDNet missed localizing small polyp regions, as illustrated in Figures 9c,d and 10c,d. In these cases, the problem was most likely one of contrast since the polyp was oversaturated. As a result, the F1 score decreased significantly. Although DC-SSDNet produced promising mAP results, it failed to detect some small polyp instances that seemed similar to portions of the colon due to lighting and contrast, resulting in a misleading bounding box and lowering the mAP and F1 scores. Even endoscopists may miss some small parts that cannot be detected by the naked eye or that are hidden from view behind a fold. However, the proposed DC-SSDNet model proved its efficiency in localizing small polyp regions at a fast detection speed while ensuring precision.

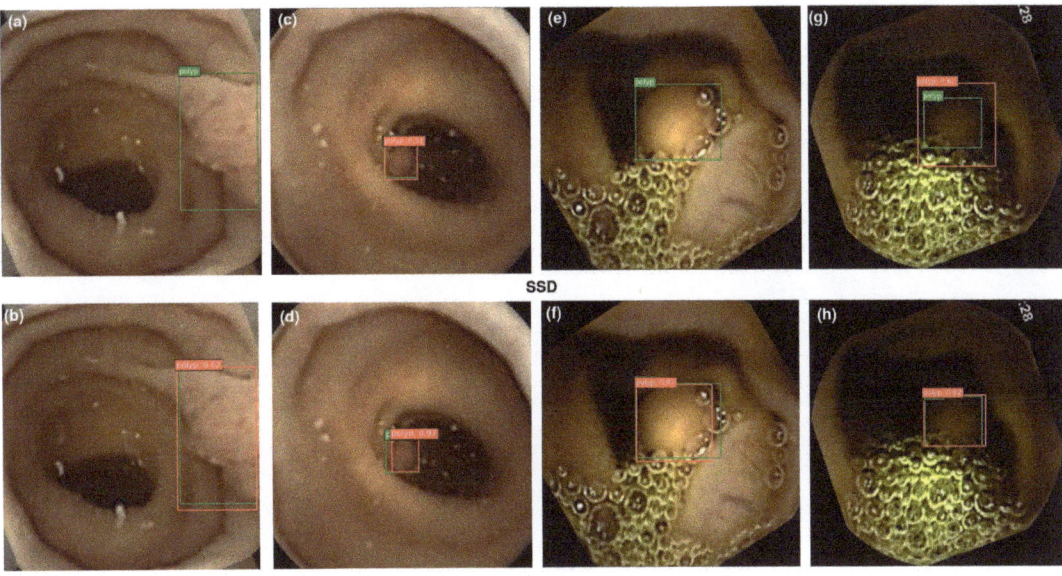

Figure 8. On the WCE test set, visualization results comparing SSD300 (**a**,**c**,**e**,**g**) and the proposed DC-SSDNet network (**b**,**d**,**f**,**h**). True bounding boxes with IoU of 0.5 or greater are drawn in green, whereas predicted bounding boxes are in red.

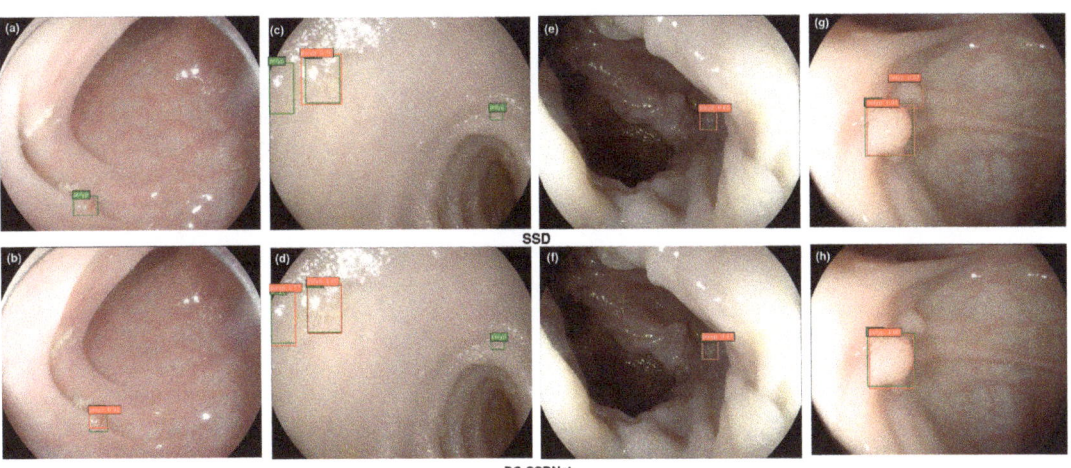

Figure 9. On the Etis-Larib test set, visualization results comparing SSD300 (**a**,**c**,**e**,**g**) and the proposed DC-SSDNet network (**b**,**d**,**f**,**h**). True bounding boxes with IoU of 0.5 or greater are drawn in green, whereas predicted bounding boxes are in red.

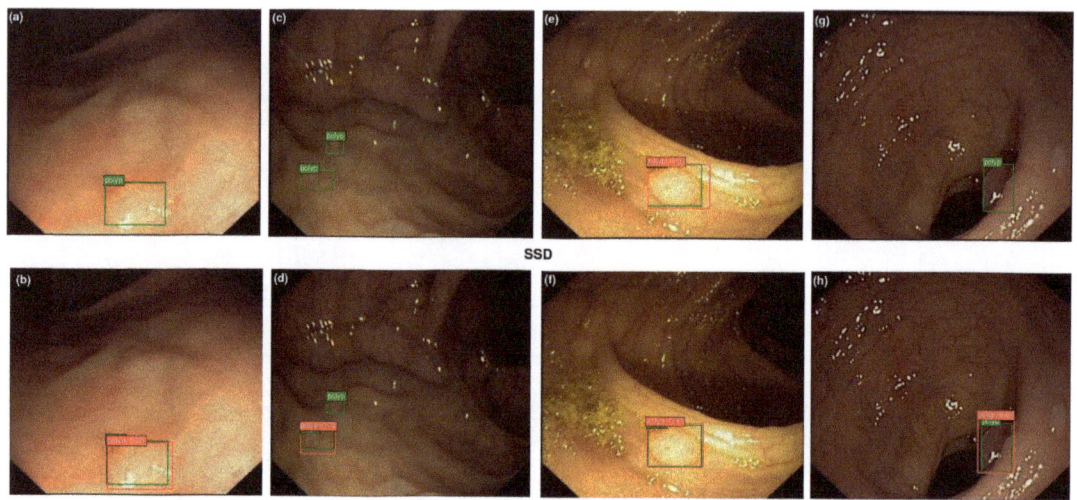

Figure 10. On the CVC-ClinicDB test set, visualization results comparing SSD300 (**a**,**c**,**e**,**g**) and the proposed DC-SSDNet network (**b**,**d**,**f**,**h**). True bounding boxes with IoU of 0.5 or greater are drawn in green, whereas predicted bounding boxes are in red.

5. Conclusions

This work suggested an improved SSD detector based on a redesigned DenseNet (DC-SSDNet) emphasizing polyp detection in the WCE, Etis-Larib, and CVC-ClinicDB datasets. Many researchers in the field use their own datasets due to medical imaging ethics and the lack of publicly available and annotated WCE polyp datasets. Thus, their results may suffer from subjectivity. The DC-SSDNet network aimed to exploit the potential of feature reuse as opposed to relearning features in later layers. The proposed approach used stacked dense and transition blocks instead of simple convolution layers with a capacity of the SSD network to be more compact while going deeper, yielding condensed models that were easy to train and highly parameter-efficient. The compact DenseNet-46 compressed unnecessary convolution layers of each dense block to reduce the amount of feature redundancy, resulting in fewer overall parameters and faster training times. The small polyp areas' visual appearance was modeled by directly connecting layers throughout the network and generating novel pyramidal feature maps. While training data from scratch, the DC-SSDNet detector achieved comparable, if not superior, performance in mAP compared to other state-of-the-art pretrained models with real-time processing speed on the WCE and public datasets (CVC-ClinicDB and Etis-Larib). Artifacts and other factors may degrade performance and negatively affect the detection process. We will conduct further studies in the future around this shortcoming while maintaining the smaller running time. Rather than proposing polyp identification tasks on WCE and colonoscopy frames, future studies will investigate hybrid architectures to present a unique detection method for video colonoscopy. Furthermore, it would be interesting to use a hybrid 2D/3D architecture and assess its performance by employing other promising backbones.

Author Contributions: Conceptualization, M.S.; Methodology, M.S.; Validation, S.L.; software, Z.K.; Formal analysis, M.E.A.; Visualization, M.E.A.; Supervision, L.K. All authors have read and agreed to the published version of the manuscript.

Funding: This work was partially supported by the Ministry of National Education, Vocational Training, Higher Education and Scientific Research, the Ministry of Industry, Trade and Green and Digital Economy, the Digital Development Agency (ADD), and the National Center for Scientific and Technical Research (CNRST). Project number: ALKHAWARIZMI/2020/20.

Data Availability Statement: Publicly available datasets were analyzed in this study. The CVC-ClinicDB datasets are publicly available here: https://polyp.grand-challenge.org/CVCClinicDB/ (accessed on 23 January 2023). The ETIS-Larib dataset is publicly available here: https://polyp.grand-challenge.org/EtisLarib (accessed on 25 January 2023).

Conflicts of Interest: The authors declare no conflict of interest.

Abbreviations

GI tract	Gastrointestinal tract
WCE	Wireless capsule endoscopy
MICCAI	Medical Image Computing and Computer Assisted Intervention
YOLO	You only look once
SSD	Single-shot multibox detector
R-CNN	Region-based convolutional neural network
R-FCN	Region-based fully convolutional network
DenseNet	Dense network
DCNN	Deep convolutional neural network
pool	pooling
ResNet	Residual network
FPN	Feature pyramid network
DSSD	Deconvolutional single-shot detector
ROI	Region of interest
Conv	Convolutional layer
DC-SSDNet	Densely connected single-shot multibox detector network
MaxPool	Max pooling
Pad	Padding
AveragePool	Average pooling
L2 Regul	L2 regularization
VCE	Video capsule endoscopy
Adam	Adaptive moment
neg-pos-ratio	negative positive ratio
mAP	Mean average precision
FPS	Frames per second
TP	True positive
FP	False positive
IoU	Intersection over union
FN	False negative
BN	Batch normalization
FSSD	Fusion single-shot multibox detector

References

1. Dulf, E.H.; Bledea, M.; Mocan, T.; Mocan, L. Automatic Detection of Colorectal Polyps Using Transfer Learning. *Sensors* **2021**, *21*, 5704. [CrossRef] [PubMed]
2. Shin, Y.; Qadir, H.A.; Aabakken, L.; Bergsland, J.; Balasingham, I. Automatic colon polyp detection using region based deep cnn and post learning approaches. *IEEE Access* **2018**, *6*, 40950–40962. [CrossRef]
3. Souaidi, M.; Abdelouahad, A.A.; El Ansari, M. A fully automated ulcer detection system for wireless capsule endoscopy images. In Proceedings of the 2017 International Conference on Advanced Technologies for Signal and Image Processing (ATSIP), Fez, Morocco, 22–24 May 2017; pp. 1–6.
4. Souaidi, M.; El Ansari, M. Automated Detection of Wireless Capsule Endoscopy Polyp Abnormalities with Deep Transfer Learning and Support Vector Machines. In *Advanced Intelligent Systems for Sustainable Development (AI2SD'2020)*; Springer: Berlin/Heidelberg, Germany, 2020; pp. 870–880.
5. Benhida, H.; Souadi, M.; El Ansari, M. Convolutional Neural Network for Automated Colorectal Polyp Semantic Segmentation on Colonoscopy Frames. In Proceedings of the 2022 9th International Conference on Wireless Networks and Mobile Communications (WINCOM), Rabat, Morocco, 26–29 October 2022; pp. 1–5.
6. Lafraxo, S.; Ansari, M.E. Regularized Convolutional Neural Network for Pneumonia Detection Trough Chest X-rays. In Proceedings of the International Conference on Advanced Intelligent Systems for Sustainable Development, Tangier, Morocco, 21–26 December 2020; pp. 887–896.

7. Souaidi, M.; El Ansari, M. Multi-scale analysis of ulcer disease detection from WCE images. *IET Image Process.* **2019**, *13*, 2233–2244. [CrossRef]
8. Nogueira-Rodríguez, A.; Domínguez-Carbajales, R.; Campos-Tato, F.; Herrero, J.; Puga, M.; Remedios, D.; Rivas, L.; Sánchez, E.; Iglesias, Á.; Cubiella, J.; et al. Real-time polyp detection model using convolutional neural networks. *Neural Comput. Appl.* **2022**, *34*, 10375–10396. [CrossRef]
9. Chen, X.; Zhang, K.; Lin, S.; Dai, K.F.; Yun, Y. Single Shot Multibox Detector Automatic Polyp Detection Network Based on Gastrointestinal Endoscopic Images. *Comput. Math. Methods Med.* **2021**, *2021*, 2144472. [CrossRef]
10. Souaidi, M.; El Ansari, M. A New Automated Polyp Detection Network MP-FSSD in WCE and Colonoscopy Images based Fusion Single Shot Multibox Detector and Transfer Learning. *IEEE Access* **2022**, *10*, 47124–47140. [CrossRef]
11. Redmon, J.; Divvala, S.; Girshick, R.; Farhadi, A. You only look once: Unified, real-time object detection. In Proceedings of the IEEE Conference on Computer Vision and Pattern Recognition, Las Vegas, NV, USA, 26 June–1 July 2016; pp. 779–788.
12. Liu, W.; Anguelov, D.; Erhan, D.; Szegedy, C.; Reed, S.; Fu, C.Y.; Berg, A.C. Ssd: Single shot multibox detector. In Proceedings of the European Conference on Computer Vision, Amsterdam, The Netherlands, 11–14 October 2016; pp. 21–37.
13. Girshick, R.; Donahue, J.; Darrell, T.; Malik, J. Rich feature hierarchies for accurate object detection and semantic segmentation. In Proceedings of the IEEE Conference on Computer Vision and Pattern Recognition, Columbus, OH, USA, 23–28 June 2014; pp. 580–587.
14. Ren, S.; He, K.; Girshick, R.; Sun, J. Faster R-CNN: Towards real-time object detection with region proposal networks. *IEEE Trans. Pattern Anal. Mach. Intell.* **2016**, *39*, 1137–1149. [CrossRef]
15. Dai, J.; Li, Y.; He, K.; Sun, J. *Object Detection via Region-Based Fully Convolutional Networks*; People's Posts and Telecommunications Press: Beijing, China, 2016.
16. Zhai, S.; Shang, D.; Wang, S.; Dong, S. DF-SSD: An improved SSD object detection algorithm based on DenseNet and feature fusion. *IEEE Access* **2020**, *8*, 24344–24357. [CrossRef]
17. Souaidi, M.; Charfi, S.; Abdelouahad, A.A.; El Ansari, M. New features for wireless capsule endoscopy polyp detection. In Proceedings of the 2018 International Conference on Intelligent Systems and Computer Vision (ISCV), Fez, Morocco, 2–4 April 2018; pp. 1–6.
18. Szegedy, C.; Liu, W.; Jia, Y.; Sermanet, P.; Reed, S.; Anguelov, D.; Erhan, D.; Vanhoucke, V.; Rabinovich, A. Going deeper with convolutions. In Proceedings of the IEEE Conference on Computer Vision and Pattern Recognition, Boston, MA, USA, 7–12 June 2015; pp. 1–9.
19. He, K.; Zhang, X.; Ren, S.; Sun, J. Deep residual learning for image recognition. In Proceedings of the IEEE Conference on Computer Vision and Pattern Recognition, Las Vegas, NV, USA, 26 June–1 July 2016; pp. 770–778.
20. Chen, B.L.; Wan, J.J.; Chen, T.Y.; Yu, Y.T.; Ji, M. A self-attention based faster R-CNN for polyp detection from colonoscopy images. *Biomed. Signal Process. Control* **2021**, *70*, 103019. [CrossRef]
21. Pacal, I.; Karaman, A.; Karaboga, D.; Akay, B.; Basturk, A.; Nalbantoglu, U.; Coskun, S. An efficient real-time colonic polyp detection with YOLO algorithms trained by using negative samples and large datasets. *Comput. Biol. Med.* **2022**, *141*, 105031. [CrossRef]
22. Hong-Tae, C.; Ho-Jun, L.; Kang, H.; Yu, S. SSD-EMB: An Improved SSD Using Enhanced Feature Map Block for Object Detection. *Sensors* **2021**, *21*, 2842.
23. Dai, K.; R-FCN, Y. Object detection via region-based fully convolutional networks. *arXiv* **2016**, arXiv:1605.06409.
24. Lin, T.Y.; Dollár, P.; Girshick, R.; He, K.; Hariharan, B.; Belongie, S. Feature pyramid networks for object detection. In Proceedings of the IEEE Conference on Computer Vision and Pattern Recognition, Honolulu, HI, USA, 21–26 July 2017; pp. 2117–2125.
25. Fu, C.Y.; Liu, W.; Ranga, A.; Tyagi, A.; Berg, A.C. Dssd: Deconvolutional single shot detector. *arXiv* **2017**, arXiv:1701.06659.
26. Jia, X.; Mai, X.; Cui, Y.; Yuan, Y.; Xing, X.; Seo, H.; Xing, L.; Meng, M.Q.H. Automatic polyp recognition in colonoscopy images using deep learning and two-stage pyramidal feature prediction. *IEEE Trans. Autom. Sci. Eng.* **2020**, *17*, 1570–1584. [CrossRef]
27. Qadir, H.A.; Shin, Y.; Solhusvik, J.; Bergsland, J.; Aabakken, L.; Balasingham, I. Polyp detection and segmentation using mask R-CNN: Does a deeper feature extractor CNN always perform better? In Proceedings of the 2019 13th International Symposium on Medical Information and Communication Technology (ISMICT), Oslo, Norway, 8–10 May 2019; pp. 1–6.
28. Tashk, A.; Nadimi, E. An innovative polyp detection method from colon capsule endoscopy images based on a novel combination of RCNN and DRLSE. In Proceedings of the 2020 IEEE Congress on Evolutionary Computation (CEC), Glasgow, UK, 19–24 July 2020; pp. 1–6.
29. Liu, M.; Jiang, J.; Wang, Z. Colonic polyp detection in endoscopic videos with single shot detection based deep convolutional neural network. *IEEE Access* **2019**, *7*, 75058–75066. [CrossRef]
30. Wang, Y.; Li, H.; Jia, P.; Zhang, G.; Wang, T.; Hao, X. Multi-scale densenets-based aircraft detection from remote sensing images. *Sensors* **2019**, *19*, 5270. [CrossRef]
31. Misawa, M.; Kudo, S.E.; Mori, Y.; Hotta, K.; Ohtsuka, K.; Matsuda, T.; Saito, S.; Kudo, T.; Baba, T.; Ishida, F.; et al. Development of a computer-aided detection system for colonoscopy and a publicly accessible large colonoscopy video database (with video). *Gastrointest. Endosc.* **2021**, *93*, 960–967. [CrossRef]
32. Jeong, J.; Park, H.; Kwak, N. Enhancement of SSD by concatenating feature maps for object detection. *arXiv* **2017**, arXiv:1705.09587.
33. Zhang, X.; Chen, F.; Yu, T.; An, J.; Huang, Z.; Liu, J.; Hu, W.; Wang, L.; Duan, H.; Si, J. Real-time gastric polyp detection using convolutional neural networks. *PLoS ONE* **2019**, *14*, e0214133. [CrossRef]

34. Wang, T.; Shen, F.; Deng, H.; Cai, F.; Chen, S. Smartphone imaging spectrometer for egg/meat freshness monitoring. *Anal. Methods* **2022**, *14*, 508–517. [CrossRef]
35. Souaidi, M.; El Ansari, M. Multi-Scale Hybrid Network for Polyp Detection in Wireless Capsule Endoscopy and Colonoscopy Images. *Diagnostics* **2022**, *12*, 2030. [CrossRef] [PubMed]
36. Prasath, V.S. Polyp detection and segmentation from video capsule endoscopy: A review. *J. Imaging* **2016**, *3*, 1. [CrossRef]
37. Bernal, J.; Sánchez, F.J.; Fernández-Esparrach, G.; Gil, D.; Rodríguez, C.; Vilariño, F. WM-DOVA maps for accurate polyp highlighting in colonoscopy: Validation vs. saliency maps from physicians. *Comput. Med. Imaging Graph.* **2015**, *43*, 99–111. [CrossRef] [PubMed]
38. We, O. ETIS-Larib Polyp DB. 2015. Available online: https://polyp.grand-challenge.org/EtisLarib/ (accessed on 27 March 2022).
39. Ma, W.; Wang, X.; Yu, J. A Lightweight Feature Fusion Single Shot Multibox Detector for Garbage Detection. *IEEE Access* **2020**, *8*, 188577–188586. [CrossRef]
40. Shen, Z.; Liu, Z.; Li, J.; Jiang, Y.G.; Chen, Y.; Xue, X. Dsod: Learning deeply supervised object detectors from scratch. In Proceedings of the IEEE International Conference on Computer Vision, Venice, Italy, 22–29 October 2017; pp. 1919–1927.
41. Liu, X.; Guo, X.; Liu, Y.; Yuan, Y. Consolidated domain adaptive detection and localization framework for cross-device colonoscopic images. *Med. Image Anal.* **2021**, *71*, 102052. [CrossRef]
42. Wang, D.; Zhang, N.; Sun, X.; Zhang, P.; Zhang, C.; Cao, Y.; Liu, B. Afp-net: Realtime anchor-free polyp detection in colonoscopy. In Proceedings of the 2019 IEEE 31st International Conference on Tools with Artificial Intelligence (ICTAI), Portland, OR, USA, 4–6 November 2019; pp. 636–643.
43. Qadir, H.A.; Shin, Y.; Solhusvik, J.; Bergsland, J.; Aabakken, L.; Balasingham, I. Toward real-time polyp detection using fully CNNs for 2D Gaussian shapes prediction. *Med Image Anal.* **2021**, *68*, 101897. [CrossRef]
44. Pacal, I.; Karaboga, D. A robust real-time deep learning based automatic polyp detection system. *Comput. Biol. Med.* **2021**, *134*, 104519. [CrossRef]
45. Krenzer, A.; Banck, M.; Makowski, K.; Hekalo, A.; Fitting, D.; Troya, J.; Sudarevic, B.; Zoller, W.G.; Hann, A.; Puppe, F. A Real-Time Polyp Detection System with Clinical Application in Colonoscopy Using Deep Convolutional Neural Networks. *J. Imaging* **2023**, *9*, 26. [CrossRef]

Disclaimer/Publisher's Note: The statements, opinions and data contained in all publications are solely those of the individual author(s) and contributor(s) and not of MDPI and/or the editor(s). MDPI and/or the editor(s) disclaim responsibility for any injury to people or property resulting from any ideas, methods, instructions or products referred to in the content.

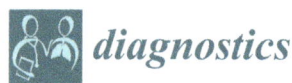

Article

Negative Samples for Improving Object Detection—A Case Study in AI-Assisted Colonoscopy for Polyp Detection

Alba Nogueira-Rodríguez [1,2,*], Daniel Glez-Peña [1,2], Miguel Reboiro-Jato [1,2] and Hugo López-Fernández [1,2]

1 CINBIO, Department of Computer Science, ESEI—Escuela Superior de Ingeniería Informática, Universidade de Vigo, 32004 Ourense, Spain
2 SING Research Group, Galicia Sur Health Research Institute (IIS Galicia Sur), SERGAS-UVIGO, 36213 Vigo, Spain
* Correspondence: alnogueira@uvigo.es

Abstract: Deep learning object-detection models are being successfully applied to develop computer-aided diagnosis systems for aiding polyp detection during colonoscopies. Here, we evidence the need to include negative samples for both (i) reducing false positives during the polyp-finding phase, by including images with artifacts that may confuse the detection models (e.g., medical instruments, water jets, feces, blood, excessive proximity of the camera to the colon wall, blurred images, etc.) that are usually not included in model development datasets, and (ii) correctly estimating a more realistic performance of the models. By retraining our previously developed YOLOv3-based detection model with a dataset that includes 15% of additional not-polyp images with a variety of artifacts, we were able to generally improve its F1 performance in our internal test datasets (from an average F1 of 0.869 to 0.893), which now include such type of images, as well as in four public datasets that include not-polyp images (from an average F1 of 0.695 to 0.722).

Keywords: colorectal cancer; deep learning; convolutional neural network (CNN); polyp detection; polyp localization

1. Introduction

Computer-aided diagnosis (CAD) systems for polyp detection are now reality, thanks to the advances in and the application of deep learning (DL). So far, many randomized control trials (RCT) have already been performed [1–6], some of them associated with commercial systems [7], and many more are being developed. The growing number of reviews on this topic demonstrates that polyp detection is much more advanced than polyp characterization [5,7–9], and a recent meta-analysis of six RCTs showed that there is an increase in both adenoma and polyp detection rates with the utilization of artificial intelligence (AI)-assisted colonoscopy [5].

In the context of the PolyDeep project (https://www.polydeep.org, accessed on 11 January 2023), we developed and reported, in 2021, a real-time polyp detection model based on a YOLOv3 pre-trained with PASCAL VOC datasets [10]. The base model was fine-tuned using a private dataset containing 941 different polyps and 28,576 images annotated by expert endoscopists [11]. The performance of this model in a bounding box-based evaluation using still images (a test partition of our private dataset) was an F1 score of 0.88 (recall = 0.87, precision = 0.89), reaching a state-of-the-art level.

In follow-up work [12], we reported, in 2022, the results of testing this model on ten public colonoscopy image datasets, which, to the best of our knowledge, was the biggest systematic evaluation of a polyp detection model without retraining. We also analyzed these results in the context of the results from another 20 state-of-the-art publications using the same public datasets. We observed that our model had an average F1 score decay of 13.65% when tested on the ten public datasets. This number may seem high, but it must be taken into account the high degree of variability in the public datasets, as

Citation: Nogueira-Rodríguez, A.; Glez-Peña, D.; Reboiro-Jato, M.; López-Fernández, H. Negative Samples for Improving Object Detection—A Case Study in AI-Assisted Colonoscopy for Polyp Detection. *Diagnostics* **2023**, *13*, 966. https://doi.org/10.3390/diagnostics13050966

Academic Editor: Eun-Sun Kim

Received: 15 January 2023
Accepted: 1 March 2023
Published: 3 March 2023

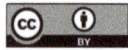

Copyright: © 2023 by the authors. Licensee MDPI, Basel, Switzerland. This article is an open access article distributed under the terms and conditions of the Creative Commons Attribution (CC BY) license (https:// creativecommons.org/licenses/by/ 4.0/).

some of them contain not-polyp images and multiple-polyp images, resulting in a slightly different scenario compared to the type of images used to develop our base model (only polyp-containing images).

Since then, we have also released an updated version of our dataset and other complementary datasets through the PIBAdb Colorectal Polyp Image Cohort (https://www.iisgaliciasur.es/home/biobanco/cohorte-pibadb, accessed on 11 January 2023), which is publicly available at the biobank of the Galicia Sur Health Research Institute (IISGS). This image cohort was created with the aim of making public the data collected during the PolyDeep project, including, mainly, images with polyps located with bounding boxes annotated by expert endoscopists, but also other colon images without polyps and the videos of colonoscopies from which the images were extracted. Notably, one of the complementary datasets published includes ~14,000 not-polyp images (the "PIBAdb Not Polyp" image gallery). These images without polyps have been extracted automatically (one image per second) from annotated videos and they may contain artifacts (e.g., instrumental, on-screen information, etc.), be blurred or very close to mucosa. This follows the general trend of the latest public datasets available, which are larger and include images without polyps.

In light of the findings of our previous works, our efforts to keep improving our model have been data-centric. In this regard, some studies have already used not-polyp images during training to improve the performance of the model [13], and, therefore, in this work we assess the usefulness of the recent not-polyp images included in the PIBAdb database to improve the performance of our previous model. Our belief is that training using these images will allow us to improve the predictive positive value of the model (precision), while maintaining its sensitivity levels (recall).

Rationale (Hypothesis)

The rationale behind the inclusion of no-object images, or negative samples, in an object detection network is guided by the fact that, when such models are implemented in a real setting, the model could face out-of-distribution samples, that is, image types that have content that was not used during the model development.

A polyp detection network trained only with polyp-containing images (at least one polyp per image) uses the outside-boxes image content as the "negative" samples, learning not to predict bounding boxes there. This may be sufficient if all the possible negative content is there, but this is not the case in endoscopies, especially during the polyp-finding phase. The normal mucosa content behind a polyp is not the only negative content to learn from. There are many other scenarios (out-of-distribution) that will arise during the exploration (e.g., medical instruments, water jets, feces, blood, excessive proximity of the camera to the colon wall, blurred images, etc.) that could lead the network to identify parts of the image as something similar to a polyp, or, at least, more similar to a polyp than to normal mucosa, producing many false positives.

With this study, we aim at exploiting this hypothesis by retraining our model with such out-of-distribution images in order to improve its positive predictive value, while maintaining its sensitivity. Moreover, we will put special focus on testing the model with this kind of image at different proportions, since test datasets that do not include them are not able to capture the real performance of detection models in the real setting. In summary, we want to move out-of-distribution samples to in-distribution samples.

2. Materials and Methods

2.1. Our Base Model for Polyp Detection

In 2021, we reported the results of a real-time colorectal polyp detection model based on YOLOv3 [11]. This model was trained and evaluated with a private dataset built using 28,576 images with located polyps from the PIBAdb cohort, both with white light (WL) and narrow-band imaging (NBI) light. This dataset includes a subset of images automatically extracted at a rate of one image per second (16,691) and a subset of images manually selected by expert endoscopists (11,885).

For the model development, the private dataset was divided into three partitions: (i) a training partition (49%; 13,873 images) for model training during the development phase, (ii) a validation partition (21%; 6045 images) for model evaluation and selecting the best model during the development phase, and (iii) a test partition (30%; 8658 images) for best model evaluation after the development phase. The resulting model, pre-trained with the PASCAL VOC 2007 and 2012 challenges and fine-tuned with the dataset comprising both the training and validation partitions, achieved an F1 score of 0.88 (recall = 0.87, precision = 0.89) and an average precision (AP) of 0.87 evaluated on the test partition. As noted in the introduction, this model was later evaluated on ten public datasets, without retraining, in order to assess its generalization capabilities [12], showing an average F1 decay of 13.65%.

2.2. Public Datasets

Table 1 shows the most relevant details of the ten public colonoscopy image datasets selected in our previous study [12], which are also the subject of this study. Regarding polyp location in the dataset images, four dataset provide it as bounding boxes (KUMC [14], SUN [13], LDPolypVideo [15], and Kvasir-SEG [16]), while seven datasets use binary masks (CVC-ClinicDB [17], CVC-ColonDB [18,19], CVC-PolypHD [18,19], ETIS-Larib [20], CVC-ClinicVideoDB [21,22], PICCOLO [23], and Kvasir-SEG [16]). As the polyp detection model evaluated in this work uses bounding boxes, it was necessary to transform the binary masks into bounding boxes in six datasets (ClinicDB [17], CVC-ColonDB [18,19], CVC-PolypHD [18,19], ETIS-Larib [20], CVC-ClinicVideoDB [21,22], and PICCOLO [23]). The process followed to perform these transformations was explained in our previous study [12], and the conversion scripts are available at https://github.com/sing-group/public-datasets-to-voc (accessed on 11 January 2023).

Table 1. Summary of the ten public colonoscopy image datasets for polyp location including: the name and publication/s related with the dataset (Dataset), the year when the dataset was published (Year), the image resolution (Resolution), the number of images in the dataset (No. of images), the method used to provide image location (Ground Truth), and whether the dataset includes images without polyps and the percentage of images with polyps in case they are included (Without polyps?).

Dataset	Year	Resolution	No. of Images	Ground Truth	Without Polyps?
CVC-ColonDB [18,19]	2012	574 × 500	300	Mask	No
ETIS-Larib [20]	2014	1225 × 966	196	Mask	No
CVC-ClinicDB [17]	2015	384 × 288	612	Mask	No
CVC-ClinicVideoDB [21,22]	2017	384 × 288	11,954	Mask	Yes (16.14%)
CVC-PolypHD [18,19]	2018	1920 × 1080	56	Mask	No
Kvasir-SEG [16]	2020	332 × 487 to 1920 × 1072	1000	Bounding box and mask	No
PICCOLO [23]	2020	854 × 480, 1920 × 1080	3433	Mask	Yes (1.25%)
KUMC [14]	2021	Various resolutions	37,899	Bounding box	Yes (5.08%)
SUN [13]	2021	1240 × 1080	49,136	Bounding box	No *
LDPolypVideo [15]	2021	560 × 480	40,186	Bounding box	Yes (15.7%)

* The SUN dataset contains 109,554 frames without polyps that were not downloaded for our experiments.

Taking into account the characteristics of the different datasets, a high degree of variability can be observed with respect to the number of images included, and whether they contain not-polyp images or not [8,24]. Nevertheless, the trend in recent years is to create increasingly larger datasets with the presence of images without polyps.

2.3. Experimental Setup

The experiments consist of training new models using the original polyp image dataset of our base model and progressively injecting it with different percentages of not-polyp images. The original dataset partitions (i.e., training, validation, and test) were augmented with not-polyp images at rates around 2%, 5%, 10%, and 15% of the initial number of images in the partition.

Starting from the images of each original partition, where each polyp only belongs to one single partition, we progressively added each percentage of images without polyps. The image injection was performed incrementally for each percentage, ensuring that the same not-polyp image was in the same partition type (training, validation, or test) and that the images found in the lower percentage datasets were part of the higher percentage datasets, creating supersets for each partition and dataset. For example, all the images in the 2% training are also included in the 5% dataset, along with an additional 3% of new not-polyp images. The number of resulting images for each partition is shown in the following, Figure 1.

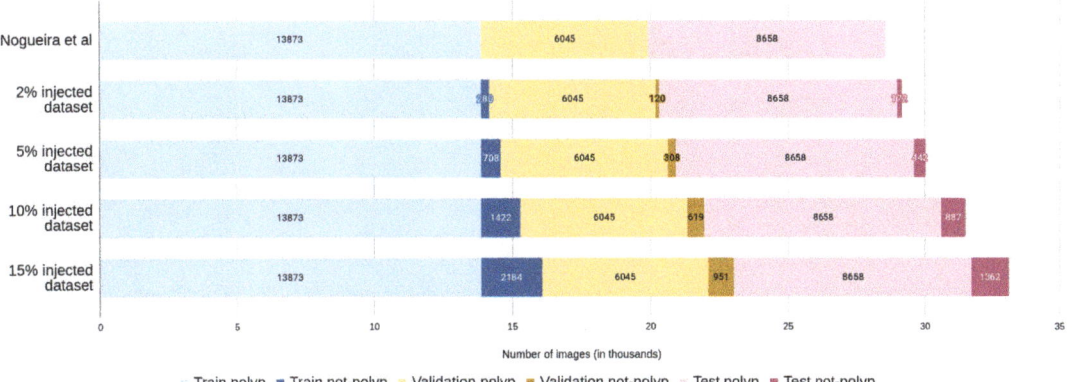

Figure 1. Not-polyp datasets created from the original polyp images dataset [11].

Figure 2 shows diverse examples of not-polyp images that have been used to train the new networks. As can be seen, these images may contain medical instruments, water jets, feces, blood, excessive proximity of the camera to the colon wall, blurred images, etc.

As in our previous works [11,12], the model development and evaluation was done using Compi [25,26] pipelines, which can be found at the GitHub repository: https://github.com/sing-group/polydeep-object-detection (accessed on 11 January 2023). Specifically, the model training was performed using the train.xml pipeline, while the model evaluation was performed using the text.xml pipeline of this repository.

Once retrained (see details in "Model development and selection"), we evaluated the performance of each new model in an (i) intra-dataset evaluation, using the test partition of the base model, as well as the not-polyp augmented test partitions, and in an (ii) inter-dataset evaluation, using the ten public colonoscopy imaging datasets selected in the previous study.

2.4. Evaluation Metrics

Since the main goal of a colorectal polyp detection model is to identify all the polyps shown on camera during a colonoscopy, we have selected recall (or sensitivity) as one of the evaluation measures. In addition, as the ability to not show detections in locations where there is no polyp is also important, because they can disturb or distract an endoscopist, we have also selected precision (or positive predictive value) as a second evaluation measure. Finally, since it acts as a summary of the two evaluation measures mentioned above, we have chosen F_1 as the main evaluation measure.

Given that the output of the detection model is a bounding box, in this work we define:
- True Positive (TP): as a predicted bounding box that is over a true bounding box.
- False Positive (FP): as a predicted bounding box that is not over a true bounding box.

- False Negative (FN): as a true bounding box where there is no predicted bounding box over it.

Taking into account these definitions, the selected performance metrics (i.e., recall, precision, and F_1) are defined as follows:

$$\text{recall(or sensitivity)} = \frac{TP}{TP + FN}$$

$$\text{precision(or positive predictive value)} = \frac{TP}{TP + FP}$$

$$F_1 = 2 \times \frac{\text{precision} \cdot \text{recall}}{\text{precision} + \text{recall}} = \frac{2 \times TP}{2 \times TP + FP + FN}$$

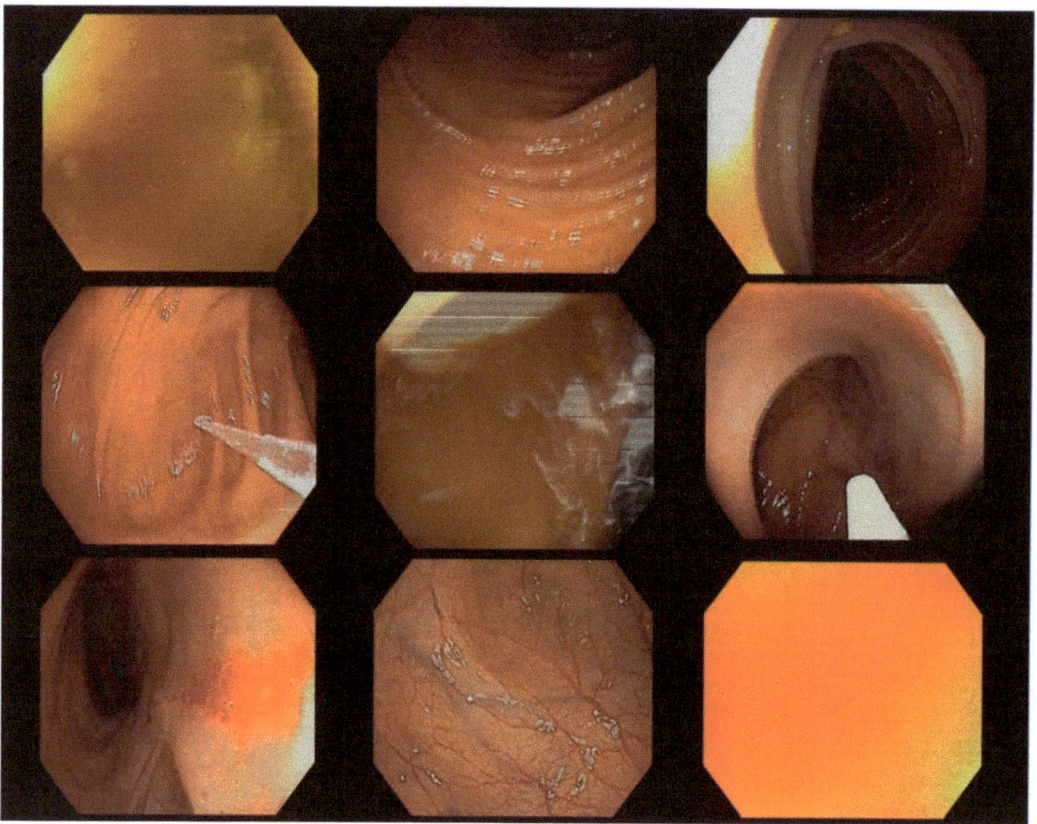

Figure 2. Random sample of the not-polyp images included in the injected datasets.

3. Results and Discussion

The experiments are focused on obtaining the performance metrics of each model in a test partition with similar images with which it was trained (intra-dataset evaluation) and, also, evaluating the models with a test partition where the images belong to public datasets (inter-dataset evaluation). The results are completed with a frame analysis to see how false positive identifications are removed.

3.1. Model Development and Selection

Following the same strategy as in our previous works [11,12], each model was retrained again, starting from the initial pre-trained YOLOv3 and using the training partition for 50 epochs. The same training parameters were used for all the models. The best model is selected by the maximum AP achieved in the validation partition during those 50 epochs. Once the best model is selected, it is configured with the confidence score threshold that maximizes the F1 score in the validation partition. Table 2 shows the metrics of the selected models with the best AP achieved in the validation partition images during the training process. AP is equivalent to the Area Under the Precision-Recall Curve (AUPRC), being the average precision at various confidence score thresholds.

Table 2. Performance metrics in each validation partition for the selected models.

	Confidence Score Threshold	Recall	Precision	F_1	AP
Nogueira et al. [11]	0.19	0.905	0.912	0.909	0.920
Model injection 2%	0.24	0.897	0.917	0.907	0.920
Model injection 5%	0.18	0.911	0.915	0.913	0.923
Model injection 10%	0.22	0.884	0.918	0.901	0.918
Model injection 15%	0.15	0.903	0.920	0.912	0.923

As a result, we have the original model ("Nogueira et al."), plus four additional models ("Model injection p", where p is the percentage of injection of not-polyp images into the dataset partitions used to develop the model).

3.2. Intra-Dataset Evaluation

First, we evaluated the models trained after the injection of not-polyp images using the test partition of the base model (Nogueira et al., i.e., without not-polyp images). The results are shown in Table 3.

Table 3. Performance metrics of each model on the original test partition of Nogueira et al., which does not contain not-polyp images.

Training Dataset	Recall	Precision	F_1
Nogueira et al. [11]	0.872	0.890	0.881
Model injection 2%	0.867	0.894	0.880
Model injection 5%	0.875	0.902	0.888
Model injection 10%	0.850	0.904	0.876
Model injection 15%	0.880	0.910	0.895

Regarding recall, all the models show a slight fluctuation, ranging from 0.85 in the model trained with the addition of 10% not-polyp images, to 0.88 in the model trained with the addition of 15% not-polyp images. On the other hand, the precision increases as the models are trained with increasing numbers of not-polyp images, and thus achieves the highest value in the model trained with the addition of 15% of not-polyp images (0.91), which also obtains the best F1 score (0.895). In comparison with the base model, the models trained with the addition of 5% and 15% not-polyp images show a slightly better F1 score, whereas the 2% and 10% models a slightly lower one. In summary, the difference is small, and no model shows a clear improvement in the original test partition.

However, as we are looking for a test scenario that better reflects the out-of-distribution samples that the models will face in a real setting, mimicked by including not-polyp images in the test partition, we also performed the evaluation with the test partitions that include different proportions of not-polyp images (also from 2% up to 15%). Since the true polyp images remain the same in all the new not-polyp-containing test partitions, the recall of any given model will remain exactly the same as shown in Table 3, but the precision, and thus the F1, are expected to be affected. Concretely, Table 4 shows the different precision metrics obtained by testing all the models with the different test partitions.

Table 4. Precision metrics obtained with different models against different not-polyp injections into the original test partition.

Model	Test Partitions (Percentage of Not-Polyp Augmentation)			
	2%	5%	10%	15%
Nogueira et al. [11]	0.882	0.871	0.852	0.836
Model injection 2%	0.890	0.886	0.879	0.871
Model injection 5%	0.899	0.895	0.888	0.881
Model injection 10%	0.902	0.901	0.897	0.895
Model injection 15%	0.909	0.907	0.904	0.901

As can be seen, precision is positively correlated with the number of not-polyp images used for training the different models, which evidences the benefit of training with not-polyp images, and it is inversely correlated with the number of not-polyp images in the test partition, which is a statistically expected effect.

Putting it all together, Figure 3 shows the recall and precision comparing two distant test partitions: the original one, which does not contain any not-polyp images, and the largest not-polyp containing test partition, which contains the addition of 15% of not-polyp images.

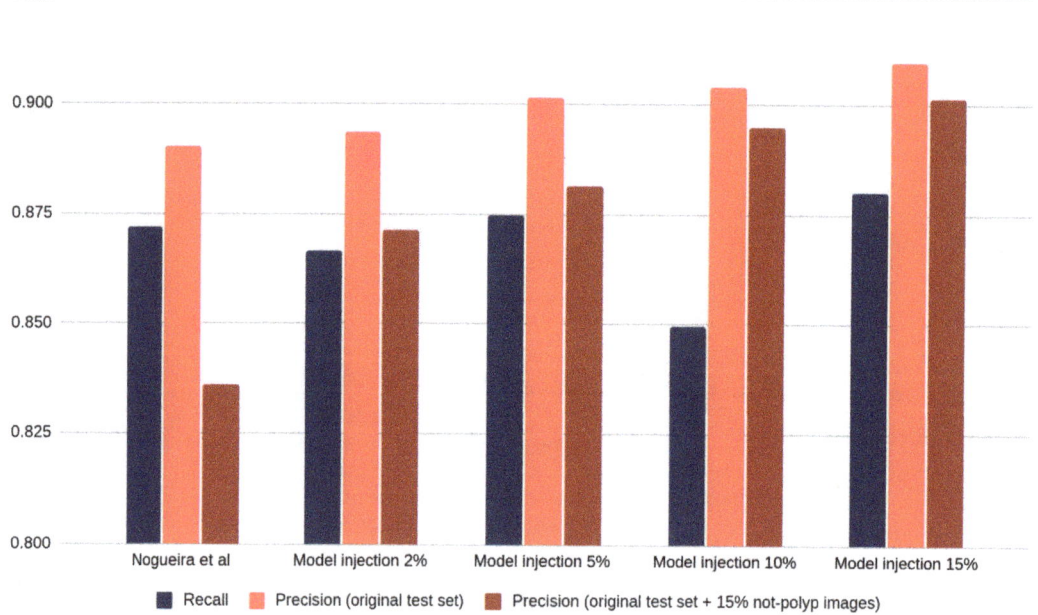

Figure 3. Recall of the five trained models (blue) and their precision in both the original test partition (pink) and the same with the addition of 15% of not-polyp images (dark red) [11].

It can be observed from Figure 3 that the precision decay of the original model is the biggest one (red bars in the leftmost column of Figure 3). However, as we create models trained with an increasing number of not-polyp images, this precision recovers (dark red bars' progression in Figure 3).

In order to compare all the models, Figure 4 shows the F1 score of all the models in both test scenarios (without not-polyp images and with the addition of 15% of not-polyp images). As it can be seen, the test partition that includes the addition of 15% of not-polyp images (dark bars in Figure 4) is more challenging, and each model attains a lower F1 score. Moreover, the addition of not-polyp images for training does not show a consistent benefit in the original test partition (light bars in Figure 4), whereas it does in the test partition that adds 15% of not-polyp images (dark bars in Figure 4). We draw attention to the lowest value obtained with the original model in the not-polyp test partition (from the original 0.88 to 0.85). Finally, in terms of the F1 score, the model trained with the highest number of not-polyp images showed the best F1 score in both test partitions (0.895 and 0.891).

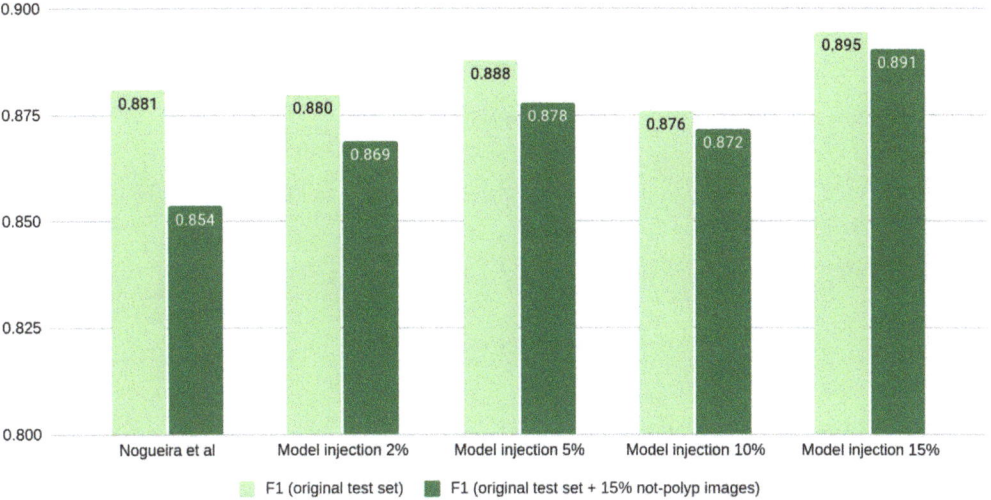

Figure 4. F1 of the five trained models in both the original test partition (light green) and the same with the addition of 15% of not-polyp images (dark green) [11].

3.3. Inter-Dataset Evaluation

Table 5 shows the performance of our five models, i.e., the baseline model presented in Nogueira et al. [11], plus the four new models trained with different percentages of not-polyp image injections, on the same public datasets analyzed in our previous work [12]. Globally, the average F1 score remains almost the same, with an F1 around 0.75 (see global averages in Table 5). As a result, we could discard an unexpected worsening in the public datasets.

However, when the testing results are divided into functions of whether the testing dataset contains not-polyp images or not, the results differ. In the case of the results obtained in the datasets that contain not-polyp images, the models trained with not-polyp images attain, on average, greater than or equal to the F1 scores of the original model, where the model with a 15% injection of not-polyp images is able to increase the F1 in the four datasets, raising the original average of 0.695 to 0.722. The behavior of the same models in the datasets that only contain polyp images is more heterogeneous, but a general decrease in the average F1 is observed, ranging from 0.749 to 0.799 in comparison with the original average of 0.800.

In order to visualize the performance changes among our four new models in each public dataset, Figure 5 compares the F1 performances obtained by our baseline model (X axis) and the F1 performances obtained by the four new models trained with not-polyp images (Y axis). The public datasets that contain not-polyp images are marked in light blue.

Table 5. F1 score of the five trained models in the 10 public datasets. Averages are provided for all datasets, datasets with both polyp and not-polyp images (4 datasets), and for datasets with only polyp images (6 datasets).

	Training Dataset				
	Nogueira et al. [11]	Not-Polyp Injection			
		2%	5%	10%	15%
Datasets with both polyp and not-polyp images					
LDPolypVideo	0.522	0.563	0.516	0.491	0.564
ClinicVideoDB	0.774	0.803	0.813	0.809	0.800
KUMC	0.818	0.811	0.819	0.762	0.831
PICCOLO	0.667	0.601	0.691	0.759	0.691
average	*0.695*	*0.694*	*0.710*	*0.705*	*0.722*
Datasets only with polyp images					
ClinicDB	0.845	0.843	0.867	0.786	0.824
ColonDB	0.826	0.848	0.883	0.689	0.797
SUN	0.805	0.764	0.738	0.765	0.746
KVASIR	0.807	0.800	0.797	0.840	0.830
Etis-Larib	0.718	0.732	0.679	0.594	0.685
PolypHD	0.800	0.729	0.826	0.820	0.820
average	*0.800*	*0.786*	*0.799*	*0.749*	*0.784*
global average	*0.758*	*0.749*	*0.763*	*0.731*	*0.759*

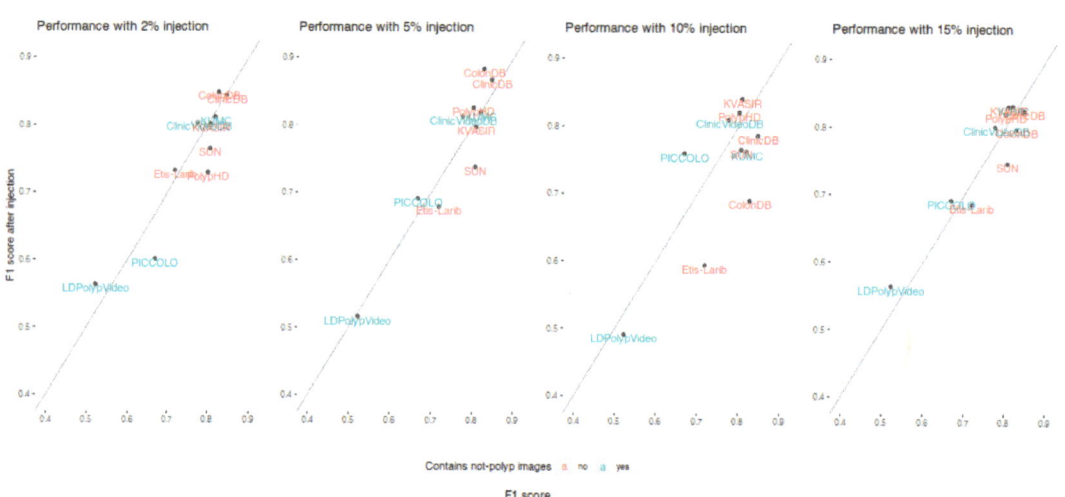

Figure 5. Comparison between the F1 performances obtained by our baseline model in the ten public datasets (X axis) and the F1 performances obtained by the four new models trained with not-polyp images (Y axis). Public datasets containing not-polyp images are marked in light blue. Points above the diagonal line represent benefit.

Focusing more on the relative variations, Figure 6 shows the relative change on F1 among all the public datasets between the models trained with not-polyp images with respect to the original model (trained without not-polyp images) in the same test dataset.

Again, we have grouped the results according to the presence or not of not-polyp images in the test partition. The left part of Figure 6 shows a general benefit in the four public datasets with not-polyp images (dark boxes). By contrast, regarding the performance in the public datasets without not-polyp images, a general worsening is observed (light boxes). When the results are disaggregated by model, the right part of Figure 6 shows that the better performance is always obtained in datasets that include not-polyp images for all the models. Finally, the model trained with 15% of additional not-polyp images attains the highest benefit in the not-polyp-containing datasets (dark box in the right-most column in Figure 6), being the only one showing a benefit of all of the four public datasets with not-polyp images.

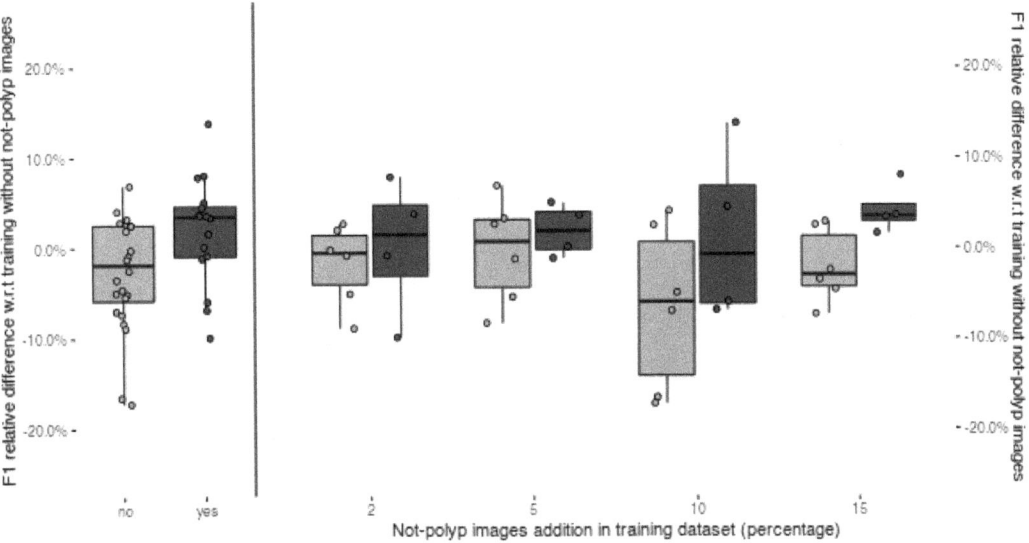

Figure 6. Relative F1 differences in the same test dataset with respect to our baseline model (trained without not-polyp images), and grouped test dataset type (i.e., containing or not containing not-polyp images).

3.4. Qualitative Analysis

To perform a qualitative analysis, the five models (the base model presented in Nogueira et al. plus the new four models trained with different percentages of not-polyp image injections) have been used to process two videos at a rate of 25 fps: (i) an 18 s video of a polyp (450 frames); and (ii) a 14 s video of normal mucosa (not-polyp) (350 frames). The two videos are provided as Supplementary Videos S1 and S2, respectively. Table 6 shows a global summary of the predictions made over the two videos.

Regarding the polyp video, in Table 6 we see a general recall of 90%, in terms of distinct frames that contain at least one emitted bounding box, and very small differences among all the models (see relative change, third column in Table 6). Regarding the not-polyp video, we see a drastic reduction in the total number of bounding boxes, with respect to the original model, which were all false positives (see relative change, last column in Table 6).

In order to give some illustrative examples within these two videos, Figure 7 contains some frames with bounding box predictions in the polyp video. As expected, the five models are able to detect the polyp correctly in almost all the frames (first row of Figure 7). However, in this specific polyp video, the new models even surpass the detection ability of the base model (slightly better recall, as shown in Table 6), where some of the false negatives (white box in the second row of Figure 7) in the original model were corrected by the not-polyp-trained models. Moreover, some false positive identifications (boxes not in the correct location of the polyp) emitted by the baseline model disappear in the not-polyp-trained models (second and third rows of Figure 7).

Table 6. Summary of the network predictions in both polyp and not-polyp videos. For the polyp video, the total number of distinct frames with at least one bounding box is reported, as a proxy of the recall (assuming that, at least one of the bounding boxes in the frame is placed over the polyp). For the not-polyp video, the total number of bounding boxes is reported, which are all false positives. Relative changes if these metrics are also reported among different models.

	Polyp Video (450 Frames)		Not-Polyp Video (350 Frames)	
	Frames with at Least One Bounding Box	Relative Change	Total Bounding Boxes (False Positives)	Relative Change
Nogueira et al. [11]	404 (89.78%)	-	90	-
Model injection 2%	418 (92.89%)	+3.47%	43	−52.22%
Model injection 5%	419 (93.11%)	+3.71%	24	−73.33%
Model injection 10%	416 (92.44%)	+2.97%	16	−82.22%
Model injection 15%	407 (90.44%)	+0.74%	63	−30.00%

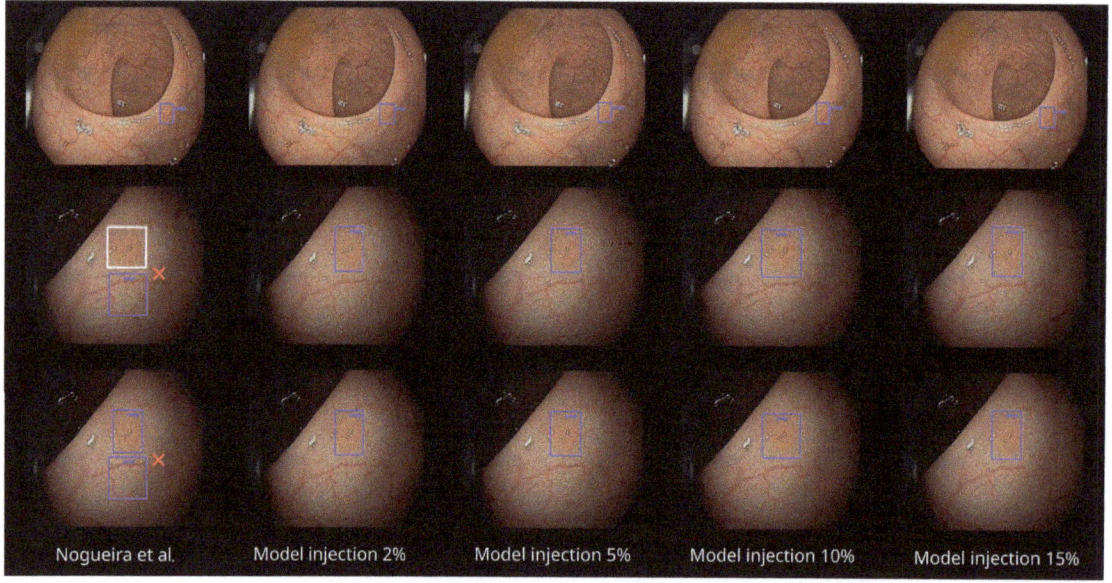

Figure 7. The five models with three sample frames of the polyp video analyzed (Supplementary Video S1). The false positive identifications are marked with red cross marks. The false negatives are marked in white boxes (added manually for illustration purposes) [11].

Regarding the not-polyp video, Figure 8 again shows three example frames. The base model produces false positive identifications in the three frames, while most of the not-polyp-trained models do not.

Focusing on the real out-of-distribution samples that we wanted to address in this study, we include two additional video clips found in two exploration videos. Figure 9 shows some frames of different situations found in two exploration videos included in the PIBAdb (provided as Supplementary Videos S3 and S4). These include, for instance, close to the wall of the colon images (first row), water jet (fourth row), or blurry images due to water (fifth row). The base model tends to produce false positives in such situations, as the first column shows, that the not-polyp-trained models tend to eliminate.

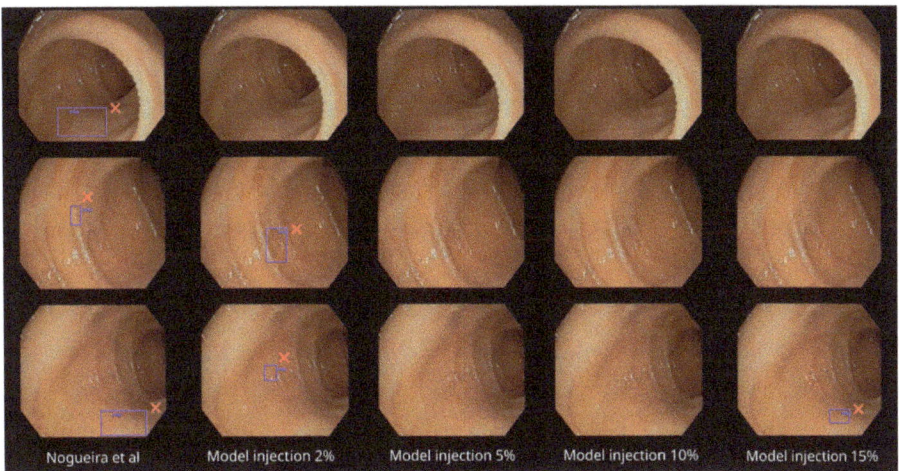

Figure 8. The five models with three sample frames of the not-polyp video segment analyzed (Supplementary Video S2). While the baseline model makes incorrect predictions (red cross marks) in the three cases, most of the not-polyp-trained models do not [11].

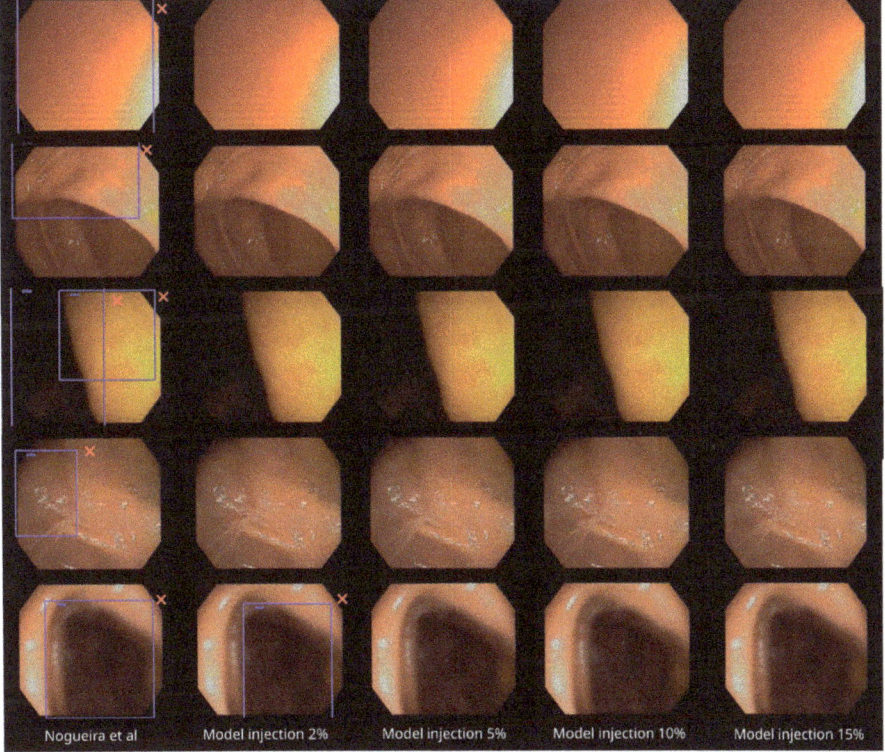

Figure 9. The five models facing different situations found in two exploration videos included in PIBAdb (provided as Supplementary Videos S3 and S4), including close to the wall of the colon (first row), water jet (fourth row), or blurry images due to water jet (fifth row). False positives are marked as red cross marks [11].

4. Conclusions

In this work, we retrained our polyp detection model with negative samples that were out-of-distribution images for our previous model in order to improve its positive predictive value (precision), while maintaining its sensitivity (recall), in the real setting. We have trained several models with different amounts of not-polyp images, incrementing our original training set from 2% up to 15% not-polyp images. We have evaluated them with both internal and public test partitions that include different amounts of such not-polyp images.

Regarding the performance of the models in our test partitions, or intra-dataset evaluation, we have observed that precision always increases as more not-polyp images are used for training the models, while recall oscillates slightly among them. The model trained with a 15% injection of not-polyp images was able to maintain the recall and reach the best precision of all the test partitions that include not-polyp images (average F1 of 0.893). Moreover, the original model was unable to maintain its original performance in the test partition that included the not-polyp images (descending from 0.881 to an average of 0.869), which illustrates the need for a test partition that includes this kind of image, which was kept out-of-distribution during the initial development.

On the other hand, we observed that the performance of the models in the public datasets containing not-polyp images also increases as more not-polyp images were used for training. Again, the model trained with a 15% injection of not-polyp images attained the best average F1 (0.722), and the biggest difference from the baseline model (average F1 of 0.695). In the public datasets with only polyp images, the results are more heterogeneous and differ depending on the dataset and model used. Altogether, the average F1 of each new model remained almost the same (~0.75), and, therefore, an unexpected worsening in the public datasets due to training with not-polyp images is discarded.

As noted before, the general trend is that the latest public datasets available include images without polyps, and our results suggest that it is worth using them (i) as negative samples for training, as it improves the performance in scenarios closer to real colonoscopies, and (ii) to correctly estimate the real performance of the detection models. The benefits are even observed when testing in datasets that only contain polyp images, although with higher variability.

Based on these observations, we think that there is room for improvement in polyp detection models using more data. Thus, future work to improve our model will be data-centric, as well. First, as the best performing model was the one trained with the highest amount of not-polyp images, also maintaining a good recall, it seems that the ceiling has not been reached in terms of the best proportion of not-polyp images to inject. More experiments in this direction could give us interesting insights. Our PIBAdb database still contains both annotated polyp images and not-polyp images that were not used to train the models, and it would be interesting to see if using more training data with both polyp and not-polyp images can increase the performance. Also, a lot of public datasets are available, and it would be interesting to see if training with some images from them (maybe the most challenging ones) can improve the performance in both our dataset and in the other public datasets.

Supplementary Materials: The following supporting information can be downloaded at: https://www.mdpi.com/article/10.3390/diagnostics13050966/s1, Supplementary Video S1 (S1_Video_polyp.mp4): an 18 s video of a polyp (450 frames). Supplementary Video S2 (S2_Video_Not_Polyp.mp4): (ii) a 14 s video of normal mucosa (not-polyp) (350 frames). Supplementary Video S3 (S3_Exploration_1.mp4): a 15 s video of an exploration from PIBAdb. Supplementary Video S4 (S4_Exploration_2.mp4): a 15 s video of an exploration from PIBAdb.

Author Contributions: Conceptualization, A.N.-R., D.G.-P. and H.L.-F.; data curation, A.N.-R.; funding acquisition, D.G.-P. and M.R.-J.; investigation, A.N.-R., D.G.-P. and H.L.-F.; methodology, A.N.-R., D.G.-P. and H.L.-F.; project administration, D.G.-P. and M.R.-J.; software, A.N.-R.; supervision, D.G.-P. and H.L.-F.; writing—original draft, A.N.-R., D.G.-P. and H.L.-F.; writing—review and editing, A.N.-R., D.G.-P., M.R.-J. and H.L.-F. All authors have read and agreed to the published version of the manuscript.

Funding: This work was partially supported by: (i) Ministerio de Ciencia y Competitividad and Ministerio de Ciencia e Innovación, Gobierno de España under the scope of the PolyDeep and PolyDeepAdvance projects (DPI2017-87494-R, PDC2021-121644-I00); (ii) by Consellería de Educación, Universidades e Formación Profesional (Xunta de Galicia) under the scope of the strategic funding ED431C2018/55-GRC and ED431C 2022/03-GRC Competitive Reference Group.

Institutional Review Board Statement: The study was conducted in accordance with the Declaration of Helsinki, and approved by Ethics Committee of Pontevedra-Vigo-Ourense research (code 2017/427 on 28 February 2018).

Informed Consent Statement: Informed consent was obtained from all subjects involved in the study.

Data Availability Statement: Publicly available datasets were analyzed in this study. Our not-polyp datasets are a subset of PIBAdb Colorectal Polyp Image Cohort, which can be requested here: https://www.iisgaliciasur.es/home/biobanco/cohorte-pibadb. Third-party datasets are available upon request to their owners.

Acknowledgments: We want to acknowledge Jorge Bernal for the support in accessing the CVC datasets and Heyato Itoh for giving access to the SUN dataset. The PICCOLO dataset included in this study was provided by the Basque Biobank (http://www.biobancovasco.org, accessed on January 2022). SING group thanks the CITI (Centro de Investigación, Transferencia e Innovación) from the University of Vigo for hosting its IT infrastructure.

Conflicts of Interest: The authors declare no conflict of interest.

References

1. Wang, P.; Berzin, T.M.; Brown, J.R.G.; Bharadwaj, S.; Becq, A.; Xiao, X.; Liu, P.; Li, L.; Song, Y.; Zhang, D.; et al. Real-time automatic detection system increases colonoscopic polyp and adenoma detection rates: A prospective randomised controlled study. *Gut* **2019**, *68*, 1813–1819. [CrossRef] [PubMed]
2. Gong, D.; Wu, L.; Zhang, J.; Mu, G.; Shen, L.; Liu, J.; Wang, Z.; Zhou, W.; An, P.; Huang, X.; et al. Detection of colorectal adenomas with a real-time computer-aided system (ENDOANGEL): A randomised controlled study. *Lancet Gastroenterol. Hepatol.* **2020**, *5*, 352–361. [CrossRef]
3. Wang, P.; Liu, X.; Berzin, T.M.; Glissen Brown, J.R.; Liu, P.; Zhou, C.; Lei, L.; Li, L.; Guo, Z.; Lei, S.; et al. Effect of a deep-learning computer-aided detection system on adenoma detection during colonoscopy (CADe-DB trial): A double-blind randomised study. *Lancet Gastroenterol. Hepatol.* **2020**, *5*, 343–351. [CrossRef]
4. Liu, W.-N.; Zhang, Y.-Y.; Bian, X.-Q.; Wang, L.-J.; Yang, Q.; Zhang, X.-D.; Huang, J. Study on detection rate of polyps and adenomas in artificial-intelligence-aided colonoscopy. *Saudi J. Gastroenterol.* **2020**, *26*, 13. [CrossRef] [PubMed]
5. Su, J.-R.; Li, Z.; Shao, X.-J.; Ji, C.-R.; Ji, R.; Zhou, R.-C.; Li, G.-C.; Liu, G.-Q.; He, Y.-S.; Zuo, X.-L.; et al. Impact of a real-time automatic quality control system on colorectal polyp and adenoma detection: A prospective randomized controlled study (with videos). *Gastrointest. Endosc.* **2020**, *91*, 415–424.e4. [CrossRef] [PubMed]
6. Repici, A.; Badalamenti, M.; Maselli, R.; Correale, L.; Radaelli, F.; Rondonotti, E.; Ferrara, E.; Spadaccini, M.; Alkandari, A.; Fugazza, A.; et al. Efficacy of Real-Time Computer-Aided Detection of Colorectal Neoplasia in a Randomized Trial. *Gastroenterology* **2020**, *159*, 512–520.e7. [CrossRef]
7. Hann, A.; Troya, J.; Fitting, D. Current status and limitations of artificial intelligence in colonoscopy. *United Eur. Gastroenterol. J.* **2021**, *9*, 527–533. [CrossRef]
8. Nogueira-Rodríguez, A.; Domínguez-Carbajales, R.; López-Fernández, H.; Iglesias, Á.; Cubiella, J.; Fdez-Riverola, F.; Reboiro-Jato, M.; Glez-Peña, D. Deep Neural Networks approaches for detecting and classifying colorectal polyps. *Neurocomputing* **2021**, *423*, 721–734. [CrossRef]
9. Viscaino, M.; Torres Bustos, J.; Muñoz, P.; Auat Cheein, C.; Cheein, F.A. Artificial intelligence for the early detection of colorectal cancer: A comprehensive review of its advantages and misconceptions. *World J. Gastroenterol.* **2021**, *27*, 6399–6414. [CrossRef]
10. Everingham, M.; Van Gool, L.; Williams, C.K.I.; Winn, J.; Zisserman, A. The Pascal Visual Object Classes (VOC) Challenge. *Int. J. Comput. Vis.* **2010**, *88*, 303–338. [CrossRef]

11. Nogueira-Rodríguez, A.; Domínguez-Carbajales, R.; Campos-Tato, F.; Herrero, J.; Puga, M.; Remedios, D.; Rivas, L.; Sánchez, E.; Iglesias, Á.; Cubiella, J.; et al. Real-time polyp detection model using convolutional neural networks. *Neural Comput. Appl.* **2021**, *34*, 10375–10396. [CrossRef]
12. Nogueira-Rodríguez, A.; Reboiro-Jato, M.; Glez-Peña, D.; López-Fernández, H. Performance of Convolutional Neural Networks for Polyp Localization on Public Colonoscopy Image Datasets. *Diagnostics* **2022**, *12*, 898. [CrossRef] [PubMed]
13. Misawa, M.; Kudo, S.; Mori, Y.; Hotta, K.; Ohtsuka, K.; Matsuda, T.; Saito, S.; Kudo, T.; Baba, T.; Ishida, F.; et al. Development of a computer-aided detection system for colonoscopy and a publicly accessible large colonoscopy video database (with video). *Gastrointest. Endosc.* **2021**, *93*, 960–967.e3. [CrossRef]
14. Li, K.; Fathan, M.I.; Patel, K.; Zhang, T.; Zhong, C.; Bansal, A.; Rastogi, A.; Wang, J.S.; Wang, G. Colonoscopy polyp detection and classification: Dataset creation and comparative evaluations. *PLoS ONE* **2021**, *16*, e0255809. [CrossRef] [PubMed]
15. Ma, Y.; Chen, X.; Cheng, K.; Li, Y.; Sun, B. LDPolypVideo Benchmark: A Large-Scale Colonoscopy Video Dataset of Diverse Polyps. In *Medical Image Computing and Computer Assisted Intervention—MICCAI 2021*; de Bruijne, M., Cattin, P.C., Cotin, S., Padoy, N., Speidel, S., Zheng, Y., Essert, C., Eds.; Springer International Publishing: Cham, Germany, 2021; Volume 12905, pp. 387–396.
16. Pogorelov, K.; Schmidt, P.T.; Riegler, M.; Halvorsen, P.; Randel, K.R.; Griwodz, C.; Eskeland, S.L.; de Lange, T.; Johansen, D.; Spampinato, C.; et al. KVASIR: A Multi-Class Image Dataset for Computer Aided Gastrointestinal Disease Detection. In Proceedings of the 8th ACM on Multimedia Systems Conference—MMSys'17, Taipei, Taiwan, 20–23 June 2017; ACM Press: Taipei, Taiwan, 2017; pp. 164–169.
17. Bernal, J.; Sánchez, F.J.; Fernández-Esparrach, G.; Gil, D.; Rodríguez, C.; Vilariño, F. WM-DOVA maps for accurate polyp highlighting in colonoscopy: Validation vs. saliency maps from physicians. *Comput. Med. Imaging Graph.* **2015**, *43*, 99–111. [CrossRef] [PubMed]
18. Bernal, J.; Sánchez, J.; Vilariño, F. Towards automatic polyp detection with a polyp appearance model. *Pattern Recognit.* **2012**, *45*, 3166–3182. [CrossRef]
19. Vázquez, D.; Bernal, J.; Sánchez, F.J.; Fernández-Esparrach, G.; López, A.M.; Romero, A.; Drozdzal, M.; Courville, A. A Benchmark for Endoluminal Scene Segmentation of Colonoscopy Images. *J. Healthc. Eng.* **2017**, *2017*, 4037190. [CrossRef]
20. Silva, J.; Histace, A.; Romain, O.; Dray, X.; Granado, B. Toward embedded detection of polyps in WCE images for early diagnosis of colorectal cancer. *Int. J. Comput. Assist. Radiol. Surg.* **2014**, *9*, 283–293. [CrossRef]
21. Angermann, Q.; Bernal, J.; Sánchez-Montes, C.; Hammami, M.; Fernández-Esparrach, G.; Dray, X.; Romain, O.; Sánchez, F.J.; Histace, A. Towards Real-Time Polyp Detection in Colonoscopy Videos: Adapting Still Frame-Based Methodologies for Video Sequences Analysis. In *Computer Assisted and Robotic Endoscopy and Clinical Image-Based Procedures*; Cardoso, M.J., Arbel, T., Luo, X., Wesarg, S., Reichl, T., González Ballester, M.Á., McLeod, J., Drechsler, K., Peters, T., Erdt, M., et al., Eds.; Springer International Publishing: Cham, Germany, 2017; pp. 29–41.
22. Bernal, J.J.; Histace, A.; Masana, M.; Angermann, Q.; Sánchez-Montes, C.; Rodriguez, C.; Hammami, M.; Garcia-Rodriguez, A.; Córdova, H.; Romain, O.; et al. Polyp Detection Benchmark in Colonoscopy Videos using GTCreator: A Novel Fully Configurable Tool for Easy and Fast Annotation of Image Databases. In Proceedings of the 32nd CARS Conference, Berlin, Germany, 20–23 June 2018.
23. Sánchez-Peralta, L.F.; Pagador, J.B.; Picón, A.; Calderón, Á.J.; Polo, F.; Andraka, N.; Bilbao, R.; Glover, B.; Saratxaga, C.L.; Sánchez-Margallo, F.M. PICCOLO White-Light and Narrow-Band Imaging Colonoscopic Dataset: A Performance Comparative of Models and Datasets. *Appl. Sci.* **2020**, *10*, 8501. [CrossRef]
24. Houwen, B.B.S.L.; Nass, K.J.; Vleugels, J.L.A.; Fockens, P.; Hazewinkel, Y.; Dekker, E. Comprehensive review of publicly available colonoscopic imaging databases for artificial intelligence research: Availability, accessibility, and usability. *Gastrointest. Endosc.* **2022**, *97*, 184–199.e6. [CrossRef]
25. López-Fernández, H.; Graña-Castro, O.; Nogueira-Rodríguez, A.; Reboiro-Jato, M.; Glez-Peña, D. Compi: A framework for portable and reproducible pipelines. *PeerJ Comput. Sci.* **2021**, *7*, e593. [CrossRef] [PubMed]
26. Nogueira-Rodríguez, A.; López-Fernández, H.; Graña-Castro, O.; Reboiro-Jato, M.; Glez-Peña, D. Compi Hub: A Public Repository for Sharing and Discovering Compi Pipelines. In Proceedings of the Practical Applications of Computational Biology & Bioinformatics, 14th International Conference (PACBB 2020), L'Aquila, Italy, 17–19 June 2020; Panuccio, G., Rocha, M., Fdez-Riverola, F., Mohamad, M.S., Casado-Vara, R., Eds.; Springer International Publishing: Cham, Germany, 2021; pp. 51–59.

Disclaimer/Publisher's Note: The statements, opinions and data contained in all publications are solely those of the individual author(s) and contributor(s) and not of MDPI and/or the editor(s). MDPI and/or the editor(s) disclaim responsibility for any injury to people or property resulting from any ideas, methods, instructions or products referred to in the content.

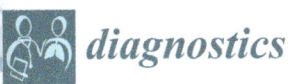

Article

Comparison of Machine Learning Models and the Fatty Liver Index in Predicting Lean Fatty Liver

Pei-Yuan Su [1,2,*], Yang-Yuan Chen [1,3], Chun-Yu Lin [4], Wei-Wen Su [1], Siou-Ping Huang [1] and Hsu-Heng Yen [1,2,5,6,7]

1. Department of Internal Medicine, Division of Gastroenterology, Changhua Christian Hospital, Changhua 500, Taiwan; 27716@cch.org.tw (Y.-Y.C.); 35301@cch.org.tw (W.-W.S.); 182972@cch.org.tw (S.-P.H.); 91646@cch.org.tw (H.-H.Y.)
2. College of Medicine, National Chung Hsing University, Taichung 400, Taiwan
3. Department of Hospitality Management, MingDao University, Changhua 500, Taiwan
4. Department of Family Medicine, Yumin Hospital, Nantou 540, Taiwan; amonslin@gmail.com
5. General Education Center, Chienkuo Technology University, Changhua 500, Taiwan
6. Department of Electrical Engineering, Chung Yuan Christian University, Taoyuan 320, Taiwan
7. Artificial Intelligence Development Center, Changhua Christian Hospital, Changhua 500, Taiwan
* Correspondence: 111252@cch.org.tw

Abstract: The reported prevalence of non-alcoholic fatty liver disease in studies of lean individuals ranges from 7.6% to 19.3%. The aim of the study was to develop machine-learning models for the prediction of fatty liver disease in lean individuals. The present retrospective study included 12,191 lean subjects with a body mass index < 23 kg/m^2 who had undergone a health checkup from January 2009 to January 2019. Participants were divided into a training (70%, 8533 subjects) and a testing group (30%, 3568 subjects). A total of 27 clinical features were analyzed, except for medical history and history of alcohol or tobacco consumption. Among the 12,191 lean individuals included in the present study, 741 (6.1%) had fatty liver. The machine learning model comprising a two-class neural network using 10 features had the highest area under the receiver operating characteristic curve (AUROC) value (0.885) among all other algorithms. When applied to the testing group, we found the two-class neural network exhibited a slightly higher AUROC value for predicting fatty liver (0.868, 0.841–0.894) compared to the fatty liver index (FLI; 0.852, 0.824–0.81). In conclusion, the two-class neural network had greater predictive value for fatty liver than the FLI in lean individuals.

Keywords: lean fatty liver; machine learning model; fatty liver index

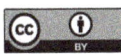

1. Introduction

Non-alcoholic fatty liver disease (NAFLD) is one of the most prevalent forms of liver disease worldwide and is associated with increased risks of cirrhosis and hepatocellular carcinoma (HCC) [1]. Incidence rates of HCC have been higher in patients with nonalcoholic steatohepatitis (NASH) cirrhosis than in those with non-cirrhotic NAFLD. In Asian populations, a Japanese study revealed a 5-year HCC incidence of 11.3% among patients with NASH cirrhosis [2]. The global prevalence of NAFLD has been reported as 25.24%, with a regional prevalence of 27.37% in Asia [3]. Fatty liver in lean individuals has similar clinical characteristics to NAFLD [4]. In fact, a Swedish registry study found that although lean individuals with NAFLD had a lower baseline fibrosis severity than did non-lean individuals, they were still at high risk for developing severe liver disease [5]. Lean individuals with NAFLD are at increased risk of developing type 2 diabetes mellitus (DM) and metabolic syndrome and increased risk of mortality from cardiovascular and liver diseases [4,6]. Lean and non-lean individuals with NAFLD share several metabolic risk factors, including hypertriglyceridemia, low high-density lipoprotein (HDL) levels, type 2 DM, hypertension, metabolic syndrome, increased body mass index (BMI) and increased waist circumference. Generic characteristics, such as the PNPLA3 G allele, also play an important role in the development of NAFLD among lean individuals. The prevalence of NAFLD in lean individuals according to different BMI criteria (23–25 kg/m^2) reportedly ranges from 7.6% to 19.3% [7]. The prevalence of NAFLD in a population with a BMI < 24 kg/m^2 from south Taiwan was reported as 18.5% [8].

NAFLD can be diagnosed by liver biopsy or image. The gold standard method for the diagnosis of steatosis is liver biopsy; however, this approach is invasive and carries some bleeding risk. Meanwhile, diagnostic imaging, such as ultrasonography, computed tomography and magnetic resonance imaging, is time-consuming, costly and not always available in remote areas. Early diagnosis of hepatic steatosis based on risk factors helps clinicians identify the adverse events of NAFLD and prescribe more lifestyle interventions to prevent them. In addition, the diagnosis of NAFLD in lean individuals can easily be missed. Several biomarkers have been investigated as predictors of fatty liver, including markers of apoptosis and oxidative stress, the BARD score and the fatty liver index (FLI) [9]. The FLI is the most validated tool for predicting hepatic steatosis in the general and lean population [10]. Artificial intelligence (AI) has also been used to predict NAFLD for several years. Electronic health records and imaging data are the two main sources of data used to develop machine-learning models [11]. The area under the receiver operating characteristic (AUROC) for predicting NAFLD was higher for AI-assisted ultrasound (0.98) compared to AI-assisted clinical data sets (0.85). Our previous report demonstrated that a machine learning model using extreme gradient boosting (XGBoost) had a greater predictive value for fatty liver [12]. However, there was limited data on using machine learning models to predict lean fatty liver in the world. The aim of our study is trying to develop machine learning models for the prediction of lean fatty liver and to compare these models with FLI in the lean population.

2. Materials and Methods

2.1. Patient Selection

This retrospective study included subjects that had received a health checkup at Changhua Christian Hospital between January 2009 and January 2019. All subjects were adults (20–80 years old) and "lean," as defined by a BMI < 23 kg/m^2. Collected clinical data and ultrasound findings were from the same day. Only subjects with complete data for all parameters, including complete blood counts and biochemistry and lipid profiles, were included in the study analysis. We excluded subjects with incomplete clinical parameters and those whose BMI was $\geq$23 kg/m^2. Initially, 45,006 subjects were enrolled. We then excluded 13,076 subjects with incomplete clinical datasets and 19,739 subjects whose BMI was $\geq$ 23 kg/m^2. Finally, a total of 12,191 subjects were included in the study (Figure 1). The present study was approved by the Ethics Committee of Changhua Christian Hospital (CCH IRB No: 191012), and informed consent was waived as all data were deidentified.

2.2. Ultrasound Imaging

Fatty liver disease was defined as moderate-to-severe fatty change on ultrasonography. All participants fasted for at least 6 h prior to ultrasound examinations. Ultrasonography was performed by three independent ultrasound operators who were blinded to clinical data. Moderate-to-severe fatty changes on ultrasound were defined as the presence of at least 3 of the following 4 features: (1) hepatorenal echo contrast, (2) liver brightness, (3) deep attenuation and (4) vascular blurring [13,14].

2.3. Model Construction and Validation

The dataset was divided into a training group (70%, 8533 subjects) and a testing group (30%, 3568 subjects) using a randomized 70–30 split. Due to the low prevalence of fatty liver among the lean individuals included in the present study, healthy controls and participants with fatty liver disease were randomized into each group using a 2:1 ratio (Figure 1). The training set and validation set were randomly selected from the training group using an 80–20 split and a 10-fold cross-validation model. The machine learning platform used in the present study was Azure Machine Learning, a cloud-based computing platform (Azure ML; Microsoft, Redmond, WA, USA). Nine 2-class classification algorithms were compared, including a neural network, averaged perceptron, a locally-deep support vector machine, logistic regression, a support vector machine, a Bayes point machine, a decision jungle, a boosted decision tree and a decision forest. After building the machine learning algorithms, the testing group was used to identify the algorithm with the greatest predictive power for fatty liver compared to the FLI.

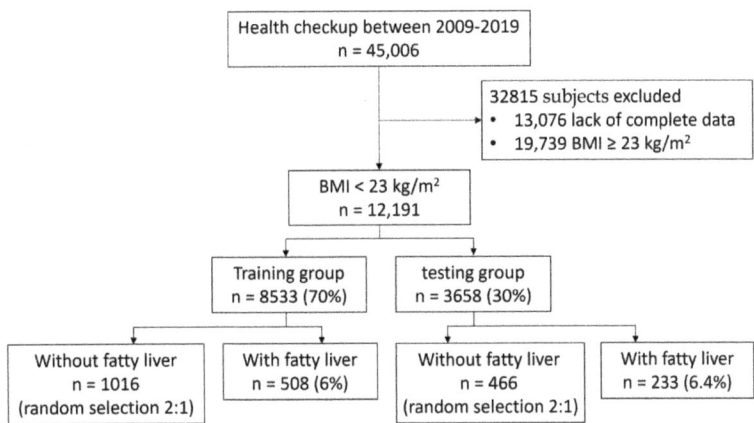

Figure 1. Participant flow chart for the training and testing groups in the present study.

2.4. Feature Selection

The clinical features included in our dataset were age, gender, height, weight, waist, BMI, systolic blood pressure (SBP), diastolic blood pressure (DBP), white blood cell count, red blood cell, hemoglobin, platelet, mean corpuscular volume, mean corpuscular hemoglobin, mean corpuscular hemoglobin concentration, red cell distribution width, aspartate aminotransferase, alanine aminotransferase (ALT), r-glutamyl transpeptidase (r-GT), total cholesterol, HDL, low-density lipoprotein, triglyceride (TG), creatinine, fasting serum glucose, Fibrosis-4 (FIB-4) score and FLI. Filter-based feature selection was used to rank each feature according to the calculated scores for each feature. Six feature scoring methods were used in the present study: Pearson's correlation, mutual information, Kendall correlation, Spearman's correlation, the chi-squared test and the Fisher score. After comparisons between ranking lists, we selected the 10 features most commonly used in clinical practice to build a prediction model.

2.5. FLI

The FLI was developed to predict hepatic steatosis in the general population by Giorgio Bedogni et al. [15] The FLI was calculated using the following equation:

$$(e^{0.953 \times \log_e (\text{triglycerides}) + 0.139 \times \text{BMI} + 0.718 \times \log_e (\text{r-GT}) + 0.053 \times \text{waist circumference} - 15.745}) / (1 + e^{0.953 \times \log_e (\text{triglycerides}) + 0.139 \times \text{BMI} + 0.718 \times \log_e (\text{r-GT}) + 0.053 \times \text{waist circumference} - 15.745}) \times 100$$

2.6. Statistical Analysis

The chi-squared test was used to compare categorical variables, and the Mann–Whitney U test was used to compare continuous variables between groups. AUROC values were calculated using optimal cut-off values identified using the Youden index test. All statistical analyses were performed using SPSS version 22.0 (IBM Corp., Armonk, NY, USA), with 2-tailed p values < 0.05 indicating statistical significance.

3. Results

3.1. Clinical Characteristics of the Participants

Of the 12191 lean subjects, 741 (6.1%) had fatty liver. The training group comprised 8533 subjects (70%), of which 508 (6%) had fatty liver. The testing group comprised 3568 subjects (30%), of which 233 (6.4%) had fatty liver. The clinical characteristics of study subjects in the training group according to the presence or absence of fatty liver are shown in Table 1. Subjects with fatty liver were older, with a male predominance, compared to subjects without fatty liver. Significant differences in waist circumference, BMI, blood pressure, white blood cell count, serum hemoglobin, platelet count, serum glucose, serum biochemistry parameters, serum lipid profiles and FLI were observed between subjects with and without fatty liver. Histogram findings for both groups are shown in Figure 2. Accordingly, the figure shows that the distribution of the FLI is skewed to the right, with a slight difference between the two groups.

Table 1. Clinical parameters in lean subjects with and without fatty liver.

	With Fatty Liver ($n = 508$)	Without Fatty Liver ($n = 1016$)	p-Value
Age (years)	52.69 ± 8.97	47.32 ± 11.17	<0.001
Gender, male	304 (59.8%)	438 (43.1%)	<0.001
Height (cm)	164.47 ± 8.11	163.52 ± 7.8	0.010
Weight (kg)	59.8 ± 6.31	56.04 ± 6.95	<0.001
Waist circumference (cm)	78.54 ± 5.1	73.14 ± 5.77	<0.001
SBP (mmHg)	127.24 ± 15.82	116.44 ± 14.57	<0.001
DBP (mmHg)	80.44 ± 9.5	74.42 ± 9.21	<0.001
BMI (kg/m^2)	22.05 ± 0.78	20.9 ± 1.48	<0.001
WBC ($\times 10^9$/L)	5.84 ± 1.49	5.18 ± 1.44	<0.001
RBC count ($\times 10^9$/L)	4.76 ± 0.54	4.58 ± 0.48	<0.001
Hb (g/dL)	14.28 ± 1.36	13.73 ± 1.48	<0.001
MCV (fL)	42.57 ± 3.82	41.06 ± 4.1	<0.001
RBC volume (fL)	90.02 ± 7.46	90.1 ± 7.32	0.568
MCH (pg)	30.23 ± 2.95	30.14 ± 2.86	0.387
MCHC (g/dL)	33.54 ± 0.95	33.41 ± 0.88	0.001
Platelet ($\times 10^3$/L)	226.59 ± 52.13	219.24 ± 49.68	0.009
RBC-RDW (%)	13.32 ± 1.04	13.51 ± 1.22	0.004
Glucose (mg/dL)	106.73 ± 31.21	91.48 ± 13.12	<0.001
AST (IU/L)	28.04 ± 15.42	23.03 ± 10.01	<0.001
ALT (IU/L)	31.36 ± 19.93	20.7 ± 12.26	<0.001
r-GT (U/L)	31.39 ± 56.94	17.68 ± 12.91	<0.001
Total cholesterol (mg/dL)	198.89 ± 37.48	190.62 ± 33.34	<0.001
HDL (mg/dL)	46.82 ± 10.66	57.06 ± 13.96	<0.001
LDL (mg/dL)	124.6 ± 34.5	115.23 ± 28.68	<0.001
Triglyceride (mg/dL)	138.14 ± 78.5	81.93 ± 45.67	<0.001
Cr (mg/dL)	0.78 ± 0.2	0.75 ± 0.18	0.001
FIB-4	1.26 ± 0.6	1.21 ± 0.63	0.014
FLI	18.66 ± 12.43	7.13 ± 6.75	<0.001

Abbreviations: SBP, systolic blood pressure; DBP, diastolic blood pressure; BMI, body mass index; WBC, white blood cell count; RBC, red blood cell; Hb, hemoglobin; MCV, mean corpuscular volume; MCH, mean corpuscular hemoglobin; MCHC, mean corpuscular hemoglobin concentration; RDW, red cell distribution width; AST, aspartate aminotransferase; ALT, alanine aminotransferase; r-GT, r-glutamyl transpeptidase; HDL, high-density lipoprotein; LDL, low-density lipoprotein; Cr, creatinine; FIB-4, fibrosis index based on four factors; FLI, fatty liver index.

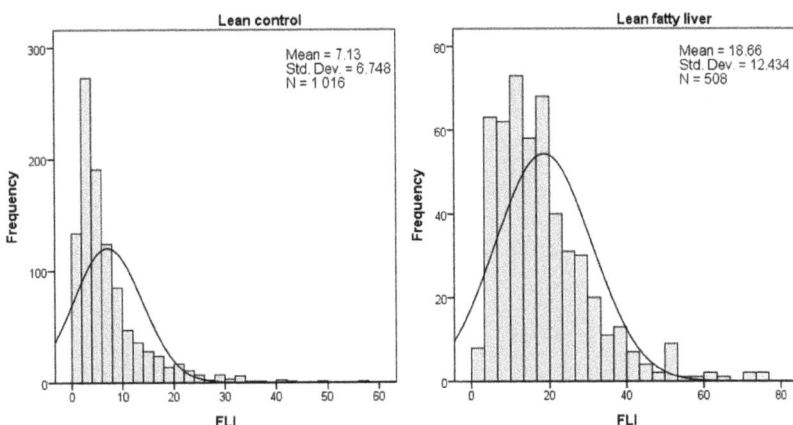

Figure 2. Histogram of fatty liver index (FLI) from lean fatty liver and control in the training group.

3.2. Feature Selection and Comparison of Classification Algorithms in the Training Set

Table 2 shows the 10 features selected by the six different scoring methods. The 10 highest scoring features were BMI, waist circumference, weight, age, serum TG, serum HDL, serum glucose, serum ALT, SBP and DBP. Table 3 shows the nine different classification algorithms of the machine learning models using the 10 selected features and all 27 features. The best predictive model was the two-class neural network using 10 features, with an AUROC value of 0.885, an accuracy of 0.816, a recall of 0.661, an F1 score of 0.72 and a precision of 0.791. (Figure 3).

Table 2. The 10 features selected by the six different scoring methods.

Method (Correlation Coefficient)	Scored Features									
Pearson correlation	Steatosis	Waist	TG	BMI	HDL	Glucose	SBP	ALT	DBP	Weight	Age
	1	0.417	0.412	0.388	0.349	0.325	0.321	0.313	0.292	0.254	0.235
Mutual information	Steatosis	TG	BMI	Waist	rGT	ALT	Glucose	HDL	SBP	DBP	Age
	1	0.105	0.097	0.094	0.089	0.086	0.078	0.067	0.055	0.045	0.039
Kendall correlation	Steatosis	TG	Waist	rGT	ALT	BMI	Glucose	HDL	SBP	DBP	AST
	1	0.364	0.348	0.341	0.334	0.325	0.310	0.297	0.264	0.243	0.212
Spearman correlation	Steatosis	TG	Waist	rGT	ALT	BMI	Glucose	HDL	SBP	DBP	Weight
	1	0.444	0.419	0.409	0.403	0.398	0.374	0.359	0.320	0.293	0.258
Chi-squared	Steatosis	TG	Waist	ALT	BMI	rGT	Glucose	HDL	SBP	DBP	AST
	1	316.830	272.800	264.647	260.506	255.513	236.273	197.071	164.514	136.655	117.880
Fisher Score	Steatosis	Waist	TG	BMI	HDL	Glucose	SBP	ALT	DBP	Weight	Age
	1	0.210	0.204	0.177	0.139	0.118	0.115	0.109	0.093	0.069	0.058

Abbreviations: TG, triglycerides; ALT, alanine aminotransferase; r-GT, r-glutamyl transpeptidase; BMI, body mass index; SBP, systolic blood pressure; DBP, diastolic blood pressure; AST, aspartate aminotransferase; HDL, high-density lipoprotein.

3.3. Comparison of Machine Learning Models and the FLI Using the Testing Set

The FLI index was calculated in the testing group and compared to the machine learning model comprising a two-class neural network. The AUROC value was higher for the machine learning model using 10 selected features (above-mentioned; 0.868, 95% CI 0.841–0.894) compared to the FLI (0.852, 95% CI 0.824–0.881) and machine learning model using four selected features (same as factors in FLI including waist, BMI, r-GT and TG) (0.851, 95% CI 0.823–0.879; Figure 4). The optimal cut-off value, according to the Youden index test for the FLI, was 9, with a sensitivity of 82.4% and specificity of 74.9%.

Table 3. Results from the nine machine learning models using the 10 selected features and all 27 features.

Model	Features	AUROC	Accuracy	Recall	F1 Score	Precision
Two-class neural network	10	0.885	0.816	0.661	0.72	0.791
	27	0.877	0.793	0.624	0.683	0.756
Two-class averaged perceptron	10	0.875	0.8	0.624	0.69	0.773
	27	0.874	0.79	0.615	0.677	0.753
Two-class locally-deep support vector machine	10	0.845	0.797	0.569	0.667	0.805
	27	0.833	0.77	0.505	0.611	0.775
Two-class logistic regression	10	0.867	0.793	0.596	0.674	0.774
	27	0.874	0.787	0.596	0.667	0.756
Two-class support vector machine	10	0.872	0.8	0.633	0.693	0.767
	27	0.866	0.793	0.642	0.69	0.745
Two-class Bayes point machine	10	0.86	0.77	0.505	0.611	0.775
	27	0.878	0.77	0.495	0.607	0.783
Two-class decision jungle	10	0.849	0.78	0.624	0.67	0.723
	27	0.851	0.784	0.578	0.656	0.759
Two-class boosted decision tree	10	0.859	0.764	0.624	0.654	0.687
	27	0.871	0.793	0.67	0.699	0.73
Two-class decision forest	10	0.852	0.784	0.56	0.649	0.772
	27	0.846	0.774	0.578	0.646	0.733

Abbreviations: AUROC, area under the receiver operating characteristic.

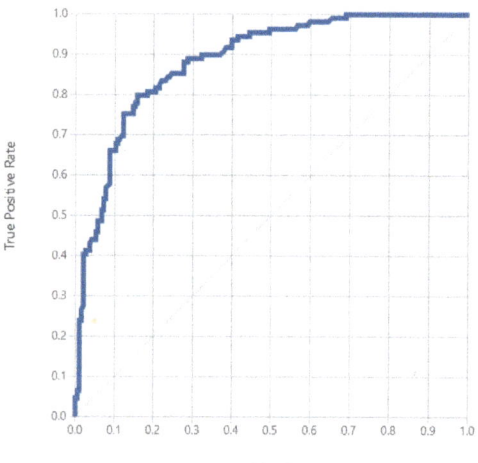

Figure 3. Area under the receiver operating characteristic curve for the machine learning model using a two-class neural network (AUROC value, 0.885).

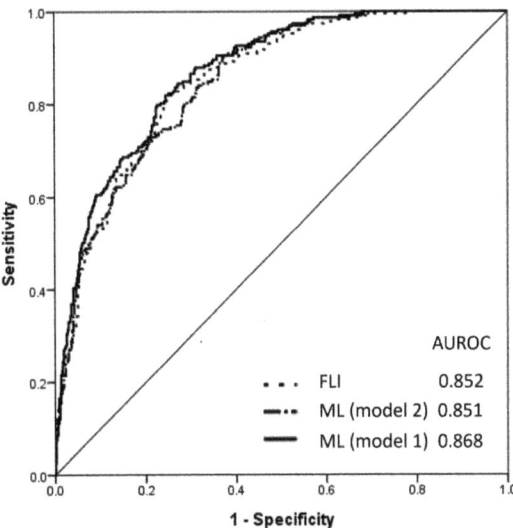

Figure 4. Area under the receiver operating characteristic (AUROC) curves of the machine learning (ML) model 1 comprising a two-class neural network using 10 selected features (body mass index, waist, weight, age, triglyceride (TG), high-density lipoprotein, glucose, alanine aminotransferase, systolic blood pressure and diastolic blood pressure), ML model 2 comprising a two-class neural network using four selected features (body mass index, waist, TG and r-glutamyl transpeptidase) and the fatty liver index (FLI) for predicting steatosis in lean individuals using the testing set.

4. Discussion

The present study is the first to use machine learning models to predict fatty liver in lean individuals. Our results demonstrate that a machine learning model had a slightly greater ability to discriminate between fatty liver and non-fatty liver in lean subjects from an Asian population compared to a conventional scoring system for predicting fatty liver (FLI). These machine learning algorithms may have utility in predicting fatty liver in regions where ultrasonography is not available and in analyzing pathophysiologic correlations with other clinical outcomes, such as cardiovascular events or mortality.

There is significant heterogeneity in the reported prevalence of fatty liver in lean individuals from previous studies due to the use of an upper limit of BMI ranging from 23 to 25 kg/m² to define "lean" individuals in different populations. Two previous meta-analyses reported an overall prevalence of NAFLD in lean populations of 10.2% and 10.6% [16,17]. A lower prevalence of NAFLD was observed when lower BMI criteria were used and in populations based on patients attending health check-ups. The definition of "lean" in the present study was a BMI < 23 kg/m², and the prevalence of fatty liver in lean individuals was 6.1%. This prevalence of NAFLD in lean individuals was lower than reported by a similar study in a Taiwanese population conducted in 2019 which reported a prevalence of NAFLD of 18.5% in individuals with a BMI < 24 kg/m² [8]. Other than differences in BMI cut-off values, criteria for diagnosing NAFLD using ultrasound may represent a further confounding factor as fatty liver was defined as moderate-to-severe fatty change on ultrasound in the present study. A similar prevalence (10.37%) of NAFLD in a non-obese population (BMI < 25 kg/m²) was reported from a study conducted in China which observed a higher prevalence of NAFLD in patients aged 50–59 years [18].

Differing factors are associated with NAFLD in lean and obese patients. The most common factors related to NAFLD in lean patients included BMI, waist circumference, serum triglyceride levels, serum HDL levels, DM, metabolic syndrome, blood pressure and serum liver enzyme levels [5]. Genetic factors are associated with the development of NAFLD in lean individuals, including patatin-like phospholipase domain-containing

3 (PNPLA3, rs738409 C > G) and transmembrane 6 superfamily member 2 (TM6SF2, rs58542926 C > T) [19,20]. The FLI contains four risk factors, including triglyceride, BMI, r-GT and waist circumference. Age is also an important risk of NAFLD in lean people. According to a meta-analysis, lean individuals with NAFLD were older than lean controls, with a mean difference of 2.87 years [21]. Sex differences have also been noted in NAFLD, such that a higher prevalence of NAFLD was found among males than among females. Liver outcomes in both sexes have been controversial, given that the effects of a dysmetabolic state might be greater in females than in males [22]. However, studies on the effects of sex on NAFLD in lean individuals have currently been limited. The present study used a cloud-based computing platform and filter-based selection to identify waist circumference, serum TG, BMI, weight, serum HDL, serum glucose, SBP, serum ALT, DBP and age as the 10 highest scoring factors. Although baseline characteristics showed male predominant in lean fatty liver, sex was not identified as an important feature in our model. These findings were similar to the results of previous studies [23,24].

AI has been used to predict NAFLD and classify the severity of liver fibrosis for many years [25]. A range of machine learning models and deep learning modules have been developed using large-scale electronic health records and images from clinical investigations, including histology, ultrasonography, computed tomography and magnetic resonance imaging [26]. Several public cloud-based platforms can be used to develop machine learning models, including Tensorflow (Google Brain Team, Menlo Park, CA, USA), WEKA (University of Waikato, Hamilton, New Zealand), the Orange Data Mining platform (Bioinformatics Lab, University of Ljubljana, Slovenia) and Azure Machine Learning (Microsoft, Redmond, WA, USA) [11]. According to a meta-analysis, AI-assisted ultrasonography had a higher area under the curve for the detection of NAFLD than an AI-assisted clinical data set (0.98 vs. 0.85) [9]. Several machine learning algorithms have been used to predict NAFLD, including extreme gradient boosting (XGBoost), neural network, support vector machine, logistic regression, decision forests and decision jungles. XGBoost is easy to interpret and has been shown to have good predictive utility in diagnosing NAFLD (AUROC, 0.882–0.931) in several studies [12,27,28]. While neural networks can address non-linear correlations and complex models, they require large computer resources and have a tendency to overfit. Meanwhile, support vector machines can handle high-dimensional data and non-linear correlations but have low efficacy due to their high computational costs. Logistic regression models are easy to train and interpret but cannot address non-linear problems. There was no available publication that used machine learning for the detection of lean NAFLD in the lean population. This is the first study to predict fatty liver in lean individuals using Azure Machine Learning which utilized nine different machine learning tools with a two-class neural network found to be the best machine learning algorithm (AUROC, 0.885). The predictive power is better in machine learning algorithms using 10 features than 27 features. The situation that performance was reduced by adding features may be explained by two possible reasons. First, when too many features are added to a machine learning model, it can lead to overfitting and influence the results from validation and test sets. Second, some features may not be useful in predicting outcomes or may be highly correlated with other features. When these features are added to the machine learning model, they can introduce noise and reduce the predictive value. After incorporating the neural network and the FLI into the testing group, we found that the neural network using 10 selected features had a slightly greater AUROC than did the FLI and neural network using four selected features (same as factors in FLI). This suggests the presence of non-linear correlations between these 10 features, which can be detected using certain specific machine learning algorithms. However, better information quality may be another possible explanation because the AUROCs are similar between the machine learning model using four features and FLI.

Scoring algorithms have been developed to predict hepatic steatosis. The FLI was developed in 2006 and had an accuracy for predicting steatosis of 0.84 [15]. Recently, the FLI has also been used to predict 10-year cardiovascular disease risks and mortality. [29] A study including a Korean population showed the individual who had a higher FLI (≥60) had a higher Framingham 10-year CVD risk (odds ratio 2.56). Another study from Korea showed that FLI could be a poor prognostic factor, particularly in the underweight population (BMI < 18.5 kg/m^2). [30] Moreover, a study from China showed that a triglyceride and glucose index (TyG) developed to predict insulin resistance could also be used to identify NAFLD, although its AUROC was not particularly good (0.782). [31] Different cut-off values for the FLI for the prediction of fatty liver have been assessed in lean populations, with a previous study conducted in Taiwan demonstrating a cut-off value of 15 had the highest discriminant ability in a lean population and a further study conducted in Turkey demonstrated a cut-off value of 5.68 had the highest AUROC (0.748) for predicting NAFLD in lean females with polycystic ovary syndrome [8,32]. In the present study, the FLI had an AUROC value of 0.852 for predicting steatosis in lean individuals using a cut-off value of 9 identified using the Youden index test. We compared FLI cut-off values of 9 and 15 using a machine learning model in the testing group, with AUROC values of 0.784 for the FLI using a cut-off value of 9, 0.752 for the two-class neural network (scored probability > 0.5) and 0.722 for the FLI using a cut-off value of 15.

The present study had some limitations. First, we did not collect data on hepatitis B and C virus status or history of alcohol consumption or diabetes. The present study comprised subjects with fatty liver on ultrasound which may have included patients with NAFLD and alcoholic fatty disease. Although patients with viral hepatitis and alcohol liver disease may have been included in the present study, further studies are required to determine the predictive ability of machine learning models in detecting steatosis in populations with a single liver disease etiology. Metabolic-associated fatty liver disease (MAFLD) is not a suitable representation of our study subjects, given that our subjects do not satisfy the diagnostic criteria for MAFLD. Second, some clinical parameters were not included in the present study, such as uric acid, HbA1C, C-reactive protein and homeostasis model assessment for insulin resistance (HOMA-IR). These parameters have been shown to be associated with lean NAFLD [21,33]. Third, we did not collect histological data from liver biopsies or other non-invasive imaging techniques, such as the controlled attenuation parameter measured by FibroScan® or magnetic resonance imaging-derived proton density fat fraction to confirm the degree of the steatosis. Our use of ultrasonography may have resulted in the underdiagnosis of hepatic steatosis in our patients relative to that using histology. Accordingly, the prevalence of fatty liver may have been underestimated in the present study. This would suggest that the machine learning model cannot be used to predict mild steatosis in the general population.

5. Conclusions

The present study describes the development of machine learning models to predict fatty liver in lean individuals, with a two-class neural network model found to have the greatest predictive ability. The AUROC value was slightly higher using the machine learning model than the FLI. In addition, the prevalence of fatty liver in lean individuals was 6.1%, and the optimal FLI cut-off value was 9 in the present study. These results can help clinicians promptly and accurately diagnose fatty liver disease in lean subjects considering that hepatic steatosis in lean populations can be easily overlooked or treated late. Further studies with larger sample sizes using other forms of clinical information and image are required to validate the utility of novel machine-learning models in predicting steatosis and fibrosis.

Author Contributions: Conceptualization and methodology of the study, H.-H.Y. and Y.-Y.C.; manuscript drafting, P.-Y.S.; data collection, C.-Y.L.; validation, S.-P.H.; revision and editing of the manuscript, W.-W.S. and H.-H.Y. All authors have read and agreed to the published version of the manuscript.

Funding: This research was funded by Changhua Christian Hospital (111-CCH-IRP-107).

Institutional Review Board Statement: The study was conducted in accordance with the Declaration of Helsinki and approved by the institutional review board of Changhua Christian Hospital (IRB Number: 191012).

Informed Consent Statement: Patient consent was waived due to all data were deidentified.

Data Availability Statement: Data are available on reasonable request.

Conflicts of Interest: The authors declare no conflict of interest.

References

1. Huang, D.Q.; El-Serag, H.B.; Loomba, R. Global epidemiology of NAFLD-related HCC: Trends, predictions, risk factors and prevention. *Nat. Rev. Gastroenterol. Hepatol.* **2021**, *18*, 223–238. [CrossRef] [PubMed]
2. Yatsuji, S.; Hashimoto, E.; Tobari, M.; Taniai, M.; Tokushige, K.; Shiratori, K. Clinical features and outcomes of cirrhosis due to non-alcoholic steatohepatitis compared with cirrhosis caused by chronic hepatitis C. *J. Gastroenterol. Hepatol.* **2009**, *24*, 248–254. [CrossRef] [PubMed]
3. Younossi, Z.M.; Koenig, A.B.; Abdelatif, D.; Fazel, Y.; Henry, L.; Wymer, M. Global epidemiology of nonalcoholic fatty liver disease—Meta-analytic assessment of prevalence, incidence, and outcomes. *Hepatology* **2016**, *64*, 73–84. [CrossRef]
4. Long, M.T.; Noureddin, M.; Lim, J.K. AGA clinical practice update: Diagnosis and management of nonalcoholic fatty liver disease in lean individuals: Expert review. *Gastroenterology* **2022**, *163*, 764–774.e1. [CrossRef] [PubMed]
5. Hagström, H.; Nasr, P.; Ekstedt, M.; Hammar, U.; Stål, P.; Hultcrantz, R.; Kechagias, S. Risk for development of severe liver disease in lean patients with nonalcoholic fatty liver disease: A long-term follow-up study. *Hepatol. Commun.* **2017**, *2*, 48–57. [CrossRef]
6. Zou, Z.Y.; Wong, V.W.S.; Fan, J.G. Epidemiology of nonalcoholic fatty liver disease in non-obese populations: Meta-analytic assessment of its prevalence, genetic, metabolic, and histological profiles. *J. Dig. Dis.* **2020**, *21*, 372–384. [CrossRef]
7. Maier, S.; Wieland, A.; Cree-Green, M.; Nadeau, K.; Sullivan, S.; Lanaspa, M.; Johnson, R.; Jensen, T. Lean NAFLD: An underrecognized and challenging disorder in medicine. *Rev. Endocr. Metab. Disord.* **2021**, *22*, 351–366. [CrossRef]
8. Hsu, C.L.; Wu, F.Z.; Lin, K.H.; Chen, Y.H.; Wu, P.C.; Chen, Y.H.; Chen, C.S.; Wang, W.W.; Ynan, G.Y.; Yu, H.C. Role of fatty liver index and metabolic factors in the prediction of nonalcoholic fatty liver disease in a lean population receiving health checkup. *Clin. Transl. Gastroenterol.* **2019**, *10*, 1–8. [CrossRef]
9. Decharatanachart, P.; Chaiteerakij, R.; Tiyarattanachai, T.; Treeprasertsuk, S. Application of artificial intelligence in non-alcoholic fatty liver disease and liver fibrosis: A systematic review and meta-analysis. *Ther. Adv. Gastroenterol.* **2021**, *14*, 17562848211062807. [CrossRef]
10. Castellana, M.; Donghia, R.; Guerra, V.; Procino, F.; Lampignano, L.; Castellana, F.; Zupo, R.; Sardone, R.; De Pergola, G.; Romanelli, F.; et al. Performance of Fatty Liver Index in Identifying Non-Alcoholic Fatty Liver Disease in Population Studies. A Meta-Analysis. *J. Clin. Med.* **2021**, *10*, 1877. [CrossRef]
11. Wong, G.L.H.; Yuen, P.C.; Ma, A.J.; Chan, A.W.H.; Leung, H.H.W.; Wong, V.W.S. Artificial intelligence in prediction of non-alcoholic fatty liver disease and fibrosis. *J. Gastroenterol. Hepatol.* **2021**, *36*, 543–550. [CrossRef] [PubMed]
12. Chen, Y.Y.; Lin, C.Y.; Yen, H.H.; Su, P.Y.; Zeng, Y.H.; Huang, S.P.; Liu, I.L. Machine-learning algorithm for predicting fatty liver disease in a Taiwanese population. *J. Pers. Med.* **2022**, *12*, 1026. [CrossRef] [PubMed]
13. Scatarige, J.C.; Scott, W.W.; Donovan, P.J.; Siegelman, S.S.; Sanders, R.C. Fatty infiltration of the liver: Ultrasonographic and computed tomographic correlation. *J. Ultrasound Med.* **1984**, *3*, 9–14. [CrossRef] [PubMed]
14. Hamaguchi, M.; Kojima, T.; Itoh, Y.; Harano, Y.; Fujii, K.; Nakajima, T.; Kato, T.; Takeda, N.; Okuda, J.; Ida, K.; et al. The severity of ultrasonographic findings in nonalcoholic fatty liver disease reflects the metabolic syndrome and visceral fat accumulation. *Am. J. Gastroenterol.* **2007**, *102*, 2708–2715. [CrossRef]
15. Bedogni, G.; Bellentani, S.; Miglioli, L.; Masutti, F.; Passalacqua, M.; Castiglione, A.; Tiribelli, C. The fatty liver index: A simple and accurate predictor of hepatic steatosis in the general population. *BMC Gastroenterol.* **2006**, *6*, 33. [CrossRef]
16. Ye, Q.; Zou, B.; Yeo, Y.H.; Li, J.; Huang, D.Q.; Yang, H.; Liu, C.; Kam, L.Y.; Tan, X.X.E.; Chien, N.; et al. Global prevalence, incidence, and outcomes of non-obese or lean non-alcoholic fatty liver disease: A systematic review and meta-analysis. *Lancet Gastroenterol. Hepatol.* **2020**, *5*, 739–752. [CrossRef]
17. Shi, Y.; Wang, Q.; Sun, Y.; Zhao, X.; Kong, Y.; Ou, X.; Jia, J.; Wu, S.; You, H. The prevalence of lean/nonobese nonalcoholic fatty liver disease: A systematic review and meta-analysis. *J. Clin. Gastroenterol.* **2020**, *54*, 378–387. [CrossRef]
18. Li, Y.; Chen, Y.; Tian, X.; Zhang, S.; Jiao, J. Comparison of clinical characteristics between obese and non-obese patients with nonalcoholic fatty liver disease (Nafld). *Diabetes Metab. Syndr. Obes.* **2021**, *14*, 2029–2039. [CrossRef]
19. Ahadi, M.; Molooghi, K.; Masoudifar, N.; Namdar, A.B.; Vossoughinia, H.; Farzanehfar, M. A review of non-alcoholic fatty liver disease in non-obese and lean individuals. *J. Gastroenterol. Hepatol.* **2021**, *36*, 1497–1507. [CrossRef]
20. Chahal, D.; Sharma, D.; Keshavarzi, S.; Arisar, F.A.Q.; Patel, K.; Xu, W.; Bhat, M. Distinctive clinical and genetic features of lean vs overweight fatty liver disease using the UK biobank. *Hepatol. Int.* **2022**, *16*, 325–336. [CrossRef]
21. Alam, S.; Eslam, M.; Hasan, N.S.; Anam, K.; Chowdhury, M.A.B.; Khan, M.A.S.; Hasan, M.J.; Mohamed, R. Risk factors of nonalcoholic fatty liver disease in lean body mass population: A systematic review and meta-analysis. *JGH Open* **2021**, *5*, 1236–1249. [CrossRef] [PubMed]

22. Fresneda, S.; Abbate, M.; Busquets-Cortés, C.; López-González, A.; Fuster-Parra, P.; Bennasar-Veny, M.; Yáñez, A.M. Sex and age differences in the association of fatty liver index-defined non-alcoholic fatty liver disease with cardiometabolic risk factors: A cross-sectional study. *Biol. Sex Differ.* **2022**, *13*, 64. [CrossRef] [PubMed]
23. Cho, H.C. Prevalence and factors associated with nonalcoholic fatty liver disease in a nonobese Korean population. *Gut Liver* **2016**, *10*, 117–125. [CrossRef] [PubMed]
24. Trifan, A.; Rotaru, A.; Stafie, R.; Stratina, E.; Zenovia, S.; Nastasa, R.; Huiban, L.; Cuciureanu, T.; Muzîca, C.; Chiriac, S.; et al. Clinical and laboratory characteristics of normal weight and obese individuals with non-alcoholic fatty liver disease. *Diagnostics* **2022**, *12*, 801. [CrossRef] [PubMed]
25. Li, Y.; Wang, X.; Zhang, J.; Zhang, S.; Jiao, J. Applications of artificial intelligence (AI) in researches on non-alcoholic fatty liver disease (NAFLD): A systematic review. *Rev. Endocr. Metab. Disord.* **2022**, *23*, 387–400. [CrossRef] [PubMed]
26. Nam, D.; Chapiro, J.; Paradis, V.; Seraphin, T.P.; Kather, J.N. Artificial intelligence in liver diseases: Improving diagnostics, prognostics and response prediction. *JHEP Rep.* **2022**, *4*, 100443. [CrossRef]
27. Pei, X.; Deng, Q.; Liu, Z.; Yan, X.; Sun, W. Machine learning algorithms for predicting fatty liver disease. *Ann. Nutr. Metab.* **2021**, *77*, 38–45. [CrossRef]
28. Liu, Y.X.; Liu, X.; Cen, C.; Li, X.; Liu, J.M.; Ming, Z.Y.; Yu, S.F.; Tang, X.F.; Zhou, L.; Yu, J.; et al. Comparison and development of advanced machine learning tools to predict nonalcoholic fatty liver disease: An extended study. *Hepatobiliary Pancreat. Dis. Int.* **2021**, *20*, 409–415. [CrossRef]
29. Chung, T.H.; Kim, J.K.; Kim, J.H.; Lee, Y.J. Fatty Liver Index as a Simple and Useful Predictor for 10-year Cardiovascular Disease Risks Determined by Framingham Risk Score in the General Korean Population. *J. Gastrointest. Liver Dis.* **2021**, *30*, 221–226. [CrossRef]
30. Chung, G.E.; Jeong, S.-M.; Cho, E.J.; Yoo, J.-J.; Cho, Y.; Na Lee, K.; Shin, D.W.; Kim, Y.J.; Yoon, J.-H.; Han, K.; et al. Association of fatty liver index with all-cause and disease-specific mortality: A nationwide cohort study. *Metabolism* **2022**, *133*, 155222. [CrossRef]
31. Zhang, S.; Du, T.; Zhang, J.; Lu, H.; Lin, X.; Xie, J.; Yang, Y.; Yu, X. The triglyceride and glucose index (TyG) is an effective biomarker to identify nonalcoholic fatty liver disease. *Lipids Health Dis.* **2017**, *16*, 15. [CrossRef] [PubMed]
32. Arıkan, D.; Önmez, A.; Aksu, E.; Taşdemir, N. Predictivity of fatty liver index for non-alcoholic fatty liver disease in lean females with polycystic ovary syndrome. *Afr. Health Sci.* **2022**, *22*, 648–656. [CrossRef] [PubMed]
33. Young, S.; Tariq, R.; Provenza, J.; Satapathy, S.K.; Faisal, K.; Choudhry, A.; Friedman, S.L.; Singal, A.K. Prevalence and profile of nonalcoholic fatty liver disease in lean adults: Systematic review and meta-analysis. *Hepatol. Commun.* **2020**, *4*, 953–972. [CrossRef] [PubMed]

Disclaimer/Publisher's Note: The statements, opinions and data contained in all publications are solely those of the individual author(s) and contributor(s) and not of MDPI and/or the editor(s). MDPI and/or the editor(s) disclaim responsibility for any injury to people or property resulting from any ideas, methods, instructions or products referred to in the content.

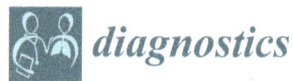 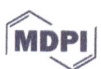

Communication

Evaluating the Utility of a Large Language Model in Answering Common Patients' Gastrointestinal Health-Related Questions: Are We There Yet?

Adi Lahat [1,*], Eyal Shachar [1], Benjamin Avidan [1], Benjamin Glicksberg [2] and Eyal Klang [3]

1. Chaim Sheba Medical Center, Department of Gastroenterology, Affiliated to Tel Aviv University, Tel Aviv 69978, Israel
2. Mount Sinai Clinical Intelligence Center, Icahn School of Medicine at Mount Sinai, New York, NY 10029, USA
3. The Sami Sagol AI Hub, ARC Innovation Center, Chaim Sheba Medical Center, Affiliated to Tel-Aviv University, Tel Aviv 69978, Israel
* Correspondence: zokadi@gmail.com

Abstract: Background and aims: Patients frequently have concerns about their disease and find it challenging to obtain accurate Information. OpenAI's ChatGPT chatbot (ChatGPT) is a new large language model developed to provide answers to a wide range of questions in various fields. Our aim is to evaluate the performance of ChatGPT in answering patients' questions regarding gastrointestinal health. Methods: To evaluate the performance of ChatGPT in answering patients' questions, we used a representative sample of 110 real-life questions. The answers provided by ChatGPT were rated in consensus by three experienced gastroenterologists. The accuracy, clarity, and efficacy of the answers provided by ChatGPT were assessed. Results: ChatGPT was able to provide accurate and clear answers to patients' questions in some cases, but not in others. For questions about treatments, the average accuracy, clarity, and efficacy scores (1 to 5) were 3.9 ± 0.8, 3.9 ± 0.9, and 3.3 ± 0.9, respectively. For symptoms questions, the average accuracy, clarity, and efficacy scores were 3.4 ± 0.8, 3.7 ± 0.7, and 3.2 ± 0.7, respectively. For diagnostic test questions, the average accuracy, clarity, and efficacy scores were 3.7 ± 1.7, 3.7 ± 1.8, and 3.5 ± 1.7, respectively. Conclusions: While ChatGPT has potential as a source of information, further development is needed. The quality of information is contingent upon the quality of the online information provided. These findings may be useful for healthcare providers and patients alike in understanding the capabilities and limitations of ChatGPT.

Keywords: OpenAI's ChatGPT; chatbot; natural language processing (NLP); medical information; gastroenterology; patients' questions

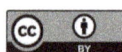

1. Introduction

Gastrointestinal (GI) complaints and symptoms account for approximately 10% of all general practice consultations [1,2] and are apparently very common in the general population. As healthcare providers specializing in this field, we are frequently called upon to answer a wide range of patients' gastrointestinal health questions. In recent years, large language models, such as OpenAI's recent release of the ChatGPT chatbot [3], have been developed to provide answers to a wide range of questions in various fields, including healthcare [4].

AI chatbots employ deep learning-based natural language processing (NLP) that evaluates natural human language input and replies accordingly in a conversational mode [5]. These models have the potential to provide patients with quick and easy access to accurate and reliable information about their gastrointestinal health with 24/7 availability, high cost-effectiveness, and potentially less bias based on patients' demographic characteristics such as gender, race, or age [6]. A recent systematic review assessing the value of AI chatbots in healthcare showed promising results in terms of the effectiveness provided [7].

The recent release of OpenAI's ChatGPT in November 2022 [3] has garnered immense popularity, as its technical abilities are believed to be superior to previous chatbot versions [8]. In a recent article [8], the chatbot was described as "astonishingly skilled at mimicking authentic writing" and was regarded as "So Good It Can Fool Humans". It was believed to have passed the ultimate" Turing test"—which states that a machine will be regarded as intelligent if its responses are indistinguishable from those given by a human comparator [9].

The effectiveness of large language models in answering patients' questions in the field of gastroenterology has not yet been thoroughly evaluated. In this paper, we aim to evaluate the performance of OpenAI's ChatGPT chatbot in answering patients' questions concerning gastrointestinal (GI) topics. This evaluation will focus on several key areas, including the accuracy and clarity of the information provided, the ability of the model to handle a wide range of questions, and the overall effectiveness of the model in addressing patients' concerns and providing them with the information they need to make informed decisions about their health.

Our evaluation aims to provide insights into the capabilities and limitations of large language models in answering patients' questions in various gastroenterology subjects. Ultimately, our goal is to contribute to the ongoing development of large language models and their use in the field of gastroenterology, with the aim of improving the quality of care and information available to patients.

2. Methods

To evaluate the performance of the newly- released large language model, OpenAI's ChatGPT chatbot, in answering patients' GI-related questions, we conducted a comprehensive study using a representative sample of real-life questions from patients in this field. The study was designed to assess the accuracy and clarity of the information provided by the chatbot, as well as its overall effectiveness in addressing patients' concerns and providing them with the information they need to make informed decisions about their health.

The study sample consisted of 110 real-life questions from patients in the field of gastroenterology, gathered from open internet sites providing medical information to diverse patients' questions. These questions were selected to cover a wide range of topics, including common symptoms, diagnostic tests, and treatments for various gastrointestinal conditions. The questions were selected to reflect the types of questions typically asked by patients in gastroenterology and to provide a representative sample of the types of questions that the chatbot would encounter in a real-world setting.

The questions were provided to the OpenAI chatbot and the answers were recorded. The answers provided by the chatbot were then assessed in consensus by three experienced gastroenterologists, each with more than 20 years of experience. All gastroenterologists work in a tertiary medical center, as well as in community clinics, and together cover all sub-specializations of gastroenterology: IBD experts, motility, hepatology, nutrition, and advanced endoscopy.

The physicians graded each chatbot answer according to a scale of 1–5 (1 the lowest score, 5 the highest) in 4 categories: accuracy, clarity, up-to-date knowledge, and effectiveness in a consensus agreement between all three gastroenterologists. Since the questions were divided according to specific topics—common symptoms, diagnostic tests, and treatments—results are shown in a separate table for every topic. (Table 1—treatments, Table 2—symptoms, Table 3—diagnostic tests.) Results are summarized visually in Figures 1–3, respectively. All questions and chatbot answers are attached in the Supplementary Materials.

Table 1. Grades of the OpenAI chatbot answers to treatment-related questions.

Question No.	Accuracy	Clarity	Up-to-Date	Efficacy	Remarks
1	3	2	3	3	
2	3	4	3	3	
3	4	3	4	3	
4	4	4	4	3	
5	4	4	3	2	
6	5	5	4	4	
7	4	4	3	2	
8	4	4	3	2	
9	4	3	4	3	
10	5	5	4	4	
11	4	4	4	3	
12	4	4	3	3	
13	3	3	3	2	
14	4	3	4	3	
15	2	4	2	2	
16	4	3	4	4	
17	4	3	4	3	
18	4	5	5	4	
19	3	3	2	2	
20	3	4	4	3	
21	2	3	2	2	
22	4	4	4	5	
23	4	2	3	2	
24	3	4	3	3	
25	4	4	5	4	
26	4	5	5	4	
27	5	5	4	4	
28	4	5	5	4	
29	4	5	4	4	
30	5	4	5	5	
31	4	5	4	4	
32	4	5	4	3	
33	5	5	5	5	
34	4	3	4	3	
35	5	4	4	4	
36	3	3	4	3	
37	2	3	2	2	
38	4	3	4	3	
39	5	4	5	5	
40	4	5	4	4	
41	5	5	5	5	
42	4	4	5	4	
Average ± SD	3.9 ± 0.8	3.9 ± 0.9	3.8 ± 0.9	3.3 ± 0.9	
Median (IQR)	4 (4–4)	4 (3–5)	4 (3–4)	3 (3–4)	

Table 2. Grades of the OpenAI chatbot answers to symptoms-related questions.

Question No.	Accuracy	Clarity	Up-to-Date	Efficacy	Remarks
1	3	4	3	3	
2	5	5	5	5	
3	3	4	3	3	
4	3	4	3	3	
5	3	4	3	3	
6	3	3	3	3	

Table 2. *Cont.*

Question No.	Accuracy	Clarity	Up-to-Date	Efficacy	Remarks
7	4	4	4	4	
8	3	4	3	3	
9	3	4	3	3	
10	4	4	4	4	
11	3	3	3	3	
12	3	3	3	3	
13	2	3	2	2	
14	3	2	3	2	
15	4	4	4	3	
16	3	4	3	3	
17	3	4	3	3	
18	4	4	3	3	
19	3	3	3	3	
20	3	4	3	3	
21	5	3	4	4	
22	3	4	3	3	
23	5	5	5	5	
Average ± SD	3.4 ± 0.8	3.7 ±0.7	3.3 ± 0.7	3.2 ± 0.7	
Median (IQR)	3 (3–4)	4 (3–4)	3 (3–3.5)	3 (3–3)	

Table 3. Grades of the OpenAI chatbot answers to diagnostic-related questions.

Question No.	Accuracy	Clarity	Up-to-Date	Efficacy	Remarks
1	5	5	5	5	
2	5	4	4	3	
3	4	5	5	5	
4	4	5	5	4	
5	5	4	5	4	
6	5	4	4	5	
7	0	0	0	0	Not found
8	5	4	5	4	
9	1	1	1	1	Mistake
10	5	5	5	5	
11	5	5	5	5	
12	4	5	4	4	
13	5	5	5	5	
14	5	5	5	4	
15	5	5	5	5	
16	5	4	5	4	
17	5	4	5	4	
18	4	4	5	4	
19	5	4	5	4	
20	4	5	4	4	
21	5	3	3	3	Asks info
22	5	5	5	5	
23	0	0	0	0	Not found
24	5	5	5	5	
25	3	4	4	3	
26	3	4	4	3	
27	4	4	4	4	
28	5	5	5	5	
29	5	5	5	5	
30	3	4	3	3	

Table 3. *Cont.*

Question No.	Accuracy	Clarity	Up-to-Date	Efficacy	Remarks
31	5	5	5	5	
32	4	5	5	4	
33	3	4	4	3	
34	5	5	4	5	
35	5	5	5	5	
36	1	1	1	1	Mistake
37	0	0	0	0	Not found
38	0	0	0	0	Not found
39	3	4	3	3	
40	4	5	4	4	
41	0	0	0	0	Not found
42	0	0	0	0	Not found
43	3	5	0	2	
44	5	5	4	5	
45	4	5	4	4	
Average ± SD	3.7 ± 1.7	3.8 ± 1.7	3.6 ± 1.8	3.5 ± 1.7	
Median (IQR)	4 (3–5)	4 (4–5)	4 (3–5)	4 (3–5)	

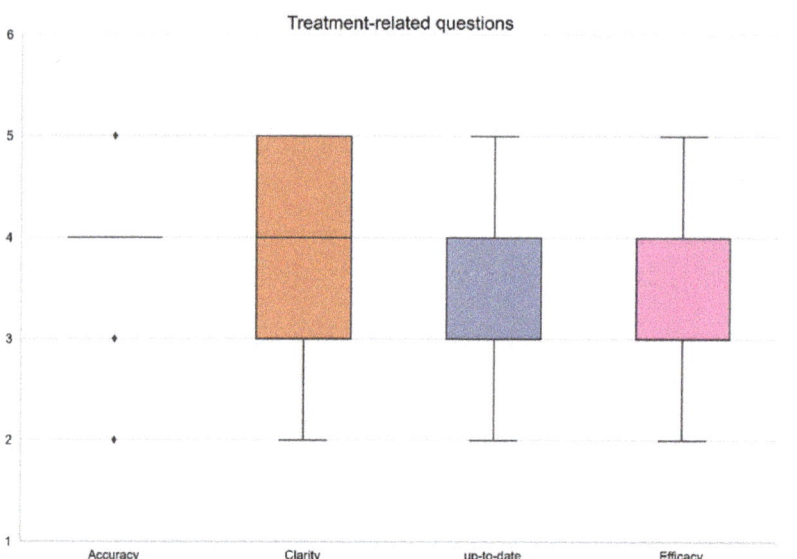

Figure 1. Graphic distribution pattern of grades assigned to the responses provided by the OpenAI chatbot in relation to treatment-related questions.

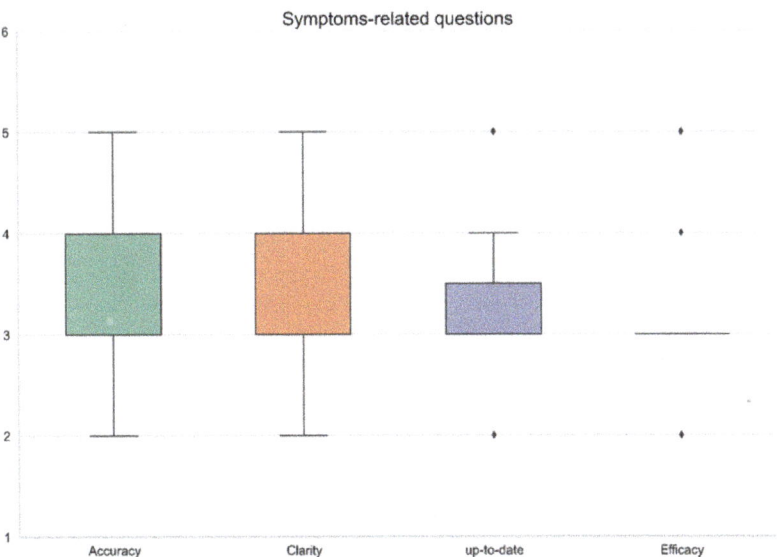

Figure 2. Graphic distribution pattern of grades assigned to the responses provided by the OpenAI chatbot in relation to symptoms-related questions.

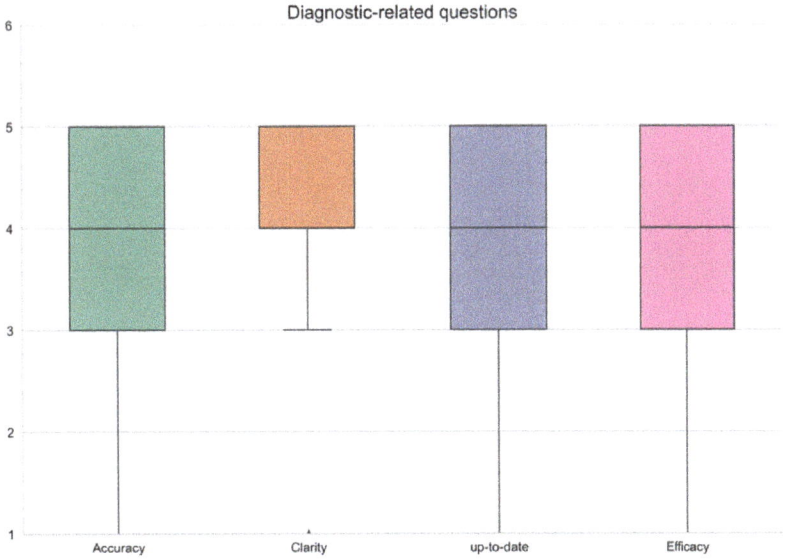

Figure 3. Graphic distribution pattern of grades assigned to the responses provided by the OpenAI chatbot in relation to diagnostic-related questions.

Statistical Analysis

Python (Ver. 3.9) was used for all statistical calculations. The average score ± standard deviation (SD) was calculated for each category and is shown in a table. A distribution graph of the answer grades for all groups by answer category was plotted. A Kruskal–Wallis one-way analysis of variance was used to determine the statistical difference between the groups.

3. Results

Overall, 110 various typical patient questions were presented to the OpenAI chatbot. Forty-two included various questions regarding treatment options in diverse gastroenterology fields. Questions were chosen to include the whole spectrum of specification from very specific questions (e.g., treatment for GI cancers according to the stage) to wider questions not referring to definite disease staging or severity (e.g., "what is the treatment for ulcerative colitis"?). All questions chosen were short and clear for better standardization. The results of the evaluation for the treatment questions are shown in Table 1.

A full list of all questions and answers is presented in the Supplementary Materials.

Overall, the OpenAI chatbot answers to the questions dealing with treatment options varied wildly between the different topics and were inconsistent in their level. Notably, at the end of almost all the answers, the patient is referred to a doctor/healthcare provider for further evaluation.

The results of the evaluation for questions related to symptoms are shown in Table 2. In the answers to the symptom-related questions, the OpenAI chatbot shows the same pattern, and the majority of answers referred the patient to consult a physician.

The results of the evaluation for questions related to diagnostic examinations are shown in Table 3.

Diversity in the quality of answers to the diagnostic examination was the highest of all groups. While many answers were correct and informative, other medical terms were simply not recognized by the chatbot (Table 3).

Figures 1–3 graphically display the distribution pattern of grades assigned to the responses provided by the OpenAI chatbot in relation to treatment, symptoms, and diagnostic-related questions, respectively.

As shown graphically in Figures 1–3, the distribution of grades by answer group in the treatment-related and symptoms-related groups are similar and relatively consistent, while the distribution of the diagnostic-related group is wide and inconsistent.

Statistical difference between the groups was shown for the subjects of accuracy ($p = 0.019$) and up-to-date ($p = 0.009$), but not for the subjects of clarity ($p = 0.071$) and efficacy ($p = 0.071$).

4. Discussion

Overall, our study provides a comprehensive evaluation of the performance of a large language model, OpenAI's ChatGPT chatbot, in answering patients' questions in the field of gastroenterology. The results of the study will hopefully be valuable for healthcare providers and patients alike, as they will provide important insights into the capabilities and limitations of these models in providing accurate and reliable information about gastrointestinal health.

Generally, the results of our evaluation of OpenAI's ChatGPT large language model, as a potential tool for answering patients' GI-related questions, are concerning. Despite the impressive capabilities of this model in other applications, our study found that it was insufficient for reliably answering patients' questions in this domain.

In our study, we presented the model with a range of common gastroenterological questions and assessed its ability to provide accurate and helpful responses. While the model could generate responses for all questions, the accuracy and helpfulness of these responses varied significantly. In many cases, the model's responses were either incomplete or entirely incorrect, indicating a lack of understanding of the subject matter.

These findings are particularly concerning given the importance of accurate information in the medical field. Patients often rely on Internet information to make decisions about their health and well-being, and inaccurate information can have serious consequences. As such, it is essential that any tool used to provide medical information to patients be able to provide accurate and reliable responses.

Interestingly, while the answers to treatment-based questions and symptom-based questions showed a similar and relatively steady quality and effectivity (Tables 1 and 2,

Figure 1), diagnostic-related results diverged between high performance to incorrect/missing data (Table 3, Figure 1). These results may improve with time as the OpenAI chatbot acquires more data.

Furthermore, our study also highlighted the limitations of OpenAI's ChatGPT chatbot in the medical domain. The ability to understand and accurately respond to complex medical questions requires a deep understanding of the subject matter, as well as the ability to process and integrate information from a variety of sources [10]. While ChatGPT is an impressive model with many capabilities, it is not yet advanced enough to fulfill this role. Notably, it should be acknowledged that the utilization of real-world questions in our study resulted in the inclusion of numerous acronyms, which could potentially pose challenges in web-based research settings. However, due to our intention to assess the effectiveness of ChatGPT in addressing authentic patient inquiries, we refrained from including the complete expressions, despite the potential difficulties associated with the acronyms.

Our results are in line with previous data assessing other artificial intelligence conversational agents in healthcare [6,7,11]. As a group, the bot's function was found to be relatively satisfactory and useful, with moderate effectiveness. It is, therefore, important to characterize specific strengths and weaknesses of the chatbot in order to maximize its benefits.

Recent data from the last months suggest that LLMs hold the potential for significant impacts in medicine [12,13].

In our previous work, we examined the utility of ChatGPT in identifying top research questions in gastroenterology. Our conclusion was that ChatGPT may be a useful tool for identifying research priorities in the field of GI, yet we noted the need to improve the originality of the research questions identified [12].

In telehealth, LLMs such as ChatGPT could improve efficiency and scalability, and provide unbiased care [14]. Despite its proficiency in generating differential diagnosis lists, ChatGPT does not surpass human physicians [15]. Moreover, LLMs can offer innovative methods in medical education [16]. Yet, it is crucial to address LLM's limitations to maintain accuracy and reliability in patient care. Furthermore, Rasmussen et al. [17] and Samaan et al. [18] evaluated the accuracy of ChatGPT in generating responses to typical questions related to vernal keratoconjunctivitis and bariatric surgery, respectively. Both found the model to be broadly accurate. Xie et al. [19] conducted a similar study using a simulated rhinoplasty consultation, and while they observed that ChatGPT provided easily comprehensible answers, it was less effective at providing detailed, personalized advice. Yeo et al. [20] tested ChatGPT on questions about cirrhosis and hepatocellular carcinoma, finding the AI capable but not comprehensive in its knowledge. Johnson et al. [21] investigated the accuracy of ChatGPT in generating responses to common cancer myths and misconceptions, concluding that it often provided accurate information. Lastly, a comprehensive pilot study on ChatGPT by Johnson et al. [22] discovered that its responses were largely accurate across a wide range of medical questions.

Significantly, it is worth mentioning that all of these studies have been published within the recent months subsequent to the initial release of the inaugural version of ChatGPT. This accumulation of research findings attests to the remarkable potential impact and significance that ChatGPT holds for the field of medicine in the foreseeable future.

Our study had a few limitations. First, the choice of questions naturally influenced the answers obtained by the OpenAI chatbot. However, the wide variety of questions and their relatively high number minimized the chance for bias. Furthermore, the answers were graded with the consensus of three physicians; there is a possibility that other physicians might have had a different point of view. Nevertheless, to minimize that risk, we chose highly experienced gastroenterologists with wide clinical experience and more than 70 years of practicing gastroenterology both in a tertiary medical center and in community practice. Lastly, there were no comparisons with other chatbots to gauge the relative merits of ChatGPT against other similar technologies, and no blinded comparison between human and chatbot answers was performed. These research directions necessitate further dedicated exploration to explore and investigate its potential in greater detail.

Importantly, our study did not include patients' comments and, therefore, is not valid in terms of assessing patients' points of view. This merits further specific research.

Overall, our study suggests that caution should be exercised when considering the use of a large language model, such as OpenAI's ChatGPT, for providing medical information to patients. While the model has the potential to be a powerful tool, it is not yet ready to be relied upon for this critical task. Further research and development are needed to improve its capabilities in the medical domain before it can be used with confidence.

Supplementary Materials: The following supporting information can be downloaded at: https://www.mdpi.com/article/10.3390/diagnostics13111950/s1, File S1: Common patient questions.

Author Contributions: A.L. and E.K. formulated the idea and designed the study. A.L., B.A. and E.S. prepared the data. B.G. performed the analysis. A.L., E.S. and B.A. provided clinical expertise. A.L., E.K., B.A. and B.G. critically reviewed the manuscript. All authors have read and agreed to the published version of the manuscript.

Funding: This research received no external funding.

Institutional Review Board Statement: Not applicable.

Informed Consent Statement: Not applicable.

Data Availability Statement: Due to data privacy regulations, the raw data of this study cannot be shared.

Conflicts of Interest: The authors declare no conflict of interest.

References

1. Seifert, B.; Rubin, G.; de Wit, N.; Lionis, C.; Hall, N.; Hungin, P.; Jones, R.; Palka, M.; Mendive, J. The management of common gastrointestinal disorders in general practice: A survey by the European Society for Primary Care Gastroenterology (ESPCG) in six European countries. *Dig. Liver Dis.* **2008**, *40*, 659–666. [CrossRef] [PubMed]
2. Holtedahl, K.; Vedsted, P.; Borgquist, L.; Donker, G.A.; Buntinx, F.; Weller, D.; Braaten, T.; Hjertholm, P.; Månsson, J.; Strandberg, E.L.; et al. Abdominal symptoms in general practice: Frequency, cancer suspicions raised, and actions taken by GPs in six European countries. Cohort study with prospective registration of cancer. *Heliyon* **2017**, *3*, e00328. [CrossRef] [PubMed]
3. Available online: https://openai.com/blog/chatgpt/ (accessed on 1 March 2023).
4. Lee, H.; Kang, J.; Yeo, J. Medical Specialty Recommendations by an Artificial Intelligence Chatbot on a Smartphone: Development and Deployment. *J. Med. Internet Res.* **2021**, *23*, e27460. [CrossRef] [PubMed]
5. Montenegro, J.L.Z.; da Costa, C.A.; Righi, R.D.R. Survey of conversational agents in health. *Expert Syst. Appl.* **2019**, *129*, 56–67. [CrossRef]
6. Palanica, A.; Flaschner, P.; Thommandram, A.; Li, M.; Fossat, Y. Physicians' Perceptions of Chatbots in Health Care: Cross-Sectional Web-Based Survey. *J. Med. Internet Res.* **2019**, *21*, e12887. [CrossRef] [PubMed]
7. Milne-Ives, M.; de Cock, C.; Lim, E.; Shehadeh, M.H.; de Pennington, N.; Mole, G.; Normando, E.; Meinert, E. The Effectiveness of Artificial Intelligence Conversational Agents in Health Care: Systematic Review. *J. Med. Internet Res.* **2020**, *22*, e20346. [CrossRef] [PubMed]
8. Available online: https://www.bloomberg.com/news/articles/2022-12-07/openai-chatbot-so-good-it-can-fool-humans-even-when-it-s-wrong (accessed on 1 March 2023).
9. Turing, A.M. Computing Machinery and Intelligence. In *Mind*; New Series; Oxford University Press on Behalf of the Mind Association: Oxford, UK, 1950; Volume 59, pp. 433–460.
10. Vayena, E.; Blasimme, A.; Cohen, I.G. Machine learning in medicine: Addressing ethical challenges. *PLoS Med.* **2018**, *15*, e1002689. [CrossRef] [PubMed]
11. Powell, J. Trust Me, I'm a Chatbot: How Artificial Intelligence in Health Care Fails the Turing Test. *J. Med. Internet Res.* **2019**, *21*, e16222. [CrossRef] [PubMed]
12. Lahat, A.; Shachar, E.; Avidan, B.; Shatz, Z.; Glicksberg, B.S.; Klang, E. Evaluating the use of large language model in identifying top research questions ingastroenterology. *Sci. Rep.* **2023**, *13*, 4164. [CrossRef] [PubMed]
13. Ge, J.; Lai, J.C. Artificial intelligence-based text generators in hepatology: ChatGPT isjust the beginning. *Hepatol. Commun.* **2023**, *7*, e0097. [CrossRef] [PubMed]
14. Lahat, A.; Klang, E. Can advanced technologies help address the global increase in demand for specialized medical care and improve telehealth services? *J. Telemed. Telecare* **2023**, 1357633X231155520. [CrossRef] [PubMed]

15. Hirosawa, T.; Harada, Y.; Yokose, M.; Sakamoto, T.; Kawamura, R.; Shimizu, T. Diagnostic Accuracy of Differential-Diagnosis Lists Generated by Generative Pretrained Transformer 3 Chatbot for Clinical Vignettes with Common Chief Complaints: A Pilot Study. *Int. J. Environ. Res. Public Health* **2023**, *20*, 3378. [CrossRef] [PubMed]
16. Eysenbach, G. The Role of ChatGPT, Generative Language Models, and Artificial Intelligence in Medical Education: A Conversation with ChatGPT and a Call for Papers. *JMIR Med. Educ.* **2023**, *9*, e46885. [CrossRef] [PubMed]
17. Rasmussen, M.L.R.; Larsen, A.C.; Subhi, Y.; Potapenko, I. Artificial intelligence-based ChatGPT chatbot responses for patient and parent questions on vernal keratoconjunctivitis. *Graefe's Arch. Clin. Exp. Ophthalmol.* **2023**. [CrossRef] [PubMed]
18. Samaan, J.S.; Yeo, Y.H.; Rajeev, N.; Hawley, L.; Abel, S.; Ng, W.H.; Srinivasan, N.; Park, J.; Burch, M.; Watson, R.; et al. Assessing the Accuracy of Responses by the Language Model ChatGPT to Questions Regarding Bariatric Surgery. *Obes. Surg.* **2023**, *33*, 1790–1796. [CrossRef] [PubMed]
19. Xie, Y.; Seth, I.; Hunter-Smith, D.J.; Rozen, W.M.; Ross, R.; Lee, M. Aesthetic Surgery Advice and Counseling from Artificial Intelligence: A Rhinoplasty Consultation with ChatGPT. *Aesthetic Plast Surg.* **2023**. [CrossRef] [PubMed]
20. Yeo, Y.H.; Samaan, J.S.; Ng, W.H.; Ting, P.S.; Trivedi, H.; Vipani, A.; Ayoub, W.; Yang, J.D.; Liran, O.; Spiegel, B.; et al. Assessing the performance of ChatGPT in answering questions regarding cirrhosis and hepatocellular carcinoma. *Clin. Mol. Hepatol.* **2023**. [CrossRef] [PubMed]
21. Johnson, S.B.; King, A.J.; Warner, E.L.; Aneja, S.; Kann, B.H.; Bylund, C.L. Using ChatGPT to evaluate cancer myths and misconceptions: Artificial intelligence and cancer information. *JNCI Cancer Spectr.* **2023**, *7*, pkad015. [CrossRef] [PubMed]
22. Johnson, D.; Goodman, R.; Patrinely, J.; Stone, C.; Zimmerman, E.; Donald, R.; Chang, S.; Berkowitz, S.; Finn, A.; Jahangir, E.; et al. Assessing the Accuracy and Reliability of AI-Generated Medical Responses: An Evaluation of the Chat-GPT Model. *Res. Sq.* **2023**, *preprint*. [CrossRef]

Disclaimer/Publisher's Note: The statements, opinions and data contained in all publications are solely those of the individual author(s) and contributor(s) and not of MDPI and/or the editor(s). MDPI and/or the editor(s) disclaim responsibility for any injury to people or property resulting from any ideas, methods, instructions or products referred to in the content.

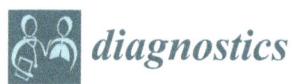

Review

Advancing Colorectal Cancer Diagnosis with AI-Powered Breathomics: Navigating Challenges and Future Directions

Ioannis K. Gallos [1,*], Dimitrios Tryfonopoulos [1], Gidi Shani [2], Angelos Amditis [1], Hossam Haick [2] and Dimitra D. Dionysiou [1,*]

[1] Institute of Communication and Computer Systems, National Technical University of Athens, Zografos Campus, 15780 Athens, Greece; d.tryfonopoulos@iccs.gr (D.T.); a.amditis@iccs.gr (A.A.)
[2] Laboratory for Nanomaterial-Based Devices, Technion—Israel Institute of Technology, Haifa 3200003, Israel; gidishani@gmail.com (G.S.); hhossam@technion.ac.il (H.H.)
* Correspondence: ioannis.gallos@iccs.gr (I.K.G.); dimitra.dionysiou@iccs.gr (D.D.D.)

Abstract: Early detection of colorectal cancer is crucial for improving outcomes and reducing mortality. While there is strong evidence of effectiveness, currently adopted screening methods present several shortcomings which negatively impact the detection of early stage carcinogenesis, including low uptake due to patient discomfort. As a result, developing novel, non-invasive alternatives is an important research priority. Recent advancements in the field of breathomics, the study of breath composition and analysis, have paved the way for new avenues for non-invasive cancer detection and effective monitoring. Harnessing the utility of Volatile Organic Compounds in exhaled breath, breathomics has the potential to disrupt colorectal cancer screening practices. Our goal is to outline key research efforts in this area focusing on machine learning methods used for the analysis of breathomics data, highlight challenges involved in artificial intelligence application in this context, and suggest possible future directions which are currently considered within the framework of the European project ONCOSCREEN.

Keywords: breathomics; colorectal cancer; volatile organic compounds; machine learning; artificial intelligence; automated diagnosis; validation; manifold learning; ONCOSCREEN

Citation: Gallos, I.K.; Tryfonopoulos, D.; Shani, G.; Amditis, A.; Haick, H.; Dionysiou, D.D. Advancing Colorectal Cancer Diagnosis with AI-Powered Breathomics: Navigating Challenges and Future Directions. *Diagnostics* 2023, 13, 3673. https://doi.org/10.3390/diagnostics13243673

Academic Editors: Eun-Sun Kim and Kwang-Sig Lee

Received: 10 November 2023
Revised: 12 December 2023
Accepted: 13 December 2023
Published: 15 December 2023

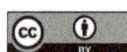

Copyright: © 2023 by the authors. Licensee MDPI, Basel, Switzerland. This article is an open access article distributed under the terms and conditions of the Creative Commons Attribution (CC BY) license (https:// creativecommons.org/licenses/by/ 4.0/).

1. Introduction

Cancer is a group of complex diseases linked to abnormal cell growth with devastating consequences for the patient. It ranks as a leading cause of death and a profound barrier to increasing life expectancy worldwide [1]. Detection of cancer in early stages along with timely and appropriate treatment is a critical component of reducing cancer-related mortality and morbidity [2]. Currently, there is a lack of reliable screening modalities for highly fatal cancers like pancreatic and gastric cancer [3]. Similarly, for highly prevalent malignancies such as breast and colorectal cancer (CRC), there is plenty of room for enhancing the existing screening practices. In particular, colonoscopy and fecal immunochemical test (FIT) are widely accepted as the cornerstones for the early detection of CRC [4]. During a colonoscopy procedure, early precancerous lesions can be detected and removed by a clinical expert. Nevertheless, colonoscopy is an invasive and costly procedure with low rates of compliance [5]. FIT serves as a complementary or alternative screening modality to colonoscopy for patients that decline the latter [4]; it is a non-invasive and low-cost test that serves as a widely adopted screening procedure for the large part of the average-risk population. Nevertheless, FIT shows modest accuracy in detecting CRC and advanced adenoma (AA), with sensitivity remaining under 70% and 50%, respectively [6]. Hence, CRC screening suffers from both low rates of adherence to the test (e.g., colonoscopy) as well as low detection rates (e.g., FIT).

In an effort to address the aforementioned problems, recent technological advances have brought up new novel non- or minimally invasive approaches such as breath, blood, and imaging-based tests [7,8]. In recent years, metabolomics has steadily gained momentum in various frontiers including disease detection and personalized medicine [9,10]. Breath volatolomics, also known as breathomics, can be seen as a branch of metabolomics, focusing on human breath. Breathomics studies volatile organic compounds (VOCs) and their metabolites that come from our respiratory system and internal organs. By simply exhaling air through a breathing device, it becomes possible to capture and analyze the profile of VOCs that are exhaled and present in the sample. Typically, a "breath biopsy" can be acquired in a non-invasive manner through the use of analytical methods like gas chromatography–mass spectrometry (GC-MS) or by utilizing sensors of various electronic nose devices [11]. Over two thousand VOCs have been reported to emanate from the human body [12], forming an inexhaustible treasure trove of biomarkers, which in turn have been linked to various diseases, including cancer [13,14]. Cancer cells undergo metabolic alterations which can result in the release of specific VOCs. For example, it has been shown that these cells tend to metabolize glucose via aerobic glycolysis rather than oxidative phosphorylation, an effect known as the Warburg effect [15]. Researchers posit the hypothesis that these VOCs are released into the bloodstream and eventually expelled through exhalation, passing through the endobronchial cavity [16]. A free web-based database, also known as the Cancer Odor Database (COD), contains comprehensive information about cancer-related VOCs, with its data being extracted directly from the scientific literature [17]. Another more general and recent database, the Human Breathomics Database (HBD) [18], contains comprehensive information about VOCs reported in 2766 publications. It provides biomedical information, underlying biochemical pathways and current scientific evidence regarding the association of each VOC with various diseases. In particular, research efforts on the determination of cancer-related VOCs have shown that some may contribute to more than five different cancer types [14,19]. For example, Nakhleh et al. utilized 13 VOCs for the detection and discrimination between 17 different disease conditions from 813 patients [14]. Despite the fact that breath analysis is still in early stages of development, analyzing breath composition holds significant potential for contributing to several subfields of cancer research such as detection [11,13], screening/monitoring [20], prognosis [21], and treatment response [11,22]. This review will focus on the relevance of volatolomics to CRC and recent theoretical and technological advancements derived from the field of breathomics in this regard.

GC-MS is undeniably the gold standard in breath analysis in terms of precision, as it enables separation, identification, and quantification of the different VOCs in the exhaled breath gas. Alternative ways such as sensor-based techniques have also been introduced with increasing interest [23]. Since GC-MS is resource-intensive, time-consuming, and requires special expertise, sensor arrays in the form of breathing electronic devices/noses (e-noses) constitute mobile, cost-effective, and user-friendly diagnostic alternatives that are capable of providing quick results. Studies employing e-noses and breath-based VOCs towards detection of CRC and AA are emerging at an increasing rate [24–28]. As a trade-off for their virtues, the latter detect mixtures of VOCs instead of identifying the actual mass of specific compounds. In other words, sensor arrays or e-noses are designed to imitate the human olfactory system with the use of chemical sensors [29]. Applications of e-nose devices in terms of odor perception are most often treated as black box models, focusing more on the accuracy of the task to be performed (e.g., diagnosis/monitoring) and less on understanding of how and why the subsequent results are derived [29].

While the use of chemical sensors holds the potential to revolutionize today's medical diagnostics on CRC breath, it also faces significant challenges and limitations [30]. First and foremost, confounding factors such as age, diet, genetics, and smoking habits can introduce variability in breath composition, threatening with inaccurate results [14]. Second, timing and method of breath sample collection are critical considerations also, as exhaled breath profiles can change rapidly with fluctuations in blood chemistry [31]. Third, standardized protocols for uniform and repeatable breath sampling are imperative. Technical sensitivity, particularly regarding sensor responses to temperature and humidity, presents obstacles that necessitate controlled and sterile environments for analysis [32]. Fourth, data analysis also poses difficulties, with the choice of statistical methods, validation, and complex modeling needing careful consideration [33]. For example, the breath signature of CRC derives from statistical procedure; one has to seek differences between hundreds of VOCs that might be present. Searching for statistically significant differences between breath profiles of CRC patients and healthy controls, one needs to take into account the multiple comparison problem to ensure no false discoveries [33]. Today, breath-based VOCs reported as biomarkers for CRC detection exhibit a substantial amount of variation in the scientific literature [8,34–44]. Fifth, achieving strong predictive values for disease diagnosis and monitoring large-scale, multicenter clinical trials with blind validation are required [30]. Sixth, special emphasis on reproducibility and adaptation to real-world clinical conditions have to be given so as to formulate widely accepted technical and clinical standards in order to accelerate research and finally integrate breath analysis into routine medical testing. A study discussing technical standards and recommendations for sample collection and analytic approaches for lung disease can be found in [45]. Addressing these challenges is crucial to establishing breath-based diagnosis in the clinical practice.

In this article we particularly focus on how advancements from the field of machine learning (ML) and artificial intelligence (AI) can be used towards useful, reliable, accurate, and reproducible research towards breath-based diagnosis. It is the first review article that exclusively focuses on AI applications for CRC detection using breathomics; it aims to present the latest findings reported on the use of AI techniques and methods targeting breath-based VOCs for CRC diagnosis and has been performed in the context of the Horizon Europe project ONCOSCREEN (https://oncoscreen.health/, accessed on 10 December 2023). The project seeks to develop novel methodologies for cancer screening and early detection, ultimately aiming to enhance citizen awareness, participation, and adherence to relevant protocols. Among the various solutions proposed by the project, CRC diagnosis using breath-based VOCs is planned to be pursued utilizing both analytical and sensor-based methodologies. As a first step, a GC-MS instrument will be used for collecting prospective breath samples from healthy controls as well as CRC-diagnosed patients, thereby establishing a VOC signature database. Subsequently, a previously developed sensor array-based breath analyzer prototype [46], originally used for the detection of gastric cancer VOCs, will be modified based on the gas biomarkers defined in the GC-MS analysis phase. The basic analytical principle of the breath analyzer is based on the activity of a gold nanoparticle sensor array. This array was made of 8 different chemistries detecting the transient effect of the breath sample on the resistance of each of these sensors for 60 s. This led to the generation of 8×60 observations for each breath sample. The recent model has been upgraded to harbor 48 sensors resulting in 48×60 time points for each breath sample to enable a richer picture best analyzed by different AI frameworks. In our opinion, this mode of VOC mixture detection and labeling best resembles the principle of smell distinction existing in the mammalian olfactory bulb. Finally, an AI module of the device will be trained on electrochemical signal responses between healthy and CRC samples. The resulting new prototype will be tested prospectively for its ability to offer a portable and quick way of early CRC diagnosis. The project foresees a comprehensive testing and validation process, including a clinical validation study involving the enrollment of 4100 patients/citizens.

The rest of the article is structured as follows: we start with a brief introduction around CRC and then we explore its breath blueprint as it is derived from past studies. We then report the capabilities of contemporary diagnosis models for CRC and, subsequently, we dive into each step of a typical AI pipeline towards the diagnosis of CRC. We place special emphasis on identifying future challenges and considerations for the extension of the existing breathomics AI toolbox against CRC. We hope that this overview forms a basis upon which the community can further elaborate towards new advances taking into consideration the current challenges. A schematic representation of the topics discussed in this work can be seen in Figure 1.

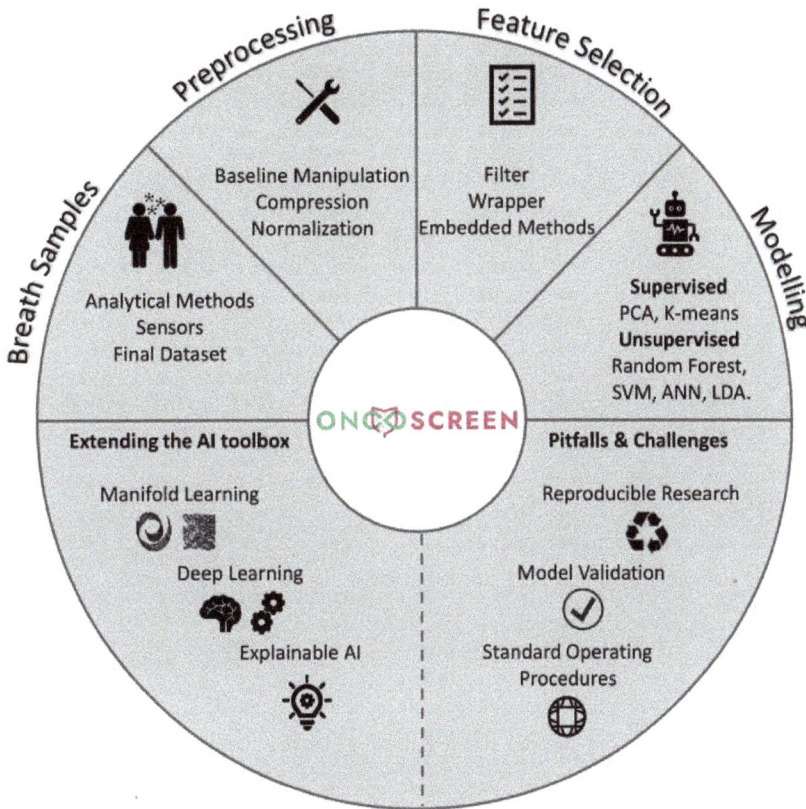

Figure 1. Schematic representation of the topics discussed within the scope of this study.

2. Colorectal Cancer

Colorectal cancer can be categorized as colon or rectal cancer depending on where it initially develops. Despite their differences, these cancers are often grouped together [47]. The majority of colorectal tumors emerge from small clusters called polyps on the inner lining of the colon or rectum. The probability of a polyp transforming into cancer varies greatly depending on its type, with some of them never turning into cancer [48]. Polyps can be widely characterized as adenomatous, hyperplastic, inflammatory, or sessile serrated [49]. Hyperplastic and inflammatory polyps are frequently detected, with the adenomatous polyps being considered precancerous [50]. Due to a higher risk of developing into CRC, polyps characterized as sessile serrated are also regarded as adenomas [51]. Certain characteristics of polyps such as the size being larger than 1 cm, the segregation of more than three of them, or the detection of dysplasia after removal are linked with elevated risk of cancer development [52,53]. Over time, some precancerous polyps progress into cancerous growths within the walls of the colon or rectum [54]. The majority of CRC cases are adenocarcinomas originating from mucus-producing cells in the inner layer that play the role of lubrication and protection for the colon and rectum [55]. Of the adenocarcinomas, signet ring cell and mucinous cancers may have a less favorable prognosis [56,57]. Finally, less common types of CRC include carcinoid and gastrointestinal tumors, lymphomas, and sarcomas [58,59]. Typically, the progression of a polyp to a malignant state takes several years [54]. In many cases, patients do not experience symptoms until the cancer has already progressed to either an early or advanced stage of development [60,61]. Therefore, early detection, diagnosis, and staging by making use of diverse biomarkers are essential for effective cancer treatment [62].

3. Breath Blueprint as Biomarker for Early Detection and Monitoring of CRC

Scientific efforts towards the discovery of a CRC blueprint in breath began in the early 2000s [44,63,64]. Overall, CRC has been consistently linked with classes of VOCs such as alcohols, alkanes, aldehydes, and ketones [65,66], with the last two commonly found in cancer metabolism [67]. Multiple studies have tried to come up with a CRC breath profile [8,14,38,42–44,64]. Typically, these studies conduct VOC analysis in breath samples using GC-MS analysis and later check for differences between groups of CRC patients and healthy controls. If statistically significant differences are found in the levels of VOC prevalence between groups, then these VOCs are suggested as potential biomarkers for the disease. However, due to several differences in methodologies, technical equipment, pre-processing routine, sample sizes, or even different cancer stages (known to affect the VOC profile), a reliable and reproducible pattern of VOCs as biomarkers for general clinical practice is yet to become available. The list of CRC breath-based VOC biomarkers that have been reported in the scientific literature can be inspected in Table 1. Their underlying biochemical pathways and functionalities are further explored in [38,65,68].

Table 1. Biomarkers reported for CRC.

Technique	Sample Size	VOC	Reference
GC-MS	CRC (15); Controls (20)	Acetone; heptanoic acid; 2,6,10-trimethyldodecane;	Śmiełowska et al., 2023 [34]
GC-MS	CRC (30); Controls (84)	2-propenoic acid ethenyl ester; lactic acid; 2,4-dimethyl-pyrrole; p-menth-3-ene; 6-methyl heptane; 2,2,4,4-tetramethylpentane; 2-methylfuran; propyl pyruvate; and 2 unknown identified VOCs	Cheng et al., 2022 [35]
GC-MS	CRC (162); Controls (1270)	propyl propionate; dimethyl sulfide; 1-penten-3-ol; 3,4-dimethyl-1,5-cyclooctadiene; 2-propenyl ester of acetic acid; branched tetradecane; 2-methyl-2-propanol; 4-ethyl-1-octyn-3-ol;2,2,4-trimethyl-3-pentanol; cyclopropane; 2-ethoxypropane; 2-phenoxy-ethanol; heptane; branched tridecane;	Woodfield et al., 2022 [36]
IMR-MS	CRC (52); Controls (45)	Dinitrogen Oxide; Nitrous Acid; 1,3-Butadiene; Acetic Acid; Unknown identified VOCs (9)	Politi et al., 2021 [37]
GC-MS	CRC (83); Controls (90)	Tetradecane; ethylbenzene; 5,9-undecadien-2-one, 6,10-dimethyl (E); decane; benzoic acid; 1,3-bis(1-methylethenyl) benzene; decanal; unidentified compound; ethyl-1-hexanol; dodecane; ethanone; 1{[}4-(1-methylethenyl)phenyl{]}; acetic acid	Altomare et al., 2020 [66]
SIFT-MS	CRLM(51); Controls (54)	(E)-2-Nonene; acetaldehyde; triethyl amine	Miller-Atkins 2020 [39]
SIFT-MS	CRC (50); Controls (100) *	Propanal	Markar et al., 2019 [40]
GC-MS	CRC (71); Controls (89)	2-ethylhexanol; 3-methylhexane; 5-ethyl-3-methyloctane; acetone; ethanol; ethyl acetate; ethylbenzene; isononane; isoprene; nonanal; styrene; toluene; undecane	Nakhleh et al., 2017 [14]

Table 1. *Cont.*

Technique	Sample Size	VOC	Reference
GC-MS	CRC(65); Controls (122)	Acetone, 6 ethyl acate, ethanol, 4-methyl octane	Amal et al., 2016 [8]
GC-MS	CRC (48); Controls (32) **	1,2-pentadiene; beta-pinene; 2-methylbutane; 1-methyl-3-(1-methylethyl)benzene; 2-methylpentane; 1-(1-methylethenyl)-2-(1-methylethyl)benzene; 5-butylnonane; methylcyclopentane; undecane; cyclohexane; heptane; nonanal; methylcyclohexane; dodecane; 4-methyl-2-pentanone; decanal; 1-methylnaphthalene; 1-ethyl-1,2,4-trimethylbenzene; 1-octene 1-ethyl-2,4,5-trimethylbenzene; octane; 2,3-dihydro-1,6-dimethyl-1H-indene; 1,2,3-trimethylbenzene; 2,3-dihydro-4,7-dimethyl-1H- indene; 1,3-dimethylbenzene; 1,3-dimethyl-5-(1-methylethyl)benzene; 1,4-dimethylbenzene; 2-methylnaphthalene; propylbenzene;	Altomare et al., 2015 [41]
GC-MS	CRC (20); Controls (20)	Cyclohexanone, 2,2-dimethyldecane; dodecane; 4-ethyl-1-octyn3-ol; ethylailine; cydoctyimethanol; trans-2-dodecen-1-ol; 3- hydroxy-2,4,4-timethylpentyl2-methyipropanoate; 6-t-buty4-2,29,9-tetramethyl-3,5-decadien-7-yne	Wang et al., 2014 [42]
GC-MS	CRC (37); Controls (41)	Nonanal; 4-methy1-2-pentanone; decanal; 2-methylbutane; 1.2-pentadiene, 2-metyipentane,3-methylpentane; methylcyclopentane; cyclohexane; methylcyclohexane; 1,3-dimethylbenzene; 4 methyloctane; 1,4-dimethylbenzene; a(4-methylundecane, rt = 11-3); b(timethyldecane, RT = 13-2)	Altomare et al., 2013 [43]
GC-MS	CRC (26); Controls (22)	1,10-(1-butenylidene)bisbenzene; 1,3-dmethy benzene; 1- iodononane; {[}(1,1-dimethyiethyl)thio{]}acetic acid; 4-(4-propylcyclohexyl)-40 cyano{[}1,10-biphenyl{]}-4-yl ester benzoic acid; 2-amino-5isopropyl-8-methyl-1-azulenecarbonitrile	Peng et al., 2010 [44]

Note: CRLM: colorectal cancer liver metastases; GC-MS: gas chromatography—mass spectrometry; SIFT-MS: selected ion flow tube mass spectrometry; IMR-MS: ion molecule reaction–mass spectrometry. * 50 of controls with normal LGI tract endoscopy and 50 found positive including inflammatory bowel diseases (IBD), diverticular disease, and polyps. ** Former patients found disease free after oncologic follow up.

Meta-analyses on the diagnosis of cancer focusing exclusively on breath-based VOCs have consistently shown optimistic results [68,69]. Specifically, on a systematic review and meta-analysis on different cancer types, Hanna et al. reported that despite a substantial variability among 63 studies, the pooled sensitivity reached 79% along with a pooled specificity of 89%. Xiang et al. further ratified previous results by focusing exclusively on gastrointestinal cancer and CRC, thus reporting pooled sensitivity of 85% and pooled specificity of 89%. They both concluded that while breath-based VOCs have the potential for clinical screening, standardized tools and protocols have to be introduced in an effort to mitigate the heterogeneity in the discriminatory VOCs reported and the subsequent diagnostic metrics. Finally, a more recent meta-analysis [23] considering 52 studies and 3677 patients with cancer, including CRC, reported 90% sensitivity and 87% specificity. The study exclusively focused on the diagnostic power of e-noses and though the authors reported optimistic results, they stated that most of the studies considered involved a small sample size and poor standardization.

Apart from meta-analyses relying only on breath-based VOCs, there have been some studies considering VOCs coming from different sources, such as fecal and urine VOCs. That being said, according to a meta-analysis on CRC screening using VOCs from different sources [70], the authors considered 10 studies spanning from 2012 to the end of 2019. The reported pooled sensitivity and specificity were found to be 82% and 79%, respectively. The results suggested that VOCs can be considered a stable and robust tool for CRC screening but not as a single and exclusive diagnostic test. Interestingly, VOCs associated with breath exhibited higher sensitivity and specificity than their counterparts (e.g., VOCs from feces and urine). Another meta-analysis from Wang. et al. [71] focused on diagnosis of neoplasms of the digestive system including CRC, using VOCs from different sources. Specifically for CRC, the authors included 16 studies (out of a total of 36 with over 3000 participants) and reported 84% pooled sensitivity and 82% specificity. Remarkably, the authors reported that breath-based VOCs behaved better (i.e., in terms of diagnostic metrics) than VOCs from other sources. Specifically, by considering only breath-based studies, the reported pooled sensitivity and specificity were both 87%. In Table 2 we present sensitivity and specificity rates reported in studies using breath-based VOCs as biomarkers for diagnosing CRC.

Table 2. Reported sensitivity and specificity on diagnosis of CRC based on exhaled VOCs.

Technique	Sample Size	Sensitivity	Specificity	Reference
Sensors	CRC (105); Controls (186)	0.79	0.53	Połaka et al., 2023 [72]
GC-MS	CRC (15); Controls (20)	0.94	1	Śmiełowska et al., 2023 [34]
GC-MS	CRC (30); Controls (84)	0.8	0.7	Cheng et al., 2022 [35]
GC-MS	CRC (162); Controls (1270)	0.79	0.86	Woodfield et al., 2022 [36]
IMR-MS	CRC (52); Controls (45)	0.96	0.73	Politi et al., 2021 [37]
GC-MS + sensors	CRC (82); Controls (87)	0.9	0.93	Altomare et al., 2020 [38]
SIFT-MS	CRLM (51); Controls (54)	0.28	0.89	Miller Atkins et al., 2020 [39]
e-nose	CRC (62) *	0.88	0.75	Steenhuis et al., 2020 [26]
e-nose	CRC (70); Controls (125)	0.95	0.64	Keulen et al., 2020 [27]
SIFT-MS	CRC (50); Controls (50) CRC (50); Controls (50) **	0.96 0.90	0.76 0.66	Markar et al., 2019 [40]
e-nose	CRC (15); Controls (15)	0.93	0.1	Altomare et al., 2016 [73]
GC-MS + sensors	CRC (65); Controls (122)	0.85	0.94	Amal et al., 2016 [8]
GC-MS	CRC (48); Controls (32) ***	1	0.98	Altomare et al., 2015 [41]
GC-MS	CRC (37); Controls (41)	0.86	0.83	Altomare et al., 2013 [43]

Note: CRLM: colorectal cancer liver metastases; GC-MS: gas chromatography—mass spectrometry; SIFT-MS: selected ion flow tube mass spectrometry; IMR-MS: ion molecule reaction–mass spectrometry. * Detection of extraluminal local recurrences or metastases in the follow-up of curatively treated CRC patients. ** Inflammatory bowel diseases (IBD), diverticular disease, and polyps. *** former Patients found disease free after oncologic follow up.

4. Applications of Machine Learning in Exhaled Breath Analysis: The Case of CRC

Machine learning (ML) can be seen as a part of AI that revolves around the development of methods aiming to enable machines to learn from data. Applications of ML span various domains, including medicine and disease diagnosis, particularly in situations where traditional algorithms are impractical and/or insufficient. Roughly speaking, ML approaches can be divided into three broad categories of learning, namely supervised, unsupervised, and reinforcement learning. The main difference between the supervised and the unsupervised learning paradigm lies in the fact that in the first case the computer is learning from labeled examples with known inputs and desired outputs. On the other hand, unsupervised learning tries to discover inherent structures from unlabeled data without explicit guidance, typically with consideration of some measure of similarity between the data entities. Finally, reinforcement learning typically involves an agent that is learning to make decisions through trial and error, receiving feedback in the form of rewards/penalties. Through an iterative process, long-term cumulative rewards are maximized based on the observed outcomes. For the rest of this review, we will focus on the supervised and the unsupervised learning paradigms.

In the following, we sketch the main pillars of the standard ML methodology in VOC analysis. Typically, the analysis pipeline starts with data acquisition, either with an analytical or a sensor-based method (for their relative advantages and disadvantages see Section 1). It continues with the pre-processing and feature extraction steps. Preprocessing is a stage where we transform the raw data into a comprehensible format to augment the downstream analysis. Feature extraction is the process of generating new values (features) from the initial measurements that are informative, non-redundant, and aid in the subsequent learning, ultimately leading to useful and informed models. The next step usually includes feature selection, a level of analysis where we choose the most discriminatory features/biomarkers present in our dataset, towards parsimonious modeling to enhance predictive and generalization capabilities. Then, we proceed to the actual modeling for discrimination between patients and healthy controls in a supervised/unsupervised manner. Finally, model validation takes place to assess the model's performance and confirm the usefulness of the model in real world applications.

In Table 3 we present the key characteristics of the pipeline used in studies considering breath-based VOCs towards the diagnosis of CRC.

Table 3. Analysis pipelines of studies using breath-based VOCs towards CRC diagnosis.

Technique	Sample Size	Preprocessing Pipeline/Feature Extraction	Feature Selection	# of Features	Classifier	Validation	Validation Type	Reference
Sensors	CRC (105); Controls (186)	Data normalization; removal of erroneous sensor signals; extraction of statistical measures	Greedy stepwise selection; evolutionary search	75 (model with best results based on accuracy reported)	Random Forest, C4.5 (decision tree classifier); Artificial Neural Network; Naïve Bayes	70–30% split training and validation set	Internal	Polaka et al., 2023 [72]
GC-MS	CRC (15); Controls (20)	Removal of artifacts; imputation using median; Shapiro–Wilk test;	Mann–Whitney U test; DFA; forward stepwise method; filtering based on certain metabolic reactions;	3	Artificial Neural Networks	10-fold Cross validation	Internal	Śmiełowska et al., 2023 [34]
GC-MS	CRC (30); Controls (84)	Noise removal; baseline correction; alignment; normalization; peak picking; scaling	Features detected in at least 20% of all classes considered	10	Isolation Forest	LOOCV	Internal	Cheng et al., 2022 [35]

Table 3. Cont.

Technique	Sample Size	Preprocessing Pipeline/Feature Extraction	Feature Selection	# of Features	Classifier	Validation	Validation Type	Reference
GC-MS	CRC (162); Controls (1270)	Log-transformation; variance stabilization; normalization	ANOVA; Random forest	-	Random Forest, alphanet, SVM, LASSO; elastic net regression;	Repeated 5-fold Cross validation	Internal	Woodfield et al., 2022 [36]
IMR-MS	CRC (52); Controls (45)	Exclusion of specific chemicals (via *t*-test with reference sample); Standardization prior to modelling;	LASSO	15 (13 VOCs, Age, Sex)	Logistic Regression	50-fold Cross validation	Internal	Politi et al., 2021 [37]
GC-MS + sensors	CRC (82); Controls (87)	-	Mann–Whitney U test; univariate analysis and ranking of features; multivariate Stepwise Logistic Regression;	15 (14 VOCs, Age)	Logistic Regression	LOOCV	Internal	Altomare et al., 2020 [38]
SIFT-MS	CRLM (51); Controls (54)	Log-transformation; PCA noise removal; imputation of missing values (mean)	-	24 (22 VOCs, Sex, Age)	Random Forest	LOOCV on 95% of the dataset. 5% as a Test set	Internal	Miller Atkins et al., 2020 [39]
e-nose	CRC (62) *	TUCKER3	-	-	Artificial Neural Networks	10-fold cross validation	Internal	Steenhuis et al., 2020 [26]
e-nose	CRC (70); Controls (125)	Standardization; TUCKER3	-	11 (components derived from TUCKER3)	Artificial Neural Networks	10-fold cross validation	Internal	Keulen et al., 2020 [27]
SIFT-MS	CRC (50); Controls (50) CRC (50); Controls (50) **	-	Univariate statistics; Multivariate Logistic Regression	1	Logistic regression	100% of data as training set	Internal	Markar et al., 2019 [40]
e-nose	CRC (15); Controls (15)	Calculation of mean response of the signal	PCA based on variance explained	2 (1st and 2nd principal component)	Probabilistic Neural Networks	LOOCV	Internal	Altomare et al., 2016 [73]
GC-MS + sensors	CRC (65); Controls (122)	-	-	1 (Canonical variable from DFA applied to all sensing features)	DFA	70–30% split training and validation set	Internal	Amal et al., 2016 [8]
GC-MS	CRC (48); Controls (32) ***	-	Mann–Whitney U test	11	Probabilistic Neural Networks	LOOCV	Internal	Altomare et al., 2015 [41]

268

Table 3. *Cont.*

Technique	Sample Size	Preprocessing Pipeline/Feature Extraction	Feature Selection	# of Features	Classifier	Validation	Validation Type	Reference
GC-MS	CRC (37); Controls (41)	-	Mann–Whitney U test	15	Probabilistic Neural Networks	LOOCV	Internal	Altomare et al., 2013 [43]

Note: GC-MS: gas chromatography—mass spectrometry; IMR-MS: ion molecule reaction–mass spectrometry; SIFT-MS: selected ion flow tube mass spectrometry; CRLM: colorectal cancer liver metastases; LOOCV: Leave one out cross validation; PCA: Principal Component Analysis; LASSO: Least absolute Shrinkage and selection operator; SVM: support vector machine. * Detection of extraluminal local recurrences or metastases in the Follow Up of curatively treated CRC patients. ** Inflammatory bowel diseases (IBD), diverticular disease, and polyps. *** former patients found disease free after oncologic follow up.

4.1. Pre-Processing and Feature Extraction

Pre-processing is the initial stage of processing raw data. Roughly speaking, pre-processing involves transforming raw data into a format that is comprehensible and augments the performance of the following steps. The most commonly applied strategies can be broadly categorized as baseline manipulation, compression, and normalization transforms [74]. The baseline manipulation refers to the transformations that attempt to correct for the baseline of the signal with the aim of suppressing the effect of sensor drifts (e.g., signal slowly deviates independently of the measured property due to changes in temperature, electronic aging of components, etc.). Compression transformations address the problem of dimensionality, effectively reducing the number of measurements trying to optimize the trade-off between an accurate representation and a reasonable size of the final dataset. Normalization transformations are commonly applied to smooth variations between sensors, such as for example an inherently higher signal magnitude of some sensor over the others. Other forms of preprocessing align more to the quality assurance of the data. Such procedures include the removal of artefacts, suppression of noise, and handling the missing values via imputation [34]. These types of transformations can also enhance the performance of ML algorithms in terms of faster convergence in the optimization process, robustness of results, and accuracy [75].

In the context of ML and pattern recognition, feature extraction plays a crucial role as it involves taking an initial set of measurements and generating new values (features) that are informative, non-redundant, and aid in the subsequent learning and generalization processes. Despite the fact that it is very difficult to categorize the different families of methodologies, feature extraction methods can be divided into three main groups, the piecemeal, the curve fitting/statistical measures, and the transformation-based techniques. Regarding the piecemeal features, these are the features that are directly computed on the sensor's response, including first and second derivatives which can be translated as the reaction rate of the sensor and the acceleration, respectively. Other features in this category involve measures such as the computation of maximum value, the rising and the falling slopes during steady state, transient response, and others [76]. In the case of the curve fitting methods, we actually fit a model on the sensor's response in order to measure specific model parameters [77]. Models that are commonly used for fitting purposes include polynomial function, exponential, and auto-regressive models. Here, we could also consider statistical measures that are computed directly on the distribution of the sensor-response such as mean, median, skewness, kurtosis, etc. Finally, there are transformation-based methods involving the conversion of our signal to the frequency domain such as the Discrete Fourier Transform (DFT) or the Discrete Wavelet Transform (DWT), which combine the virtues of DFT but also preserves temporal information. An example of successful application of DWT can be found in [78]. The authors pre-processed their data using DWT and later applied Principal Component Analysis (PCA) trying to discriminate between the different odors.

Since the preprocessing routine plays a significant role in the subsequent steps of a long pipeline, it is particularly important to be reported in detail, so as to have a common ground and the diverse results reported by different authors can be compared. In Table 3 the reader can inspect the different preprocessing pipelines used in studies considering breath-based VOCs towards CRC diagnosis. It is remarkable that for 5 out of 14 studies included in Table 3, we did not manage to find comprehensible information on the preprocessing pipeline applied by the authors.

4.2. Feature Selection

Distinct from feature extraction, feature selection focuses on choosing a subset of existing features rather than creating new ones. Overall, feature selection plays a crucial role in enhancing the efficiency and effectiveness of data analysis. It aims to simplify models, reduce computational times, increase accuracy, robustness of learning, and enable the interpretability of the final model (such as suggesting a few biomarkers that are probably connected to a disease) [79]. The rationale/hypothesis behind feature selection is that the data usually contain redundant and/or irrelevant features that can be eliminated without significant information loss. While the simplest approach involves testing each possible subset to minimize the error rate, this exhaustive search is computationally impractical for large feature sets. The feature selection algorithms are divided into three broad categories: filter, wrapper, and embedded methods [24].

Filter methods are computationally efficient and capture the usefulness of the features based on statistical measures such as correlation but are not tuned to a specific model. For example, there is no complex predictive model involved and, thus, no parameter selection is needed. Instead, these methods may measure the degree of association between the target and the independent variables (e.g., in our case, how the healthy population differs from the diseased; with respect to which features?). They tend to produce more general feature sets but they usually score lower in prediction performance than wrappers or embedded methods. Examples of such methods and their applications include the Analysis Of Variance (ANOVA) [36,40], Welch's *t*-test [8], and the Mann–Whitney U test [41,43]. Wrapper methods use a predictive model to score feature subsets. Each subset is used to train and test a model with its error rate, producing a final score. While computationally intensive, wrapper methods are most likely to produce better results than filter methods. Examples and applications include stepwise selection [38,72], the recursive feature elimination process [21], and the evolutionary search [72]. Embedded methods incorporate feature selection as part of the model construction process. Examples of such methods and their applications include the Least Absolute Shrinkage and Selection Operator (LASSO), which penalizes regression coefficients using L1 norm regularization [37,80], ridge regression (L2 norm regularization), Elastic Net regularization [36] (which combines L1 and L2 norm regularization), and Random Forests which utilize the Gini impurity index or information gain/entropy for ranking features by relative importance [36,39]. These methods offer a balance between filters and wrappers in terms of computational complexity.

4.3. Modeling and Classification

The most relevant features considered in the previous steps constitute the final feature set that is naturally used for modeling and classification. This can be performed in either a supervised or unsupervised manner. The latter does not involve class labels and tries to blindly find statistical similarities between data points with the ultimate goal of finding associations or distinct clusters of similar data points in a sample. A popular algorithm for data-driven modeling in an unsupervised manner is the Principal Component Analysis (PCA) [73,81], which can be used in conjunction with the K-means clustering algorithm for classification purposes. K-means have been utilized in cancer research including CRC [82,83]. On the other hand, supervised learning uses class labels as ground truth to train a model performing over specific tasks. Applications of supervised learning include algorithms such as Random Forests [35,39], Support Vector Machines (SVM) [36], Logistic Regression [37,38,40], Artificial Neural Networks (ANN) [26,27,41,43,73], and Linear discriminant Analysis (LDA) [8]. Despite the fact that supervised learning is more extensively used in disease diagnosis, unsupervised learning is particularly helpful for visualizing the data through clustering and gaining insights into the nature of a particular phenomenon or disease.

It should be noted that every algorithm has its own strengths and weaknesses and no consensus on the general use of specific algorithms exists in the literature. The algorithms can be further divided into linear and non-linear. The non-linear algorithms assume a nonlinear relationship between the target variable and predictors used for classification. In the linear case, separation between groups can be achieved through a linear combination of the explanatory variables and, in simplifying terms, this can be thought of as a straight line on a 2D plane. The nonlinear case involves nonlinear relationships among predictors to achieve separation. Despite the conceptual superiority of non-linear algorithms and the often better predictive performance, they are more complex and therefore often hinder the ability to interpret the final model [84,85]. Explainability in the context of AI applications refers to our ability to explain why and under which circumstances a decision is made by a trained model. For example, in a clinical setting, medical experts are interested in the clinical inference, which in turn plays a crucial role in the diagnosis, staging, or following of a specific curative treatment [86]. Finally, other factors to consider when it comes to the selection of a specific algorithm are the computational complexity and the proneness to overfitting which must be assessed thoroughly through the process of model validation [87].

4.4. Model Training and Validation

Model training and validation can be seen as two distinct parts towards modelling. Training refers to the process of fitting the best combination of parameters to the model using a training set, while validation refers to the evaluation of performance using a validation set (e.g., to tune hyperparameters) and a test set. In practice, in order to develop an AI model, multiple models are fitted and we ultimately choose the best candidate (with specific parameters and hyperparameters) judging by its performance on the validation set. If we incorrectly assess a model's performance, then we might choose a useless configuration. Naturally, the validation strategy affects both the internal parameters (such as weights and biases, which are parameters automatically derived during the training process) and hyperparameters (which are essential for optimizing the model and are externally set by the researcher) of a model. In cases where we consider a feature selection process during training (i.e., candidate models consider different feature sets), insufficient validation may affect the suggested biomarkers [88–90]. That said, model validation is involved whenever training occurs, either only to estimate (e.g., in an unbiased manner) prediction performance (e.g., accuracy, sensitivity, specificity, etc.) or to tune parameters with respect to them. At last, the final error estimate is obtained when the best candidate model is finally applied on unseen test samples. Of course, we expect that the model scores more or less the same as when applied to the validation data. In a case where the test error is much larger than the validation error, overfitting can occur. Hence, model validation gives us a hint of the expected test error while testing aims for an unbiased estimate of the model's performance in a real clinical setting, battling the well-known phenomenon of overfitting [88,91]. The test dataset should be independent of the training and validation sets.

Commonly applied validation strategies for both tuning AI algorithms and estimation of performance are the Hold-out strategy (e.g., splitting into train, validation, and test set) and CV. The Hold-out strategy splits the data into training, validation, and test sets and follows the procedure described above. CV divides data into k subsets. The model is trained and evaluated repeatedly k times, each time using different subsets leaving one subset out for validation and the rest for training purposes. Next, performance metrics are obtained and averaged with the aim of providing estimates of the model's prediction error. When k matches the number of samples in the data set, the method is called Leave One Out Cross Validation (LOOCV). The main difference between the two approaches is that cross-validation utilizes the entire dataset enabling all data to be incorporated in model training and validation. CV may help in reducing the variance in model performance estimates induced by a specific split into training and testing data [91]. The last step is again to test the best candidate model (e.g., based on CV score) on an unseen and independent testing dataset.

Finally, the validation strategy can be characterized as internal or external depending on the cohorts/datasets used for validation. Internal validation refers to the validity of the model inside a single cohort, while external validation refers to the validity of the model spanning external cohorts. External validation is much more powerful than internal in the sense that the model is capable of performing as intended even when there are substantial differences among data sources. For a diagnosis model on CRC, external validation would mean to test the ability of the model to diagnose the disease in cohorts of hospitals in different countries, for patient populations with different demographics, etc. Here, we have to note that none of the 14 studies included in Table 3 used an external dataset to validate findings. Moreover, most of the time the authors reported the validation error (e.g., mainly due to the fact of using limited samples) since the cross validation is applied on the entirety of the available datasets (Table 3).

5. Future Considerations: Extending the AI Toolbox towards Disease Diagnosis

This section delves into future considerations that extend the AI toolbox currently in use, regarding breath-based diagnosis of CRC. These forward-looking directions are framed within the context of the ONCOSCREEN project's ongoing advancements and developments. We explore three key axes: manifold learning, deep learning, and explainable AI, each representing a critical dimension in the quest to enhance the understanding and performance of the contemporary models on diagnosis of CRC.

Over the past years, linear data-driven approaches such as PCA and LDA have become part of the conventional breath analysis research towards preprocessing, dimensionality reduction, visualization, and modelling in terms of a few "dominant", discriminatory variables [8,73,81]. In the context of dimensionality reduction, nonlinear alternatives of the aforementioned methodologies have been introduced like the kernel Principal Component Analysis (kPCA), ISOmetric feature MAPping (ISOMAP), Locally linear Embedding (LLE), and Diffusion Maps [92–95]. Originating from the field of manifold learning, the fundamental assumption is based on the manifold hypothesis, suggesting that high-dimensional data often lie on or near a lower-dimensional manifold within the high-dimensional space. In simpler terms, it is assumed that the data can be effectively represented in a lower-dimensional space taking into account nonlinear (or locally linear) measures (such as the geodesic distance between data points [90]) of similarity between data points. By exploring and leveraging the intrinsic structure of high-dimensional data, one can enhance not only the diagnostic capabilities of a model, but also uncover subtle patterns and relationships within complex datasets. For example, given a number of features resembling either a sensor's resistance or the levels (e.g., abundance) of VOCs in the breath samples, we can find eigenvectors that capture non-linear combinations of our initial feature set and tentatively follow the intrinsic geometry of the underlying manifold. This may allow for visualization and exploration of non-trivial and subtle properties. Such techniques have been successful in various fields where big, complex data and non-linear phenomena are involved. Applications include the diagnosis of schizophrenia with the use of functional magnetic resonance imaging data [90,96], classification of images of handwritten digits [92], forecasting of brain signals [97] and financial time series [98], bifurcation analysis from spatio-temporal data produced by lattice Boltzmann simulations [99], and others. Specifically, Gallos et al. [96] used a variety of manifold learning techniques to construct (embedded) brain connectivity networks (e.g., by mapping correlation matrices in the low dimensional space prior to network construction), utilizing graph theoretic measures towards diagnosis of schizophrenia. Diffusion Maps outperformed their linear counterparts in terms of diagnostic capability. In a follow up study [90], ISOMAP was also applied to demonstrate that learning and feature selection on the low dimensional space was again beneficial in simplifying and raising the predictive performance of the model, ultimately leading to the discovery of a few informative biomarkers for the disease.

Beyond the classic ML methodologies, a subset of ANN-based frameworks also known as deep learning (DL) led to breakthroughs in several fields such as medical image processing [100] and medical diagnosis [101]. DL's ability to process large scale data enables the analysis of raw data even without pre-processing, frequently with high precision [24,102]. In particular, applications on breath-based VOCs towards cancer diagnosis have been introduced [103] and frameworks have been suggested. These include time series stemming from e-nose devices [104]. Specifically, for CRC, the efforts have targeted colonoscopic [105], endoscopic [106] and histopathological [107] images, mostly by using Convolutional Neural Networks (CNN), an architecture designed for analyzing visual data. These types of ANNs utilize convolutional layers to automatically extract meaningful features and have achieved remarkable success in computer vision tasks such as image recognition and object detection. A review can be found in [108]. Within the context of DL, different architectures exist. These include Autoencoders, which utilize a bottleneck layer to extract meaningful features or reduce the dimensionality [103]. An additional method is Recurrent Neural Networks (RNN), which consist of recurrent connections to preserve information across time steps, hence allowing for them to capture temporal dependencies. The latter are also suitable for time series analysis and have been applied towards the optimization of e-nose systems [109] and odor classification [110]. Despite their merits, DL frameworks have their own limitations and challenges. Typically, they need vast amounts of data in order to reach their full potential, they are computationally expensive, have elevated probabilities of overfitting, and are accompanied by high complexity and low interpretability. A comprehensive discussion can be found in [111].

In an effort to address the interpretability of the AI models, remarkable advancements have been made towards the establishment of tools and frameworks that provide understandable explanations regarding outputs and decisions made by the AI models [112–114]. In the literature, the predominant terminology for this field is Explainable AI (XAI) [115]. A characteristic framework is the so-called Shapley additive explanations (SHAP), an approach originating from game theory that attempts to explain the output of AI models. The Shapley values can be used in a model agnostic way [116], thus serving as a useful tool that may accompany various machine learning algorithms. Conceptually, it can be regarded as an extension of the Local Interpretable Model-agnostic Explanations (LIME) approach [117]. In simple terms, the absolute Shapley value reflects how each feature contributes to the final outcome as it is derived from an AI model [113]. However, only a few studies have considered such frameworks on CRC [112]. For example [112], tried to classify CRC patients based on the gut microbiome, and managed to both find CRC-associated bacteria and explore subgroups of CRC patients based on PCA that was imposed on SHAP values. Other frameworks include Gradient-weighted Class activation mapping (Grad-Cams), and these can be applied to CNN-based models to provide transparency and visual explanations [118]. Applications on the diagnosis of CRC include the diagnostic evaluation from colonoscopy images [105] and, more recently, CRC diagnosis and grading utilizing histopathological images [107]. Since this methodology is compatible with CNN-based models, it is natural that it can also be used on time series data employing 1D CNN models [119,120] or even encoding (multivariate) time series data (e.g., one univariate time series per sensor of an e-nose) into two-dimensional images (e.g., a correlation matrix or a dissimilarity matrix in general) towards classification/diagnosis (e.g., CRC patients and healthy controls) via pattern recognition [121].

6. Challenges and Pitfalls in the Use of AI Modelling towards Diagnosis

While the use of AI and especially ML towards diagnosis has been predominant in the past years, one has to put a significant emphasis on model validation to ensure their model generalizes into new unseen data [91]. Estimation of the true capabilities of the contemporary AI models should not be taken lightly. First of all, in cases where the dataset is imbalanced, something very common in disease diagnosis, splits of the dataset (e.g., into training and test splits) should be performed in a stratified manner. This means to practically keep the same percentages of classes in each split. Second, in order to avoid data leakage, transformations such as standardization of data or PCA should consider only the training data. This applies because we do not want our model to be trained using information contained on the unseen test dataset, for this would strongly bias our estimates of performance and likely the true capabilities of the model. Third, it is of paramount importance that wherever a CV procedure is used (with the exception for LOOCV), the estimated performance of the model should be reported in terms of average and standard deviation, which reflect the variability of the model's performance [89]. For even better/refined estimates of model performance or parameter tuning, repeats of CV can also be beneficial [122]. Fourth, even a loop of CV may not be enough to come up with an unbiased estimate of the model's performance, especially when feature selection is taking place at the same time inside the same loop [90,123]. Fifth, feature selection should be used in conjunction with CV (especially when embedded methods are used), as the opposite has been shown to strongly overestimate model's performance [122]. To put it simply, it is crucial that the feature selection process does not "see" all data and then use the optimal feature set to evaluate the performance of a model on the same set. Hence, it is strongly advised that the validation of AI models should take place in the form of a nested CV consisting of an inner loop for optimizing hyperparameters and an outer loop of CV for evaluating performance. Sixth, it is highly recommended to always test the final model on an unseen test dataset (i.e., that is not considered during the model construction phase) after estimating the predicted performance of using a CV scheme. Specifically, Varma et al. [123] reported that the difference between the single CV error estimate and the true error was in some cases greater than 20%, which can be dramatically significant, especially in cases where the classification rates are moderate. Finally, it should be made clear that a CV for assessing a model's performance produces an estimation of prediction error and by no means can this be considered the true test error, which can only be inducted by using sufficiently large unseen test samples (i.e., external validation). This is a common misconception in the scientific community [122,124].

7. Conclusions

This article focused on AI/ML methods used for the analysis of breathomics data in the context of CRC. The needs for improved CRC screening and monitoring were highlighted in parallel with the reported shortcomings of the contemporary standard protocols. VOCs that have been identified as potential biomarkers in previous studies have been presented. Further, we presented the diagnostic performances of contemporary models along the AI pipelines. We explored the main steps of typical AI pipelines in breath analysis for both analytical and sensor-based techniques. The latter are promising methods holding several potential advances over analytical methods in terms of cost, time, portability, and ease of use. Next, we stated future considerations and challenges with a view on extending the AI toolbox that is currently used towards CRC diagnosis via breathomics. The review discusses new potentials in the use of AI, such as the applications of non-linear dimensionality reduction/manifold learning algorithms, DL frameworks, and XAI sets of tools. These tools can potentially enhance diagnostic performance, explore non-linear and complex relationships among features, and provide insights into a "finer" choice of biomarkers with contribution to diagnosis. Despite the optimistic results of breath-based diagnosis in terms of sensitivity and specificity, there is substantial variability among studies and a reliable device and/or pipeline is yet to be developed. In this direction, model training and validation procedures have to be strictly defined and the model's capabilities need to be reported in terms of both internal and external validation. Finally, preprocessing pipelines should be reported transparently and in more detail towards reproducible research.

Author Contributions: Conceptualization, I.K.G. and D.D.D.; investigation, I.K.G. and D.T.; writing—original draft preparation, I.K.G. and D.T.; writing—review and editing, I.K.G., D.D.D., D.T. and G.S.; supervision, A.A. and H.H.; project administration, D.D.D. and A.A.; funding acquisition, A.A. and D.D.D. All authors have read and agreed to the published version of the manuscript.

Funding: This research has been funded by the European Union's Horizon Europe research and innovation program under grant agreement No. 101097036 (ONCOSCREEN). Views and opinions expressed are, however, those of the author(s) only and do not necessarily reflect those of the European Union or the European Health and Digital Executive Agency. Neither the European Union nor the granting authority can be held responsible for them.

Data Availability Statement: This study did not generate or analyze any novel data; thus, data sharing does not apply.

Acknowledgments: The authors would like to thank all partners of the ONCOSCREEN Consortium for the insightful collaboration throughout the project activities.

Conflicts of Interest: The authors declare that the research was conducted in the absence of any commercial or financial relationships that could be construed as a potential conflict of interest.

References

1. Sung, H.; Ferlay, J.; Siegel, R.L.; Laversanne, M.; Soerjomataram, I.; Jemal, A.; Bray, F. Global Cancer Statistics 2020: GLOBOCAN Estimates of Incidence and Mortality Worldwide for 36 Cancers in 185 Countries. *CA Cancer J. Clin.* **2021**, *71*, 209–249. [CrossRef]
2. Schwartzberg, L.; Broder, M.S.; Ailawadhi, S.; Beltran, H.; Blakely, L.J.; Budd, G.T.; Carr, L.; Cecchini, M.; Cobb, P.; Kansal, A.; et al. Impact of Early Detection on Cancer Curability: A Modified Delphi Panel Study. *PLoS ONE* **2022**, *17*, e0279227. [CrossRef]
3. Krilaviciute, A.; Heiss, J.A.; Leja, M.; Kupcinskas, J.; Haick, H.; Brenner, H. Detection of Cancer through Exhaled Breath: A Systematic Review. *Oncotarget* **2015**, *6*, 38643. [CrossRef]
4. Rex, D.K.; Boland, C.R.; Dominitz, J.A.; Giardiello, F.M.; Johnson, D.A.; Kaltenbach, T.; Levin, T.R.; Lieberman, D.; Robertson, D.J. Colorectal Cancer Screening: Recommendations for Physicians and Patients from the US Multi-Society Task Force on Colorectal Cancer. *Gastroenterology* **2017**, *153*, 307–323. [CrossRef] [PubMed]
5. Gimeno Garcia, A.Z. Factors Influencing Colorectal Cancer Screening Participation. *Gastroenterol. Res. Pract.* **2012**, *2012*, 483417. [CrossRef] [PubMed]
6. Mo, S.; Dai, W.; Wang, H.; Lan, X.; Ma, C.; Su, Z.; Xiang, W.; Han, L.; Luo, W.; Zhang, L.; et al. Early Detection and Prognosis Prediction for Colorectal Cancer by Circulating Tumour DNA Methylation Haplotypes: A Multicentre Cohort Study. *EClinicalMedicine* **2023**, *55*, 101717. [CrossRef] [PubMed]
7. Shaukat, A.; Levin, T.R. Current and Future Colorectal Cancer Screening Strategies. *Nat. Rev. Gastroenterol. Hepatol.* **2022**, *19*, 521–531. [CrossRef]
8. Amal, H.; Leja, M.; Funka, K.; Lasina, I.; Skapars, R.; Sivins, A.; Ancans, G.; Kikuste, I.; Vanags, A.; Tolmanis, I.; et al. Breath Testing as Potential Colorectal Cancer Screening Tool. *Int. J. Cancer* **2016**, *138*, 229–236. [CrossRef]
9. Gowda, G.A.N.; Zhang, S.; Gu, H.; Asiago, V.; Shanaiah, N.; Raftery, D. Metabolomics-Based Methods for Early Disease Diagnostics. *Expert. Rev. Mol. Diagn.* **2008**, *8*, 617–633. [CrossRef]
10. Jacob, M.; Lopata, A.L.; Dasouki, M.; Abdel Rahman, A.M. Metabolomics toward Personalized Medicine. *Mass. Spectrom. Rev.* **2019**, *38*, 221–238. [CrossRef]
11. Vadala, R.; Pattnaik, B.; Bangaru, S.; Rai, D.; Tak, J.; Kashyap, S.; Verma, U.; Yadav, G.; Dhaliwal, R.S.; Mittal, S.; et al. A Review on Electronic Nose for Diagnosis and Monitoring Treatment Response in Lung Cancer. *J. Breath. Res.* **2023**, *17*, 024002. [CrossRef]
12. Drabińska, N.; Flynn, C.; Ratcliffe, N.; Belluomo, I.; Myridakis, A.; Gould, O.; Fois, M.; Smart, A.; Devine, T.; Costello, B.D.L. A Literature Survey of All Volatiles from Healthy Human Breath and Bodily Fluids: The Human Volatilome. *J. Breath. Res.* **2021**, *15*, 34001. [CrossRef]
13. van der Schee, M.; Pinheiro, H.; Gaude, E. Breath Biopsy for Early Detection and Precision Medicine in Cancer. *Ecancermedicalscience* **2018**, *12*, ed84. [CrossRef] [PubMed]
14. Nakhleh, M.K.; Amal, H.; Jeries, R.; Broza, Y.Y.; Aboud, M.; Gharra, A.; Ivgi, H.; Khatib, S.; Badarneh, S.; Har-Shai, L.; et al. Diagnosis and Classification of 17 Diseases from 1404 Subjects via Pattern Analysis of Exhaled Molecules. *ACS Nano* **2017**, *11*, 112–125. [CrossRef] [PubMed]
15. Koppenol, W.H.; Bounds, P.L.; Dang, C.V. Otto Warburg's Contributions to Current Concepts of Cancer Metabolism. *Nat. Rev. Cancer* **2011**, *11*, 325–337. [CrossRef] [PubMed]
16. Hakim, M.; Broza, Y.Y.; Barash, O.; Peled, N.; Phillips, M.; Amann, A.; Haick, H. Volatile Organic Compounds of Lung Cancer and Possible Biochemical Pathways. *Chem. Rev.* **2012**, *112*, 5949–5966. [CrossRef]
17. Janfaza, S.; Banan Nojavani, M.; Khorsand, B.; Nikkhah, M.; Zahiri, J. Cancer Odor Database (COD): A Critical Databank for Cancer Diagnosis Research. *Database* **2017**, *2017*, bax055. [CrossRef] [PubMed]
18. Kuo, T.-C.; Tan, C.-E.; Wang, S.-Y.; Lin, O.A.; Su, B.-H.; Hsu, M.-T.; Lin, J.; Cheng, Y.-Y.; Chen, C.-S.; Yang, Y.-C.; et al. Human Breathomics Database. *Database* **2020**, *2020*, baz139. [CrossRef] [PubMed]

19. Janfaza, S.; Khorsand, B.; Nikkhah, M.; Zahiri, J. Digging Deeper into Volatile Organic Compounds Associated with Cancer. *Biol. Methods Protoc.* **2019**, *4*, bpz014. [CrossRef]
20. Keogh, R.J.; Riches, J.C. The Use of Breath Analysis in the Management of Lung Cancer: Is It Ready for Primetime? *Curr. Oncol.* **2022**, *29*, 7355–7378. [CrossRef]
21. Wang, C.; Long, Y.; Li, W.; Dai, W.; Xie, S.; Liu, Y.; Zhang, Y.; Liu, M.; Tian, Y.; Li, Q.; et al. Exploratory Study on Classification of Lung Cancer Subtypes through a Combined K-Nearest Neighbor Classifier in Breathomics. *Sci. Rep.* **2020**, *10*, 5880. [CrossRef] [PubMed]
22. De Vries, R.; Muller, M.; Van Der Noort, V.; Theelen, W.; Schouten, R.D.; Hummelink, K.; Muller, S.H.; Wolf-Lansdorf, M.; Dagelet, J.W.F.; Monkhorst, K.; et al. Prediction of Response to Anti-PD-1 Therapy in Patients with Non-Small-Cell Lung Cancer by Electronic Nose Analysis of Exhaled Breath. *Ann. Oncol.* **2019**, *30*, 1660–1666. [CrossRef] [PubMed]
23. Scheepers, M.H.M.C.; Al-Difaie, Z.; Brandts, L.; Peeters, A.; van Grinsven, B.; Bouvy, N.D. Diagnostic Performance of Electronic Noses in Cancer Diagnoses Using Exhaled Breath: A Systematic Review and Meta-Analysis. *JAMA Netw. Open* **2022**, *5*, e2219372. [CrossRef] [PubMed]
24. Rangarajan, M.; Pandya, H.J. Breath VOC Analysis and Machine Learning Approaches for Disease Screening: A Review. *J. Breath. Res.* **2023**, *17*, 024001.
25. Oakley-Girvan, I.; Davis, S.W. Breath Based Volatile Organic Compounds in the Detection of Breast, Lung, and Colorectal Cancers: A Systematic Review. *Cancer Biomark.* **2018**, *21*, 29–39. [CrossRef]
26. Steenhuis, E.G.M.; Schoenaker, I.J.H.; de Groot, J.W.B.; Fiebrich, H.B.; de Graaf, J.C.; Brohet, R.M.; van Dijk, J.D.; van Westreenen, H.L.; Siersema, P.D. Feasibility of Volatile Organic Compound in Breath Analysis in the Follow-up of Colorectal Cancer: A Pilot Study. *Eur. J. Surg. Oncol.* **2020**, *46*, 2068–2073. [CrossRef]
27. van Keulen, K.E.; Jansen, M.E.; Schrauwen, R.W.M.; Kolkman, J.J.; Siersema, P.D. Volatile Organic Compounds in Breath Can Serve as a Non-Invasive Diagnostic Biomarker for the Detection of Advanced Adenomas and Colorectal Cancer. *Aliment. Pharmacol. Ther.* **2020**, *51*, 334–346. [CrossRef]
28. Van De Goor, R.; Leunis, N.; Van Hooren, M.R.A.; Francisca, E.; Masclee, A.; Kremer, B.; Kross, K.W. Feasibility of Electronic Nose Technology for Discriminating between Head and Neck, Bladder, and Colon Carcinomas. *Eur. Arch. Oto-Rhino-Laryngol.* **2017**, *274*, 1053–1060. [CrossRef]
29. Liu, T.; Guo, L.; Wang, M.; Su, C.; Wang, D.; Dong, H.; Chen, J.; Wu, W. Review on Algorithm Design in Electronic Noses: Challenges, Status, and Trends. *Intell. Comput.* **2023**, *2*, 12. [CrossRef]
30. Amor, R.E.; Nakhleh, M.K.; Barash, O.; Haick, H. Breath Analysis of Cancer in the Present and the Future. *Eur. Respir. Rev.* **2019**, *28*, 190002. [CrossRef]
31. Haick, H.; Broza, Y.Y.; Mochalski, P.; Ruzsanyi, V.; Amann, A. Assessment, Origin, and Implementation of Breath Volatile Cancer Markers. *Chem. Soc. Rev.* **2014**, *43*, 1423–1449. [CrossRef]
32. Konvalina, G.; Haick, H. Sensors for Breath Testing: From Nanomaterials to Comprehensive Disease Detection. *Acc. Chem. Res.* **2014**, *47*, 66–76. [CrossRef] [PubMed]
33. Broadhurst, D.I.; Kell, D.B. Statistical Strategies for Avoiding False Discoveries in Metabolomics and Related Experiments. *Metabolomics* **2006**, *2*, 171–196. [CrossRef]
34. Śmiełowska, M.; Ligor, T.; Kupczyk, W.; Szeliga, J.; Jackowski, M.; Buszewski, B. Screening for Volatile Biomarkers of Colorectal Cancer by Analyzing Breath and Fecal Samples Using Thermal Desorption Combined with GC-MS (TD-GC-MS). *J. Breath. Res.* **2023**, *17*, 47102. [CrossRef] [PubMed]
35. Cheng, H.R.; van Vorstenbosch, R.W.R.; Pachen, D.M.; Meulen, L.W.T.; Straathof, J.W.A.; Dallinga, J.W.; Jonkers, D.M.A.E.; Masclee, A.A.M.; van Schooten, F.-J.; Mujagic, Z.; et al. Detecting Colorectal Adenomas and Cancer Using Volatile Organic Compounds in Exhaled Breath: A Proof-of-Principle Study to Improve Screening. *Clin. Transl. Gastroenterol.* **2022**, *13*, e00518. [CrossRef] [PubMed]
36. Woodfield, G.; Belluomo, I.; Laponogov, I.; Veselkov, K.; Lin, G.; Myridakis, A.; Ayrton, O.; Španěl, P.; Vidal-Diez, A.; Romano, A.; et al. Diagnostic Performance of a Noninvasive Breath Test for Colorectal Cancer: COBRA1 Study. *Gastroenterology* **2022**, *163*, 1447–1449. [CrossRef] [PubMed]
37. Politi, L.; Monasta, L.; Rigressi, M.N.; Princivalle, A.; Gonfiotti, A.; Camiciottoli, G.; Perbellini, L. Discriminant Profiles of Volatile Compounds in the Alveolar Air of Patients with Squamous Cell Lung Cancer, Lung Adenocarcinoma or Colon Cancer. *Molecules* **2021**, *26*, 550. [CrossRef] [PubMed]
38. Altomare, D.F.; Picciariello, A.; Rotelli, M.T.; De Fazio, M.; Aresta, A.; Zambonin, C.G.; Vincenti, L.; Trerotoli, P.; De Vietro, N. Chemical Signature of Colorectal Cancer: Case–Control Study for Profiling the Breath Print. *BJS Open* **2020**, *4*, 1189–1199. [CrossRef]
39. Miller-Atkins, G.; Acevedo-Moreno, L.-A.; Grove, D.; Dweik, R.A.; Tonelli, A.R.; Brown, J.M.; Allende, D.S.; Aucejo, F.; Rotroff, D.M. Breath Metabolomics Provides an Accurate and Noninvasive Approach for Screening Cirrhosis, Primary, and Secondary Liver Tumors. *Hepatol. Commun.* **2020**, *4*, 1041–1055. [CrossRef]
40. Markar, S.R.; Chin, S.-T.; Romano, A.; Wiggins, T.; Antonowicz, S.; Paraskeva, P.; Ziprin, P.; Darzi, A.; Hanna, G.B. Breath Volatile Organic Compound Profiling of Colorectal Cancer Using Selected Ion Flow-Tube Mass Spectrometry. *Ann. Surg.* **2019**, *269*, 903–910. [CrossRef]

41. Altomare, D.F.; Di Lena, M.; Porcelli, F.; Travaglio, E.; Longobardi, F.; Tutino, M.; Depalma, N.; Tedesco, G.; Sardaro, A.; Memeo, R.; et al. Effects of Curative Colorectal Cancer Surgery on Exhaled Volatile Organic Compounds and Potential Implications in Clinical Follow-Up. *Ann. Surg.* **2015**, *262*, 862–867. [CrossRef]
42. Wang, C.; Ke, C.; Wang, X.; Chi, C.; Guo, L.; Luo, S.; Guo, Z.; Xu, G.; Zhang, F.; Li, E. Noninvasive Detection of Colorectal Cancer by Analysis of Exhaled Breath. *Anal. Bioanal. Chem.* **2014**, *406*, 4757–4763. [CrossRef] [PubMed]
43. Altomare, D.F.; Di Lena, M.; Porcelli, F.; Trizio, L.; Travaglio, E.; Tutino, M.; Dragonieri, S.; Memeo, V.; De Gennaro, G. Exhaled Volatile Organic Compounds Identify Patients with Colorectal Cancer. *J. Br. Surg.* **2013**, *100*, 144–150. [CrossRef] [PubMed]
44. Peng, G.; Hakim, M.; Broza, Y.Y.; Billan, S.; Abdah-Bortnyak, R.; Kuten, A.; Tisch, U.; Haick, H. Detection of Lung, Breast, Colorectal, and Prostate Cancers from Exhaled Breath Using a Single Array of Nanosensors. *Br. J. Cancer* **2010**, *103*, 542–551. [CrossRef] [PubMed]
45. Horváth, I.; Barnes, P.J.; Loukides, S.; Sterk, P.J.; Högman, M.; Olin, A.-C.; Amann, A.; Antus, B.; Baraldi, E.; Bikov, A.; et al. A European Respiratory Society Technical Standard: Exhaled Biomarkers in Lung Disease. *Eur. Respir. J.* **2017**, *49*, 1600965. [CrossRef] [PubMed]
46. Leja, M.; Kortelainen, J.M.; Polaka, I.; Turppa, E.; Mitrovics, J.; Padilla, M.; Mochalski, P.; Shuster, G.; Pohle, R.; Kashanin, D.; et al. Sensing Gastric Cancer via Point-of-Care Sensor Breath Analyzer. *Cancer* **2021**, *127*, 1286–1292. [CrossRef] [PubMed]
47. Paschke, S.; Jafarov, S.; Staib, L.; Kreuser, E.-D.; Maulbecker-Armstrong, C.; Roitman, M.; Holm, T.; Harris, C.C.; Link, K.-H.; Kornmann, M. Are Colon and Rectal Cancer Two Different Tumor Entities? A Proposal to Abandon the Term Colorectal Cancer. *Int. J. Mol. Sci.* **2018**, *19*, 2577. [CrossRef]
48. Smith, R.A.; Fedewa, S.; Siegel, R. Early Colorectal Cancer Detection—Current and Evolving Challenges in Evidence, Guidelines, Policy, and Practices. *Adv. Cancer Res.* **2021**, *151*, 69–107. [PubMed]
49. Perea García, J.; Arribas, J.; Cañete, Á.; García, J.L.; Álvaro, E.; Tapial, S.; Narváez, C.; Vivas, A.; Brandáriz, L.; Hernández-Villafranca, S.; et al. Association of Polyps with Early-Onset Colorectal Cancer and throughout Surveillance: Novel Clinical and Molecular Implications. *Cancers* **2019**, *11*, 1900. [CrossRef]
50. Kim, M.; Vogtmann, E.; Ahlquist, D.A.; Devens, M.E.; Kisiel, J.B.; Taylor, W.R.; White, B.A.; Hale, V.L.; Sung, J.; Chia, N.; et al. Fecal Metabolomic Signatures in Colorectal Adenoma Patients Are Associated with Gut Microbiota and Early Events of Colorectal Cancer Pathogenesis. *mBio* **2020**, *11*, e03186-19. [CrossRef]
51. Murakami, T.; Sakamoto, N.; Nagahara, A. Endoscopic Diagnosis of Sessile Serrated Adenoma/Polyp with and without Dysplasia/Carcinoma. *World J. Gastroenterol.* **2018**, *24*, 3250. [CrossRef]
52. Eichenseer, P.J.; Dhanekula, R.; Jakate, S.; Mobarhan, S.; Melson, J.E. Endoscopic Mis-Sizing of Polyps Changes Colorectal Cancer Surveillance Recommendations. *Dis. Colon. Rectum* **2013**, *56*, 315–321. [CrossRef]
53. Alecu, M.; Simion, L.; Straja, N.D.; Brătucu, E. Multiple Polyps and Colorectal Cancer. *Chirurgia* **2014**, *109*, 342–346.
54. Waldum, H.; Fossmark, R. Gastritis, Gastric Polyps and Gastric Cancer. *Int. J. Mol. Sci.* **2021**, *22*, 6548. [CrossRef] [PubMed]
55. Coleman, O.I.; Haller, D. Microbe–Mucus Interface in the Pathogenesis of Colorectal Cancer. *Cancers* **2021**, *13*, 616. [CrossRef] [PubMed]
56. Steel, M.J.; Bukhari, H.; Gentile, L.; Telford, J.; Schaeffer, D.F. Colorectal Adenocarcinomas Diagnosed Following a Negative Faecal Immunochemical Test Show High-Risk Pathological Features in a Colon Screening Programme. *Histopathology* **2021**, *78*, 710–716. [CrossRef] [PubMed]
57. Zhang, J.; Xie, X.; Wu, Z.; Hu, H.; Cai, Y.; Li, J.; Ling, J.; Ding, M.; Li, W.; Deng, Y. Mucinous Adenocarcinoma Predicts Poor Response and Prognosis in Patients with Locally Advanced Rectal Cancer: A Pooled Analysis of Individual Participant Data from 3 Prospective Studies. *Clin. Color. Cancer* **2021**, *20*, e240–e248. [CrossRef]
58. Nitsche, U.; Zimmermann, A.; Späth, C.; Müller, T.; Maak, M.; Schuster, T.; Slotta-Huspenina, J.; Käser, S.A.; Michalski, C.W.; Janssen, K.-P.; et al. Mucinous and Signet-Ring Cell Colorectal Cancers Differ from Classical Adenocarcinomas in Tumor Biology and Prognosis. *Ann. Surg.* **2013**, *258*, 775. [CrossRef]
59. Hu, X.; Li, Y.-Q.; Li, Q.-G.; Ma, Y.-L.; Peng, J.-J.; Cai, S. Mucinous Adenocarcinomas Histotype Can Also Be a High-Risk Factor for Stage II Colorectal Cancer Patients. *Cell. Physiol. Biochem.* **2018**, *47*, 630–640. [CrossRef]
60. Park, E.J.; Baek, J.-H.; Choi, G.-S.; Park, W.C.; Yu, C.S.; Kang, S.-B.; Min, B.S.; Kim, J.H.; Kim, H.R.; Lee, B.H.; et al. The Role of Primary Tumor Resection in Colorectal Cancer Patients with Asymptomatic, Synchronous, Unresectable Metastasis: A Multicenter Randomized Controlled Trial. *Cancers* **2020**, *12*, 2306. [CrossRef]
61. Chow, J.S.; Chen, C.C.; Ahsan, H.; Neugut, A.I. A Population-Based Study of the Incidence of Malignant Small Bowel Tumours: SEER, 1973–1990. *Int. J. Epidemiol.* **1996**, *25*, 722–728. [CrossRef] [PubMed]
62. Ogunwobi, O.O.; Mahmood, F.; Akingboye, A. Biomarkers in Colorectal Cancer: Current Research and Future Prospects. *Int. J. Mol. Sci.* **2020**, *21*, 5311. [CrossRef] [PubMed]
63. Probert, C.S.J.; Khalid, T.; Ahmed, I.; Johnson, E.; Smith, S.; Ratcliffe, N.M. Volatile Organic Compounds as Diagnostic Biomarkers in Gastrointestinal and Liver Diseases. *J. Gastrointest. Liver Dis.* **2009**, *18*, 337–343.
64. Vernia, F.; Valvano, M.; Fabiani, S.; Stefanelli, G.; Longo, S.; Viscido, A.; Latella, G. Are Volatile Organic Compounds Accurate Markers in the Assessment of Colorectal Cancer and Inflammatory Bowel Diseases? A Review. *Cancers* **2021**, *13*, 2361. [CrossRef] [PubMed]
65. Chung, J.; Akter, S.; Han, S.; Shin, Y.; Choi, T.G.; Kang, I.; Kim, S.S. Diagnosis by Volatile Organic Compounds in Exhaled Breath from Patients with Gastric and Colorectal Cancers. *Int. J. Mol. Sci.* **2022**, *24*, 129. [CrossRef]

66. De Vietro, N.; Aresta, A.; Rotelli, M.T.; Zambonin, C.; Lippolis, C.; Picciariello, A.; Altomare, D.F. Relationship between Cancer Tissue Derived and Exhaled Volatile Organic Compound from Colorectal Cancer Patients. Preliminary Results. *J. Pharm. Biomed. Anal.* **2020**, *180*, 113055. [CrossRef]
67. Dima, A.C.; Balaban, D.V.; Dima, A. Diagnostic Application of Volatile Organic Compounds as Potential Biomarkers for Detecting Digestive Neoplasia: A Systematic Review. *Diagnostics* **2021**, *11*, 2317. [CrossRef]
68. Xiang, L.; Wu, S.; Hua, Q.; Bao, C.; Liu, H. Volatile Organic Compounds in Human Exhaled Breath to Diagnose Gastrointestinal Cancer: A Meta-Analysis. *Front. Oncol.* **2021**, *11*, 606915. [CrossRef]
69. Hanna, G.B.; Boshier, P.R.; Markar, S.R.; Romano, A. Accuracy and Methodologic Challenges of Volatile Organic Compound–Based Exhaled Breath Tests for Cancer Diagnosis: A Systematic Review and Meta-Analysis. *JAMA Oncol.* **2019**, *5*, e182815. [CrossRef]
70. Zhou, W.; Tao, J.; Li, J.; Tao, S. Volatile Organic Compounds Analysis as a Potential Novel Screening Tool for Colorectal Cancer: A Systematic Review and Meta-Analysis. *Medicine* **2020**, *99*, e20937. [CrossRef]
71. Wang, L.; Li, J.; Xiong, X.; Hao, T.; Zhang, C.; Gao, Z.; Zhong, L.; Zhao, Y. Volatile Organic Compounds as a Potential Screening Tool for Neoplasm of the Digestive System: A Meta-Analysis. *Sci. Rep.* **2021**, *11*, 23716. [CrossRef] [PubMed]
72. Poļaka, I.; Mežmale, L.; Anarkulova, L.; Kononova, E.; Vilkoite, I.; Veliks, V.; Leščinska, A.M.; Stonāns, I.; Pčolkins, A.; Tolmanis, I.; et al. The Detection of Colorectal Cancer through Machine Learning-Based Breath Sensor Analysis. *Diagnostics* **2023**, *13*, 3355. [CrossRef]
73. Altomare, D.F.; Porcelli, F.; Picciariello, A.; Pinto, M.; Di Lena, M.; Caputi Iambrenghi, O.; Ugenti, I.; Guglielmi, A.; Vincenti, L.; De Gennaro, G. The Use of the PEN3 E-Nose in the Screening of Colorectal Cancer and Polyps. *Tech. Coloproctol.* **2016**, *20*, 405–409. [CrossRef] [PubMed]
74. Gutierrez-Osuna, R.; Nagle, H.T. A Method for Evaluating Data-Preprocessing Techniques for Odour Classification with an Array of Gas Sensors. *IEEE Trans. Syst. Man Cybern. (Cybern.)* **1999**, *29*, 626–632. [CrossRef] [PubMed]
75. Sola, J.; Sevilla, J. Importance of Input Data Normalization for the Application of Neural Networks to Complex Industrial Problems. *IEEE Trans. Nucl. Sci.* **1997**, *44*, 1464–1468. [CrossRef]
76. Yan, J.; Guo, X.; Duan, S.; Jia, P.; Wang, L.; Peng, C.; Zhang, S. Electronic Nose Feature Extraction Methods: A Review. *Sensors* **2015**, *15*, 27804–27831. [CrossRef]
77. Carmel, L.; Levy, S.; Lancet, D.; Harel, D. A Feature Extraction Method for Chemical Sensors in Electronic Noses. *Sens. Actuators B Chem.* **2003**, *93*, 67–76. [CrossRef]
78. Agustika, D.K.; Triyana, K. Application of Principal Component Analysis and Discrete Wavelet Transform in Electronic Nose for Herbal Drinks Classification. In *Proceedings of the AIP Conference Proceedings, Yogyakarta, Indonesia, 11–13 November 2015*; AIP Publishing: New York, NY, USA, 2016; Volume 1755, p. 170012.
79. Guyon, I.; Elisseeff, A. An Introduction to Variable and Feature Selection. *J. Mach. Learn. Res.* **2003**, *3*, 1157–1182.
80. Ranstam, J.; Cook, J.A. LASSO Regression. *J. Br. Surg.* **2018**, *105*, 1348. [CrossRef]
81. Jollife, I.T. *Principal Component Analysis*, 2nd ed.; Springer: Berlin, Germany, 2002.
82. Florensa, D.; Mateo-Fornés, J.; Solsona, F.; Pedrol Aige, T.; Mesas Julió, M.; Piñol, R.; Godoy, P. Use of Multiple Correspondence Analysis and K-Means to Explore Associations between Risk Factors and Likelihood of Colorectal Cancer: Cross-Sectional Study. *J. Med. Internet Res.* **2022**, *24*, e29056. [CrossRef]
83. Dubey, A.K.; Gupta, U.; Jain, S. Analysis of K-Means Clustering Approach on the Breast Cancer Wisconsin Dataset. *Int. J. Comput. Assist. Radiol. Surg.* **2016**, *11*, 2033–2047. [CrossRef]
84. Ouyang, F.; Guo, B.; Ouyang, L.; Liu, Z.; Lin, S.; Meng, W.; Huang, X.; Chen, H.; Qiu-Gen, H.; Yang, S. Comparison between Linear and Nonlinear Machine-Learning Algorithms for the Classification of Thyroid Nodules. *Eur. J. Radiol.* **2019**, *113*, 251–257. [CrossRef]
85. Ebrahim, M.; Sedky, A.A.H.; Mesbah, S. Accuracy Assessment of Machine Learning Algorithms Used to Predict Breast Cancer. *Data* **2023**, *8*, 35. [CrossRef]
86. Zhang, Y.; Weng, Y.; Lund, J. Applications of Explainable Artificial Intelligence in Diagnosis and Surgery. *Diagnostics* **2022**, *12*, 237. [CrossRef]
87. Uddin, S.; Khan, A.; Hossain, M.E.; Moni, M.A. Comparing Different Supervised Machine Learning Algorithms for Disease Prediction. *BMC Med. Inform. Decis. Mak.* **2019**, *19*, 281. [CrossRef]
88. Diaz-Uriarte, R.; de Lope, E.; Giugno, R.; Fröhlich, H.; Nazarov, P.V.; Nepomuceno-Chamorro, I.A.; Rauschenberger, A.; Glaab, E. Ten Quick Tips for Biomarker Discovery and Validation Analyses Using Machine Learning. *PLoS Comput. Biol.* **2022**, *18*, e1010357. [CrossRef] [PubMed]
89. Rafało, M. Cross Validation Methods: Analysis Based on Diagnostics of Thyroid Cancer Metastasis. *ICT Express* **2022**, *8*, 183–188. [CrossRef]
90. Gallos, I.K.; Gkiatis, K.; Matsopoulos, G.K.; Siettos, C. ISOMAP and Machine Learning Algorithms for the Construction of Embedded Functional Connectivity Networks of Anatomically Separated Brain Regions from Resting State FMRI Data of Patients with Schizophrenia. *AIMS Neurosci.* **2021**, *8*, 295. [CrossRef] [PubMed]
91. Vazquez-Zapien, G.J.; Mata-Miranda, M.M.; Garibay-Gonzalez, F.; Sanchez-Brito, M. Artificial Intelligence Model Validation before Its Application in Clinical Diagnosis Assistance. *World J. Gastroenterol.* **2022**, *28*, 602. [CrossRef] [PubMed]

92. Tenenbaum, J.B.; De Silva, V.; Langford, J.C. A Global Geometric Framework for Nonlinear Dimensionality Reduction. *Science* **2000**, *290*, 2319–2323. [CrossRef] [PubMed]
93. Roweis, S.T.; Saul, L.K. Nonlinear Dimensionality Reduction by Locally Linear Embedding. *Science* **2000**, *290*, 2323–2326. [CrossRef] [PubMed]
94. Schölkopf, B.; Smola, A.; Müller, K.-R. Kernel Principal Component Analysis. In *Proceedings of the Artificial Neural Networks—ICANN'97: 7th International Conference, Lausanne, Switzerland, 8–10 October 1997*; Springer: Berlin/Heidelberg, Germany, 2005; pp. 583–588.
95. Coifman, R.R.; Lafon, S. Diffusion Maps. *Appl. Comput. Harmon. Anal.* **2006**, *21*, 5–30. [CrossRef]
96. Gallos, I.K.; Galaris, E.; Siettos, C.I. Construction of Embedded FMRI Resting-State Functional Connectivity Networks Using Manifold Learning. *Cogn. Neurodyn* **2021**, *15*, 585–608. [CrossRef] [PubMed]
97. Gallos, I.K.; Lehmberg, D.; Dietrich, F.; Siettos, C. Data-Driven Modelling of Brain Activity Using Neural Networks, Diffusion Maps, and the Koopman Operator. *arXiv* **2023**, arXiv:2304.11925.
98. Papaioannou, P.G.; Talmon, R.; Kevrekidis, I.G.; Siettos, C. Time-Series Forecasting Using Manifold Learning, Radial Basis Function Interpolation, and Geometric Harmonics. *Chaos Interdiscip. J. Nonlinear Sci.* **2022**, *32*, 83113. [CrossRef]
99. Galaris, E.; Fabiani, G.; Gallos, I.; Kevrekidis, I.; Siettos, C. Numerical Bifurcation Analysis of Pdes from Lattice Boltzmann Model Simulations: A Parsimonious Machine Learning Approach. *J. Sci. Comput.* **2022**, *92*, 34. [CrossRef]
100. Razzak, M.I.; Naz, S.; Zaib, A. Deep Learning for Medical Image Processing: Overview, Challenges and the Future. *Classif. BioApps Autom. Decis. Mak.* **2018**, *26*, 323–350.
101. Litjens, G.; Sánchez, C.I.; Timofeeva, N.; Hermsen, M.; Nagtegaal, I.; Kovacs, I.; Hulsbergen-Van De Kaa, C.; Bult, P.; Van Ginneken, B.; Van Der Laak, J. Deep Learning as a Tool for Increased Accuracy and Efficiency of Histopathological Diagnosis. *Sci. Rep.* **2016**, *6*, 26286. [CrossRef]
102. Ye, Z.; Liu, Y.; Li, Q. Recent Progress in Smart Electronic Nose Technologies Enabled with Machine Learning Methods. *Sensors* **2021**, *21*, 7620. [CrossRef]
103. Aslam, M.A.; Xue, C.; Chen, Y.; Zhang, A.; Liu, M.; Wang, K.; Cui, D. Breath Analysis Based Early Gastric Cancer Classification from Deep Stacked Sparse Autoencoder Neural Network. *Sci. Rep.* **2021**, *11*, 4014. [CrossRef]
104. Längkvist, M.; Karlsson, L.; Loutfi, A. A Review of Unsupervised Feature Learning and Deep Learning for Time-Series Modeling. *Pattern Recognit. Lett.* **2014**, *42*, 11–24. [CrossRef]
105. Zhou, D.; Tian, F.; Tian, X.; Sun, L.; Huang, X.; Zhao, F.; Zhou, N.; Chen, Z.; Zhang, Q.; Yang, M.; et al. Diagnostic Evaluation of a Deep Learning Model for Optical Diagnosis of Colorectal Cancer. *Nat. Commun.* **2020**, *11*, 2961. [CrossRef] [PubMed]
106. Park, H.-C.; Kim, Y.-J.; Lee, S.-W. Adenocarcinoma Recognition in Endoscopy Images Using Optimized Convolutional Neural Networks. *Appl. Sci.* **2020**, *10*, 1650. [CrossRef]
107. Zhou, P.; Cao, Y.; Li, M.; Ma, Y.; Chen, C.; Gan, X.; Wu, J.; Lv, X.; Chen, C. HCCANet: Histopathological Image Grading of Colorectal Cancer Using CNN Based on Multichannel Fusion Attention Mechanism. *Sci. Rep.* **2022**, *12*, 15103. [CrossRef] [PubMed]
108. Li, Z.; Liu, F.; Yang, W.; Peng, S.; Zhou, J. A Survey of Convolutional Neural Networks: Analysis, Applications, and Prospects. *IEEE Trans. Neural Netw. Learn. Syst.* **2021**, *33*, 6999–7019. [CrossRef] [PubMed]
109. Zou, Y.; Lv, J. Using Recurrent Neural Network to Optimize Electronic Nose System with Dimensionality Reduction. *Electronics* **2020**, *9*, 2205. [CrossRef]
110. Fukuyama, K.; Matsui, K.; Omatsu, S.; Rivas, A.; Corchado, J.M. Feature Extraction and Classification of Odor Using Attention Based Neural Network. In *Distributed Computing and Artificial Intelligence, 16th International Conference*; Springer: Cham, Switzerland, 2020; pp. 142–149.
111. Alzubaidi, L.; Zhang, J.; Humaidi, A.J.; Al-Dujaili, A.; Duan, Y.; Al-Shamma, O.; Santamaría, J.; Fadhel, M.A.; Al-Amidie, M.; Farhan, L. Review of Deep Learning: Concepts, CNN Architectures, Challenges, Applications, Future Directions. *J. Big Data* **2021**, *8*, 53. [CrossRef]
112. Rynazal, R.; Fujisawa, K.; Shiroma, H.; Salim, F.; Mizutani, S.; Shiba, S.; Yachida, S.; Yamada, T. Leveraging Explainable AI for Gut Microbiome-Based Colorectal Cancer Classification. *Genome Biol.* **2023**, *24*, 21. [CrossRef]
113. Massafra, R.; Fanizzi, A.; Amoroso, N.; Bove, S.; Comes, M.C.; Pomarico, D.; Didonna, V.; Diotaiuti, S.; Galati, L.; Giotta, F.; et al. Analyzing Breast Cancer Invasive Disease Event Classification through Explainable Artificial Intelligence. *Front. Med.* **2023**, *10*, 1116354. [CrossRef]
114. Sabol, P.; Sinčák, P.; Hartono, P.; Kočan, P.; Benetinová, Z.; Blichárová, A.; Verbóová, L.; Štammová, E.; Sabolová-Fabianová, A.; Jašková, A. Explainable Classifier for Improving the Accountability in Decision-Making for Colorectal Cancer Diagnosis from Histopathological Images. *J. Biomed. Inform.* **2020**, *109*, 103523. [CrossRef]
115. Gunning, D.; Stefik, M.; Choi, J.; Miller, T.; Stumpf, S.; Yang, G.-Z. XAI—Explainable Artificial Intelligence. *Sci. Robot.* **2019**, *4*, eaay7120. [CrossRef] [PubMed]
116. Rodríguez-Pérez, R.; Bajorath, J. Interpretation of Compound Activity Predictions from Complex Machine Learning Models Using Local Approximations and Shapley Values. *J. Med. Chem.* **2019**, *63*, 8761–8777. [CrossRef] [PubMed]
117. Ribeiro, M.T.; Singh, S.; Guestrin, C. "Why Should i Trust You?" Explaining the Predictions of Any Classifier. In Proceedings of the 22nd ACM SIGKDD International Conference on Knowledge Discovery and Data Mining, San Francisco, CA, USA, 13–17 August 2016; pp. 1135–1144.

118. Selvaraju, R.R.; Cogswell, M.; Das, A.; Vedantam, R.; Parikh, D.; Batra, D. Grad-Cam: Visual Explanations from Deep Networks via Gradient-Based Localization. In Proceedings of the IEEE International Conference on Computer Vision, Venice, Italy, 22–29 October 2017; pp. 618–626.
119. Garg, P.; Davenport, E.; Murugesan, G.; Wagner, B.; Whitlow, C.; Maldjian, J.; Montillo, A. Automatic 1D Convolutional Neural Network-Based Detection of Artifacts in MEG Acquired without Electrooculography or Electrocardiography. In Proceedings of the 2017 International Workshop on Pattern Recognition in Neuroimaging (PRNI), Toronto, ON, Canada, 21–23 June 2017; pp. 1–4.
120. Zhao, X.; Wen, Z.; Pan, X.; Ye, W.; Bermak, A. Mixture Gases Classification Based on Multi-Label One-Dimensional Deep Convolutional Neural Network. *IEEE Access* **2019**, *7*, 12630–12637. [CrossRef]
121. Yang, C.-L.; Chen, Z.-X.; Yang, C.-Y. Sensor Classification Using Convolutional Neural Network by Encoding Multivariate Time Series as Two-Dimensional Colored Images. *Sensors* **2019**, *20*, 168. [CrossRef]
122. Krstajic, D.; Buturovic, L.J.; Leahy, D.E.; Thomas, S. Cross-Validation Pitfalls When Selecting and Assessing Regression and Classification Models. *J. Cheminform.* **2014**, *6*, 10. [CrossRef]
123. Varma, S.; Simon, R. Bias in Error Estimation When Using Cross-Validation for Model Selection. *BMC Bioinform.* **2006**, *7*, 91. [CrossRef]
124. Hastie, T.; Tibshirani, R.; Friedman, J.H.; Friedman, J.H. *The Elements of Statistical Learning: Data Mining, Inference, and Prediction*; Springer: Berlin/Heidelberg, Germany, 2009; Volume 2.

Disclaimer/Publisher's Note: The statements, opinions and data contained in all publications are solely those of the individual author(s) and contributor(s) and not of MDPI and/or the editor(s). MDPI and/or the editor(s) disclaim responsibility for any injury to people or property resulting from any ideas, methods, instructions or products referred to in the content.

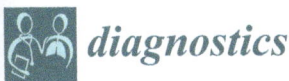 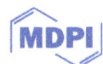

Article

Gastro-BaseNet: A Specialized Pre-Trained Model for Enhanced Gastroscopic Data Classification and Diagnosis of Gastric Cancer and Ulcer

Gi Pyo Lee [1], Young Jae Kim [2], Dong Kyun Park [3], Yoon Jae Kim [3], Su Kyeong Han [4] and Kwang Gi Kim [2,*]

[1] Department of Health Sciences and Technology, Gachon Advanced Institute for Health Sciences and Technology (GAIHST), Gachon University, Incheon 21565, Republic of Korea; jeju5582@gmail.com

[2] Department of Biomedical Engineering, Gachon University Gil Medical Center, College of Medicine, Gachon University, Incheon 21565, Republic of Korea; kimyj10528@gmail.com

[3] Division of Gastroenterology, Department of Internal Medicine, Gachon University Gil Medical Center, College of Medicine, Gachon University, Incheon 21565, Republic of Korea; pdk66@gilhospital.com (D.K.P.); yoonjaemed@gmail.com (Y.J.K.)

[4] Health IT Research Center, Gachon University Gil Medical Center, Incheon 21565, Republic of Korea; skhan1211@naver.com

* Correspondence: kimkg@gachon.ac.kr

Abstract: Most of the development of gastric disease prediction models has utilized pre-trained models from natural data, such as ImageNet, which lack knowledge of medical domains. This study proposes Gastro-BaseNet, a classification model trained using gastroscopic image data for abnormal gastric lesions. To prove performance, we compared transfer-learning based on two pre-trained models (Gastro-BaseNet and ImageNet) and two training methods (freeze and fine-tune modes). The effectiveness was verified in terms of classification at the image-level and patient-level, as well as the localization performance of lesions. The development of Gastro-BaseNet had demonstrated superior transfer learning performance compared to random weight settings in ImageNet. When developing a model for predicting the diagnosis of gastric cancer and gastric ulcers, the transfer-learned model based on Gastro-BaseNet outperformed that based on ImageNet. Furthermore, the model's performance was highest when fine-tuning the entire layer in the fine-tune mode. Additionally, the trained model was based on Gastro-BaseNet, which showed higher localization performance, which confirmed its accurate detection and classification of lesions in specific locations. This study represents a notable advancement in the development of image analysis models within the medical field, resulting in improved diagnostic predictive accuracy and aiding in making more informed clinical decisions in gastrointestinal endoscopy.

Keywords: gastroscopy; transfer learning; deep learning; Gastro-BaseNet; ImageNet; endoscopy

Citation: Lee, G.P.; Kim, Y.J.; Park, D.K.; Kim, Y.J.; Han, S.K.; Kim, K.G. Gastro-BaseNet: A Specialized Pre-Trained Model for Enhanced Gastroscopic Data Classification and Diagnosis of Gastric Cancer and Ulcer. *Diagnostics* **2024**, *14*, 75. https://doi.org/10.3390/diagnostics14010075

Academic Editors: Eun-Sun Kim and Kwang-Sig Lee

Received: 29 November 2023
Revised: 25 December 2023
Accepted: 26 December 2023
Published: 28 December 2023

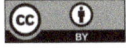

Copyright: © 2023 by the authors. Licensee MDPI, Basel, Switzerland. This article is an open access article distributed under the terms and conditions of the Creative Commons Attribution (CC BY) license (https://creativecommons.org/licenses/by/4.0/).

1. Introduction

According to 2020 GLOBOCAN statistics, gastric cancer is the most common malignancy among men and women, with more than 1 million new cases worldwide and the fifth highest incidence (5.6%) and fourth highest mortality (7.7%) among men and women combined. The highest incidence of gastric cancer in the world is in East Asia and Eastern Europe [1]. Gastric cancer is diagnosed through endoscopy, which visually confirms the location and type of tumor in the stomach. Histologic confirmation through biopsy is necessary to make a final diagnosis [2]. However, gastroscopy misses gastric cancer between 4.6% and 14.3% of the time because it requires the examiner to detect the lesion with the naked eye [3].

Recently, researchers have been applying artificial intelligence (AI) and convolutional neural networks (CNN) to detect advanced gastric cancer and early gastric cancer. Lee et al. [4] developed a malignancy prediction model with an accuracy of 96.49% (normal and gastric cancer classification) and 77.12% (gastric cancer and gastric ulcer) using CNN-based models of ResNet50, InceptionV3, and VGG16. Ma et al. [5] developed an early gastric cancer classification model with an accuracy of 98.84% and an F1 score of 98.18% using GAIN-ResNet50 using attention maps. Wei et al. [6] developed a DCNN model using VGG16 and ResNet50 to classify non-malignant mucosa (normal) and gastric cancer, with an accuracy of 92.50% and a sensitivity of 94%. In particular, both senior and novice endoscopists showed higher accuracy and performance. Teramoto et al. [7] developed a gastric cancer prediction model based on VGG, DenseNet, InceptionV3, and ResNet; the DenseNet121 model showed the highest performance with a sensitivity of 97.0% and a specificity of 99.4%. Yuan et al. [8] trained a diagnostic model using the YOLO architecture to determine the most predicted results as the final diagnosis, with a classification accuracy of 93.5%, sensitivity of 59.2%, and specificity of 99.3% for early gastric cancer and a classification accuracy of 98.4%, sensitivity of 100ss%, and specificity of 98.1% for advanced gastric cancer. Cho et al. [9] developed a binary classification model to classify cancer and non-cancer using InceptionResNetV2, with an accuracy of 76% and an AUC of 0.706.

Those previous studies developed a CNN model for detecting and predicting the diagnosis of both early and advanced stages of gastric cancer. This did not involve training a new model with randomly assigned weight values. Instead, a pre-trained model was fine-tuned on a large dataset using the weights of the initial model, referred to as transfer learning. The widely used dataset for pretraining models was ImageNet [10], and its weights were utilized during the transfer learning process. However, ImageNet was an image dataset of a thousand classes for various objects and was pre-trained with images from a completely different environment than gastroscopy images. This study presented the development of a pre-trained model called Gastro-BaseNet, which utilized gastroscopic images to classify normal and abnormal diagnoses, such as gastric cancer and ulcers. During the pre-training phase, Gastro-BaseNet acquired information about the characteristics of abnormal gastric lesions as opposed to those found in a normal stomach. This pre-trained knowledge in endoscopic images formed the basis of our pre-trained information and enhanced training efficiency compared to other pre-trained models such as ImageNet, which relied on knowledge from other natural image domains.

Our study involved the development of Gastro-BaseNet through the training of model layers and weights, specifically for the classification of abnormal gastric diseases. This model proved valuable in predicting specific gastric diagnoses and replaced pre-trained models in more specialized studies that involve gastroscopic images. Therefore, we utilized Gastro-BaseNet to classify gastric cancer and ulcers, comparing its performance with a predictive model that employed the weights of pre-trained models to confirm the feasibility of using an optimized model for research on endoscopic datasets.

2. Materials and Methods

2.1. Data Acquation

We constructed a training database for Gastro-BaseNet to predict abnormal gastric lesions utilizing gastroscopic image data. We had examined the medical and pathology records of patients who visited Gachon University Gil Hospital (IRB No. GBIRB 2021-383) between January 2019 and December 2022 and underwent gastroscopy to establish their final diagnosis (Table 1). We selected a total of 1902 patients, 1135 men and 767 women, with a mean age of 68.03 ($\pm$12.00), and divided into three categories: 1070 patients diagnosed with gastric cancer, 720 men and 350 women, with a mean age of 70.45 ($\pm$11.05), 532 patients diagnosed with gastric ulcer, 317 men and 215 women, with a mean age of 67.19 ($\pm$12.61), and 300 patients with normal patients with no abnormal findings, 98 men and 202 women, with a mean age of 60.86 ($\pm$11.09), based on the pathology results. The images collected from patients consisted of frozen images manually captured from the screen during gastroscopy by a gastrointestinal specialist. For patients with a diagnosis, only images containing regions of cancer or ulcer were collected, while for normal patients, all images taken during the examination were collected. Therefore, the number of images collected for each patient varies by disease. The average number of frozen images collected per patient, by diagnosis, was approximately 5.76 (±3.48) of gastric cancer, 6.20 (±4.15) of ulcers, and 33.52 (±10.65) of normal cases. Finally, the dataset consisted of a total of 19,518 images and consisted of 6164 images of gastric cancer, 3297 images of gastric ulcers, and 10,057 images of normal regions.

Table 1. Number of datasets built for training Gastro-BaseNet and datasets for deep learning training.

	Normal	Abnormal		Total
		Gastric Cancer	Gastric Ulcer	
Train	7297	4476	2409	14,182
Validation	738	493	263	1494
Test	2022	1195	625	3842
Total (Number of patients)	10,057 (300)	6164 (1070)	3297 (532)	19,518 (1902)

Then, we constructed another dataset to verify the performance of transfer learning by Gastro-BaseNet. We collected still images of patients diagnosed with gastric cancer and gastric ulcers through histologic examination from June 2018 to November 2021 who visited Gachon University Gil Hospital. When selecting the patient's data for evaluating transfer learning according to a model pre-trained by gastroscopic data, the patients collected for training Gastro-BaseNet were excluded. To evaluate the efficiency of the transfer learning on Gastro-BaseNet, additional studies were conducted to develop diagnostic models for two types of gastric lesions: gastric cancer (study 1) and gastric ulcers (study 2). In Table 2, we selected a total of 1033 patients, 660 men and 373 women, with a mean age of 65.56 (±13.00), and divided them into three categories: 707 patients diagnosed with gastric cancer used for study 1484 men and 223 women, with a mean age of 68.01 (±11.82), 178 patients diagnosed with gastric ulcer used for study 2121 men and 57 women, with a mean age of 62.45 (±14.52), and 148 patients with normal patients that had nothing abnormal findings, 55 men and 93 women, with a mean age of 57.62 (±12.56), based on the pathology results. The average number of frozen images collected per patient, by diagnosis, was approximately 5.27 (±3.09) of gastric cancer, 6.31 (±3.98) of gastric ulcers, and 34.82 (±11.24) of normal cases. Finally, the dataset consisted of a total of 10,001 images and consisted of 3724 images of gastric cancer, 1124 images of gastric ulcers, and 5153 images of normal regions.

Table 2. Number of patients and image datasets for training models to classify gastric cancers (study 1) or gastric ulcers (study 2) by using transfer learning based on Gastro-BaseNet.

	Study 1: Gastric Cancer			Study 2: Gastric Ulcer		
	Normal	Gastric Cancer	Total	Normal	Gastric Ulcer	Total
Train	3662	2671	6333	3617	789	4406
Validation	416	273	689	461	92	553
Test	1075	780	1855	1075	243	1318
Total (Number of patients)	5153 (148)	3724 (707)	8877 (855)	5153 (148)	1124 (178)	6277 (326)

All images were captured in the white-light imaging mode. The image was extracted into JPG format, and the resolution of the original image was very varied, ranging from 187 × 186 to 1350 × 1062 pixels.

2.2. Study Environment

The system environment for deep learning employed an IBM Power System AC922 8335-GTH (IBM, Armonk, NY, USA) with a single NVIDIA Tesla V100-SXM2 32 GB (NVIDIA, Santa Clara, CA, USA). The operating system used was Ubuntu 18.04.5. We used Python (version 3.7.10) with TensorFlow frameworks (version 2.6.0) and Keras (version 2.6.0) for training and evaluating models. For image processing, the OpenCV (version 4.6.0) libraries were used.

2.3. Data Preprocess

Freeze image, captured screen in esophagogastroduodenoscopy, included useless information about patient name, patient ID, study date, endoscopy device, etc. These were located outside of the video frame in most of the images. To extract a valid area of gastroscopy video, we applied a frame-extraction algorithm and cropped the images of a valid region to train models from them (Figure 1). In a few images, some areas of marked information invaded the valid frame. However, these data included the training dataset because it improved the generality of the trained model as a result of noise and prevented the loss of clear cancer or ulcer areas.

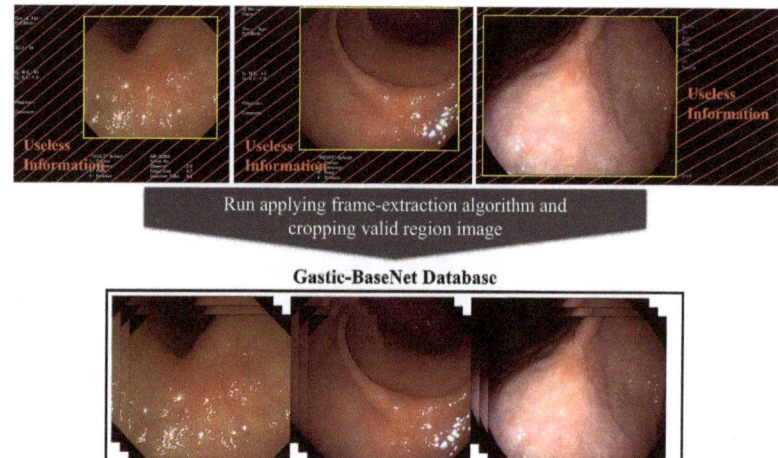

Figure 1. The process of cropping useless information regions from the initial collected gastroscopic images and building an image database.

To train deep learning models, we resized the collected images with the ImageNet dataset to the image size of the pre-trained models' input shape. The pre-trained models used in this study were ResNet50 and EfficientNetB0, both with a resolution of 224 × 224.

2.4. Transfer Learning

Transfer learning is a training technique that transfers the processing ability of a pre-trained model to solve one task and utilizes it to solve another task [11,12]. By using a large amount of data, the feature extraction phase of a well-trained model is recalled and transferred to learn the new task. In this case, the training time is reduced, and the trained model's performance is improved. Transfer learning trains the weights in two different ways, according to the users' objectives [13]. One is called freeze mode, which freezes the feature extraction phase of the pre-trained model and allows only the new classifier part to be trained. This is used when the pre-trained model and the new training dataset have a similar problem or domain image. The other is called fine-tune mode through the pre-trained model, and the new training dataset has completely different problems or domain images; both feature extraction and classifiers are trained and tuned [14]. This can be carried out by training all layers of the feature extraction part, or by freezing some layers (lower layer part) that extract general features and training the rest of the layers (upper layer part) that extract problem-specific features.

For transfer learning, the fully connected (FC) layer responsible for the classifier of the existing trained CNN model is removed, and new FC layers are connected to adjust the weights through training for our purpose [15]. Gastro-BaseNet was used a pre-trained model from the ImageNet database to classify normal or abnormal (including gastric cancer and ulcers) in gastroscopic images to transfer learning. To develop a predictive model for gastric cancer or ulcer, we used two pre-trained models (ImageNet, which is generally used, and Gastro-BaseNet, which is trained by a gastroscopic database) and compared their performance (Figure 2).

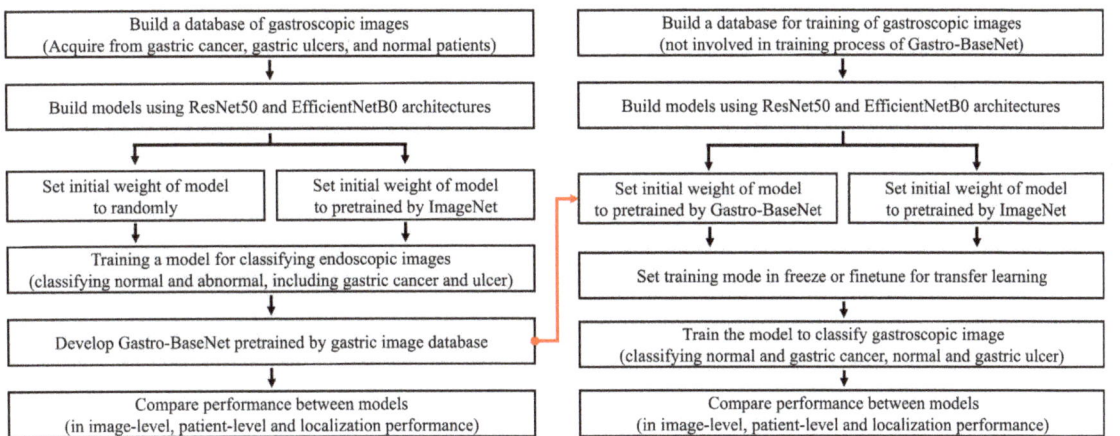

Figure 2. Flowchart of the process for developing Gastro-BaseNet, a pretraining model used for gastroscopic images, and validating the training results with the pretraining model; the red line means the developed pretrained Gastro-BaseNet was used for the initial weight setting.

In this study, ResNet50 [16] and EfficientNetB0 [17] were used as base architectures. These CNN models were built with a base architecture and applied with pre-trained weights open to the public. These were built by removing the existing FC layers and adding layers for global average pooling, batch normalization, and a new FC layer for binary classification. Models were fine-tuned to predict gastric diseases using a newly constructed training and validation dataset.

2.5. Setting Model Training Hyperparameters

Pre-trained models used for diagnosing gastric cancer or gastric ulcers were trained based on ResNet50 and EfficientNetB0 architectures (Figure 3). The layers from model architectures and the weight were loaded, and the top block that functions as a classifier was removed. The training model was built by connecting the feature extraction part, excluding the removed block, and a new classifier block for binary classification of normal and gastric lesions. The new classifier block consisted of global average pooling, a batch normalization layer, and an FC layer for predicting the final classified result. For the training model using transfer learning, two model training methods were used: fine-tune mode, which adjusts the weights of all layers, and freeze mode, which adjusts the weights of the classifier only. The hyperparameters for training were set to stochastic gradient descent (SGD), momentum 0.9, decay 0.0001, learning rate 0.0001, batch size 256, and epoch 1000, with an early stopping setting to terminate training if learning did not improve in 60 epochs. All model training was performed with the same settings. For training models using transfer learning, two model training methods were used: fine-tune mode, which adjusts the weights of all layers, and freeze mode, which adjusts the weights of the classifier only. The hyperparameters for training were set to stochastic gradient descent (SGD), momentum 0.9, decay 0.0001, learning rate 0.0001, batch size 256, and epoch 1000, with an early stopping setting to terminate training if learning did not improve in 60 epochs. All model training was performed with the same settings.

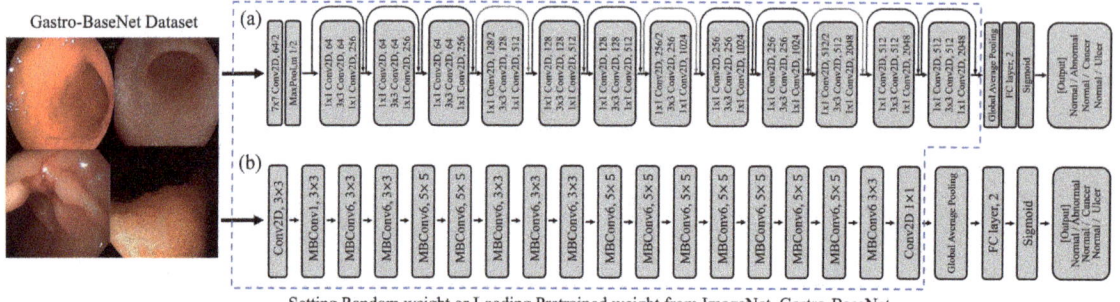

Figure 3. The architectures of the models used for deep learning training are (**a**) ResNet50 and (**b**) EfficientNetB0.

2.6. Statistical Analysis

2.6.1. Image-Level Performance

To evaluate the performance of the trained CNN model based on Gastro-BaseNet, performance metrics were calculated and compared with the results obtained with ImageNet. A new, unseen image (not involved at all in the training stage) was applied to the training model to predict whether the image was a gastric cancer or a gastric ulcer for each purpose. The predicted diagnosis was compared to the label (ground truth, GT) and represented according to a confusion matrix. Based on indications including true positive (TP), true negative (TN), false positive (FP), and false negative (FN) calculated by the confusion matrix, classification performance indicators with accuracy, sensitivity, specificity, and F1 score were calculated. Receiver operating characteristic (ROC) analysis [18] and area under the curve (AUC) were conducted to compare transfer-learned performance based on Gastro-BaseNet and ImageNet.

2.6.2. Patient-Level Performance

The collected image dataset was built by acquiring multiple frozen images from a single patient. However, the performance evaluation at the image level performed earlier calculated performance indications for every result as an independent event, even if they were the same lesions from the same patient.

Thus, we conducted patient-level analysis, and the predicted diagnosis result with the largest number of images diagnosed by the AI model was regarded as the final diagnosis for that patient case. At this time, if the number of counts for each decision diagnosed as normal or abnormal by the AI system was the same in the same patient, the patient's final diagnosis was considered undetermined and excluded from the evaluation metric calculation.

2.6.3. Localization Performance

Grad-CAM is a proposed method for explainable AI that uses a heatmap to represent weights to explain what the model is looking at and making decisions about [19]. Grad-CAM extracted from the model classifying as diagnosis highlighted the areas in red color with a high probability of localizing a lesion. Using this, a thresholding algorithm can be applied to specify the location of the lesion as predicted by the AI model.

In this study, we set a threshold value for localization to 0.5 in grad-CAM and set the area above the threshold value as the location of the lesion predicted by the model. We calculated the sensitivity of the detected location by comparing the interaction over union

(IoU) score with the lesion location manually labeled and determining the case above 0.3 of the IoU as TP. These processes were introduced in Figure 4.

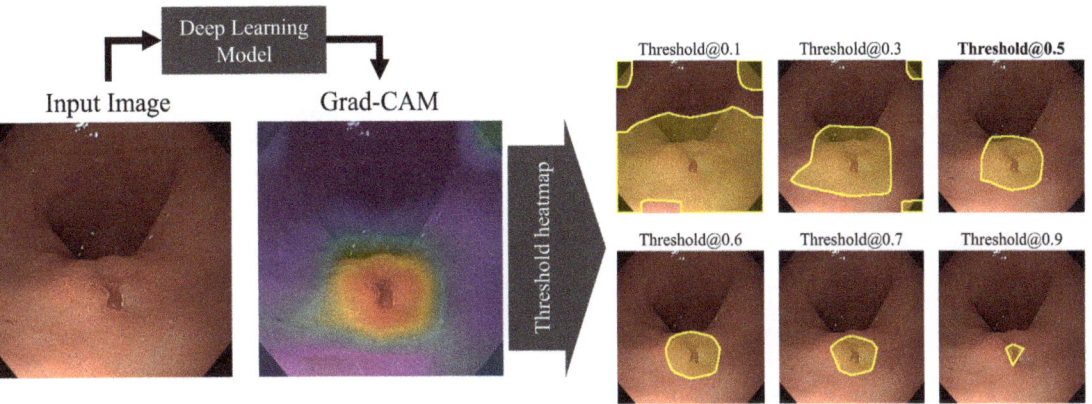

Figure 4. The evaluation process for calculating localization performance based on Grad-CAM; yellow line: the location of the lesion predicted by the model, the bolded threshold: the value used for localization in this study.

3. Results

3.1. Gastro-BaseNet

We developed a pre-trained model, Gastro-BaseNet, based on gastroscopic images. Gastro-BaseNet was trained to classify and predicted normal cases and abnormal cases, including stomach cancer and stomach ulcers. We developed Gastro-BaseNet by comparing the performance of the model trained by setting the initial weight randomly and the pre-trained weight with ImageNet as the initial weight, based on the ResNet50 and EfficientNetB0 model architectures (Table 3). In the two models using ResNet50 and EfficientNetB0, the model trained by tuning the weights of the entire network through fine-tune mode from the pre-trained weight as the ImageNet dataset showed the highest performances with accuracy of 91.88% and 91.93% and sensitivity of 90.38% and 91.26% in image-level performance. Then it showed accuracy of 95.42% and 95.92% in each model architecture in patient-level performance and the highest sensitivity performance of 82.19% in localization performance when trained with the ResNet50 architecture. The ROC analysis and pairwise comparison of ROC curves were conducted on the predicted performance of the model. Figure 5 showed the comparison of ROC curves for two model architectures. In both cases, models trained through fine-tune mode based on ImageNet pre-trained models exhibited the highest performance with AUCs of 96.54% and 96.95%, and the differences were statistically significant compared to training from random initial weights and freeze mode. The p-values for all results of the pairwise comparison of ROC curves was lower than 0.0001.

Table 3. Result of Gastro-BaseNet performance, a classification model for abnormalities indicative of gastric lesions, by pretrained weights and training mode.

Model Architecture	Hyperparameters		Image-Level Performance (%)					Patient-Level Performance (%)			Localization Performance (%)
	Training Mode	Pretrained Weight	Accuracy	Sensitivity	Specificity	F1 Score	AUC	Accuracy	Sensitivity	Specificity	Sensitivity
ResNet50	fine-tune	Random	83.91	87.42	80.76	84.09	89.57	88.38	90.06	79.31	41.23
	freeze	ImageNet	88.50	87.09	89.76	89.15	92.39	92.68	91.61	98.31	58.11
	fine-tune	ImageNet	91.88	90.38	93.22	92.36	96.54	95.42	94.53	100.0	82.19

Table 3. Cont.

Model Architecture	Hyperparameters		Image-Level Performance (%)					Patient-Level Performance (%)			Localization Performance (%)
	Training Mode	Pretrained Weight	Accuracy	Sensitivity	Specificity	F1 Score	AUC	Accuracy	Sensitivity	Specificity	Sensitivity
EfficientNetB0	fine-tune	Random	79.54	84.29	75.27	79.48	86.10	83.11	85.94	68.33	63.43
	freeze	ImageNet	87.79	87.25	88.28	88.39	91.44	92.43	91.94	95.00	61.52
	fine-tune	ImageNet	91.93	91.26	92.53	92.35	96.95	95.92	95.13	100.0	70.74

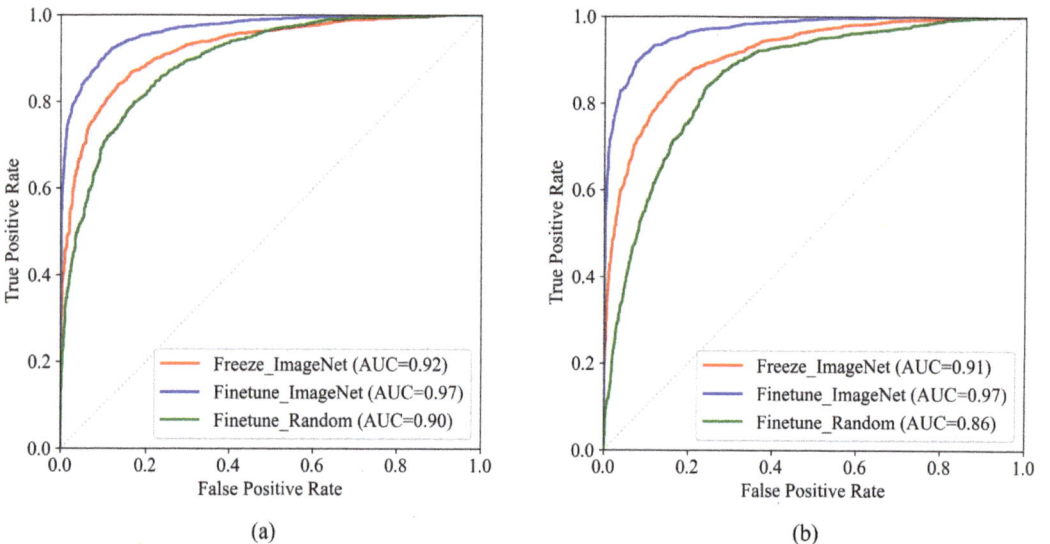

Figure 5. Comparison of ROC curves for normal and abnormal classification models: (**a**) comparison of model performance by training method based on ResNet50 architecture. (**b**) comparison of model performance by training method based on EfficientNetB0 architecture.

3.2. Models Trained on Transfer Learning Based on Gastro-BaseNet

We used a gastroscopic dataset to develop a model to predict normal and abnormal diagnosis, including gastric cancer and gastric ulcers. Using the developed Gastro-BaseNet for classifying abnormal diagnosis as a pre-trained weight, we applied transfer learning techniques to develop training models to predict the diagnosis of gastric cancer and gastric ulcer, respectively. We compared the performance differences of the training models with the traditional ImageNet weights.

3.2.1. Gastric Cancer Classification Trained by Gastro-BaseNet

We developed classification models that predict the presence of gastric cancer disease in input images of endoscopy through transfer learning based on Gastro-BaseNet. Except for the pre-trained model for transfer learning, the rest of the training environment was set the same. In training using the ResNet50 architecture, the performance of the model with transfer learning using Gastro-BaseNet was 94.07% in freeze mode and 94.72% in fine-tune mode, and the accuracy was improved by 3.61% and 4.05% compared to the performance of the model with transfer learning using ImageNet in the same training mode (Table 4). However, in training with the EfficientNetB0 architecture, the performance of the model trained with ImageNet showed higher accuracy than Gastro-BaseNet. Nevertheless, the sensitivity performance of the model using Gastro-BaseNet is 98.97%, which is an improvement of 10.39% and 5.64% in each mode compared to that using ImageNet, and the AUC score of the model using Gastro-BaseNet is improved by 3.06% when trained in freeze mode for image-level performance. The results of the ROC comparison analysis using the

ResNet50 architecture are presented in Figure 6a. Transfer learning using Gastro-BaseNet with the ResNet50 architecture demonstrated the highest performance, with AUC scores of 97.90% and 97.43% in fine-tune and freeze training modes, respectively. According to Table 5, there was a statistically significant difference with training by ImageNet in both freeze and fine-tune modes (p-values were lower than 0.0001). Figure 6b shows the ROC curves using the EfficientNetB0 architecture. The model performance using Gastro-BaseNet in fine-tune mode showed an AUC of 96.42%. The result of the pairwise comparison of ROC curves in Table 5 between Gastro-BaseNet and ImageNet in freeze mode revealed a p-value lower than 0.0001, indicating a statistically significant difference.

Table 4. Results of gastric cancer classification model performance trained by Gastro-BaseNet and ImageNet by pretrained weights and training mode.

Model Architecture	Hyperparameters		Image-Level Performance (%)					Patient-Level Performance (%)			Localization Performance (%)
	Training Mode	Pretrained Weight	Accuracy	Sensitivity	Specificity	F1 Score	AUC	Accuracy	Sensitivity	Specificity	Sensitivity
ResNet50	freeze	ImageNet	90.46	90.26	90.60	91.67	94.81	96.99	96.32	100.0	80.26
	fine-tune	ImageNet	90.67	92.44	89.40	91.74	96.22	95.29	94.29	100.0	82.94
	freeze	Gastro-BaseNet	94.07	93.72	94.33	94.86	97.43	97.66	97.16	100.0	83.99
	fine-tune	Gastro-BaseNet	94.72	94.10	95.16	95.43	97.90	97.66	97.16	100.0	87.19
EfficientNetB0	freeze	ImageNet	88.79	87.82	89.49	90.24	91.73	92.26	91.37	96.55	67.15
	fine-tune	ImageNet	94.02	93.33	94.51	94.82	97.05	97.66	97.16	100.0	68.54
	freeze	Gastro-BaseNet	85.71	98.21	76.65	86.15	97.01	95.32	99.29	7667	75.72
	fine-tune	Gastro-BaseNet	83.45	98.97	72.19	83.49	96.42	95.88	100.0	7667	78.50

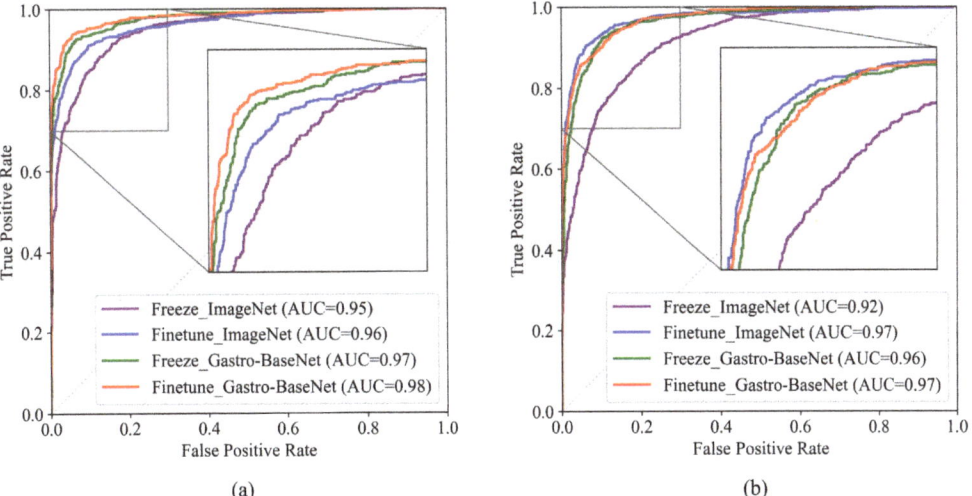

Figure 6. Comparison of ROC curves for normal and gastric cancer classification models using Gastro-BaseNet: (**a**) comparison of model performance by training method based on ResNet50 architecture; (**b**) comparison of model performance by training method based on EfficientNetB0 architecture.

In patient-level performance, the model using ResNet50 architecture-based Gastro-BaseNet showed higher accuracy and sensitivity than ImageNet. In the EfficientNetB0 model, the accuracy of the model using Gastro-BaseNet increased by more than 10%, and the sensitivity was higher than that of using ImageNet. In addition, the localization performance shows that the model using transfer learning with Gastro-BaseNet has superior location detection performance.

Table 5. Results of pairwise comparison of ROC curves of the gastric cancer classification model trained by Gastro-BaseNet and ImageNet by pretrained weights and training mode.

Model Architecture	Variable 1		Variable 2		p-Value
	Training Mode	Pretrained Weight	Training Mode	Pretrained Weight	
ResNet50	ImageNet	freeze	ImageNet	fine-tune	0.0006
	ImageNet	freeze	Gastro-BaseNet	freeze	<0.0001
	ImageNet	freeze	Gastro-BaseNet	fine-tune	<0.0001
	ImageNet	fine-tune	Gastro-BaseNet	freeze	0.0002
	ImageNet	fine-tune	Gastro-BaseNet	fine-tune	<0.0001
	Gastro-BaseNet	fine-tune	Gastro-BaseNet	freeze	<0.0001
EfficientNetB0	ImageNet	freeze	ImageNet	fine-tune	<0.0001
	ImageNet	freeze	Gastro-BaseNet	freeze	<0.0001
	ImageNet	freeze	Gastro-BaseNet	fine-tune	<0.0001
	ImageNet	fine-tune	Gastro-BaseNet	freeze	0.0981
	ImageNet	fine-tune	Gastro-BaseNet	fine-tune	0.8909
	Gastro-BaseNet	fine-tune	Gastro-BaseNet	freeze	0.0270

3.2.2. Gastric Ulcer Classification Trained by Gastro-BaseNet

To develop a deep learning model to diagnose gastric ulcers, we trained the model by transferring weights based on Gastro-BaseNet. In terms of image-level performance (Table 6), the ResNet50 architecture was used to improve the accuracy from 92.03% to 92.72% and the F1 score of 95.14% and 95.62% in two learning modes using Gastro-BaseNet as pre-trained weights compared to ImageNet weights, showing an increase of about 4% and a 2.5% increase in performance. The highest accuracy of 92.31% and sensitivity of 85.71% were achieved in training in freeze mode using Gastro-BaseNet on patient-level performance. In terms of localization performance, training in freeze mode using Gastro-BaseNet showed the highest detection accuracy, with a detection sensitivity of 90.80%. In image-level performance using the EfficientNetB0 architecture, the learning performance of the model using ImageNet weights was higher than that of the model using Gastro-BaseNet, with 88.54% and 88.62% of accuracy and 93.06% and 93.11% of F1 scores. However, in other performances about the diagnosis of gastric ulcer, the AUC scores of the model using Gastro-BaseNet were 90.84% and 90.04%, which showed higher performance than the model using ImageNet, especially in patient-level performance, with higher accuracy of 89.39% and 88.89%. In terms of localization performance, the freeze training mode using Gastro-BaseNet showed 81.82% localization performance. Figure 7 shows the results of predicting the location of lesions extracted by grad-CAM and manually labeling the lesion location as GT. Compared to ImageNet, the model trained on Gastro-BaseNet focused on detecting regions that were very similar to the GT regions. In particular, the model trained on EfficientNetB0 found similar locations for two lesions that were missed by all other training models.

In the ResNet50 architecture, the highest AUC score of 93.82% was achieved using Gastro-BaseNet in fine-tune mode, as shown in Figure 8a. According to the pairwise comparison results of the ROC curves in Table 7, there is a p-value of 0.0005 in the freeze mode and a p-value of 0.0004 in the fine-tune mode. While in the EfficientNetB0 architecture (Figure 8b), both training modes showed a p-value lower than 0.0001 in pairwise comparison results, indicating a significant difference in the training using Gastro-BaseNet.

Table 6. Results of gastric ulcer classification model performance trained by Gastro-BaseNet and ImageNet by pretrained weights and training mode.

Model Architecture	Hyperparameters		Image-Level Performance (%)					Patient-Level Performance (%)			Localization Performance (%)
	Training Mode	Pretrained Weight	Accuracy	Sensitivity	Specificity	F1 Score	AUC	Accuracy	Sensitivity	Specificity	Sensitivity
ResNet50	freeze	ImageNet	88.24	71.19	92.09	92.74	88.95	87.50	76.47	100.0	68.21
	fine-tune	ImageNet	88.54	63.79	94.14	93.06	88.90	87.50	76.47	100.0	64.52
	freeze	Gastro-BaseNet	92.03	76.54	95.53	95.14	92.76	92.31	85.71	100.0	80.11
	fine-tune	Gastro-BaseNet	92.72	71.60	97.49	95.62	93.82	88.89	78.79	100.0	90.80
EfficientNetB0	freeze	ImageNet	88.54	63.79	94.14	93.06	83.65	87.50	76.47	100.0	64.52
	fine-tune	ImageNet	88.62	63.79	94.23	93.11	81.97	85.71	72.73	100.0	72.90
	freeze	Gastro-BaseNet	74.51	95.06	69.86	81.72	90.84	89.39	100.0	76.67	81.82
	fine-tune	Gastro-BaseNet	83.76	76.54	85.40	89.56	90.04	88.89	78.79	100.0	68.28

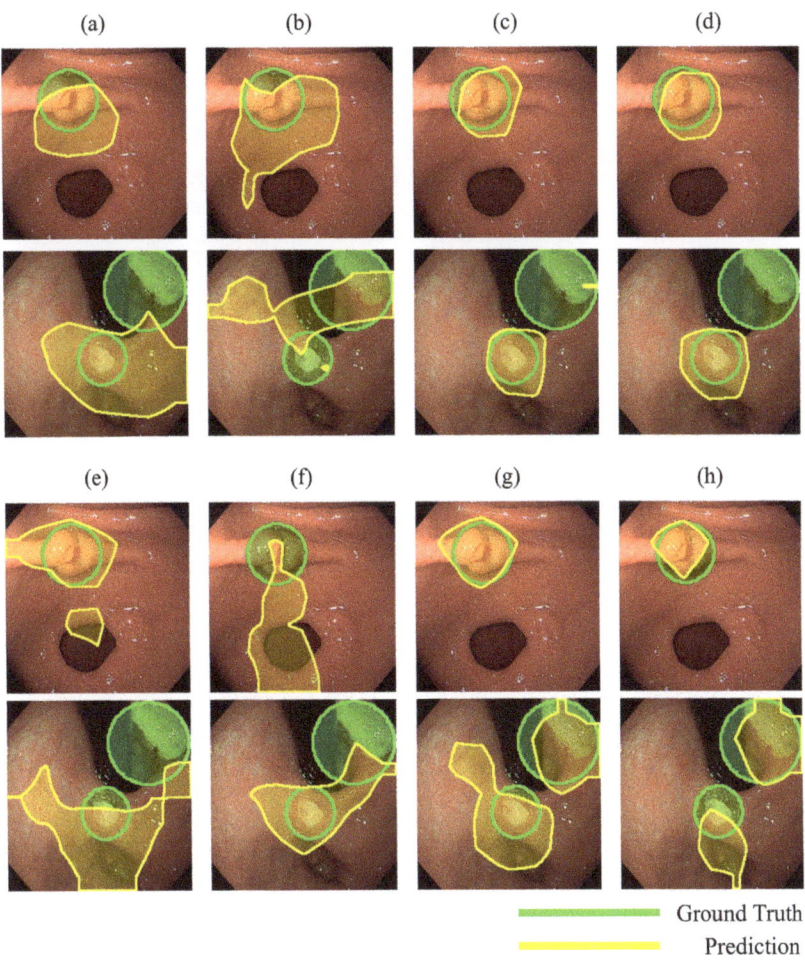

Figure 7. Results of evaluating localization performance based on Grad-CAM; transfer-learned on ResNet50 architecture (**a**) by ImageNet and freeze mode; (**b**) by ImageNet and fine-tune mode; (**c**) by Gastro-BaseNet and freeze mode; (**d**) by Gastro-BaseNet and fine-tune mode and transfer-learned on EfficientNetB0 architecture; (**e**) by ImageNet and freeze mode; (**f**) by ImageNet and fine-tune mode; (**g**) by Gastro-BaseNet and freeze mode; (**h**) by Gastro-BaseNet and fine-tune mode.

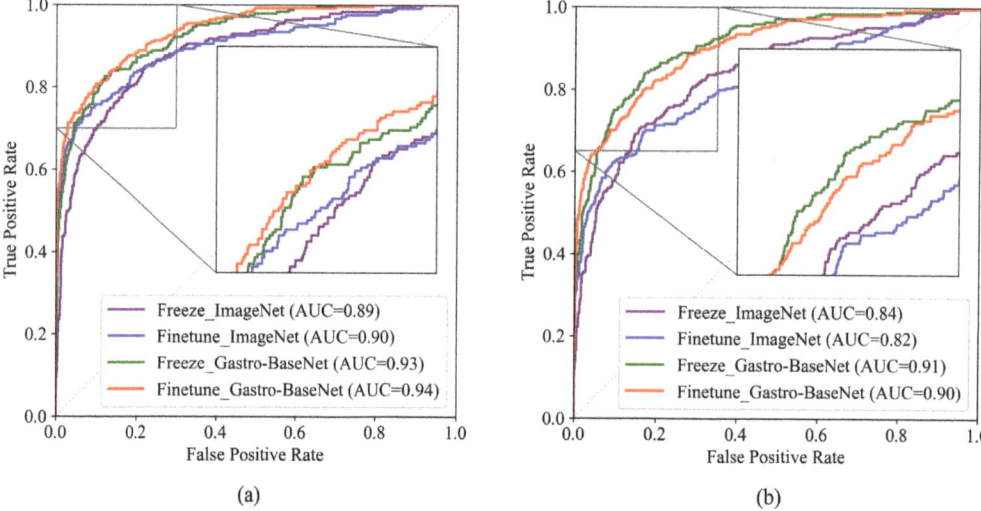

Figure 8. Comparison of ROC curves for normal and gastric ulcer classification models using Gastro-BaseNet: (**a**) comparison of model performance by training method based on ResNet50 architecture; (**b**) comparison of model performance by training method based on EfficientNetB0 architecture.

Table 7. Results of pairwise comparison of ROC curves of the gastric ulcer classification model trained by Gastro-BaseNet and ImageNet by pretrained weights and training mode.

Model Architecture	Variable 1		Variable 2		p-Value
	Training Mode	Pretrained Weight	Training Mode	Pretrained Weight	
ResNet50	ImageNet	freeze	ImageNet	fine-tune	0.4423
	ImageNet	freeze	Gastro-BaseNet	freeze	0.0005
	ImageNet	freeze	Gastro-BaseNet	fine-tune	<0.0001
	ImageNet	fine-tune	Gastro-BaseNet	freeze	0.0165
	ImageNet	fine-tune	Gastro-BaseNet	fine-tune	0.0004
	Gastro-BaseNet	fine-tune	Gastro-BaseNet	freeze	0.0280
EfficientNetB0	ImageNet	freeze	ImageNet	fine-tune	0.3943
	ImageNet	freeze	Gastro-BaseNet	freeze	<0.0001
	ImageNet	freeze	Gastro-BaseNet	fine-tune	<0.0001
	ImageNet	fine-tune	Gastro-BaseNet	freeze	<0.0001
	ImageNet	fine-tune	Gastro-BaseNet	fine-tune	<0.0001
	Gastro-BaseNet	fine-tune	Gastro-BaseNet	freeze	0.4122

4. Discussion

In this study, we developed a pre-trained model using gastroscopic data and used it to train a deep learning model to predict gastric cancer or gastric ulcer; these compared the performance of the model trained with ImageNet, which is widely used [20]. Then, it generated Gastro-BaseNet, a model more optimized for gastroscopic images. These showed higher performance than the model performance that was transfer-learned by ImageNet. To develop a pre-trained model using gastroscopic data, we trained classification on images of abnormal lesions, including gastric cancer and gastric ulcer. To demonstrate the training effectiveness in general transfer learning, some experiments were conducted: first, we trained the initial model weights set at random. Second, the model was trained in freeze mode, using the weights of the pre-trained model like ImageNet to train only a part of the classifier. At last, the model was trained in fine-tune mode, and the entire network was tuned with small changes. To verify the performance of the trained model, we fed the model with a test dataset that was not involved in training and compared the prediction results. Two evaluation metrics were introduced and compared: image-level, which evaluates the total number of images as independent cases, and patient-level, which extracts individual results for images collected from the same patient and evaluates the most frequent prediction as the final result. Additionally, we compared the localization performance based on the location information extracted using grad-CAM, which was generated from models trained with abnormal data containing gastric lesions.

The pre-trained model to classify the abnormal classes of gastroscopic images showed an accuracy of 91.88% and 91.93% in the studies using ResNet50 and Efficient-NetB0, respectively, using transfer learning in fine-tune mode based on ImageNet, with AUC scores of 96.54% and 96.95%, and a sensitivity to localization of 82.19% in ResNet50 and 70.74% in EfficientNetB0 for very high performance in classification and localization. This indicates that it has been learned to identify the features of gastric cancer or gastric ulcer at the correct location. This confirms that models that were trained by ImageNet performed faster and better than learning weights from random models, despite training endoscopic information from completely different domains.

Next, we developed a diagnostic prediction model for gastric cancer or ulcer through transfer learning using Gastro-BaseNet. The model trained on a dataset with the domain of gastroscopy based on Gastro-BaseNet proved the prediction performance of using a pre-trained model that trained on images with a similar domain by comparing the results of transfer learning with ImageNet.

In the training of the gastric cancer classification model, the transfer learning method in fine-tune mode using Gastro-BaseNet based on the ResNet50 architecture showed the highest performance with 94.72% of accuracy, 94.10% of sensitivity, and an AUC score of 97.90%. Additionally, the localization performance was also excellent, with a sensitivity to localization 87.19%. In the training based on the EfficientNetB0 architecture, transfer learning using Gastro-BaseNet showed lower specificity compared to ImageNet (94.51% and 72.19%, respectively, in fine-tune mode). However, the sensitivity for classification of gastric cancer was the highest at 98.97% in fine-tune mode training using Gastro-BaseNet, and the accuracy was 95.88% in patient-level performance evaluation. Furthermore, performance in localization was 78.50%, which was 10.04% higher than ImageNet. In the classification model for gastric ulcers, the performance of the model using Gastro-BaseNet in the ResNet50 architecture was the highest, with an accuracy of 92.72%, an F1 score of 95.62%, and an AUC score of.93.82%. In the localization performance, especially, the sensitivity to localization in fine-tune mode based on Gastro-BaseNet showed a very high indication at 90.80%. Also, similarly to the gastric cancer classification model trained on the EfficientNetB0 architecture, it had lower accuracy and specificity compared to ImageNet. Nevertheless, it showed high performance at a sensitivity of 95.06% in freeze mode, and localization performance also showed a high sensitivity of 81.82%.

Until now, most of the training methods for developing deep learning models based on medical images (especially classification training for diagnostic prediction) have been performed based on transfer learning. The pre-trained model used at this time brought up and used the weight values of the model using ImageNet, and it showed excellent performance [14,21]. However, ImageNet-based pre-trained models did not have prior learning knowledge of medical domains. Studies about pre-trained models based on data from medical domains were not active due to many limitations on data collection, personal information protection, etc. Therefore, our study created a pre-trained model with knowledge gained through collecting various patients and images and learning about gastroscopy data that trained them, named Gastro-BaseNet.

The first limitation of our study is that we set the entire layer to be trained without proper adjustment over the number of trainable layers in the pre-trained model. The trans-fer learning may adjust the number of layers to be trained according to the domain of the training data of the pre-trained model and the domain of the training data of the newly trained model. In addition, some studies have stated that transfer learning using natural data such as ImageNet on medical data only speeds up the convergence of learning and does not affect performance improvement [22–24]. In this study, the performance improvement of the new learning model was demonstrated by a model pre-trained with gastroscopy data compared to the existing ImageNet, but it showed very high sensitivity in training based on the EfficientNetB0 model but also reduced accuracy and specificity performance.

The second limitation of our study is that we trained only on two kinds of model architectures. It may lead to a lack of diversity and limitations for use in various studies that can be conducted later. Also, we developed a pre-trained model using data collected from one medical institution and identified a diagnostic prediction model using it. Gastro-BaseNet used more than 10k images, but the diversity may be somewhat reduced due to the inclusion of many images taken from the same patient. This resulted in higher predictive performance than ImageNet without prior knowledge of the medical domain, but the lack of generalization of the model may lead to poor classification performance for collected gastroscopic images in new environments (other endoscopic devices, imaging systems, etc.).

The third limitation of our study is that we have learned the deep learning model only from the collected data without obtaining and performing more training data through data augmentation [25,26]. Deep learning requires a large amount of data, and in general, the more learning data, the higher the training performance. Although we have collected and trained large amounts of data compared to other previous studies, we can achieve performance improvements by training additional data together through image processing techniques or generative adversarial network techniques [27], etc.

The fourth limitation of our study is the lack of a more detailed analysis of the evaluation of localization. Generally, specialized architectural models for detection, such as YOLO [28] and SSD [29], are employed to predict the location of gastric lesions, offering the advantage of real-time prediction [30]. In this study, the evaluation of the localization level involved calculating the sensitivity performance for detection based on the IoU value. This can serve as a detection algorithm because the Gastro-BaseNet-based transfer-learned model demonstrates a significant difference compared to other trained models. For a quantitative comparison with results based on existing detection models, an analysis of new performance indicators such as mean average precision (mAP) and frames per second (FPS) is required. However, when using the classification model, extracting detection results through Grad-CAM involves additional steps. Consequently, we anticipate that the FPS performance, indicating the rate at which detection results are obtained, will differ significantly compared to typical detection models.

In future studies, we will secure various pre-trained models using gastroscopic image domains through training using more CNN model architectures. The secured pre-trained model will be widely used not only for various gastroscopy-related studies in the future but also for training various endoscopic medical data such as colonoscopy and esophageal endoscopy. In addition, through multicenter research, we want to build an image database captured and stored in various environments and improve the generality of the deep learning model through additional studies using it. In addition, studies are being actively conducted to develop a deep learning model that combines machine learning to predict models through selected features by applying feature fusion and selection algorithms based on extracted image features rather than classifier methods through FC layers [31]. We will explore various ensemble techniques and machine learning algorithms combined to enhance model performance and aim to compare and validate the results obtained through the application of transfer learning.

5. Conclusions

This study represents a significant stride forward in the development of diagnostic prediction fields for gastric diseases by developing pre-trained models specialized in medical image domains, especially gastroscopic images, rather than conventional natural data for deep learning models. Additionally, models pre-trained on data from a similar domain have exhibited substantial improvements in their localization performance on objects, indicating a high potential for use as a detection algorithm. Specifically, it implies that a state-of-the-art classification learning model based on the transformer algorithm, such as Vision Transformer (ViT) [32] or DeiT [33], has the capability to perform detection concurrently. The results verified through our studies will accelerate the development of advanced deep learning techniques that can be utilized in various endoscopic image-based artificial intelligence areas. With the recent advent of foundation models [34], transfer learning has emerged as an approach to improve training efficiency and reduce data requirements. This study attempts to emphasize the need to develop more specialized pre-trained models or foundation models. The final goal is to contribute to the improvement of predictive capabilities for the diagnosis of gastric diseases, enabling direct use in the actual clinical environment and paving the way for the future development of artificial intelligence technology in the field of gastrointestinal endoscopy as an early diagnosis and assistance system.

Author Contributions: Conceptualization and methodology, Y.J.K. (Young Jae Kim), D.K.P., Y.J.K. (Yoon Jae Kim) and K.G.K.; Methodology, G.P.L., Y.J.K. (Young Jae Kim) and K.G.K.; Software and formal analysis, G.P.L.; Data curation, D.K.P., Y.J.K. (Yoon Jae Kim) and S.K.H.; writing—original draft, G.P.L.; writing—review and editing, Y.J.K. (Young Jae Kim) and K.G.K. All authors have read and agreed to the published version of the manuscript.

Funding: This work was supported by the National IT Industry Promotion Agency (NIPA) grant funded by the Korea government (MSIT) (No. S0252-21-1001, Development of AI Precision Medical Solution (Doctor Answer 2.0).

Institutional Review Board Statement: The study was conducted in accordance with the Declaration of Helsinki and approved by the Institutional Review Board of Gachon University Gil Medical Center (IRB No. GBIRB 2021-383).

Informed Consent Statement: Not applicable.

Data Availability Statement: The data are not publicly available due to restrictions, e.g., privacy or ethical.

Conflicts of Interest: The authors declare no conflicts of interest.

References

1. Sung, H.; Ferlay, J.; Siegel, R.L.; Laversanne, M.; Soerjomataram, I.; Jemal, A.; Bray, F. Global Cancer Statistics 2020: GLOBOCAN Estimates of Incidence and Mortality Worldwide for 36 Cancers in 185 Countries. *CA Cancer J. Clin.* **2021**, *71*, 209–249. [CrossRef]
2. Smyth, E.C.; Nilsson, M.; Grabsch, H.I.; van Grieken, N.C.T.; Lordick, F. Gastric cancer. *Lancet* **2020**, *396*, 635–648. [CrossRef]
3. Hernanz, N.; Rodríguez de Santiago, E.; Marcos Prieto, H.M.; Jorge Turrión, M.Á.; Barreiro Alonso, E.; Rodríguez Escaja, C.; Jiménez Jurado, A.; Sierra, M.; Pérez Valle, I.; Volpato, N.; et al. Characteristics and consequences of missed gastric cancer: A multicentric cohort study. *Dig. Liver Dis.* **2019**, *51*, 894–900. [CrossRef] [PubMed]
4. Lee, J.H.; Kim, Y.J.; Kim, Y.W.; Park, S.; Choi, Y.-i.; Kim, Y.J.; Park, D.K.; Kim, K.G.; Chung, J.-W. Spotting malignancies from gastric endoscopic images using deep learning. *Surg. Endosc.* **2019**, *33*, 3790–3797. [CrossRef] [PubMed]
5. Ma, L.; Su, X.; Ma, L.; Gao, X.; Sun, M. Deep learning for classification and localization of early gastric cancer in endoscopic images. *Biomed. Signal Process. Control* **2023**, *79*, 104200. [CrossRef]
6. Wei, W.; Wan, X.; Jun, Z.; Lei, S.; Shan, H.; Qianshan, D.; Ganggang, M.; Anning, Y.; Xu, H.; Jun, L.; et al. A deep neural network improves endoscopic detection of early gastric cancer without blind spots. *Endoscopy* **2019**, *51*, 522–531. [CrossRef]
7. Teramoto, A.; Shibata, T.; Yamada, H.; Hirooka, Y.; Saito, K.; Fujita, H. Detection and characterization of gastric cancer using cascade deep learning model in endoscopic images. *Diagnostics* **2022**, *12*, 1996. [CrossRef] [PubMed]
8. Yuan, X.-L.; Zhou, Y.; Liu, W.; Luo, Q.; Zeng, X.-H.; Yi, Z.; Hu, B. Artificial intelligence for diagnosing gastric lesions under white-light endoscopy. *Surg. Endosc.* **2022**, *36*, 9444–9453. [CrossRef] [PubMed]

9. Cho, B.-J.; Bang, C.S.; Park, S.W.; Yang, Y.J.; Seo, S.I.; Lim, H.; Shin, W.G.; Hong, J.T.; Yoo, Y.T.; Hong, S.H. Automated classification of gastric neoplasms in endoscopic images using a convolutional neural network. *Endoscopy* **2019**, *51*, 1121–1129. [CrossRef] [PubMed]
10. Deng, J.; Dong, W.; Socher, R.; Li, L.-J.; Li, K.; Fei-Fei, L. Imagenet: A large-scale hierarchical image database. In Proceedings of the 2009 IEEE Conference on Computer Vision and Pattern Recognition, Miami, FL, USA, 20–25 June 2009; pp. 248–255.
11. Kora, P.; Ooi, C.P.; Faust, O.; Raghavendra, U.; Gudigar, A.; Chan, W.Y.; Meenakshi, K.; Swaraja, K.; Plawiak, P.; Rajendra Acharya, U. Transfer learning techniques for medical image analysis: A review. *Biocybern. Biomed. Eng.* **2022**, *42*, 79–107. [CrossRef]
12. Rawat, W.; Wang, Z. Deep Convolutional Neural Networks for Image Classification: A Comprehensive Review. *Neural Comput.* **2017**, *29*, 2352–2449. [CrossRef] [PubMed]
13. Pan, S.J.; Yang, Q. A Survey on Transfer Learning. *IEEE Trans. Knowl. Data Eng.* **2010**, *22*, 1345–1359. [CrossRef]
14. Kim, H.E.; Cosa-Linan, A.; Santhanam, N.; Jannesari, M.; Maros, M.E.; Ganslandt, T. Transfer learning for medical image classification: A literature review. *BMC Med. Imaging* **2022**, *22*, 69. [CrossRef] [PubMed]
15. Kaur, R.; Kumar, R.; Gupta, M. Review on Transfer Learning for Convolutional Neural Network. In Proceedings of the 2021 3rd International Conference on Advances in Computing, Communication Control and Networking (ICAC3N), Greater Noida, India, 17–18 December 2021; pp. 922–926.
16. He, K.; Zhang, X.; Ren, S.; Sun, J. Deep residual learning for image recognition. In Proceedings of the IEEE Conference on Computer Vision and Pattern Recognition, Las Vegas, NV, USA, 27–30 June 2016; pp. 770–778.
17. Tan, M.; Le, Q. Efficientnet: Rethinking model scaling for convolutional neural networks. In Proceedings of the International Conference on Machine Learning, Long Beach, CA, USA, 9–15 June 2019; pp. 6105–6114.
18. Fawcett, T. An introduction to ROC analysis. *Pattern Recognit. Lett.* **2006**, *27*, 861–874. [CrossRef]
19. Selvaraju, R.R.; Cogswell, M.; Das, A.; Vedantam, R.; Parikh, D.; Batra, D. Grad-cam: Visual explanations from deep networks via gradient-based localization. In Proceedings of the IEEE International Conference on Computer Vision, Venice, Italy, 22–29 October 2017; pp. 618–626.
20. Hussain, M.; Bird, J.J.; Faria, D.R. *A Study on CNN Transfer Learning for Image Classification*; Springer: Cham, Switzerland, 2019; pp. 191–202.
21. Morid, M.A.; Borjali, A.; Del Fiol, G. A scoping review of transfer learning research on medical image analysis using ImageNet. *Comput. Biol. Med.* **2021**, *128*, 104115. [CrossRef] [PubMed]
22. Raghu, M.; Zhang, C.; Kleinberg, J.; Bengio, S. Transfusion: Understanding transfer learning for medical imaging. *Adv. Neural Inf. Process. Syst.* **2019**, *32*, 1–22.
23. He, K.; Girshick, R.; Dollár, P. Rethinking imagenet pre-training. In Proceedings of the IEEE/CVF International Conference on Computer Vision, Seoul, Republic of Korea, 27 October–2 November 2019; pp. 4918–4927.
24. Reverberi, C.; Rigon, T.; Solari, A.; Hassan, C.; Cherubini, P.; Antonelli, G.; Awadie, H.; Bernhofer, S.; Carballal, S.; Dinis-Ribeiro, M.; et al. Experimental evidence of effective human–AI collaboration in medical decision-making. *Sci. Rep.* **2022**, *12*, 14952. [CrossRef]
25. Park, Y.R.; Kim, Y.J.; Chung, J.-W.; Kim, K.G. Convolution Neural Network Based Auto Classification Model Using Endoscopic Images of Gastric Cancer and Gastric Ulcer. *J. Biomed. Eng. Res.* **2020**, *41*, 101–106.
26. Kim, Y.-j.; Cho, H.C.; Cho, H.-c. Deep learning-based computer-aided diagnosis system for gastroscopy image classification using synthetic data. *Appl. Sci.* **2021**, *11*, 760. [CrossRef]
27. Garcea, F.; Serra, A.; Lamberti, F.; Morra, L. Data augmentation for medical imaging: A systematic literature review. *Comput. Biol. Med.* **2023**, *152*, 106391. [CrossRef]
28. Jin, T.; Jiang, Y.; Mao, B.; Wang, X.; Lu, B.; Qian, J.; Zhou, H.; Ma, T.; Zhang, Y.; Li, S.; et al. Multi-center verification of the influence of data ratio of training sets on test results of an AI system for detecting early gastric cancer based on the YOLO-v4 algorithm. *Front. Oncol.* **2022**, *12*, 953090. [CrossRef]
29. Ikenoyama, Y.; Hirasawa, T.; Ishioka, M.; Namikawa, K.; Yoshimizu, S.; Horiuchi, Y.; Ishiyama, A.; Yoshio, T.; Tsuchida, T.; Takeuchi, Y.; et al. Detecting early gastric cancer: Comparison between the diagnostic ability of convolutional neural networks and endoscopists. *Dig. Endosc.* **2021**, *33*, 141–150. [CrossRef] [PubMed]
30. Hirasawa, T.; Aoyama, K.; Tanimoto, T.; Ishihara, S.; Shichijo, S.; Ozawa, T.; Ohnishi, T.; Fujishiro, M.; Matsuo, K.; Fujisaki, J. Application of artificial intelligence using a convolutional neural network for detecting gastric cancer in endoscopic images. *Gastric Cancer* **2018**, *21*, 653–660. [CrossRef] [PubMed]
31. Yacob, Y.M.; Alquran, H.; Mustafa, W.A.; Alsalatie, M.; Sakim, H.A.M.; Lola, M.S. *H. pylori* Related Atrophic Gastritis Detection Using Enhanced Convolution Neural Network (CNN) Learner. *Diagnostics* **2023**, *13*, 336. [CrossRef] [PubMed]
32. Dosovitskiy, A.; Beyer, L.; Kolesnikov, A.; Weissenborn, D.; Zhai, X.; Unterthiner, T.; Dehghani, M.; Minderer, M.; Heigold, G.; Gelly, S. An image is worth 16 × 16 words: Transformers for image recognition at scale. *arXiv* **2020**, arXiv:2010.11929.
33. Touvron, H.; Cord, M.; Douze, M.; Massa, F.; Sablayrolles, A.; Jégou, H. Training Data-Efficient Image Transformers & Distillation through Attention. In Proceedings of the International Conference on Machine Learning, Virtual, 18–24 July 2021; pp. 10347–10357.
34. Zhuang, F.; Qi, Z.; Duan, K.; Xi, D.; Zhu, Y.; Zhu, H.; Xiong, H.; He, Q. A Comprehensive Survey on Transfer Learning. *Proc. IEEE* **2021**, *109*, 43–76. [CrossRef]

Disclaimer/Publisher's Note: The statements, opinions and data contained in all publications are solely those of the individual author(s) and contributor(s) and not of MDPI and/or the editor(s). MDPI and/or the editor(s) disclaim responsibility for any injury to people or property resulting from any ideas, methods, instructions or products referred to in the content.

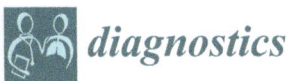 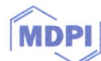

Article

Polypoid Lesion Segmentation Using YOLO-V8 Network in Wireless Video Capsule Endoscopy Images

Ali Sahafi [1,*,†], Anastasios Koulaouzidis [2,3,4,5] and Mehrshad Lalinia [1,†]

1. Department of Mechanical and Electrical Engineering, Digital and High-Frequency Electronics Section, University of Southern Denmark, 5230 Odense, Denmark; melal@sdu.dk
2. Surgical Research Unit, Odense University Hospital, 5000 Svendborg, Denmark; anastasios.koulaouzidis@rsyd.dk
3. Department of Clinical Research, University of Southern Denmark, 5230 Odense, Denmark
4. Department of Medicine, OUH Svendborg Sygehus, 5700 Svendborg, Denmark
5. Department of Social Medicine and Public Health, Pomeranian Medical University, 70204 Szczecin, Poland
* Correspondence: alisa@sdu.dk
† These authors contributed equally to this work.

Abstract: Gastrointestinal (GI) tract disorders are a significant public health issue. They are becoming more common and can cause serious health problems and high healthcare costs. Small bowel tumours (SBTs) and colorectal cancer (CRC) are both becoming more prevalent, especially among younger adults. Early detection and removal of polyps (precursors of malignancy) is essential for prevention. Wireless Capsule Endoscopy (WCE) is a procedure that utilises swallowable camera devices that capture images of the GI tract. Because WCE generates a large number of images, automated polyp segmentation is crucial. This paper reviews computer-aided approaches to polyp detection using WCE imagery and evaluates them using a dataset of labelled anomalies and findings. The study focuses on YOLO-V8, an improved deep learning model, for polyp segmentation and finds that it performs better than existing methods, achieving high precision and recall. The present study underscores the potential of automated detection systems in improving GI polyp identification.

Keywords: polypoid lesion identification; polypoid lesion segmentation; YOLO-V8; WCE images; gastrointestinal disorders; colorectal cancer; artificial intelligence

1. Introduction

Gastrointestinal (GI) tract disorders present a significant public healthcare issue in Europe, resulting in around 1 million deaths annually; aside from considerable mortality, GI pathology imposes a substantial burden on healthcare macroeconomics [1]. With a global ageing trend, it is expected that the impact of these conditions will steadily increase in the future [2]. Typically, GI tract cancers initiate as small, benign growths known as polyps, which have the potential to progress into cancer over time. Small-bowel tumours (SBTs) are relatively rare, representing around 5% of GI tract neoplasms with a variable incidence [3]. Although the prevalence varies [4], the non-specific, subtle clinical presentation of SBTs often makes their diagnosis challenging. Timely identification of SBTs is crucial for improving prognosis, considering that a conclusive diagnosis often involves employing a combination of diagnostic methods, such as wireless capsule endoscopy (WCE). Conversely, Colorectal Cancer (CRC) stands out as a widespread yet preventable form of cancer. The prognosis of cancer patients hinges on a multitude of factors, exhibiting variability contingent upon the stage and site of the malignancy, usually ranging from 48.6% to 59.4% [5]. As stated previously, the majority of CRC cases develop slowly from polyps, specifically adenomatous polyps, as depicted in Figure 1. The prompt removal of these polyps can efficiently prevent the advancement of cancer and decrease cancer-related mortality by as much as 70%. However, there is a considerable range in the adenoma detection rate (varying from 7% to 53%) owing to differences in situational awareness, technical skill, and detection aptitude among endoscopists.

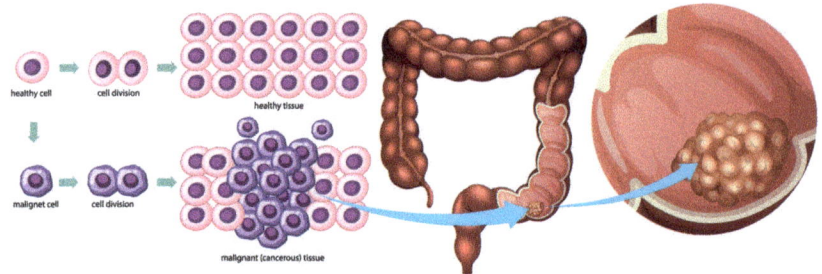

Figure 1. Progression of CRC [6].

WCE is a relatively new development in GI endoscopy. The modality involves utilising a swallowable miniature imaging device to capture digital images of the GI tract [7]. These images are transmitted to a portable recording device, downloaded with the assistance of relevant software, and subsequently scrutinised by gastroenterologists for pathology. A typical WCE session generates tens of thousands of images based on a working battery life of 8–12 h. Therefore, an effective and precise automated identification method would alleviate clinicians from the onerous task of analysing a large volume of images per patient. Computer-aided technologies, notably computer vision, offer a means of automating the analysis of WCE videos, leading to reduced processing time and examination efforts for physicians. The present research has primarily concentrated on addressing two key challenges pertinent to the analysis of GI endoscopic images: the identification and differentiation of malignant tissue. The former pertains to the identification of malignant abnormalities within the intestinal tract, encompassing conditions such as tumours, polyps, ulcers, and other manifestations primarily bleeding.

The present investigation represents an important leap forward in the domain of polypoid segmentation within WCE images. Employing artificial intelligence, particularly leveraging the innovative YOLO-V8 methodology, this study addresses the critical demand for heightened precision and efficiency in detecting polypoid lesions. It introduces a valuable clinical tool with the objective of minimising overlooked diagnoses, facilitating early identification, and contributing significantly to cancer prevention. The evaluation of the YOLO-V8 spans its diverse iterations, denoted as YOLO-V8 n, s, m, l, and x. Our results, revealing exceptional precision, recall, and mean average precision, underscore the effectiveness of this approach compared to other cutting-edge deep learning-based models. Beyond its current influence, this study establishes the foundation for forthcoming investigations into identifying and segmenting polypoid lesions. In the swiftly changing realm of computer vision, creating a benchmark dataset is increasingly recognised as a crucial requirement.

The subsequent sections of this paper are structured as follows: Section 2 explores the related works, providing an overview of relevant studies. Section 3 presents the materials used and the applied methodology. Experimental results and discussions are elaborated upon in Section 4. Finally, Section 5 serves as the conclusion, summarising the key findings and insights of the paper.

2. Related Studies

In the subsequent section, we embark on a comprehensive examination of prevailing methodologies for the analysis of WCE images, specifically focusing on their efficacy in detecting and identifying gastrointestinal issues, particularly polyps, as elucidated within the existing body of literature.

Polypoid lesion detection methods involve identifying frames that contain polypoid lesions (these frames may encompass more than one lesion without distinguishing between single or multiple ones in a given image), and segmentation, which entails segmenting the mucosal area within a frame that contains lesion(s).

In the realm of image classification, deep learning has achieved significant success due to its capacity to autonomously acquire potent feature representations from data. Despite its widespread application in natural images, the deployment of deep learning in the diagnosis of WCE images has been comparatively limited.

In the domain of polyp segmentation, recent strides have been made, exemplified by the Feedback Attention Network (FANet). Extending the advancements in polyp segmentation, Tomar et al. introduce a groundbreaking approach termed FANet [8]. This innovative architecture leverages the insights gained from each training epoch to refine subsequent predictions. FANet unifies the prior epoch's mask with the feature map of the current training epoch, implementing hard attention at various convolutional layers. Notably, the model enables iterative rectification of predictions during test time. Tomar et al. demonstrate the efficacy of FANet through substantial improvements in segmentation metrics across seven publicly available biomedical imaging datasets. The integration of feedback mechanisms in FANet showcases its potential to enhance the precision and robustness of biomedical image segmentation. Polyp segmentation poses significant challenges due to the diversity in size, colour, and texture, compounded by indistinct boundaries between polyps and mucosa. A notable solution in recent literature is the Parallel Reverse Attention Network (PraNet), proposed by Fan et al. [9]. PraNet employs a Parallel Partial Decoder (PPD) to aggregate features, generating a global map for guidance. The Reverse Attention (RA) module mines boundary cues, fostering recurrent cooperation between areas and boundaries, thereby enhancing segmentation accuracy. The efficacy of PraNet, positions it as a promising approach in advancing precise polyp segmentation in colonoscopy images. Additionally, the model integrates a parallel-partial decoder to boost its performance, a concept that has been implemented in various innovative architectures such as AMNet [10]. AMNet builds upon the edge-detection capabilities originally employed in PraNet, further improving the segmentation process.

Another noteworthy attention-based approach is illustrated in GMSRF-Net. In this model, multiple-resolution scales are uniformly fused throughout the architecture, presenting a novel method for attention. Multi-scale approaches have been explored in the context of polyp segmentation, including MSNet [11]. While the initial success of MSNet was noteworthy, recent progress has significantly refined its performance. For polyp segmentation, ensemble methods have gained traction in recent years, leading to the evolution of dual-encoder and/or dual-decoder architectures, as evidenced by Galdran et al. [12]. The study highlights the promising outcomes achieved with a dual encoder-decoder approach. However, it is crucial to note that the implementation followed a sequential structure for the dual model, where the output of one encoder-decoder acted as the input for the subsequent one. Additionally, the reliance on existing pretrained architectures limited the introduction of novel components in the network design [12].

Yang et al. developed a colon polyp detection and segmentation algorithm based on an improved MRCNN, involving training large-scale datasets, extracting the initial model, and retraining it with smaller private datasets from patients [13]. In the pursuit of lightweight network structures with high classification accuracy, Wang et al. combined VGGNets and ResNets models with global average pooling, leading to the development of two new models, VGGNets gap and ResNets gap, featuring reduced parameters without compromising performance [14]. Manouchehri et al. presented a novel convolutional neural network designed for polyp frame detection, based on the VGG network. Moreover, they introduced a comprehensive convolutional network coupled with an efficient post-processing algorithm for polyp segmentation [15].

In the pursuit of refining polyp detection effectiveness, several algorithms rooted in the YOLO series were created. Guo et al. introduced an automated polyp detection algorithm that incorporates the YOLO-V3 structure along with active learning [16]. Similarly, Cao et al. contribute a novel approach to gastric polyp detection by introducing a feature extraction and fusion module integrated with the YOLOv3 network [17]. Their methodology surpasses alternative approaches, particularly excelling in the detection of small polyps. This effectiveness is attributed to the module's capacity to seamlessly combine semantic information from high-level feature maps with low-level feature maps, thereby enhancing the detection capabilities for smaller polyps. This study underscores the significance of feature extraction and fusion in optimising deep neural networks for improved gastric polyp detection. Nogueira-Rodriguez et al. introduced a deep learning model designed for automatic polyp detection based on YOLO-V3, including an object tracking step to mitigate false positives. Model performance was augmented through training with a specialized dataset featuring a substantial number of polyp images [18]. Hoang et al. introduced a capsule endoscope system designed for small bowel and colon applications, featuring 5D position sensing and real-time automatic polyp detection. This system utilizes a YOLO-V3-based algorithm for the detection of real-time polyps, achieving an average precision of 85% [19].

In the contribution to real-time polyp detection, Pacal and Karaboga elevate the YOLOv4 algorithm by integrating Cross Stage Partial Networks (CSPNet), switching from Mish to Leaky ReLu activation, and adopting Complete Intersection over Union (CIoU) loss over Distance Intersection over Union (DIoU) [20]. Beyond algorithmic modifications, diverse architectural structures like ResNet, VGG, DarkNet53, and Transformers enhance YOLOv3 and YOLOv4 performance. Augmenting the method's effectiveness, the study employs various data augmentation techniques, an ensemble learning model, and NVIDIA TensorRT for post-processing. To ensure objective comparisons, only public datasets are utilised, aligning with the MICCAI Sub-Challenge on Automatic Polyp Detection in Colonoscopy. This study presents a comprehensive approach, yielding substantial improvements in real-time polyp detection. In a related context, Lee et al., contribute to colon polyp detection using YOLOv4, emphasising its multiscale learning capability [21]. They enhance this feature by introducing additional scales and optimising the activation function, leading to continuous feature extraction during layer weight updates. The comprehensive approach results in a significant performance boost, achieving a mean Average Precision (mAP) of 98.36. This study highlights effective strategies for refining network structure and employing data augmentation to improve colon polyp detection.

Wan and colleagues proposed a YOLO-V5-based model designed for real-time polyp detection [22]. Their approach integrates a self-attention mechanism, enhancing relevant features while diminishing less pertinent ones, ultimately leading to improved performance. In a comprehensive experimental investigation, Pacal et al. examined innovative datasets, SUN and PICCOLO, employing the Scaled YOLO-V4 algorithm [23]. The results showcased remarkable success in polyp detection for both the SUN and PICCOLO datasets, positioning the Scaled YOLO-V4 algorithm as one of the most suitable object detection methods for large-scale datasets. Souaidi et al. introduced a hybrid method based on SSDNet for polyp detection, focusing on modelling the visual appearance of small polyp areas [24]. Notably, this method incorporated modified initial-A modules instead of simple convolution layers to enhance intermediate feature maps. Experimental validation of the proposed method's polyp detection performance was conducted using public datasets. In the work by Karaman and Pacal [25], they enhance YOLO-based object detection through the utilisation of the ABC algorithm. This optimisation results in a 3% enhancement in real-time polyp detection using YOLO-V5 on the SUN and PICCOLO datasets. The research presents an adaptable and personalised methodology that is applicable to diverse datasets and any YOLO-based algorithm [26].

In reviewing the existing studies on the analysis of WCE images, it becomes evident that while numerous methodologies exhibit progress, certain gaps and limitations persist in the current body of literature. Some models, though initially showing promise, require further refinement and validation across diverse datasets to establish their generalizability.

Moreover, the overall assessment indicates a need for more comprehensive investigations into real-time capabilities, dataset adaptability, and potential limitations in various clinical scenarios. These research gaps present opportunities for future studies to address and enhance the effectiveness of methodologies for detecting and identifying GI issues in WCE images.

Table 1 presents a summary of the aforementioned prevailing methodologies for the analysis of WCE images, specifically focusing on their efficacy in detecting and identifying GI issues.

Table 1. Recent related studies.

Study	Year	Method
Song et al. [10]	2022	AMNet
Tomar et al. [8]	2022	FANet
Zhao et al. [11]	2021	MSNet
Galdran et al. [12]	2021	Double Encoder-Decoder Network
Yang et al. [13]	2020	MRCNN
Wang et al. [14]	2020	VGGNet + ResNet
Haj-Manouchehri et al. [15]	2020	CNN + VGGNet
Guo et al. [16]	2022	YOLO-V3
Cao et al. [17]	2021	YOLO-V3
Nogueira et al. [18]	2022	YOLO-V3
Hoang et al. [19]	2021	YOLO-V3
Pacal et al.[20]	2021	YOLO-V4
Lee et al. [21]	2022	YOLO-V4
Wan et al. [22]	2021	YOLO-V5
Pacal et al. [23]	2022	Scaled YOLO-V4
Souaidi et al. [24]	2022	SSDNet
Karaman et al. [25]	2023	ABC algorithm with YOLO-based
Karaman et al. [26]	2023	YOLO Algorithms

3. Material and Applied Method

3.1. Network Configuration

The models were created using the PyTorch version 2.1.0, with all training and inference processes running on the Google Colab cloud server, equipped with an NVIDIA T4 GPU (16 GB RAM), an Intel Xeon CPU at 2.20 GHz, 12 GB of RAM, and a high-speed SSD.

3.2. Dataset

We have used KID Dataset which is an accessible repository aimed at catalysing the development and assessment of innovative MDSS solutions [27–29]. Designated as KID Dataset 2, this compilation comprises meticulously annotated WCE images, captured throughout the GI tract using a MiroCam capsule endoscope with a resolution of 360 × 360 pixels. The dataset features a comprehensive array of anomalies, categorised into 303 images of vascular anomalies (small bowel angiectasias, lymphangiectasias, and luminal blood), 44 images of polypoid anomalies (lymphoid nodular hyperplasia, lymphoma, and Peutz-Jeghers polyps), 227 images of inflammatory anomalies (ulcers, aphthae, mucosal breaks with surrounding erythema, cobblestone mucosa, luminal stenoses and/or fibrotic strictures, and mucosal/villous edema), and 1778 normal images derived from the oesophagus, stomach, small bowel, and colon. The strength of the dataset lies not only in its breadth but also in the collaborative efforts of the KID working group, consisting of six centres that have contributed anonymised, annotated Capsule Endoscopy (CE) images and videos from various CE models. This collaborative endeavour has resulted in a comprehensive repository exceeding 2500 annotated CE images and 47 videos, covering diverse categories such as normal CE, vascular lesions, inflammatory lesions, lymphangiectasias, and polypoid lesions [28]. To ensure standardised representation, lesion categorisation adheres to the CE Structured Terminology (CEST), providing a robust foundation for the utility of the dataset [30]. The dataset maintains a commitment to high-quality original resolution, avoiding distortions introduced by additional compression. Image formats align with ISO/IEC 15948 [31] PNG standards, a platform-independent, lossless compression format, with alternative acceptable standards including ISO/IEC 14496-12 [32], MPEG-4, AVC (Advanced Video Coding), and H.264 for videos, encompassing F4V and FLV (Flash video) formats. To facilitate the training and evaluation of models, we performed a split of the dataset into training (70%), validation (15%), and test (15%) sets. This split ensures that our models are trained on a diverse range of data, validated for generalisation, and tested on unseen samples. The split was conducted randomly while maintaining the distribution of anomaly and normal images across the sets. Facilitating the annotation process is the integration of software tools for video manipulation and image annotation on the KID website. Annotations are supported by an open-access, platform-independent tool called Ratsnake, enabling both semantic and graphic annotations [33]. Semantic annotation utilises textual labels and adheres to standard web ontology language description logics (OWL DL) [34].

3.3. Framework and Methodology

Our main focus in enhancing our segmentation strategy revolves around amplifying segmentation capabilities, specifically targeting polypoid lesions in WCE images. To attain this objective, we harness the power of YOLO-V8 [35], an advanced iteration of the original YOLO [36].

3.3.1. YOLO-V8 Architecture

YOLO-V8 has attained cutting-edge performance by refining the model structure, incorporating both anchor box and anchor-free schemes, and integrating a diverse array of data augmentation techniques. Our deep learning framework is structured around five distinct-sized versions of YOLO-V8, labelled as n, s, m, l, and x, each characterised by varying channel depth and filter numbers as outlined in Table 2 [35]. In the backbone architecture, all five models are employed, capitalising on their balanced blend of segmentation accuracy and processing speed. Integrating YOLO-V8 into our computer vision project brings forth several advantages, with heightened accuracy emerging as a primary asset compared to its predecessors within the YOLO model lineage. YOLO-V8 extends its support to a spectrum of tasks, encompassing object segmentation, instance segmentation, and image classification, thereby enhancing its versatility for diverse applications. Positioned as the latest evolution in YOLO's object segmentation paradigm, YOLO-V8 places a central emphasis on augmenting both accuracy and efficiency relative to its forerunners. This version brings comprehensive improvements, such as an advanced network design, a new take on anchor boxes, and an updated loss function, all contributing to significantly better segmentation accuracy.

The superiority of YOLO-V8 shines through its exceptional accuracy, making it a competitive choice among cutting-edge object segmentation frameworks. Engineered with efficiency at its core, YOLO-V8 is tailored for seamless execution on standard hardware, making it a practical and feasible choice for various object segmentation tasks, including those involving edge computing scenarios. The incorporation of anchor boxes in YOLO-V8 serves to align predicted bounding boxes with ground-truth bounding boxes, thereby further enhancing the overall accuracy of the object segmentation process.

Table 2. Model specifications.

Model	d (depth_multiple)	w (width_multiple)	r (Ratio)
YOLO-V8 n	0.33	0.25	2.0
YOLO-V8 s	0.33	0.50	2.0
YOLO-V8 m	0.67	0.75	1.5
YOLO-V8 l	1.00	1.00	1.0
YOLO-V8 x	1.00	1.25	1.0

The training process of YOLO-V8 is set to achieve significantly faster speed when compared to two-stage object segmentation models, presenting it as an efficient option for projects with stringent time constraints. Diverging from the structure seen in ultralytics/YOLO-V5 [37], substantial modifications were applied to the system's backbone. This involved the replacement of C3 with C2f and the integration of the ELAN principle from YOLO-V7 [38]. Notably, the initial 6 × 6 convolution in the stem was replaced with a 3 × 3 convolution, augmenting the model's capability to capture more comprehensive gradient flow information.

The C3 module consists of three ConvModules and n DarknetBottleNecks, while the C2f module is made up of two ConvModules and n DarknetBottleNecks, which are interconnected via Split and Concat operations. The ConvModule follows a Conv-BN-SiLU activation sequence, with 'n' representing the number of bottleneck units. In the C2f module, the outputs from the Bottleneck, which includes two 3 × 3 convolutional layers with residual connections, are merged [1].

Deviating from the YOLO-V5 architecture, which incorporates a linked head, this methodology introduces a separated head, distinctly isolating the classification and segmentation elements. Significantly, the model eliminates the objectness branch, maintaining only the classification and regression branches. Anchor-Base utilises numerous anchors within the image to calculate the four offsets representing the regression object's location in relation to the anchors. This mechanism enhances the accurate determination of the object's location by employing corresponding anchors and offsets. The architectural representation of the model can be observed in Figure 2.

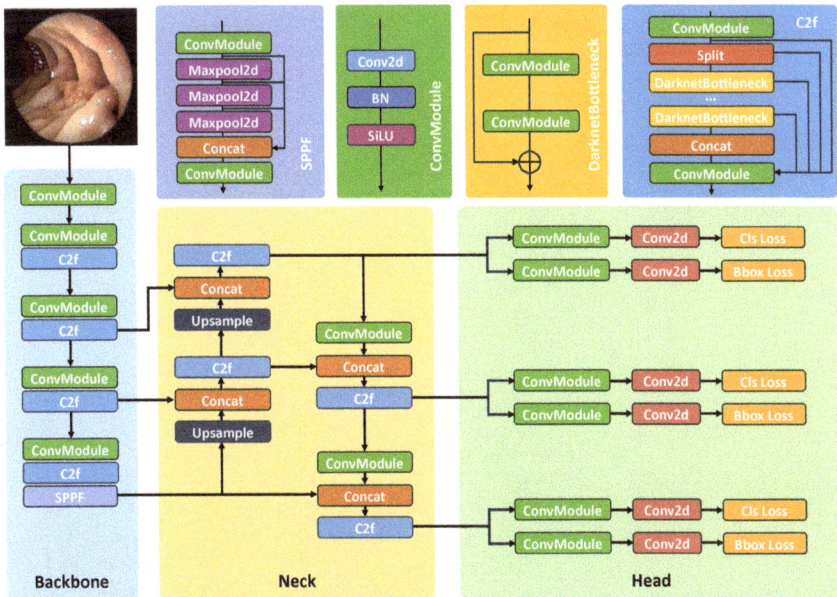

Figure 2. Architecture of YOLO-V8 with backbone and head components.

3.3.2. Training the Model

In the training phase of the model, the Task Aligned Assigner from Task-aligned One-stage Object Detection (TOOD) [39] has been employed to assign positive and negative samples. This method selects positive samples through an assessment that combines the weighted scores from both classification and regression, as detailed in Equation (1).

$$t = s^{\alpha} \cdot u^{\beta} \tag{1}$$

In this context, s represents the predicted score associated with the identified class, and u represents the Intersection over Union (IoU) between the predicted and the actual bounding box. Moreover, the model incorporates branches for classification and regression. The classification branch employs the Binary Cross-Entropy (BCE) Loss, as depicted by the subsequent equation:

$$\text{Loss}_n = -w[y_n \log(x_n) + (1 - y_n) \log(1 - x_n)] \tag{2}$$

where w represents the weight, y_n represents the labelled value, and x_n is the predicted value generated by the model.

Regarding the regression branch, Distribute Focal Loss (DFL) [40] and Complete Intersection over Union (CIoU) Loss [41] have been utilised. DFL is employed to widen the probability distribution around the object y, and its equation is expressed as follows:

$$\text{DFL}(S_n, S_{n+1}) = -((y_{n+1} - y) \log(S_n) + (y - y_n) \log(S_{n+1})) \tag{3}$$

Here, the equations for S_n and S_{n+1} are presented below:

$$S_n = \left(\frac{y_{n+1} - y}{y_{n+1} - y_n}\right), \quad S_{n+1} = \left(\frac{y - y_n}{y_{n+1} - y_n}\right) \tag{4}$$

The $CIoU_{Loss}$ introduces an influential factor into the $Distance\ IoU(DIoU)$ Loss [42], considering the aspect ratio of both the prediction and the ground truth bounding box. The equation is as follows:

$$CIoU_{Loss} = 1 - IoU + \frac{Distance_2^2}{Distance_C^2} + \frac{v^2}{(1 - IoU + v)} \tag{5}$$

where, v stands for the parameter that measures the consistency of the aspect ratio [42].

Figure 3 illustrates the training results diagrams for the applied method, encompassing five iterations of distinct versions of YOLO-V8. These plots, designated as 'n', 's', 'm', 'x', and 'l', represent distinct versions or settings of the YOLO model. Starting with YOLO-V8(n), both training and validation losses exhibit a consistent decrease over time, indicative of effective learning and good generalisation, as the validation loss closely mirrors the training loss. YOLO-V8(s) follows a similar trend, with initial volatility settling into convergence. YOLO-V8(m) exhibits initial extreme volatility, with a sudden spike in loss followed by stabilisation, potentially signalling an issue with early epochs. YOLO-V8(l) and YOLO-V8(x) share a pattern of initial spikes, yet stabilise, with their training and validation losses converging. The bottom right bar plot provides a summarised view of average or final loss values for each model version, revealing 'n' and 'l' as top performers and 'x' with the highest loss. Analysing initial spikes, convergence patterns, and potential overfitting, it is apparent that despite the initial challenges, all models eventually converge without signs of overfitting. Choosing the optimal model involves considering both final loss values and loss curves, prioritising stability and lower validation loss for robust generalisation to unseen data.

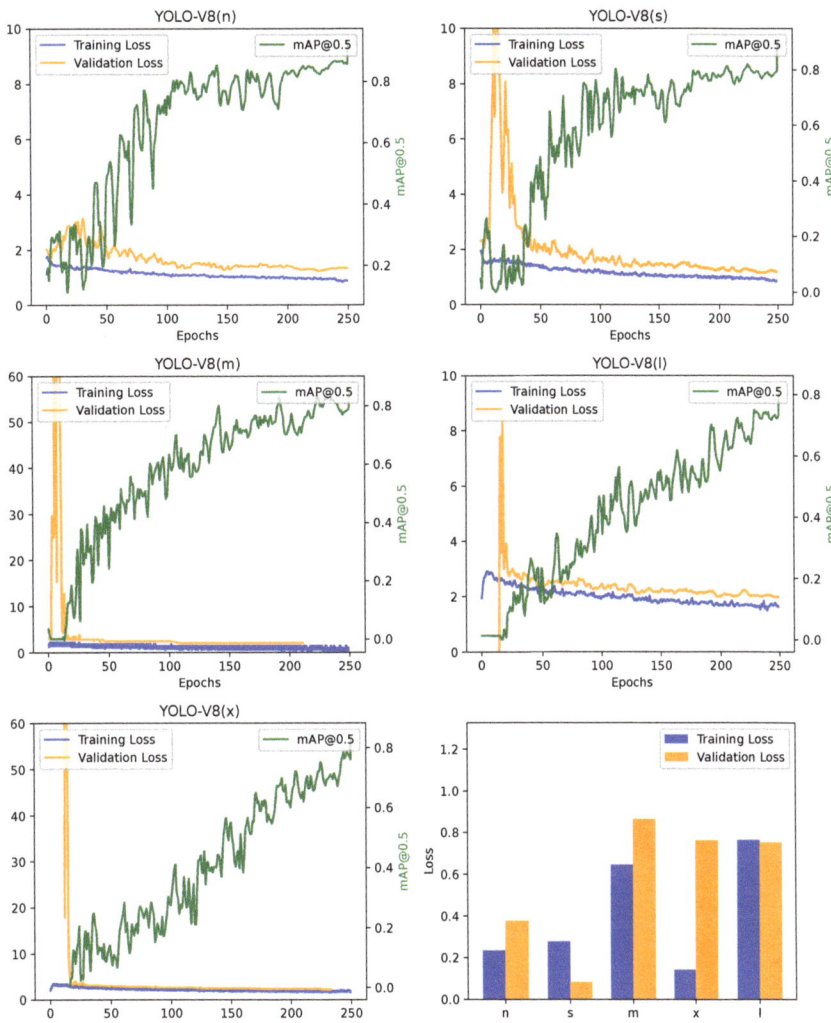

Figure 3. Training and Validation results diagrams of applied methods in 5 versions of YOLO-V8.

4. Results and Discussion

4.1. Evaluation Metrics

This paper evaluates the performance of the algorithm in segmenting polypoid lesions using three key metrics: Precision, Recall, and Dice score. The equations for these metrics are provided below:

$$Precision = \frac{TP}{TP + FP} \quad (6)$$

$$Recall = \frac{TP}{TP + FN} \quad (7)$$

$$Dice\ score = \frac{2 \times TP}{2 \times TP + FP + FN} \quad (8)$$

Within these indicators, TP (true positives) refers to the number of points correctly identified as part of polypoid lesions, indicating precise detection and labelling. FN (false negatives) denotes the number of points where polypoid lesions were present but not accurately detected, highlighting missed lesion areas. TN (true negatives) encompasses points correctly identified as not being part of polypoid lesions, contributing to the model's specificity assessment. Finally, FP (false positives) represents points incorrectly classified as part of polypoid lesions, indicating areas mistakenly identified as lesions. Together, these metrics offer a comprehensive assessment of the model's performance in distinguishing between polypoid and non-polypoid lesions, crucial for evaluating its overall effectiveness and reliability.

Precision evaluates the proportion of accurately labelled polypoid lesions among all the predicted occurrences of such lesions. It functions as a metric that gauges the precision of predictions. In polypoid lesion segmentation, precision signifies the level of confidence in correctly identifying a positive segmentation. A heightened precision value proves beneficial by minimising the occurrence of false alarms, subsequently alleviating financial and psychological stress for patients. Precision(B) (Bounding Box Precision) specifically assesses precision at an IoU (Intersection over Union) threshold of 0.5 for bounding boxes. It measures how accurately the model identifies polypoid lesions within bounding boxes, considering cases where there is at least 50% overlap with the ground truth bounding boxes.Precision(M) (Multiple IoU Precision) evaluates precision performance across a range of IoU thresholds, typically 0.5, 0.75, etc. This provides a thorough evaluation of the model's accuracy in identifying objects that have different levels of spatial intersection with the actual data, providing an understanding of its consistency in various situations.

Conversely, Recall signifies the portion of detected objects. In the context of polypoid lesion segmentation, this metric holds substantial importance, as a higher recall guarantees that a greater number of patients undergo timely follow-up examinations and receive suitable treatment. As a result, this could lead to diminished mortality rates and prevent unwarranted costs for patients. Recall quantifies the ratio of identified polypoid lesions from all images containing such lesions. Recall (B) typically stands for Recall at IoU (Intersection over Union) threshold of 0.5 for bounding boxes. It measures how well the model is able to recall (detect) objects with bounding boxes that have at least 50% overlap with the ground truth bounding boxes. Recall (M) often stands for Recall at multiple IoU thresholds, usually 0.5, 0.75, etc. It means evaluating recall performance across a range of IoU thresholds, providing a more comprehensive assessment of the model's ability to detect objects.

mAP50 (B) stands for mean Average Precision at 50% IoU threshold for bounding boxes. Average Precision (AP) is a metric that considers both precision and recall at different confidence thresholds. mAP50 (B) specifically looks at the average precision when considering bounding boxes with at least 50% overlap with the ground truth. mAP (M) stands for mean Average Precision at multiple IoU thresholds. It is a broader evaluation that looks at the average precision across a range of IoU thresholds, providing a more complete picture of the model's performance. Notably, mAP50-95 (B) stands out as a significant metric, capturing the model's performance across a broader range of detection thresholds, akin to the mAP50 measure.

Dice score measures the overlap between predicted and ground truth masks, offering a concise and intuitive measure of segmentation accuracy in the context of polypoid lesions. It ranges from 0 to 1, with 1 indicating a perfect match, making it valuable for assessing the precision of delineating regions of interest in medical image analysis.

4.2. Performance of the Applied Method

Table 3 elaborated on the hyperparameter setting by providing the key metrics of each model's performance on the validation dataset. The results presented in Table 3 underscore the outstanding performance achieved by various versions of YOLO-V8 in tasks associated with polypoid lesion segmentation.

Table 3. Training and deploying the five iterations of YOLO-V8: Evaluating performance and outcomes.

YOLO Type	Precision (B)	Recall (B)	mAP50 (B)	mAP50-95 (B)	Precision (M)	Recall (M)	mAP50 (M)	mAP50-95 (M)	Dice score	Parameters (M)	Image Segmentation Time on CPU (s)	Image Segmentation Time on T4 GPU (s)
YOLO-V8 n	98.8	81.8	93.1	73.6	98.8	81.8	93.1	70.7	89.57	3	0.3322	0.0284
YOLO-V8 s	96.3	91.8	90.3	91.8	96.3	91.8	91.05	88.8	93.99	11	1.0768	0.0388
YOLO-V8 m	98	97.9	86.04	86.3	98	97.9	86.03	83.5	97.94	27	2.0339	0.055
YOLO-V8 l	92.4	93.6	82.7	86.07	80.3	80.6	80.9	83.7	92.99	45	3.8540	0.0652
YOLO-V8 x	85.2	80.6	84.4	86.6	85.2	80.6	83.9	85.6	82.78	71	5.8717	0.1045

As a concluding step, we assessed the efficacy of our approach on the KID dataset, contrasting its outcomes with those obtained from other state-of-the-art methodologies. We utilised the generated dataset to evaluate different state-of-the-art models. Table 4 shows the evaluation results of different algorithms. This table presents a comprehensive comparison of various detection methods, evaluating their performance in terms of precision, recall, and dice score. Notably, the Resnet family exhibits high performance. This suggests their efficiency in achieving a balance between model complexity and performance. NanoNet-A, NanoNet-B, and NanoNet-C demonstrate competitive results, particularly NanoNet-B, which achieves impressive recall with a significantly lower number of parameters, making it a compelling choice for resource-efficient applications.

Visual outcomes of the applied method, along with the detected polypoid lesions and their corresponding outlines, are illustrated in Figure 4.

Table 4. Comparative analysis of different algorithms: performance results.

Study	Dataset	Architecture	Precision	Recall	Dice Score
Delagah et al. [43]	Kvasir-Capsule	SVM	99.5%	97.5%	98.47
Amiri et al. [44]	Kvasir-Capsule	Fast ROI	94.3%	90.9%	92.56
Sornapudi et al. [45]	Mayo Clinic	Resnet-101(Pre-TrainedWeights:COCO)	94.03%	94.03%	94.03
Sornapudi et al. [45]	Mayo Clinic	Resnet-101(Pre-TrainedWeights:ImageNet)	82.05%	95.52%	87.40
Sornapudi et al. [45]	Mayo Clinic	Resnet-101(Pre-TrainedWeights:Balloon)	98.46%	95.52%	96.96
Sornapudi et al. [45]	Mayo Clinic	Resnet-50(Pre-TrainedWeights:COCO)	94.12%	95.52%	94.82
Sornapudi et al. [45]	Mayo Clinic	Resnet-50(Pre-TrainedWeights:COCO)	92.06%	86.57%	89.21
Sornapudi et al. [45]	Mayo Clinic	Resnet-50(Pre-TrainedWeights:Balloon)	90%	94.03%	91.96
Goel et al. [46]	AIIMS	DICR-CNN	90%	92%	91.43
Goel et al. [46]	KID	DICR-CNN	91%	95%	92.93
Souaidi et al. [24]	KID	Hyb-SSDNet	93.29%	89.4%	91.29
Jha et al. [47]	Kvasir-Capsule	NanoNet-A	93.2%	96.9%	94.04
Jha et al. [47]	Kvasir-Capsule	NanoNet-B	93%	98.8%	95.87
Jha et al. [47]	Kvasir-Capsule	NanoNet-C	92.3%	97.5%	94.85
Our Study	KID	YOLO-V8 m	98%	97.9%	97.94

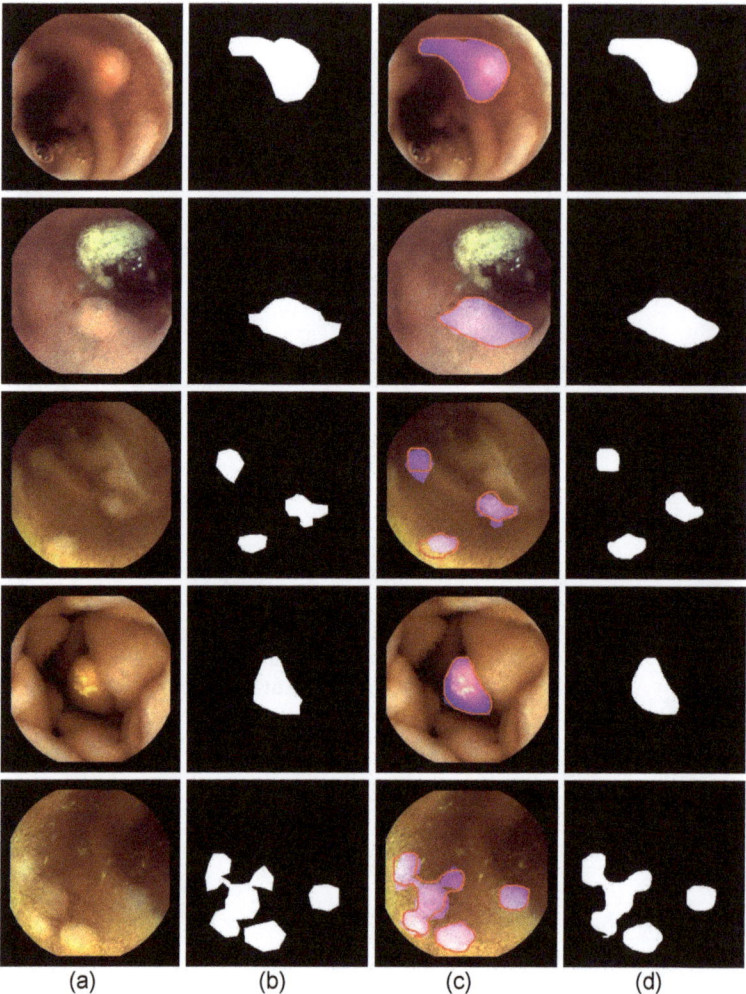

Figure 4. Segmentation results from YOLO-V8 m showcase subsets for single and multi-polypoid lesion instances in our dataset's test images: (**a**) Original Images; (**b**) Ground Truth Binary Mask; (**c**) Segmented polypoid lesion(s) outlined in red contour with the ground truth depicted in purple; and (**d**) Segmented polypoid lesion(s) Binary Mask.

4.3. Discussion

Incorporating YOLO-V8 into computer vision projects provides heightened accuracy compared to preceding YOLO models, rendering it a versatile solution for tasks such as object segmentation, instance segmentation, and image classification. This latest iteration emphasises the enhancement of accuracy and efficiency through optimised network architecture, a revamped anchor box implementation, and a modified loss function. YOLO-V8 showcases superior accuracy, establishing itself as a robust contender among state-of-the-art object detection models. Engineered for efficiency, it operates seamlessly on standard hardware, rendering it a practical choice for real-time object segmentation tasks.

This study underscores the critical importance of early detection and prevention in the context of GI tract disorders, particularly SBTs and CRC, and introduces and evaluates the YOLO-V8 deep learning model for automated polypoid lesion segmentation, addressing the pressing need for efficient and accurate computer-aided diagnosis.

The YOLO-V8 method exhibits diverse performance across its iterations (n, s, m, l, x), with YOLO-V8 m notably standing out due to its exceptional precision (98%) and recall (97.9%), making it a promising choice for accurate polypoid lesion segmentation, as indicated in Table 3. Comparatively, our study using YOLO-V8 m surpasses the performance of various state-of-the-art segmentation algorithms, as illustrated in Table 4. YOLO-V8 m outperforms other architectures in terms of precision, recall, and dice score, showcasing its effectiveness in lesion detection. When considering application-specific requirements, Resnets are recognised for their efficiency with fewer parameters, while NanoNet-B excels in resource efficiency without compromising performance. Despite YOLO-V8 m's impressive metrics, it comes with a larger model size (27 M parameters). This emphasises the need to carefully balance model complexity and performance when selecting a segmentation method tailored to a particular use case, highlighting the comprehensive insights.

The YOLO-V8 architecture has been intricately designed to facilitate optimal information flow, adeptly capturing intricate features relevant to the segmentation of polypoid lesions while minimising unnecessary computational burden. This carefully crafted design ensures smooth processing without compromising accuracy, placing a strong emphasis on attending to various scales and resolutions present in the input image. YOLO-V8 effectively addresses the multiscale nature inherent in polypoid lesions, allowing for detailed discernment at different levels and significantly contributing to heightened precision and recall compared to larger, less adaptable models. Moreover, the study's reliance on the KID Dataset, validated by the KID working group, not only enhances the credibility of the findings but also underscores the versatility of YOLO-V8 in adapting to a wide array of datasets.

By incorporating advanced training strategies and data augmentation techniques, YOLO-V8 is adeptly designed to learn from diverse datasets, a critical feature for polypoid lesion detection where size, shape, and appearance vary widely. Its adaptability significantly boosts the model's generalisation capabilities and robustness, leading to enhanced performance on previously unseen data. YOLO-V8 marks a significant evolution from its predecessor, YOLO-V5, through crucial updates and modifications that sharpen its accuracy. These advancements enable YOLO-V8 to outperform older, more resource-heavy models, showcasing its superiority in the field.

4.4. Limitations and Future Scopes

The approach presented signifies a substantial leap beyond its predecessors in the realm of YOLO algorithms, showcasing notable enhancements in hyperparameter optimisation while addressing both temporal and financial constraints. However, the study's broader impact was limited by the lack of a comprehensive public dataset. Despite achieving positive outcomes, specific datasets from existing literature were omitted because of the limited availability of polyp images and a constrained patient pool, underscoring the essential dependence on robust datasets for deep learning approaches and the imperative need for diverse and expansive datasets to showcase optimal performance. Nevertheless, the methodology has made substantial progress in improving the speed and efficiency of real-time detection, outperforming existing methods and previous iterations of YOLO. Efforts are ongoing to leverage these advancements in clinical applications by integrating available datasets. Nonetheless, an acknowledgement exists regarding the importance of datasets encompassing a more extensive range of WCE images, reflecting varied patient demographics and geographical origins [48]. In our forthcoming research, we aim to broaden our investigative scope to facilitate more comprehensive statistical evaluations. Our strategy includes the implementation of sophisticated statistical tests to delve into the relationships between model characteristics and performance metrics, with a specific emphasis on comparing models such as YOLO-V8 using advanced methodologies. This approach seeks to furnish a more profound and accurate assessment of their effectiveness.

5. Conclusions

In this study, we addressed the pressing issue of identification of polypoid lesions in WCE images, a critical aspect of preventing cancer. We introduced a detection system utilising YOLO-V8 models to aid gastroenterologists in identifying and categorising polypoid lesions accurately and efficiently. We highlighted the significance of timely polypoid lesion segmentation and removal in reducing cancer-related mortality. To this end, we harnessed the potential of WCE technology, which offers an innovative approach to diagnosing GI conditions without resorting to invasive procedures.

The KID dataset, a comprehensive repository of video capsule endoscopy images, served as the foundation for our research. We curated this dataset to focus on the polypoid lesion class, generating corresponding ground truth masks for precise segmentation tasks.

The YOLO-V8 model emerged as our chosen deep learning architecture due to its state-of-the-art accuracy, versatility, and efficiency. Our meticulous data augmentation techniques ensured the diversity and robustness of the training dataset, further enhancing the model's performance. Upon evaluating the applied approach, we achieved impressive results, demonstrating the capability of our model in polypoid lesion segmentation. The metrics of precision, recall, and mean average precision were utilised for the assessment of the different types of applied models. Among the variants and other models, YOLO-V8 m stands out with a precision of 98%, recall of 97.9% and also strikes a balance between accuracy and computational efficiency, making it a promising choice.

This research has the potential to serve as a foundational reference for future studies on polypoid lesion segmentation and classification. Given the rapid advancements in the field of computer vision in recent years, the creation of a benchmark dataset becomes crucial. Our aspiration is that the dataset generated in this study will significantly accelerate the progress of computer-aided cancer diagnosis.

Author Contributions: A.S.: Conceptualisation, Methodology, Visualisation, Formal Analysis, Project Administration, Supervision, Writing—Review & Editing. A.K.: Critical review, Writing—Review & Editing. M.L.: Conceptualisation, Methodology, Investigation, Formal Analysis, Visualisation, Writing Original Draft—Review & Editing. All authors have read and agreed to the published version of the manuscript.

Funding: This research received no external funding.

Institutional Review Board Statement: Not applicable, as this study was conducted using images sourced from KID databases, as referenced in [29].

Informed Consent Statement: Not applicable, as this study was conducted using images sourced from KID databases, as referenced in [29].

Data Availability Statement: The KID dataset (https://mdss.uth.gr/datasets/endoscopy/kid/) accessed on 12 November 2023, used in this study is not publicly available. However, interested researchers can request access to the dataset by directly contacting the dataset providers.

Conflicts of Interest: The authors declare no conflicts of interest.

References

1. Lalinia, M.; Sahafi, A. Colorectal polyp detection in colonoscopy images using YOLO-V8 network. In *Signal, Image and Video Processing*; Springer: London, UK, 2023; pp. 1–12.
2. Sahafi, A.; Wang, Y.; Rasmussen, C.; Bollen, P.; Baatrup, G.; Blanes-Vidal, V.; Herp, J.; Nadimi, E. Edge artificial intelligence wireless video capsule endoscopy. *Sci. Rep.* **2022**, *12*, 13723. [CrossRef]
3. Pan, S.Y.; Morrison, H. Epidemiology of cancer of the small intestine. *World J. Gastrointest. Oncol.* **2011**, *3*, 33–42. [CrossRef]
4. Vlachou, E.; Koffas, A.; Toumpanakis, C.; Keuchel, M. Updates in the diagnosis and management of small-bowel tumors. *Best Pract. Res. Clin. Gastroenterol.* **2023**, *64–65*, 101860. [CrossRef]
5. Lewis, J.; Cha, Y.J.; Kim, J. Dual encoder–decoder-based deep polyp segmentation network for colonoscopy images. *Sci. Rep.* **2023**, *13*, 1183. [CrossRef]
6. Image Designed by Freepik. Available online: https://www.freepik.com/ (accessed on 2 December 2023).
7. Li, Z.; Liao, Z.; McAlindon, M. *Handbook of Capsule Endoscopy*; Springer: Berlin/Heidelberg, Germany, 2014. Available online: https://link.springer.com/content/pdf/10.1007/978-94-017-9229-5.pdf (accessed on 25 November 2023).

8. Tomar, N.K.; Jha, D.; Riegler, M.A.; Johansen, H.D.; Johansen, D.; Rittscher, J.; Halvorsen, P.; Ali, S. Fanet: A feedback attention network for improved biomedical image segmentation. *IEEE Trans. Neural Networks Learn. Syst.* **2022**, *34*, 9375–9388. [CrossRef]
9. Fan, D.P.; Ji, G.P.; Zhou, T.; Chen, G.; Fu, H.; Shen, J.; Shao, L. Pranet: Parallel reverse attention network for polyp segmentation. In Proceedings of the International Conference on Medical Image Computing and Computer-Assisted Intervention, Lima, Peru, 4–8 October 2020; pp. 263–273.
10. Song, P.; Li, J.; Fan, H. Attention based multi-scale parallel network for polyp segmentation. *Comput. Biol. Med.* **2022**, *146*, 105476. [CrossRef]
11. Zhao, X.; Zhang, L.; Lu, H. Automatic polyp segmentation via multi-scale subtraction network. In Proceedings of the Medical Image Computing and Computer Assisted Intervention–MICCAI 2021: 24th International Conference, Strasbourg, France, 27 September–1 October 2021; Proceedings, Part I 24; Springer: Berlin/Heidelberg, Germany, 2021; pp. 120–130.
12. Galdran, A.; Carneiro, G.; Ballester, M.A.G. Double encoder-decoder networks for gastrointestinal polyp segmentation. In Proceedings of the Pattern Recognition, ICPR International Workshops and Challenges, Virtual Event, 10–15 January 2021; Proceedings, Part I; Springer: Berlin/Heidelberg, Germany, 2021; pp. 293–307.
13. Yang, X.; Wei, Q.; Zhang, C.; Zhou, K.; Kong, L.; Jiang, W. Colon polyp detection and segmentation based on improved MRCNN. *IEEE Trans. Instrum. Meas.* **2020**, *70*, 1–10. [CrossRef]
14. Wang, W.; Tian, J.; Zhang, C.; Luo, Y.; Wang, X.; Li, J. An improved deep learning approach and its applications on colonic polyp images detection. *BMC Med. Imaging* **2020**, *20*, 1–14. [CrossRef] [PubMed]
15. Haj-Manouchehri, A.; Mohammadi, H.M. Polyp detection using CNNs in colonoscopy video. *IET Comput. Vis.* **2020**, *14*, 241–247. [CrossRef]
16. Guo, Z.; Zhang, R.; Li, Q.; Liu, X.; Nemoto, D.; Togashi, K.; Niroshana, S.I.; Shi, Y.; Zhu, X. Reduce false-positive rate by active learning for automatic polyp detection in colonoscopy videos. In Proceedings of the 2020 IEEE 17th International Symposium on Biomedical Imaging (ISBI), Iowa City, IA, USA, 3–7 April 2020; pp. 1655–1658.
17. Cao, C.; Wang, R.; Yu, Y.; Zhang, H.; Yu, Y.; Sun, C. Gastric polyp detection in gastroscopic images using deep neural network. *PLoS ONE* **2021**, *16*, e0250632. [CrossRef] [PubMed]
18. Nogueira-Rodríguez, A.; Domínguez-Carbajales, R.; Campos-Tato, F.; Herrero, J.; Puga, M.; Remedios, D.; Rivas, L.; Sánchez, E.; Iglesias, A.; Cubiella, J.; et al. Real-time polyp detection model using convolutional neural networks. *Neural Comput. Appl.* **2022**, *34*, 10375–10396. [CrossRef]
19. Hoang, M.C.; Nguyen, K.T.; Kim, J.; Park, J.O.; Kim, C.S. Automated bowel polyp detection based on actively controlled capsule endoscopy: Feasibility study. *Diagnostics* **2021**, *11*, 1878. [CrossRef] [PubMed]
20. Pacal, I.; Karaboga, D. A robust real-time deep learning based automatic polyp detection system. *Comput. Biol. Med.* **2021**, *134*, 104519. [CrossRef] [PubMed]
21. Lee, J.N.; Chae, J.W.; Cho, H.C. Improvement of colon polyp detection performance by modifying the multi-scale network structure and data augmentation. *J. Electr. Eng. Technol.* **2022**, *17*, 3057–3065. [CrossRef]
22. Wan, J.; Chen, B.; Yu, Y. Polyp detection from colorectum images by using attentive YOLOv5. *Diagnostics* **2021**, *11*, 2264. [CrossRef]
23. Pacal, I.; Karaman, A.; Karaboga, D.; Akay, B.; Basturk, A.; Nalbantoglu, U.; Coskun, S. An efficient real-time colonic polyp detection with YOLO algorithms trained by using negative samples and large datasets. *Comput. Biol. Med.* **2022**, *141*, 105031. [CrossRef] [PubMed]
24. Souaidi, M.; El Ansari, M. Multi-scale hybrid network for polyp detection in wireless capsule endoscopy and colonoscopy images. *Diagnostics* **2022**, *12*, 2030. [CrossRef]
25. Karaman, A.; Karaboga, D.; Pacal, I.; Akay, B.; Basturk, A.; Nalbantoglu, U.; Coskun, S.; Sahin, O. Hyper-parameter optimization of deep learning architectures using artificial bee colony (ABC) algorithm for high performance real-time automatic colorectal cancer (CRC) polyp detection. *Appl. Intell.* **2023**, *53*, 15603–15620. [CrossRef]
26. Karaman, A.; Pacal, I.; Basturk, A.; Akay, B.; Nalbantoglu, U.; Coskun, S.; Sahin, O.; Karaboga, D. Robust real-time polyp detection system design based on YOLO algorithms by optimizing activation functions and hyper-parameters with artificial bee colony (ABC). *Expert Syst. Appl.* **2023**, *221*, 119741. [CrossRef]
27. Iakovidis, D.K.; Koulaouzidis, A. Software for enhanced video capsule endoscopy: challenges for essential progress. *Nat. Rev. Gastroenterol. Hepatol.* **2015**, *12*, 172–186. [CrossRef]
28. Koulaouzidis, A.; Iakovidis, D.K.; Yung, D.E.; Rondonotti, E.; Kopylov, U.; Plevris, J.N.; Toth, E.; Eliakim, A.; Johansson, G.W.; Marlicz, W.; et al. KID Project: an internet-based digital video atlas of capsule endoscopy for research purposes. *Endosc. Int. Open* **2017**, *5*, E477–E483. [CrossRef]
29. Data, M.; Signal Processing Laboratory, U.o.T. Kid—Medical Data and Signal Processing Laboratory. Available online: https://mdss.uth.gr/datasets/endoscopy/kid/ (accessed on 12 November 2023).
30. Korman, L.; Delvaux, M.; Gay, G.; Hagenmuller, F.; Keuchel, M.; Friedman, S.; Weinstein, M.; Shetzline, M.; Cave, D.; De Franchis, R.; et al. Capsule endoscopy structured terminology (CEST): Proposal of a standardized and structured terminology for reporting capsule endoscopy procedures. *Endoscopy* **2005**, *37*, 951–959. [CrossRef]
31. ISO/IEC 15948:2004; Information technology—Computer Graphics and Image Processing—Portable Network Graphics (PNG): Functional Specification. International Organization for Standardization: Geneva, Switzerland, 2004.

32. *ISO/IEC 14496-12:2022*; Information Technology—Coding of Audio-Visual Objects—Part 12: ISO Base Media File Format. International Organization for Standardization: Geneva, Switzerland, 2022.
33. Iakovidis, D.K.; Goudas, T.; Smailis, C.; Maglogiannis, I. Ratsnake: A versatile image annotation tool with application to computer-aided diagnosis. *Sci. World J.* **2014**, *2014*, 286856. [CrossRef]
34. Freitas, F.; Schulz, S.; Moraes, E. Survey of current terminologies and ontologies in biology and medicine. *Reciis* **2009**, *3*, 7–18. [CrossRef]
35. Ultralytics. 2013. Available online: https://github.com/ultralytics/ultralytics (accessed on 7 October 2023).
36. Redmon, J.; Divvala, S.; Girshick, R.; Farhadi, A. You only look once: Unified, real-time object detection. In Proceedings of the IEEE Conference on Computer Vision and Pattern Recognition, Honolulu, HI, USA, 21–26 July 2016; pp. 779–788.
37. Ge, Z.; Liu, S.; Wang, F.; Li, Z.; Sun, J. Yolox: Exceeding yolo series in 2021. *arXiv* **2021**, arXiv:2107.08430.
38. Wang, C.Y.; Bochkovskiy, A.; Liao, H.Y.M. YOLOv7: Trainable bag-of-freebies sets new state-of-the-art for real-time object detectors. In Proceedings of the IEEE/CVF Conference on Computer Vision and Pattern Recognition, Vancouver, BC, Canada, 18–22 June 2023; pp. 7464–7475.
39. Feng, C.; Zhong, Y.; Gao, Y.; Scott, M.R.; Huang, W. Tood: Task-aligned one-stage object detection. In Proceedings of the 2021 IEEE/CVF International Conference on Computer Vision (ICCV), Montreal, BC, Canada, 11–17 October 2021; pp. 3490–3499.
40. Li, X.; Wang, W.; Wu, L.; Chen, S.; Hu, X.; Li, J.; Tang, J.; Yang, J. Generalized focal loss: Learning qualified and distributed bounding boxes for dense object detection. *Adv. Neural Inf. Process. Syst.* **2020**, *33*, 21002–21012.
41. Zheng, Z.; Wang, P.; Ren, D.; Liu, W.; Ye, R.; Hu, Q.; Zuo, W. Enhancing geometric factors in model learning and inference for object detection and instance segmentation. *IEEE Trans. Cybern.* **2021**, *52*, 8574–8586. [CrossRef]
42. Zheng, Z.; Wang, P.; Liu, W.; Li, J.; Ye, R.; Ren, D. Distance-IoU loss: Faster and better learning for bounding box regression. In Proceedings of the AAAI Conference on Artificial Intelligence, New York, NY, USA, 7–12 February 2020; Volume 34, pp. 12993–13000.
43. Delagah, B.; Hassanpour, H. Feature Extraction for Polyp Detection in Wireless Capsule Endoscopy Video Frames. *J. Healthc. Eng.* **2023**, *2023*, 6076514. [CrossRef]
44. Amiri, Z.; Hassanpour, H.; Beghdadi, A. A computer-aided method for digestive system abnormality detection in WCE images. *J. Healthc. Eng.* **2021**, *2021*, 1–11. [CrossRef] [PubMed]
45. Sornapudi, S.; Meng, F.; Yi, S. Region-based automated localization of colonoscopy and wireless capsule endoscopy polyps. *Appl. Sci.* **2019**, *9*, 2404. [CrossRef]
46. Goel, N.; Kaur, S.; Gunjan, D.; Mahapatra, S. Dilated CNN for abnormality detection in wireless capsule endoscopy images. *Soft Comput.* **2022**, *26*, 1231–1247. [CrossRef]
47. Jha, D.; Tomar, N.K.; Ali, S.; Riegler, M.A.; Johansen, H.D.; Johansen, D.; de Lange, T.; Halvorsen, P. Nanonet: Real-time polyp segmentation in video capsule endoscopy and colonoscopy. In Proceedings of the 2021 IEEE 34th International Symposium on Computer-Based Medical Systems (CBMS), Aveiro, Portugal, 7–9 June 2021; pp. 37–43.
48. Dray, X.; Toth, E.; de Lange, T.; Koulaouzidis, A. Artificial intelligence, capsule endoscopy, databases, and the Sword of Damocles. *Endosc. Int. Open* **2021**, *9*, E1754–E1755. [CrossRef] [PubMed]

Disclaimer/Publisher's Note: The statements, opinions and data contained in all publications are solely those of the individual author(s) and contributor(s) and not of MDPI and/or the editor(s). MDPI and/or the editor(s) disclaim responsibility for any injury to people or property resulting from any ideas, methods, instructions or products referred to in the content.

MDPI
St. Alban-Anlage 66
4052 Basel
Switzerland
www.mdpi.com

Diagnostics Editorial Office
E-mail: diagnostics@mdpi.com
www.mdpi.com/journal/diagnostics

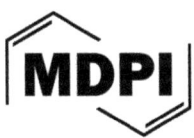

Disclaimer/Publisher's Note: The statements, opinions and data contained in all publications are solely those of the individual author(s) and contributor(s) and not of MDPI and/or the editor(s). MDPI and/or the editor(s) disclaim responsibility for any injury to people or property resulting from any ideas, methods, instructions or products referred to in the content.

www.ingramcontent.com/pod-product-compliance
Lightning Source LLC
LaVergne TN
LVHW070051120526
838202LV00102B/2021